INTERLEUKINS IN CANCER BIOLOGY

INTERLEUKINS IN CANCER BIOLOGY
Their Heterogeneous Role

ARSENIY E. YUZHALIN
Oxford, UK

ANTON G. KUTIKHIN
Kemerovo, Russia

Amsterdam • Boston • Heidelberg • London
New York • Oxford • Paris • San Diego
San Francisco • Singapore • Sydney • Tokyo

Academic Press is an imprint of Elsevier

ELSEVIER

Academic Press is an imprint of Elsevier
32 Jamestown Road, London NW1 7BY, UK
225 Wyman Street, Waltham, MA 02451, USA
525 B Street, Suite 1800, San Diego, CA 92101-4495, USA

Notice
No responsibility is assumed by the publisher for any injury and/or damage to persons
or property as a matter of products liability, negligence or otherwise, or from any use or
operation of any methods, products, instructions or ideas contained in the material herein.
Because of rapid advances in the medical sciences, in particular, independent verification of
diagnoses and drug dosages should be made

British Library Cataloguing-in-Publication Data
A catalogue record for this book is available from the British Library

Library of Congress Cataloging-in-Publication Data
A catalog record for this book is available from the Library of Congress

ISBN: 978-0-12-810325-8

For information on all Academic Press publications
visit our website at www.store.elsevier.com

Typeset by TNQ Books and Journals
www.tnq.co.in

Printed and bound in United States of America
15 16 17 18 19   10 9 8 7 6 5 4 3 2 1

Working together
to grow libraries in
developing countries

www.elsevier.com • www.bookaid.org

DEDICATION

For my brother.

—Arseniy E. Yuzhalin, Oxford, 2014

CONTENTS

Long standing data implicate interleukins as major mediators of innate and adaptive immune response. Their functions are incredibly diverse: promoting differentiation, proliferation, and maturation of immune cells, facilitating communication between them, regulating the expression of numerous genes, controlling transcription factors, and finally, governing the inflammatory process and secretion of antibodies. Interleukins provide coordinated interactions between white blood cells, thereby granting proper and effective immune response against numerous diseases, including cancer. There is a huge amount of evidence indicating that interleukins play a key role in the battle of the organism against cancer cells. Sometimes their role is ambiguous, showing both tumor-promoting and anticancer effects. On the one hand, interleukins markedly stimulate immune cells to recognize and eliminate cancer cells; on the other hand, they may also cause prolonged inflammation, angiogenesis, formation of prometastatic niche, and immune escape of tumors. Almost 40 representatives of interleukins have been discovered to date, not including multiple isoforms, receptors, and accessory proteins. Such diversity often creates confusion in the clear understanding of the functioning of interleukins as a unified network of cellular mediators capable of performing various biological effects depending on current state of the organism. Moreover, the amount of published information on this issue is extremely large, which significantly hampers the understanding of the topic. Current monograph was written with the aim to clearly sort all interleukins on their role in cancer and bring clarity to this problem. We herein summarize and discuss existing facts on the impact of all known interleukins in occurrence, development, and progression of cancer.

This book focuses on interleukins and cancer nothing more, nothing less. Using this book, the reader will find comprehensive and exhaustive information on a particular molecule in one place. We tried to make the content understandable and clear. Multiple illustrations are aimed to help to realize and remember the most important moments, and attention to subtle details is maintained in spite of the breadth of the topic. In addition, at the end of each paragraph, we offer the most promising targets for future research, which may help the investigators to develop the experimental design. Despite the fact that we try to present the material relatively simply, it is expected that the readers already have a basic knowledge in the fields of oncology, molecular biology and immunology. This book will be interesting and helpful to a wide audience, particularly biologists, immunologists, oncologists, molecular biologists, cellular biologists, pathologists, general practitioners, and other health care professionals engaged in cancer research. Interleukins on Cancer Biology: Their Heterogenous Role is advisable for graduate students of biomedical faculties studying the appropriate course and their lecturers as well.

CHAPTER 1

Introduction: Basic Concepts

*Nothing has such power to broaden the mind as the ability to investigate
systematically and truly all that comes under thy observation in life.*
Marcus Aurelius, Roman emperor (121–180 AC)

1.1 A BRIEF OVERVIEW OF CANCER PHENOMENON

1.1.1 What is Cancer?

Cancer is a disease that has always been a part of the human life. References
to cancer have been found in numerous early sources, some of which are
thousands of years old. The most ancient descriptions of tumors and cancer
treatment methods are the ancient Egyptian papyruses dated roughly to
1600 BC (Bozzone, 2009). From this source, we know that the Egyptians
used cauterizing ointments containing arsenic for the treatment of superficial tumors. Similar descriptions were found in the manuscripts of ancient
India, which described surgical removal of tumors and the use of arsenic
ointments (Bozzone, 2009). The term "cancer" itself was introduced by
Hippocrates, who described and investigated various tumors, including
those of breast, stomach, skin, cervix, rectum, and throat (Figure 1.1). Hippocrates noticed that all the cancers have a visual similarity to a crab (Greek,
karkinos) because of characteristic outgrowths aimed in opposite directions.
Regarding the treatment of cancer, Hippocrates proposed the surgical
removal of available tumors followed by treatment of postoperative wounds
with ointments containing either plant poisons or arsenic, which were supposed to kill the remaining cancer cells. In cases of internal tumors, Hippocrates suggested to give up any kind of treatment, because he believed
that the consequences of such a complex operation will kill the patient
faster than the tumor itself.

Nowadays, we understand cancer as a pathological condition of the body
where cells grow and reproduce in an uncontrollable manner. Alternatively,
cancer is referred to as a large group of diseases characterized by disorga-
nized and unregulated cell division. To date, more than 200 different cancers
are known. Importantly, almost every cell of an organism may give rise to
cancer; therefore, cancer is rather regarded as a disease of a cell than a disease

Interleukins in Cancer Biology
http://dx.doi.org/10.1016/B978-0-12-801121-8.00001-4

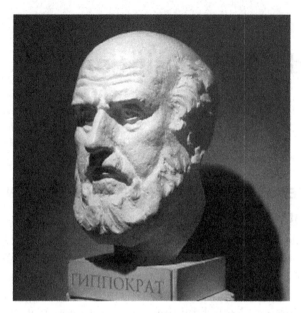

Figure 1.1 Hippocrates of Cos (460–370 BC) was an ancient Greek physician and philosopher.

of an organ. Cancer cells grow and form tumors, which are classified according to their clinical and morphological features in two main groups, namely, benign and malignant tumors. Benign tumors are characterized by a slow expansive growth, the absence of metastases, and no overall effect on the body; thus, they are regarded as noncancerous. Instead, malignant tumors are highly cancerous, which means they have several typical features, such as rapid progression, tendency to infiltration, high metastatic potential, and frequency of recurrence. In everyday practice, the term "cancer" is commonly used as a synonym for malignant tumor, and it should also be mentioned that in our book we will consider malignant tumors only. The overall effect of malignant tumors is often manifested by significant weight loss, various metabolic disturbances, skin changes, fatigue, fever, pain, and, ultimately, development of cachexia. Other general symptoms and signs may also include bleeding, indigestion, and emergence of unusual thickenings or lumps.

1.1.2 Cancer Statistics

Cancer is one of the most hazardous public health problems nowadays. According to the data of International Agency for Research on Cancer, more than 12.4 millions of new cancer cases, 7.6 millions of cancer-caused deaths, and 28 millions of cancer survivors were registered in 2008 world-wide (Jemal et al., 2010, 2011; Siegel et al., 2012). About half of cancer cases and two-thirds of cancer deaths occur in low- and middle-income countries (Jemal et al., 2010, 2011; El-Basmy et al., 2012; Kutikhin et al., 2012a; Zhivotovskiy et al., 2012; Baade et al., 2013; Krishnan et al., 2013; Krishna Rao et al., 2013; Moore, 2013; Pandey and Chandravati, 2013; Perez-Santos and Anaya-Ruiz, 2013; Zhang, 2013). Despite this scary statistics, annual death rates have been decreasing gradually since 1990 in men and since 1991 in women (Jemal et al., 2011). This progress is largely as a result of intensive development of modern preventative measures against cancer, the efficacy of which is growing every year. Obviously, prevention of a disease is much easier than its treatment, and so the problem of cancer prevention is one of the most basic issues when combating the burden of the disease.

1.1.3 Carcinogenesis and Cancer Risk

Carcinogenesis is a sophisticated multistep process of initiation, development, and progression of cancer. The key feature of this process is that it leads to a fundamental reorganization of the normal cells of the body. The occurrence of cancer is associated with an impaired proliferation and differentiation of cells due to genetic alterations. One of the most common genetic alterations is a mutation. In order to provoke cancer, the mutation must occur in a specific gene, called proto-oncogene. The proto-oncogenes are a class of genes that encode proteins and enzymes involved in the regulation of cell cycle, as well as cell differentiation, and proliferation. The proto-oncogenes are often engaged in multiple signal transduction pathways of mitosis regulation; hence, their proper functioning is extremely important for the normal cell development and homeostasis. It is important to underline that the proto-oncogenes are entirely normal genes, but occasionally they may initiate cancer development due to acquisition of genetic alterations within their structure. A single error in the proto-oncogene converts it to the oncogene, which is able to give rise to the malignant transformation (Weinberg, 2007). The oncogene is characterized as a proto-oncogene expressed at inappropriate (i.e., significantly high) levels. As a consequence, excessively high expression of the oncogene leads to an increase in protein expression and stability of its mRNA. This, in turn, alters numerous metabolic processes within a cell and ultimately results in cancer development. Currently, oncogenes are regarded as a broad class of genes that includes numerous transcription factors, receptor or cytoplasmic tyrosine kinases, mitogens, growth factors, and GTPases (Weinberg and Robert, 2007).

Apart from carcinogenesis itself, other important points we should mention are cancer risk factors and individual cancer susceptibility. A risk factor is a chance that a person will have a disease or recurrence. Some do not get cancer. Some do, and we have nothing to do with that. Why do not we all develop this disease? What is the lifetime risk for getting cancer or dying from cancer? These questions have been investigated for decades as hundreds and thousands of epidemiological studies were performed. Large-scale investigations of cancer incidence and mortality revealed that the risk of getting this disease is largely due to the possession of specific risk factors. In other words, this means any risky behavior that might provoke massive damage to genome, thereby initiating malignant transformation. So far, a huge number of factors determining the likelihood of acquiring cancer throughout life have been established. Most of them include lifestyle factors, such as excessive alcohol consumption, tobacco smoking, overweight and obesity, and lack of physical activity, and unhealthy diet (Weinberg and Robert, 2007). The above-mentioned factors are common for all malignancies; however, some types of cancer have their own risk factors. For example, prolonged exposure to UV rays and getting multiple sunburns greatly increase skin cancer risk (de Gruijl, 1999; Dummer and Maier, 2002; Rigel, 2002). The other case in the point is that long-term estrogen therapy is associated with an increased risk of breast cancer in postmenopausal women (Lumachi et al., 2011; Rozenberg et al., 2013; Williams and Lin, 2013). According to recent research, even blood group is to be considered as a risk factor for certain cancers (Xie et al., 2010; Khalili et al., 2011; Yuzhalin and Kutikhin, 2012a; Liumbruno and Franchini, 2013).

Of course, possessing a particular risk factor does not mean that a person will definitely get a disease. On the other hand, not having any risk factors does not guarantee total absence of cancer throughout life. But one thing is certain—the accumulation of risk factors is directly proportional to the probability of the occurrence of the disease.

The good thing about lifestyle factors is that they can be easily avoided, i.e., can be controlled. We can give up with pernicious habits and lead a healthy life to live without illnesses. It is estimated that up to 40% of cancers could be prevented by lifestyle changes. However, we are unfortunately not able to change our genetic predisposition to cancer. Due to differences in our genomes, some individuals are especially prone to malignant transformation and at first glance there is nothing we can do about it. However, it is well known that early defined, most of the cancers have a good cure rate. Therefore, early prevention and diagnosis based on genetic counseling are the most basic issues when combating the burden of the disease (Yuzhalin and Kutikhin, 2012b). The Human Genome Project has laid the groundwork for the understanding of the roles of genes and their inherited variations (especially single nucleotide polymorphisms) in the etiopathogenesis of cancer (Sachidanandam et al., 2001; Tsigris et al., 2007; Yuzhalin, 2011; Yuzhalin and Kutikhin, 2012c,d,e; Kutikhin and Yuzhalin, 2012a,b,c; Kutikhin et al., 2014). Importantly, some examples of personalized cancer management are applicable even today. For instance, testing for mutations involved in the development of familial breast and ovarian cancer prompts individualized prophylactic therapy including mastectomy and oophorectomy (Wang et al., 2012).

Yet another uncontrollable risk factor for cancer is age. Moreover, growing older is the biggest risk factor for developing tumors. It is well known that cancer is primarily a disease of older people, and incidence rates increase with age for most malignancies. During the twentieth century, a dramatic increase in average life expectancy has been observed; therefore, even 100 years ago the problem of cancer was not as acute as it is today. Longer lifespan is essentially associated with a higher number of accumulated mutations within the genome, which in turn increases the share of mutations within the proto-oncogenes. Much research is being performed to investigate mediators that are supposed to connect cancer and aging. For example, tumor suppressor protein p53 has a considerable influence on both general aging and cancer development; currently, multiple therapeutic approaches are being developed to ameliorate or delay aging and simultaneously prevent tumor formation (reviewed by Hasty and Christy, 2013).

1.1.4 General Mechanisms of Carcinogenesis

It is important to note that carcinogenic mutations as well as all other mutations are caused by a wide range of substances called *carcinogens*. All known mechanisms of human tumorigenesis may be divided into three main groups, namely, physical, chemical, and biological. So far, many important features of carcinogenesis are not well understood and therefore we here give only a brief insight on the existing knowledge about carcinogens and their types.

- *Physical carcinogens* are extremely variable in their nature and sources. The term "physical carcinogen" includes the following agents: ionizing radiation (all types, including X-rays, γ rays, neutrons, radon gas, and UV light), leather dust, talc, coal soot, wood dust, asbestos, erionite, and other natural and man-made mineral fibers and respirable dusts (Maltoni et al., 2000).

Plenty of experiments on mice models demonstrated that dusts and fibers cause cancer when inhaled for a long time. It was also revealed that intra-tissue implantations of hard and soft metallic or synthetic materials in the form of films, disks, squares, and foams are associated with cancer development as well (Maltoni et al., 1980; Maltoni and Sinibaldi, 1982). In addition, numerous nonfibrous particulate materials, such as crystalline silica and metallic nickel, are also regarded as carcinogens (Hueper, 1955). The mechanisms of physical carcinogenesis are well studied. Physical carcinogens are believed to have a nonspecific irritative effect on cells, which significantly violates various metabolic processes and leads to an excessive DNA damage, which results in cancer development. Generally, physical carcinogens require many years of exposure after getting inside the body to develop cancer. It has been long discovered that lung cancer is fairly frequent among industrial workers who are exposed to prolonged inhalation of asbestos, talc, or coal soot (Falk and Jurgelski, 1979; Wild, 2006; Lenters et al., 2011). With regard to radiation, it is well known that UV rays directly damage cell DNA and therefore are responsible for most cases of skin cancer. Regular use of tanning lamps and prolonged indoor tanning have long been established as important risk factors for skin cancer (Narayanan et al., 2010). The list of the most common physical carcinogens is represented in Table 1.1.

• *Chemical carcinogenesis* is characterized by the modification of the molecular structure of the DNA by various chemical compounds. Importantly, chemical carcinogens are responsible for about 80–90% of all human cancers. The most evident example of chemical carcinogenesis is the association between smoking and lung cancer (Risser, 1996). Virtually all the chemical carcinogens are ubiquitous, i.e., they can be found in the general environment, like prepared food, tobacco smoke, engine exhausts, paints, alcoholic beverages, etc. Some of the chemical carcinogens are regarded as occupational carcinogens, i.e., they can be found in specific work locations only. Importantly, many chemical substances are not carcinogenic themselves, but they convert to the carcinogenic products within the body; therefore, they are termed pro-carcinogens. It is interesting to note that cancer may also be initiated by the metabolism of endogenous chemicals as well. For example, products of lipid peroxidation and estrogens are known to produce DNA adducts as well as excessive DNA damage (Chung et al., 1996; Bolton et al., 1998). Table 1.2 includes the list of the most dangerous chemical carcinogens.

Table 1.1 Physical Carcinogens According to the International Agency for Research on Cancer List

Carcinogen	Source	Associated Cancer Type
Arsenic	Nonferrous metal smelting, electrical and semiconductor devices	Lung, skin, liver
Asbestos	Asbestos industry, fire-resistant textiles	Lung, larynx
Beryllium	Aircraft and aerospace industry, nuclear reactors	Lung
Cadmium	Various dyes and pigments, batteries, industrial paints, metal coatings	Lung
Chromium	Steel and copper alloys, tanning agent, magnetic tape coatings, abrasive, refractory materials	Lung
Diesel particulate matter (ash particulates, metallic abrasion particles, silicates)	Diesel engines' exhaust	Lung, bladder
Erionite	Sewage and agricultural waste. Used in waste treatment and in air pollution control systems	Mesothelium
Ionizing radiation	Ubiquitous. Risk occupations are radiologists, nuclear workers, underground miners, plutonium workers	Blood, bone, lung
Nickel	Nickel smelting and refining	Lung
Silica and crystalline	Granite, ceramics, and stone industries	Lung
Talc	Manufacture of cosmetics, pottery, paper	Mesothelium, lung
Wood dust	Wood industry	Nasal cavity

Siemiatycki et al. (2004).

- *Biological carcinogenesis* is referred to as a cancer that is driven by infectious agents, such as viruses, bacteria, fungi, protozoa, and helminths. As compared to previous mechanisms, biological carcinogenesis is the least studied, and numerous discrepancies may be found in the current literature on this issue. Biological carcinogenesis is the most curious one, and we will describe this in more detail. So far, the four main mechanisms of biological carcinogenesis can be proposed.

Table 1.2 Some Chemical Carcinogens According to the International Agency
for Research on Cancer List

Carcinogen	Sources	Associated Cancer Type
Aflatoxin	Food industry	Liver
Aromatic amine dyes	Dye and pigment industry	Bladder
Benzene	Light fuel oil, solvents, rubber, printing industry	Blood
Coal tars and pitches	Production of refined chemicals	Skin
Ethylene oxide	Rocket propellant, ripening agent for crops	Blood
Isopropylalcohol	Fuel additives, medical disinfecting pads, solvents	Nasal cavity
Mustard gas	Military forces	Lung, larynx, pharynx
Polycyclic aromatic hydrocarbons	Atmospheric pollutants, cooked food	All sites
Tetrachlorodibenzo-*para*-dioxin	Waste incineration, paper bleaching	All sites
Components of tobacco smoke (>30)	Tobacco	Lung
Vinyl chloride	Refrigerant	Liver

Siemiatycki et al. (2004).

- Viral mechanisms

    The phenomenon of viral carcinogenesis is remarkable. The point is that in very rare cases malignant transformation could be induced by so-called oncogenic viruses, which carry oncogenes in their own genome. Integration of the viral genome into the host chromosome is followed up by multiple transcription and translation of viral genes, including oncogenes (Weinberg and Robert, 2007). Nowadays, more than 12% of human cancers can be attributed to a viral infection (Carrillo-Infante et al., 2007). For instance, the association between human papillomavirus and cervical cancer has long been established. In extremely rare cases, viruses possessing no oncogenes in their structure may promote cancer by inserting their genome adjacent to cellular proto-oncogenes, thereby causing their expression. Due to the fact that in this case viral genome insertion is not specific and requires more time to get near the oncogene, these viruses are called slowly transforming viruses (Weinberg and Robert, 2007).

- Immune mechanisms

  It is well known that chronic inflammation caused by infectious agents greatly increases the risk of cancer occurrence in the surrounding cells. In particular, inflammation induces mutations and epigenetic alterations by means of the formation of free radicals and DNA damage, inhibition of apoptosis, and promotion of cell proliferation (Kutikhin et al., 2013). This type of mechanisms is possessed by virtually all the known biological carcinogens. In this regard, an excellent example is the *Helicobacter pylori* infection, which is a major cause of gastric cancer (Pritchard and Crabtree, 2006). Furthermore, the parasite-driven modulation of the host immune response may sometimes lead to the deregulation of tumor immune surveillance, thereby increasing risk of malignant tumor formation.

- Metabolic mechanisms

  There is accumulating evidence that infectious agents may participate in modification, degradation, biotransformation, and detoxification of chemical compounds entering the gastrointestinal tract after consumption of food and drink eventually metabolizing them to chemical carcinogens. Numerous representatives of gut and oral microbiota have shown these activities in multiple studies (Kutikhin et al., 2012b, 2013). Additionally, human gastrointestinal microbiota can also have an influence on weight gain and promote obesity hence elevating the risk of obesity-associated cancers (Robles Alonso and Guarner, 2013).

- Toxin-mediated mechanisms

  Certain bacteria and protozoa are able to produce toxins that are contained in their cell wall. Some of the toxins were demonstrated to possess carcinogenic activity by violating cell–cell interactions, proliferation, intracellular signal transduction, and cell growth and differentiation (Kutikhin et al., 2012b, 2013). In addition, several toxins were found to induce resistance to multiple mechanisms of apoptosis, thereby contributing to cancer development as well.

1.1.5 Further Cancer Development

An established tumor violates various metabolic processes within the cell and acquires partial independence from the regulatory systems of the body. The organism tries to get rid of cancer cells by means of immune response, which is not always effective. The cohesion between cancer cells is low, and therefore the development of a tumor is accompanied by the penetration of some cancer cells through the blood vessels, and the consequent spread of these cells to the other locations in the body (Weinberg and Robert, 2007). This leads to the generation of new malignancies termed metastatic tumors. Cancers develop progressively, and metastatic cancer is the terminal stage of tumor growth. The most common metastasis locations are the liver, lungs, brain, and bones (Bacac and Stamenkovic, 2008). A spread of metastases greatly decreases a patient's chance of survival; hence, most cancer deaths nowadays are due to malignancies that have spread from their primary site to other organs.

1.2 INTERLEUKINS AND THEIR SIGNIFICANCE

1.2.1 Cancer and Immunity

There is a huge amount of evidence indicating that the immune system plays a key role in the battle of the organism against cancer. In the middle of the twentieth century, it was discovered that immune cells act as sentinels in recognizing and eliminating cancer cells (Burnet, 1957). Subsequently, numerous experiments on mice testified in favor of the existence of tumor-associated antigens and immune surveillance for protection from trans-formed cells in the host (Burnet, 1971; Herberman and Holden, 1978; Thomas, 1982). Based on these findings, the model of process that inhibits carcinogenesis and maintains regular cellular homeostasis was suggested, and it was termed cancer immune surveillance (Kim et al., 2007). In the 1990s, it was hypothesized that immune surveillance is a part of more general process of cancer immunoediting, which underlies the elimination of the tumors (Dunn et al., 2002). According to the modern concept of cancer immunoediting, there are three essential phases of interaction of host and tumor cells: elimination, equilibrium, and escape, which are designated the "three E's" (Kim et al., 2007). The elimination phase consists of the recognition of a growing tumor, which is due to the fact that cancer cells express their own antigens, which cause immune cells to recognize them, and causes a subsequent infiltration of immune effector cells such as natural killer (NK) cells, to the tumor. These cells produce multiple cytokines, such as interleukins (ILs), which contribute to cancer death, or C-X-C motif chemokines (CXCLs), which inhibit angiogenesis. Subsequently, cancer cells, which have survived the elimination phase, enter the equilibrium phase, where lymphocytes exert a selection pressure on tumor cells, which are genetically unstable and rapidly mutating. The equilibrium phase results in the immune selection of tumor cells with decreased immunogenicity. Importantly, these cells are more likely to survive in an immunocompetent host, which may explain the paradox of cancer occurrence in immunologically intact patients. In the final phase, tumor cells that have acquired resistance to the immune system continue to grow and expand in an uncontrolled manner and may eventually lead to malignancies (Kim et al., 2007).

Notably, in recent years, there has been significant increase in an accumulation of scientific evidence for the concept of cancer immunosurveillance and immunoediting based on protection against development of spontaneous and chemically induced tumors in animal models, and identification of targets for immune recognition of human cancer (Dunn et al., 2002).

1.2.2 ILs and Their Effects on Cancer

The immune system operates with thousands of various proteins and enzymes that are necessary for a proper immune response. In the last decades, a large number of studies devoted to the investigation of the impact of ILs on cancer development have emerged, as they are believed to play a crucial role in anticancer defense (Lippitz, 2013). ILs are a diverse, multifunctional group of proteins that facilitate communication between various immune cells, control gene expression in these cells; operate the intensity and magnitude of an inflammatory response, and control differentiation, proliferation, and secretion of antibodies (Lodish et al., 2007). ILs proved to be extremely active agents with maximal responses, often able to be triggered with the concentration of the nanogram range. The harmonious, coordinated, and smooth functioning of ILs in many respects determines the effectiveness of the anticancer immune response. There is multiple evidence from biological, epidemiological, and clinical studies showing that impaired functioning of certain cytokines (often caused by under or overexpression of cytokine genes) may favor cancer development. For example, it was repeatedly demonstrated that a shift in a delicate balance between the activity of pro- and antiinflammatory ILs may result in prolonged inflammation, and consequently, lead to tumor formation (McLean and El-Omar, 2011; Neurath and Finotto, 2011). Certain ILs may possess both tumor-promoting and anticancer effects. For instance, it is known that IL-17 is able to reduce angiostasis and promote the secretion of angiogenic CXCLs; therefore, increased expression of IL-17 may promote a massive blood supply to the tumor (Murugaiyan and Saha, 2009). Another example is that IL-12 stimulates interferon-gamma (IFN-γ) production by T cells and NK cells, and at the same time, inhibits IL-4-mediated suppression of IFN-γ synthesis; therefore, it is believed to play a crucial role in the antitumor immune response (Del Vecchio et al., 2007).

ILs implement cell coordination by creating specific signals in a para-crine or autocrine manner. Most of them direct cell interaction through Janus kinase-signal transducer and activator of transcription signaling pathway. The impact of ILs on a cell is a complex multistep process. First of all, it is necessary to mention that each IL has a corresponding ligand-dependent receptor (IL-R), which is expressed on the surface of the target cell and participates in signaling directly. An average human cell often has no more than several hundred IL receptors on its surface. These receptors are characterized as membrane glycoproteins, which consist of an external immunoglobulin-like domain, a transmembrane region, and a cytoplasmic domain (McMahan et al., 1991). The family of IL receptors are subdivided according to the distinctive characteristic structural motifs in their extra-cellular domains (Stahl and Yancopoulos, 1993; Taniguchi, 1995). Currently, it is believed that all the receptors are split into five main subtypes, including the IL-2 receptor family, the growth hormone family, the IFN family, the gp130 family, and the gp140 family. The first step in the activa-tion of the receptor starts with binding of the IL to the corresponding receptor on the cell surface. As a result, they form a single complex, which leads to conformational changes in IL-R, bringing the Janus kinases very close to each other in order to autophosphorylate themselves. Secondly, autophosphorylation of JAKs induces a conformational change in its own structure, enabling it to further phosphorylate and activate STATs. Finally, activated STATs dissociate from the receptor and form dimers before translocating to the cell nucleus, where they regulate the transcription of selected gene clusters.

Much research has been done in the last few decades to assess the role of ILs in cancer biology. Nowadays, ILs are considered as one of the most significant agents involved in human carcinogenesis. Their impact on tumor development is ambiguous and sometimes unexplainable. On the one hand, ILs are able to stimulate the immune system to attack cancer cells and eliminate tumors; on the other hand, they may also cause pro-longed inflammation, stimulate malignant neovascularization, metastasis formation, and immune escape of tumors. Even though many peculiarities of the influence of ILs on cancer development have been understood in recent years, numerous problems on this issue still remain unsolved. The main goal of this monograph is to summarize the state of the art of the role of ILs in cancer biology and propose further directions of the research on this topic.

REFERENCES

Baade, P.D., Youlden, D.R., Cramb, S.M., Dunn, J., Gardiner, R.A., 2013. Epidemiology of prostate cancer in the Asia-Pacific region. Prostate Int. 1 (2), 47–58.

Bacac, M., Stamenkovic, I., 2008. Metastatic cancer cell. Annu. Rev. Pathol. 3, 221–247.

Bolton, J.L., Pisha, E., Zhang, F., Qiu, S., 1998. Role of quinoids in estrogen carcinogenesis. Chem. Res. Toxicol. 11 (10), 1113–1127.

Bozzone, D.M., 2009. Chapter 2. The History of Cancer and Leukemia. The Biology of Cancer: Leukemia. Chelsea House Publishers, New York 23–35.

Burnet, F.M., 1971. Immunological surveillance in neoplasia. Transplant. Rev. 7, 3–25.

Burnet, M., 1957. Cancer; a biological approach. I. The processes of control. Br. Med. J. 1 (5022), 779–786.

Carrillo-Infante, C., Abbadessa, G., Bagella, L., Giordano, A., 2007. Viral infections as a cause of cancer (review). Int. J. Oncol. 30 (6), 1521–1528.

Chung, F.L., Chen, H.J., Nath, R.G., 1996. Lipid peroxidation as a potential endogenous source for the formation of exocyclic DNA adducts. Carcinogenesis 17 (10), 2105–2111.

de Gruijl, F.R., 1999. Skin cancer and solar UV radiation. Eur. J. Cancer 35 (14), 2003–2009.

Del Vecchio, M., Bajetta, E., Canova, S., Lotze, M.T., Wesa, A., Parmiani, G., Anichini, A., 2007. Interleukin-12: biological properties and clinical application. Clin. Cancer Res. 13 (16), 4677–4685.

Dunn, G.P., Bruce, A.T., Ikeda, H., Old, L.J., Schreiber, R.D., 2002. Cancer immunoediting: from immunosurveillance to tumor escape. Nat. Immunol. 3, 991–998.

Dummer, R., Maier, T., 2002. UV protection and skin cancer. Recent Results Cancer Res. 160, 7–12.

El-Basmy, A., Al-Mohannadi, S., Al-Awadi, A., 2012. Some epidemiological measures of cancer in Kuwait: national cancer registry data from 2000–2009. Asian Pac. J. Cancer Prev. 13 (7), 3113–3118.

Falk, H.L., Jurgelski Jr, W., 1979. Health effects of coal mining and combustion: carcinogens and cofactors. Environ. Health Perspect. 33, 203–226.

Hasty, P., Christy, B.A., 2013. p53 as an intervention target for cancer and aging. Pathobiol. Aging Age. Relat. Dis. 8, 3.

Herberman, R.B., Holden, H.T., 1978. Natural cell-mediated immunity. Adv. Cancer Res. 27, 305–377.

Hueper, W.C., 1955. Experimental studies in metal carcinogenesis. IV. Cancer produced by parenterally introduced metallic nickel. J. Natl. Cancer Inst. 16, 55.

Jemal, A., Bray, F., Center, M.M., Ferlay, J., Ward, E., Forman, D., 2011. Global cancer statistics. Ca Cancer J. Clin. 61 (2), 69–90.

Jemal, A., Center, M.M., DeSantis, C., Ward, E.M., 2010. Global patterns of cancer incidence and mortality rates and trends. Cancer Epidemiol. Biomarkers Prev. 19 (8), 1893–1907.

Khalili, H., Wolpin, B.M., Huang, E.S., Giovannucci, E.L., Kraft, P., Fuchs, C.S., Chan, A.T., 2011. ABO blood group and risk of colorectal cancer. Cancer Epidemiol. Biomarkers Prev. 20 (5), 1017–1020.

Kim, R., Emi, M., Tanabe, K., 2007. Cancer immunoediting from immune surveillance to immune escape. Immunology 121 (1), 1–14.

Krishna Rao, S.V., Mejia, G., Roberts-Thomson, K., Logan, R., 2013. Epidemiology of oral cancer in Asia in the past decade – an update (2000–2012). Asian Pac. J. Cancer Prev. 14 (10), 5567–5577.

Krishnan, M., Temel, J.S., Wright, A.A., Bernacki, R., Selvaggi, K., Balboni, T., 2013. Predicting life expectancy in patients with advanced incurable cancer: a review. J. Supportive Oncol. 11 (2), 68–74.

Kutikhin, A.G., Yuzhalin, A.E., 2012a. Are Toll-like receptor gene polymorphisms associated with prostate cancer? Cancer Manage. Res. 4, 23–29.

Kutikhin, A.G., Yuzhalin, A.E., 2012b. C-type lectin receptors and RIG-I-like receptors: new points on the oncogenomics map. Cancer Manage. Res. 4, 39–53.

Kutikhin, A.G., Yuzhalin, A.E., 2012c. Inherited variation in pattern recognition receptors and cancer: dangerous liaisons? Cancer Manage. Res. 4, 31–38.

Kutikhin, A.G., Yuzhalin, A.E., Brailovskiy, V.V., Zhivotovskiy, A.S., Magarill, Y.A., Brusina, E.B., 2012a. Analysis of cancer incidence and mortality in the industrial region of South-East Siberia from 1991 through 2010. Asian Pac. J. Cancer Prev. 13 (10), 5189–5193.

Kutikhin, A.G., Yuzhalin, A.E., Brusina, E.B., Briko, N.I., 2012b. Role of infectious agents in the emergence of malignant tumors. Zh. Mikrobiol. Epidemiol. Immunobiol. (5), 104–114.

Kutikhin, A.G., Yuzhalin, A.E., Brusina, E.B., 2013. Infectious Agents and Cancer. Springer, Netherlands.

Kutikhin, A.G., Yuzhalin, A.E., Volkov, A.N., Zhivotovskiy, A.S., Brusina, E.B., 2014. Correlation between genetic polymorphisms within IL-1B and TLR4 genes and cancer risk in a Russian population: a case-control study. Tumour Biol. 35 (5), 4821–4830.

Lenters, V., Vermeulen, R., Dogger, S., Stayner, L., Portengen, L., Burdorf, A., Heederik, D., 2011. A meta-analysis of asbestos and lung cancer: is better quality exposure assessment associated with steeper slopes of the exposure-response relationships? Environ. Health Perspect. 119 (11), 1547–1555.

Lippitz, B.E., 2013. Cytokine patterns in patients with cancer: a systematic review. Lancet Oncol. 14 (6), e218–228.

Liumbruno, G.M., Franchini, M., November 15, 2013. Hemostasis, cancer, and ABO blood group: the most recent evidence of association. J. Thromb. Thrombolysis. [Epub ahead of print].

Lodish, H., Berk, A., Kaiser, C.A., Krieger, M., Scott, M.P., Bretscher, A., Ploegh, H., Matsudaira, P., 2007. Molecular Biology of the Cell, sixth ed. WH Freeman, New York, NY.

Lumachi, F., Luisetto, G., Basso, S.M., Basso, U., Brunello, A., Camozzi, V., 2011. Endocrine therapy of breast cancer. Curr. Med. Chem. 18 (4), 513–522.

Maltoni, C., Minardi, F., Holland, J.F., 2000. Physical carcinogens. In: Bast, R.C., Kufe, D.W., Pollock, R.E., Weichselbaum, R.R., Holland, F.J., Frei, E. (Eds.), Holland-Frei Cancer Medicine, fifth ed. BC Decker, Hamilton, ON, p. 2000.

Maltoni, C., Sinibaldi, C., Morisi, L., 1980. Carcinogenicity of vitallium. Long-term bioassays on Sprague-Dawley rats and Swiss mice by subcutaneous implantation. Acta Oncol. 1, 11.

Maltoni, C., Sinibaldi, C., 1982. Carcinogenicity of acrylic resins (polymethyl methacrylate) used in dentistry. Long-term bioassays on Sprague-Dawley rats by subcutaneous implantation. Acta Oncol. 3, 13.

McLean, M.H., El-Omar, E.M., 2011. Genetics of inflammation in the gastrointestinal tract and how it can cause cancer. Recent Results Cancer Res. 185, 173–183.

McMahan, C.J., Slack, J.L., Mosley, B., Cosman, D., Lupton, S.D., Brunton, L.L., Grubin, C.E., Wignall, J.M., Jenkins, N.A., Brannan, C.I., 1991. A novel IL-1 receptor, cloned from B cells by mammalian expression, is expressed in many cell types. EMBO J. 10, 2821–2832.

Moore, M.A., 2013. Overview of cancer registration research in the Asian Pacific from 2008–2013. Asian Pac. J. Cancer Prev. 14 (8), 4461–4484.

Murugaiyan, G., Saha, B., 2009. Protumor vs antitumor functions of IL-17. J. Immunol. 183, 4169–4175.

Narayanan, D.L., Saladi, R.N., Fox, J.L., 2010. Ultraviolet radiation and skin cancer. Int. J. Dermatol. 49 (9), 978–986.

Neurath, M.F., Finotto, S., 2011. IL-6 signaling in autoimmunity, chronic inflammation and inflammation-associated cancer. Cytokine Growth Factor Rev. 22, 83–89.

Pandey, S., Chandravati, 2013. Breast screening in north India: a cost-effective cancer prevention strategy. Asian Pac. J. Cancer Prev. 14 (2), 853–857.

Perez-Santos, J.L., Anaya-Ruiz, M., 2013. Mexican breast cancer research output, 2003-2012. Asian Pac. J. Cancer Prev. 14 (10), 5921–5923.

Pritchard, D.M., Crabtree, J.E., 2006. *Helicobacter pylori* and gastric cancer. Curr. Opin. Gastroenterol. 22 (6), 620–625.

Rigel, D.S., 2002. The effect of sunscreen on melanoma risk. Dermatol. Clin. 20 (4), 601–606.

Risser, N.L., 1996. Prevention of lung cancer: the key is to stop smoking. Semin. Oncol. Nurs. 12 (4), 260–269.

Robles Alonso, V., Guarner, F., 2013. Linking the gut microbiota to human health. Br. J. Nutr. 109 (Suppl. 2), S21–S26.

Rozenberg, S., Vandromme, J., Antoine, C., 2013. Postmenopausal hormone therapy: risks and benefits. Nat. Rev. Endocrinol. 9 (4), 216–227.

Sachidanandam, R., Weissman, D., Schmidt, S.C., Kakol, J.M., Stein, L.D., Marth, G., 2001. A map of human genome sequence variation containing 1.42 million single nucleotide polymorphisms. Nature 409, 928–933.

Siegel, R., Naishadham, D., Jemal, A., 2012. Cancer statistics, 2012. Ca Cancer J. Clin. 62 (1), 10–29.

Siemiatycki, J., Richardson, L., Straif, K., Latreille, B., Lakhani, R., Campbell, S., Rousseau, M.C., Boffetta, P., 2004. Listing occupational carcinogens. Environ. Health. Perspect. 112 (15), 1447–1459.

Stahl, N., Yancopoulos, G.D., 1993. The alphas, betas, and kinases of cytokine receptor complexes. Cell 74, 587–590.

Taniguchi, T., 1995. Cytokine signaling through nonreceptor protein tyrosine kinases. Science 268, 251–255.

Thomas, L., 1982. On immunosurveillance in human cancer. Yale J. Biol. Med. 55, 329–333.

Tsigris, C., Chatzitheofylaktou, A., Xiromeritis, C., Nikiteas, N., Yannopoulos, A., 2007. Genetic association studies in digestive system malignancies. Anticancer Res. 27, 3577–3587.

Wang, F., Fang, Q., Ge, Z., Yu, N., Xu, S., Fan, X., 2012. Common BRCA1 and BRCA2 mutations in breast cancer families: a meta-analysis from systematic review. Mol. Biol. Rep. 39 (3), 2109–2118.

Weinberg, R.A., 2007. The Biology of Cancer. Garland Science, New York. Print.

Wild, P., 2006. Lung cancer risk and talc not containing asbestiform fibres: a review of the epidemiological evidence. Occup. Environ. Med. 63 (1), 4–9.

Williams, C., Lin, C.Y., 2013. Oestrogen receptors in breast cancer: basic mechanisms and clinical implications. Ecancermedicalscience 7, 370.

Xie, J., Qureshi, A.A., Li, Y., Han, J., 2010. ABO blood group and incidence of skin cancer. PLoS One 5 (8), e11972.

Yuzhalin, A., 2011. The role of interleukin DNA polymorphisms in gastric cancer. Hum. Immunol. 72 (11), 1128–1136.

Yuzhalin, A.E., Kutikhin, A.G., 2012a. ABO and Rh blood groups in relation to ovarian, endometrial and cervical cancer risk among the population of South-East Siberia. Asian Pac. J. Cancer Prev. 13 (10), 5091–5096.

Yuzhalin, A.E., Kutikhin, A.G., 2012b. Integrative systems of genomic risk markers for cancer and other diseases: future of predictive medicine. Cancer Manage. Res. 4, 131–135.

Yuzhalin, A.E., Kutikhin, A.G., 2012c. Interleukin-12: clinical usage and molecular markers of cancer susceptibility. Growth Factors 30 (3), 176–191.

Yuzhalin, A.E., Kutikhin, A.G., 2012d. Inherited variations in the SOD and GPX gene families and cancer risk. Free Radical Res. 46 (5), 581–599.

Yuzhalin, A.E., Kutikhin, A.G., 2012e. Common genetic variants in the myeloperoxidase and paraoxonase genes and the related cancer risk: a review. J. Environ. Sci. Health, C Environ. Carcinog. Ecotoxicol. Rev. 30 (4), 287–322.

Zhang, Y., 2013. Epidemiology of esophageal cancer. World J. Gastroenterol. 19 (34), 5598–5606.

Zhivotovskiy, A.S., Kutikhin, A.G., Azanov, A.Z., Yuzhalin, A.E., Magarill, Y.A., Brusina, E.B., 2012. Colorectal cancer risk factors among the population of South-East Siberia: a case-control study. Asian Pac. J. Cancer Prev. 13 (10), 5183–5188.

CHAPTER 2

Interleukin-1 Superfamily and Cancer

Perfect as the wing of a bird may be, it will never enable the bird to fly if unsupported by the air. Facts are the air of science. Without them a man of science can never rise.

Ivan Pavlov, Russian physiologist (1849–1936)

2.1 INTERLEUKIN-1

2.1.1 Historical Background: Discovery of Interleukins

The marvelous story of interleukin (IL) discovery is associated with a succession of intriguing findings that were made over several decades. It has long been known that living cells are able to produce soluble factors that affect activity of other cells. In the early 1940s, Eli Menkin and Paul Beeson incubated pus cells collected from the peritoneal cavity of rabbits exposed to sterile irritant (Dinarello, 2009). The researchers demonstrated that injection of incubated pus to trained rabbits caused fever. Further investigations revealed that this fever-inducing substance was a protein, and it was named "pyrexin" or "granulocyte pyrogen" (Dinarello, 2009). This important finding provoked a plethora of active investigations of cell-derived mediators and their biological effects on the organism. A series of graceful experiments conducted by David et al. (1964) and Bloom and Bennett (1966) resulted in the discovery of a substance that significantly reduces the migration of macrophages, which now is known as macrophage migration inhibitory factor. In (Ruddle and Waksman, 1968) characterized a lymphocyte-derived factor with cytotoxic activities, currently known as lymphotoxin. Major breakthroughs in the fields of immunology and leukocyte biology have occurred every single year.

In 1971, Igal Gery and colleagues were performing experiments on human thymocytes and a mitogen phytohemagglutinin (PHA); surprisingly, they observed that white blood cells (WBCs) stimulated the mitotic activity of thymocytes in the absence of PHA (Gery et al., 1971; Oppenheim and Gery, 1993). The authors found their results reproducible and proposed that

Interleukins in Cancer Biology
http://dx.doi.org/10.1016/B978-0-12-801121-8.00002-6

this strange effect may be due to an unknown soluble factor released by WBCs. The term "lymphocyte-activating factor" (LAF) was coined for this hypothetical substance, although it was not purified and cloned yet. In order to detect the source of LAF, the authors performed the gradient separation of lymphocytes and repeated the experiment (Oppenheim and Gery, 1993). Unexpectedly, the activity proceeded from monocyte-macrophage subpopulation, not from T or B cells (Oppenheim and Gery, 1993). Further research demonstrated that production and release of LAF was activated by bacterial lipopolysaccharide (LPS), PHA, and concanavalin A (Gery et al., 1972). Moreover, LAF was reported to stimulate antigen-presenting cells and enhance allogenic mixed lymphocyte reactions (Oppenheim and Gery, 1993).

At the same time, another research group headed by Charles Dinarello was performing challenging in vivo experiments in order to investigate the previously unidentified molecule that induced fever in the studies by Menkin and Beeson (Dinarello et al., 1974; Dinarello and Wolff, 1978). By that time, the "granulocyte pyrogens" was known as "endogenous pyrogen" (EP) or "leukocytic pyrogen" (Dinarello, 2009). Their research group was able to purify EP and reveal that it acts as a thymocyte mitogen, thereby showing a similarity with LAF (Rosenwasser et al., 1979). In addition, production of EP by leukocytes was found to be activated by LPS, similarly to LAF (Oppenheim and Gery, 1993). The later finding that the two molecules are identical made it possible to expand the study and to identify its major role in numerous biological processes (Dinarello, 1996, 2009). The final name of the LAF-EP molecule was coined at the Second International Lymphokine Workshop held in Interlaken, Switzerland (Oppenheim and Gery, 1993). Dr Vern Paetkau proposed the term "interleukin" in honor of a place where that meeting took place.

A detailed understanding of the biology of IL-1 in early 1980s was connected with many difficulties. It was not easy to detect and sort out the abundance of biological effects of IL-1 on different cells. Moreover, IL-1 had shown molecular heterogeneity across series of experiments and in addition, several researchers discovered molecules that were homologous to IL-1, thereby suggesting that this agent has isoforms. Finally, it was unclear how 31 kDa precursor molecule proIL-1 transforms into mature 15 kDa protein.

2.1.2 Brief Description of IL-1

Today, IL-1 cytokine superfamily includes 11 representatives possessing similar genetic structure and wide array of functions (Nicklin et al., 2002). The most recognized and well-studied member of this superfamily is IL-1, which has a wide range of functions, upregulating numerous cytokines and acute phase enzymes, provoking inflammatory response, and activating leukocytes to implement immune reactions (Lie et al., 2012). IL-1 exists in two forms, namely, IL-1α and IL-1β. These isoforms have been first circumstantially investigated and described by March and colleagues in 1985 (March et al., 1985). Both are soluble peptides with highly pronounced proinflammatory and pyrogenic activities. IL-1α and IL-1β are predominantly expressed by fibroblasts, monocytes, neutrophils, macrophages, epithelial, dendritic, and endothelial cells, and they are also known to be synthesized by natural killer (NK) and B cells rarely. IL-1α and IL-1β derive from different precursor proteins, proIL-1α and proIL-1β, respectively, which have similar molecular weight approximately of 31 kDa. Upon synthesizing, proIL-1α and proIL-1β precursors undergo proteolytic cleavage via caspase-1 or calcium-activated protease, respectively, to take their mature form. Although IL-1α and IL-1β share only 22% homology, they bind to the same receptor, IL-1 receptor (IL-1R), and have a similar functional impact. Upon binding, the ligand–receptor complex assembles with a specific adaptor protein called IL-1R accessory protein (IL-1RAcP). Upon dimerization, the final complex activates the conserved intracellular domain of IL-1R, termed Toll–interleukin-1 (TIR) domain. The activated TIR domain recruits intracellullar adaptor protein Myd88, which consequently triggers plenty of transcription factors, such as nuclear factor kappa beta (NF-κB) and many others. These factors then travel to the nucleus where they activate the transcription of numerous genes involved in proinflammatory immune response.

A question may immediately arise: what is the point of the existence of two similar isoforms of the same molecule that exert similar functional activities? This issue was clarified by Stephen Eisenberg and colleagues, who revealed that, in fact, IL-1α and IL-1β evolutionarily diverged from a common ancestor precursor approximately 270–300 million years ago, when a duplication of an *IL-1* gene predecessor occurred. In addition, although IL-1α and IL-1β seem almost identical, they have several significant differences. First, IL-1β is a secreted cytokine, i.e., it is released by immune cells into the microenvironment in order to provide paracrine or autocrine regulation. It was found that IL-1β release is due to the formation of functional inflammasome as a mechanism (Okamoto et al., 2010). On the contrary, IL1-α is rarely secreted. In fact, IL1-α generally acts as either intracellular or membrane-bound agent and almost never leaves the cell where it was synthesized (Apte and Voronov, 2002). Moreover, several findings indicated that IL1-α may act as a nuclear factor, activating transcription of certain proinflammatory genes (Maier et al., 1994; Werman et al., 2004). Second, it is believed that IL-1β is produced only after external stimulation. For instance, a signal from pattern recognition receptors, which include Toll-like receptors (TLRs), C-type lectin receptors (CLRs), RIG-I-like receptors, and nucleotide-binding oligomerization domain receptors, is known to activate the expression of the *IL-1β* gene. In contrast, almost all types of cells producing IL-1α constantly contain a certain amount of this cytokine in the cytosol; therefore, IL-1α is frequently found in healthy tissues unlike IL-1β. Third, there is strong evidence that IL-1α may expeditiously compete immunostimulation induced by IL-1β due to interaction with the IL-1R; in other words, IL-1α may behave as a downregulator of the IL-1β activity (Boraschi et al., 1990). And fourth, it was observed that IL-1α and IL-1β act not consistently in tumor cells (Marhaba et al., 2008), and moreover, in the discussion below, we will refer to the fact that their role in cancer development is totally different.

2.1.3 IL-1-Driven Carcinogenesis

Since it has become clear that IL-1 possesses proinflammatory, immunostimulatory, and antiinfection properties, this cytokine became an attractive candidate for possible clinical application in the treatment of various diseases, including cancer. Surprisingly, the plethora of subsequent investigations aimed to shed light on the impact of IL-1 on carcinogenesis revealed that this cytokine is not a guardian angel at all. In 1992, Smith et al. performed a phase I trial study, in which subjects with advanced solid tumors were intravenously injected with IL-1α consecutively for 7 days. The authors indicated significant and potentially beneficial hematopoietic effects, including elevated cellularity of bone marrow, increased levels of thyroid-stimulating hormone, triglycerides, C-reactive protein, cortisol, and decreased levels of protein-C testosterone, and cholesterol; however, they did not observe any direct antitumor effects. In 1990, Giavazzi et al. examined whether IL-1 is a major factor for metastasis formation. The authors observed that recombinant IL-1β greatly elevated the metastatic activity of the human A375M melanoma in the nude mice lungs in a concentration-dependent manner. Several years later, the research group headed by Vidal-Vanaclocha (1994) injected recombinant human IL-1β (rHuIL-1β) into C57BL/6J mice prior to intrasplenic injection of murine B16 melanoma cells in order to investigate possible influence of IL-1 on occurrence of hepatic metastases. The authors demonstrated that mice pretreated with rHuIL-1β had significantly elevated number of tumor foci in comparison with cytokine-untreated control mice (46 versus 27, respectively). Later, Vidal-Vanaclocha et al. (2000)

replicated their previous findings, demonstrating that (1) metastatic activity was significantly reduced in the liver of *IL-1β*-deficient mice and that (2) metastasis did not develop at all in mice that were deficient in caspase-1, an IL-1β-converting enzyme. In 1996, Chirivi et al. introduced the *IL-1α* gene into the human melanoma cell line in order to evaluate the impact of this cytokine on cancer; further injection of these cells into nude mice elevated the expression of vascular cell adhesion molecule 1 (VCAM-1) on lung microvascular endothelial cells; therefore, the adhesiveness for tumor cells was increased. In 2003, Voronov et al. discovered that mice deficient in either *IL-1α* or *IL-1β* genes showed slower or no cancer development and blood vessel growth in three different tumor models as compared to wild-type mice (B16 melanoma, DA/3 mammary adenocarcinoma in BALB/e mice, and prostate cancer cell lines injected into C57Bl6 mice). Based on their results, the authors suggested that environmental IL-1 may somehow contribute to angiogenesis and invasiveness of tumors. Interestingly, the authors noticed that the contribution of IL-1α and IL-1β was different; the latter cytokine demonstrated significantly more invasive and severe pattern. Elaraj et al. (2006) observed that the mRNA of IL-1 was overexpressed in the majority of investigated metastatic human tumor samples among which are melanoma, non-small-cell lung carcinoma, and colorectal adenocarcinoma specimens. Later, Song et al. (2003) replicated these results in fibrosarcoma cell lines, showing that the reduction of tumorigenicity was associated with IL-1α-driven anticancer immune response. At the same time, the authors observed that IL-1β stimulated angiogenesis, invasiveness, and immune suppression.

To summarize, all these observations revealed that in fact, IL-1 does not possess any antitumor activities that may stimulate the organism to fight cancer; oppositely, this cytokine, in particular, IL-1β, contributes to development and progression of malignant tumors. Nevertheless, some anticancer activities of IL-1α were demonstrated. An interesting study was conducted in 2007 by Krelin et al. who investigated 3-methylcholanthrene-induced carcinogenesis in mice with *IL-1α*, *IL-β*, or simultaneous *IL-1α* and *IL-1β* gene knockout. The authors demonstrated that cancer development rate was significantly inhibited in *IL-1β*-deficient mice, while it was similar in IL-1α-deficient and wild-type mice. In some cases, *IL-1β*-deficient mice did not develop cancer at all. This observation indicates a greater role of IL-1β in cancer development as compared to IL-1α. Importantly, this study was the first evidence of different impacts of IL-1α and IL-1β in oncogenesis, and moreover, it revealed that, although some antitumor activities of IL-1α were previously observed (Song et al., 2003), this isoform is nevertheless able to stimulate cancer growth.

There is also accumulating evidence that IL-1 plays a great role in tumor angiogenesis. In 1995, Ben-Av et al. discovered that IL-1 activates the expression of vascular endothelial growth factor (VEGF) in synovial fibroblasts in patients with rheumatoid arthritis. Later, several reports revealed that IL-1β is able to stimulate the production of matrix metalloproteinases (MMPs) 3 and 9, which in turn activate synthesis and release of basic fibroblast growth factor (bFGF) (Hutchinson et al., 1992; Lefebvre et al., 1991; Sasaki et al., 1998). As known, both VEGF and bFGF are strong proangiogenic factors that have been numerously reported to stimulate the excessive tumor vasculature (reviewed by Claesson-Welsh and Welsh, 2013; Farhat et al., 2012; Kos and Dabrowski, 2002). The detailed mechanism of bFGF-induced angiogenesis was investigated by Sasaki et al. (1998), who demonstrated that IL-1 triggers the expression of inducible isoform of nitric oxide synthase (iNOS), which in turn dramatically increases the production of nitric oxide (NO) from L-arginine. Elevated concentrations of NO subsequently stimulate synthesis of MMPs and eventually, production of proangiogenic factor bFGF. Furthermore, NO is believed to maintain vessel integrity and regulate vascular permeability in tumors (Fukumura et al., 1997; Murohara et al., 1998). Additionally, it should also be noted that NO may exert a significant carcinogenic effect by itself, as recently reviewed by Korde Choudhari et al. (2012).

The above-mentioned experiments demonstrated that IL-1 may provide massive blood supply to the tumor and therefore active investigations in this field have been continued. In 2002, Saijo et al. introduced *IL-1β* gene into the mouse Lewis lung carcinoma (LLC) cell culture. As compared to wild-type LLC cells, the investigated cell line showed twofold increase in the amount of VEGF. Additionally, it was found that the amount of macrophage-inflammatory protein-2 (CXCL2, MIP-2) was increased more than 10 times in comparison with control cell culture. Of note, CXCL2 is a chemokine that has been shown to contribute to tumor angiogenesis in series of experiments (Porta et al., 2007; Nakao et al., 2005; Kujawaski et al., 2008). Furthermore, similar results were obtained by Voronov et al. (2003), who confirmed the previous report indicating that IL-1α-deficient and *IL-1β*-deficient mice have less pronounced expression of VEGF as compared to wild-type mice. Additionally, the authors indicated that IL-1 is able to stimulate VEGF expression in cancer cells in vitro (2003).

Parallel studies by Carmeliet et al. (1998), and Haddad et al. (2002) revealed that IL-1 is able to induce nuclear transportation and activation of hypoxia-inducible factor-1α (HIF-1α), an enzyme that is responsible for survival of the organism during the lack of oxygen. Overexpression of HIF-1α has been reported to cause excessive vascularization due to upregulation of VEGF, and in addition, it has also been associated with increased tumor growth and metastasis (Semenza, 2007). Recent study by Carmi et al. (2009) showed that angiogenesis induced by supernatants of LPS-stimulated hypoxic and normoxic macrophages from mice administered either with anti-IL-1β antibodies or anti-IL-1α and anti-IL-1β antibodies was totally prevented. Similarly, *IL-1β*-deficient mice did not develop angiogenesis, unlike IL-1α-deficient ones, which had angiogenesis in the condition of hypoxia. Moreover, the authors indicated that IL-1 was associated with dramatic increase in VEGF levels as well. Finally, findings by Weiss et al. (2009) showed that IL-1β promotes significant tumor growth by inducing myeloid-derived suppressor cell and regulatory T-cell expansion.

To conclude, the following fundamental mechanisms are known to promote IL-1-mediated cancer development:

- Initiation and development of severe inflammatory response due to pro-inflammatory and pyrogenic activity (Okamoto et al., 2010).
- Activation of macrophages and other immune cells to produce mutagenic reactive oxygen species during the respiratory burst.
- Stimulation of iNOS-dependent synthesis of NO, which possesses pro-carcinogenic activities (Fukumura et al., 1997; Murohara et al., 1998).
- Development of angiogenesis due to (1) recruitment of inflammatory cells to the tumor, (2) upregulation of VEGF and bFGF, and triggering of HIF-1α (Ben-Av et al., 1995; Sasaki et al., 1998; Semenza, 2007).
- Triggering the expression of adhesion molecules on endothelial and malignant cells, which subsequently leads to the transfer of cancer cells into the circulation and their further distribution over the body (Chirivi et al., 1996).

2.1.4 IL-1Ra Restrains IL-1

The third important member of the IL-1 family is the IL-1R antagonist (IL-1Ra), which was independently discovered by Jean-Michel Dayer and William Arend in 1984 (Arend and Dayer, 1990). It possesses 19% amino acid homology to IL-1α and 26% amino acid homology to IL-1β; therefore, all these molecules are quite similar. IL-1Ra represents a 25 kDa glycoprotein that acts as natural inhibitor of the activities of IL-1α and IL-β. Binding of IL-1Ra to IL-1R does not cause signal triggering because it binds to the receptor with only one binding site, unlike IL-1α and IL-1β, which establish the formation of a ligand–receptor complex with two binding sites. Simultaneous presence of agonist molecules IL-1α and IL-1β and receptor antagonist IL-1Ra within the body establishes constant competition between them for receptor occupancy; therefore, the ratio of the concentrations of these cytokines determines whether the inflammatory process will be driven or not. Interestingly, it has been reported that 17 kDa nonglycosylated precursor form of IL-1Ra is also able to inhibit IL-1α and IL-1β activity as well (Eisenberg, 1990; Carter, 1990). Notwithstanding its completely opposite effect on the organism, IL-1Ra has close structural similarity with both IL-1α and IL-β; it was found that the gene for IL-1Ra was the first to diverge from the common ancestor of IL-1 family between 350 and 360 million years ago. Apparently, the regulation of *IL-1Ra* gene expression involves several transcriptional factors, including NF-κB, PU.1, and GA-binding protein (Smith et al., 1998). Recently, it was also discovered that CC chemokine receptor type 5 signaling significantly affects production of IL-1Ra as well (Song et al., 2012).

Taking into account multiple tumor-promoting effects of IL-1, it has become clear that usage of the natural inhibitor of this cytokine may be an effective therapeutic approach to treat cancer. Indeed, numerous studies devoted to the investigation of the role of IL-1Ra in cancer development have revealed its powerful ability to restrain adverse protumorigenic activities of IL-1. Vidal-Vanaclocha et al. (1996) revealed that intraperitoneal administration of 5 mg/kg of rHuIL-1Ra 1 h before injection of rHuIL-1β substantially reduces augmentation in hepatic metastasis in C57BL/6J mice injected with B16 melanoma cell line (p < 0.01). Moreover, the authors demonstrated that mice pretreated with 1 μg/mL rHuIL-1Ra did not experience the adherence of melanoma cells to hepatic sinusoidal endothelial (HSE) cells after 6 h of exposure to bacterial LPS as compared to untreated mice. Interestingly, the addition of 1 ng/mL rHuIL-1Ra to normal sinusoidal endothelium did not change the basal adherence of B16 melanoma cells, suggesting that IL-1 does not mediate HSE responses in unstimulated endothelium, unlike LPS-treated tissue. In addition, further in-depth analysis based on previous experience (Vidal-Vanaclocha et al., 1993; Asumendi et al., 1995) allowed the authors to explain the observed results. It is known that IL-1 upregulates the expression of HSE cell mannose receptors, a type of CLR presented on the surface of macrophages and dendritic cells (DCs), which recognize microorganisms that possess mannose on their surface, and activate pathways of the complement system. Activation of HSE-specific mannose receptors is critical for the initiation of the adherence between

HSE cells and B16 melanoma cells (Vidal-Vanaclocha et al., 1993), which eventually results in metastatic process. Therefore, aside from contributing to cancer development per se, IL-1 may indirectly affect the occurrence of metastasis. The authors obtained that IL-1Ra-induced blockade of IL-1R prevented LPS-driven activation of HSE-specific mannose receptors, thereby reducing cell adherence (Vidal-Vanaclocha et al., 1996). Another research group found that IL-1Ra inhibited the augmented expression of the intracellular VCAM-1 and E-selectin induced by IL-1 on endothelial cells, thereby preventing the formation of metastasis in athymic nude mice (Chirivi et al., 1993). These findings discovered the first important property of IL-1Ra, namely, prevention of metastasis development.

Other important properties of IL-1Ra are antiproliferative and antiangiogenic activities. In 2002, Coxon et al. demonstrated that dose-dependent injection of IL-1Ra blocks bFGF- and VEGF-driven corneal angiogenesis in rats with induced arthritis, and interestingly, the effect was the same during the noninflammatory conditions. Furthermore, Weinreich et al. (2003) and Elaraj et al. (2006) found that administration of recombinant IL-1Ra (drug named anakinra) in athymic nude mice injected with melanoma cells significantly decreased tumor growth and its metastatic potential. Moreover, Elaraj et al. (2006) indicated that relative mRNA levels of IL-8 and VEGF were significantly decreased in anakinra-treated mice. This observation may indicate yet another anticancer mechanism of IL-1Ra-mediated anticancer response, as IL-8 and VEGF play a central role in tumor growth and angiogenesis. Furthermore, Konishi et al. (2005) revealed that environmental IL-1Ra inhibited IL-1β-induced VEGF expression by 87% in 65 subjects with colorectal cancer, thereby confirming the previous suggestions regarding the antiangiogenic activities of IL-1Ra. Further studies devoted to this issue finally confirmed that IL-1Ra inhibits cancer-related angiogenesis in vivo (Bar et al., 2004; Voronov et al., 2003).

Notably, yet another interesting study was recently conducted by Krelin et al. (2007), who observed that IL-1Ra-deficient mice developed cancer faster than mice deficient either in IL-1α or IL-1β genes, which is consistent with the hypothesis of IL-1-mediated cancer progression. Furthermore, supernatants of cell lines derived from IL-1Ra-deficient mice demonstrated a higher angiogenic potential as compared to supernatants of cell lines derived from both IL-1α-deficient and IL-1β-deficient mice. This finding indicates that IL-1Ra plays a key role in cancer development. Finally, Harnack et al. (2011) demonstrated that injection of anakinra into nonimmunized mice with macroscopic tumor greatly decreased levels of IL-6 and did not inhibit tumor growth. Nevertheless, administration of anakinra to preimmunized mice with palpable tumors resulted in significant regression of tumors without decrease in IL-6 levels.

Importantly, increased levels of IL-1Ra were observed in numerous malignancies, including colorectal cancer (Iwagaki et al., 1997; Ito and Miki, 1999; Kaminska et al., 2000), multiple myeloma (Gherardi et al., 1996), ovarian cancer (Mustea et al., 2008), leukemia (Barak et al., 1998), cervical carcinoma (Fujiwaki et al., 2003), pancreatic cancer (Ebrahimi et al., 2004; Poch et al., 2007), uveal melanoma (Lee et al., 2012), prostate cancer (Parekh et al., 2007), breast cancer (Lv et al., 2011), and thyroid cancer (Niedźwiecki et al., 2008). It is interesting that elevated concentrations of IL-1Ra were associated either with greater (Iwagaki et al., 1997; Ito and Miki, 1999; Kaminska et al., 2000; Fujiwaki et al., 2003; Parekh et al., 2007; Niedźwiecki et al., 2008) or lesser (Gherardi et al., 1996; Parekh et al., 2007; Poch et al., 2007) disease severity. On the contrary, several studies reported that intratumoral levels of IL-1Ra were significantly decreased (Pantschenko et al., 2003; Ricote et al., 2004). All these indications may indicate clinical importance of IL-1Ra as a marker of cancer.

To summarize, IL-1Ra is an anticancer agent constraining the destructive behavior of IL-1β within the body. Three main mechanisms of IL-1Ra-mediated antitumor response include: (1) blockade of IL-1 signaling, (2) inhibition of metastasis formation due to reduction of adherence between tumor and endothelial cells, and (3) suppression of angiogenesis in tumors (Figure 2.1). Charles Dinarello suggested treating cancer with anakinra-mediated IL-1β blockade (Dinarello, 2010). Indeed, anakinra is a safe, effective, and well-tolerated drug possessing significant clinical effectiveness in treatment of numerous diseases, including rheumatoid arthritis, familial Mediterranean fever, Castleman's disease, asbestosis, type 2 diabetes, impairments of blood–brain barrier, Behcet's disease, and juvenile idiopathic arthritis (Pascual et al., 2005; Fleischmann et al., 2006; Larsen et al., 2007; Calligaris et al., 2008; Botsios et al., 2008; El-Osta et al., 2010; Librizzi et al., 2012). In this regard, it is also necessary to mention an interesting study by Qian et al. (2013) who demonstrated that pretreatment with anakinra significantly decreased chemotherapy-induced peripheral blood injury in mice. Moreover, experiments on beagle dogs indicated that incidence and severity of neutropenia was also significantly decreased after administration of anakinra during the chemotherapy (Qian et al., 2013). Furthermore, it was found that administration of anakinra together with docetaxel and temozolomide chemotherapy showed more effective anticancer response in

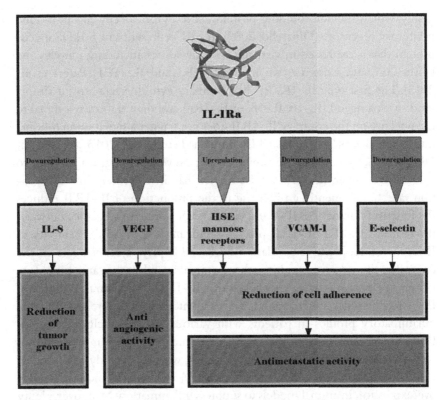

Figure 2.1 Anticancer activities of interleukin (IL)-1Ra. VEGF, vascular endothelial growth factor; VCAM-1, vascular cell adhesion molecule 1; HSE, hepatic sinusoidal endothelial. (For color version of this figure, the reader is referred to the online version of this book).

B16 melanoma mice. Thereby, chemoprotective activity of rHuIL-1Ra may also be very advantageous in regard of possible application of rHuIL-1Ra for cancer treatment.

According to all the above-mentioned investigations, it could be suggested that IL-1Ra-mediated blockade of the IL-1β activity may significantly inhibit growth and development of malignant tumors. Hopefully, subsequent research in this field will supplement and clarify existing data on the biology of IL-1Ra in tumor models in order to substantiate the application of this cytokine for further therapeutic treatment interventions.

2.1.5 IL-1 Receptors and their Relation to Cancer

Finally, a couple of words should be mentioned about IL-1R. Formally, IL-1R does not belong to the IL-1 family; in fact, it forms its own IL-1R family, which includes binding proteins, coreceptors, decoy receptors, and inhibitory receptors (Dinarello, 2009). IL-1R represents an 80 kDa glycoprotein that is expressed in virtually all body tissues, including muscles and epithelium, and exists in two forms, IL-1RI and IL-1RII (Peters et al., 2013). The first type IL-1R acts like ordinary cytokine receptor; it simply binds with a ligand (IL-1α, IL-1β, or IL-1Ra) and then transmits a signal to the nucleus; on the contrary, IL-1RII does not trigger a signal upon binding due to the lack of intracellular TIR domain (Peters et al., 2013). In fact, IL-1RII acts like a competitive inhibitor that prevents IL-1 from binding to IL-1RI; moreover, IL-1/IL-1RII complex has an extremely low dissociation rate. Consequently, an increase in the production of IL-1RII reduces the functional activity of IL-1 and vice versa. So, the subtle balance between the ratios of IL-1RI/IL-1RII plays a significant role in cells' receptivity to IL-1; therefore, negative regulation by IL-1RII plays a crucial role in the control of the organism under such a formidable and, at the same time dangerous, weapon as IL-1. It is believed that IL-1RII, as a natural inhibitor of IL-1, may be successfully applied as a therapeutic agent for creation of anti-inflammatory profiles in patients with various diseases, including cancer. Rauschmayr et al. (1997) observed that chronic inflammation induced by a well-characterized IL-1-dependent stimulus, was significantly inhibited in IL-1RII transgenic animals. Bessis et al. (2000) were able to induce IL-1RII overexpression in animal models to suppress inflammation. Moreover, plenty of agents, such as acetylsalicylic acid, glucocorticoids, prostaglandins, dexamethasone, and a plethora of ILs, including IL-4, IL-13, and IL-27, have been reported to upregulate expression of IL-1RII in vitro (Daun et al., 1999; Colotta et al., 1993; Spriggs et al., 1992; Re et al., 1994; Kalliolias et al., 2010). However, there is a lack of studies devoted to investigation of the role of IL-1R and cancer. It was found that green tea antioxidant epigallocatechin gallate is able to downregulate IL-1RI and therefore suppress IL-1-induced tumorigenic factors in human pancreatic adenocarcinoma cells (Hoffmann et al., 2011). Keita et al. (2011) revealed that endometrioid ovarian cancer cells exhibit the decrease in the expression of IL-1RII, which may indicate a probable relationship between malfunction of IL-1 inhibitor, prolonged IL-1-driven inflammation, and cancer occurrence.

However, there are two limiting factors that may restrict the potential application of IL-1RII as a therapeutic agent. First, it is known that the affinity of IL-1RII to IL-1β is 100 times higher than to IL-1α; therefore it cannot sequester the latter as good as the former. Second, in order to properly carry out its functions, IL-1RII requires the presence of the soluble form of the coreceptor, which is the alternative splice transcript of the membrane IL-1RAcP (Smeets et al., 2005). Thus, these two issues should be taken into account when developing possible therapeutic strategies based on IL-1RII.

Notably, both IL-1RI and IL-1RII have soluble isoforms, which can be detected in a small amount across various body fluids, including blood and urine (Sims et al., 1994). It is believed that these soluble isoforms are yielded by shedding of the extracellular domain of membrane-bound IL-1R by unidentified metalloproteases (Giri et al., 1990; Symons et al., 1991). Alternatively, it has been reported that in patients with autoimmune inner ear disease soluble forms of IL-1R can be produced by alternative splicing (Vambutas et al., 2009). It is interesting that along with "decoy" receptor IL-1R, soluble IL-1Rs may possess clinical significance by isolating IL-1, thereby preventing it from binding to IL-1RI and exerting a proinflammatory effect. Moreover, there is increasing evidence that soluble IL-1R is of great importance in disease development, as its concentration was found increased in patients with sepsis (Pruitt et al., 1996; Giri et al., 1994), Alzheimer disease (Garlind et al., 1999), and during IL-2 therapy (Vannier et al., 1999). Simeoni et al. successfully used soluble IL-1RII gene transfer to inhibit attenuate cardiac allograft rejection in a rat model (Simeoni et al., 2007). However, a phase I clinical trial conducted by Bernshtein et al. (1999) did not show any response to treatment of acute myeloid leukemia by recombinant IL-R.

2.1.6 Inherited Variations within the *IL-1β* Gene and Cancer

It is well known that variations in human genome may affect the susceptibility to various diseases, including cancer. Much research has been done in the last decade to explore the role of gene polymorphisms within the IL genes and cancer (Lundström et al., 2012; Yuzhalin and Kutikhin, 2012; Xu et al., 2013; Kutikhin et al., 2014; Yao et al., 2014). A particularly large number of such studies have been devoted to the *IL-1β* gene. It is out of the scope of this book to describe all the studies investigating the impact of the *IL-1β* gene polymorphisms on cancer development; however, it is worthwhile to illustrate here a reliable correlation between these polymorphisms and gastric cancer, which has been established not long ago (reviewed by Yuzhalin, 2011).

There are three most intensively investigated polymorphisms within the *IL-1β* gene that affect its expression: −511 (C > T, rs16944), −31 (T > C, rs1143627), and +3954 (C > T, rs1143634). Four comprehensive meta-analyses on the *IL-1β* gene were chosen to assess the role of these single-nucleotide polymorphisms (SNPs) in gastric cancer. Researchers have been studying the T allele of the −511 SNP for a long time. First, Camargo et al. (2006) demonstrated that −511TT carriers had increased gastric cancer risk in comparison with CC wild-type genotype carriers in 14 studies (odds ratio (OR) = 1.21). The effect was more evident for T allele carriers with non-cardiac and intestinal gastric cancer subtypes (OR = 1.66 and 1.80, respectively) among Caucasians. Interestingly, there were no correlations among Asian populations. An analysis of 39 case–control studies conducted by Wang et al. (2006) revealed similar results; the T allele of −511 was more frequent among patients with gastric cancer (OR = 1.26). Histopathologic stratification revealed that the association was stronger for patients with intestinal subtype (OR = 1.76) but not with diffuse type (OR = 1.16), which confirmed the results of Camargo et al. (2010). The authors also indicated that there was no impact of ethnicity and HP status on cancer risk in this study. The results of Xue et al. (2010) also confirmed the findings of previous authors; the T allele correlated with higher intestinal and noncardiac gastric cancer risk in 18 studies versus CC genotype (OR = 1.55 and 1.33, respectively). Interestingly, these significant results were also obtained among Caucasians but not in Asian or Hispanic populations (OR = 1.33). The fourth meta-analysis, which included 28 studies, was performed by Kamangar et al. (2006). They reported an absence of correlations between CT/TT genotypes and the gastric cancer genotype in comparison with the CC wild-type genotype (OR = 1.07 and 1.16, respectively). Ethnic stratification also indicated a lack of significant differences, as well as analysis of histopathology or tumor site.

These contradictory results could be explained by possible differences in study design, inclusion criteria of investigations, errors during the statistical analysis, differences in stratification, sample size, and chance.

However, an overwhelming majority of studies characterize the T allele of the IL1B_−511 polymorphism as frequent among Caucasian individuals with noncardiac gastric cancer, preferably for the intestinal subtype of this cancer. Therefore, it is feasible to suggest this SNP as a potential predictive marker for gastric cancer.

Investigations of the IL1B_−31 TATA-box polymorphism continue to be controversial even after several meta-analyses have been carried out. Camargo et al. (2006) revealed a slight nonsignificant connection between the C variant allele and gastric cancer risk compared with TT homozygotes (OR = 1.04) in 14 studies. Similarly, there was no association among Asian populations (OR = 0.91) as compared to either Hispanic or Caucasian populations (OR = 0.91, 1.52, and 1.11, respectively). Histologic stratification indicated a moderate increase in intestinal gastric cancer subtype among C allele carriers in Caucasian populations (OR = 1.61), but this statement was not true for the diffuse subtype of gastric cancer.

No associations were observed in the studies of Wang et al. (2006), Xue et al. (2010), and Kamangar et al. (2006; OR = 1.00, 0.97, and 0.99, respectively). Subgroup analysis did not indicate any correlations.

Investigations on the IL1B_+3954 SNP have indicated discordant results. Camargo et al. (2006) indicated a slight nonsignificant increase in gastric cancer risk among T mutant allele carriers compared with CC individuals (OR = 1.26), and the effect was more evident among Asian populations (OR = 1.73). However, the small number of studies and the deficiency of T and CT allele carriers in some studies could distort the results.

Wang et al. (2006) also determined that the T allele of the +3954 gene polymorphism contributes to cancer risk (OR = 1.37) in comparison with the CC genotype, although no analyses of HP status, tumor location, or subtype were performed. Xue et al. (2010) reported a lack of association between the +3954 polymorphism and gastric cancer.

A small number of studies on the IL-1B_+3954C/T polymorphism have been conducted. A correlation of the T allele with gastric cancer was identified, which indicates a potential role in gastric carcinogenesis.

Recently, Lee et al. (2004) discovered a new promoter IL1B_−1473G to C (rs1143623) polymorphism and reported an association between its G allele and increased risk of the intestinal type of gastric cancer (OR = 1.8 for the CG genotype and 2.1 for the GG genotype) among a Korean population. The significance of this finding should be proven by further functional and genetic association studies.

It is important not to overlook the fact that the above-mentioned meta-analyses (Camargo et al., 2006; Wang et al., 2006; Kamangar et al., 2006; Xue et al., 2010) are mostly composed of the same original studies, and therefore some degree of overlap exists. First, meta-analyses devoted to the IL1B_−511C/T polymorphism are composed of materials from 10 same case–control studies. Materials from 11 studies were included in the above-mentioned meta-analyses on the IL1B_−31T/C SNP and data from seven papers were involved in the meta-analyses on the IL1B_+3954C gene polymorphism. Such overlapping of data creates sufficient difficulties in comparison of these meta-analyses among each other, although the main trends and relations could be defined. The role of the T allele of the IL1B_−511 polymorphism may be defined as cancer predictive. The impact of the −31C allele remains unclear based on contradictory results. Several epidemiologic studies have reported that the T allele of the IL1B_−31 SNP is associated with vulnerable to persistent HP infection, which can be modified by smoking (Hamajima et al., 2001), but according to case–control studies, this allele apparently does not play a role in the development of gastric cancer, even taking into account the fact that some studies confirm this link. Finally, it should be noted that further investigation of the poorly studied IL1B_+3954 and IL1B_−1473 genetic polymorphisms is necessary.

The authors would note that this section was borrowed from their article on this issue (Yuzhalin, 2011).

2.1.7 Summary

Summarized findings obtained in the last two decades allow highlighting the considerable importance of IL-1 in cancer biology. Among the mechanisms involved in IL-1-driven carcinogenesis are: (1) strong proinflammatory activity, (2) stimulation of iNOS-dependent synthesis of NO, (3) proangiogenic activities, and triggering the expression of adhesion molecules on the surface of endothelial and malignant cells, which can lead to the development of metastasis.

Undoubtedly, further in-depth research in the field of IL-1 and its receptors may open up yet unexplored areas of cancer biology and eventually lead to a significant decrease in morbidity and mortality from cancer. For further reading, the authors highly recommend a plethora of well-written review articles by Charles Dinarello (Dinarello, 1994; Dinarello, 2006; Dinarello, 2011), which contain exhaustive data on the biology of IL-1α, IL-1β, IL-1Ra, and IL-1R.

2.2 INTERLEUKIN-18

IL-18 is an important member of the IL-1 superfamily, and although it has structural and functional relationship with IL-1, it possesses a number of specific characteristics. IL-18 was described in 1995 by Okamura et al., and initially was named interferon-gamma inducing factor for its ability to stimulate NK cells and T cells to produce and release interferon-γ (IFN-γ) in the presence of IL-12. It was found that the novel molecule's molecular weight is 18 kDa, and it is formed due to proteolytic cleavage of a 24 kDa precursor molecule named proIL-18. Subsequent studies devoted to the biology of this cytokine demonstrated that its functions are not limited to simple upregulation of IFN-γ. In fact, IL-18 upregulates the expression of numerous cytokines, such as IL-1β, granulocyte macrophage colony-stimulating factor, IL-8, soluble Fas ligand, and tumor necrosis factor alpha (TNF-α) (Robertson et al., 2006). IL-18-dependent triggering of the above-mentioned molecules leads to the activation of Th1 differentiation, suppression of osteoclast proliferation, and stimulation of NK-mediated cytotoxicity (Ushio et al., 1996; Udagawa et al., 1997; Robertson et al., 2006). Due to its extensive effects on immune cells, IL-18 plays a critical role in regulation of both innate and adaptive immunity. IL-18 is known to be produced not only by Th1 cells and NK cells, but also by macrophages, DCs, astrocytes, and microglial cells (Okamura et al., 1995; Udagawa et al., 1997; Stoll et al., 1998; Takeda et al., 1998; Conti et al., 1999). The expression of *IL-18* gene is generally triggered by IL-10, IL-1, IL-6, and TNF-α in response to the presence of an infectious agent within the body (Dinarello and Fantuzzi, 2003). The impact of IL-18 on a cell is a multistep process. First, IL-18 binds to the membrane-bound IL-18 receptor alpha (IL-18Rα) and forms a dimer. Upon dimerization, the ligand–receptor complex recruits an additional accessory protein IL-18β, which is necessary for further transduction of the signal (Born et al., 1998). As a result, the complex comprising three subunits activates the TIR domain of IL-18R, which in turn triggers the intracellullar adaptor molecule Myd88 and several interleukin-1 receptor activating kinases (IRAKs). Subsequently, these agents activate transcription factor NF-κB, which eventually lead to the expression of numerous genes. In addition, it was found that IL-18 production may be activated via alternative signaling mechanisms, involving WNT pathway, p38 mitogen-activated protein kinase (MAPK), and c-Jun N-terminal kinase (Mo et al., 2012; Zhang et al., 2013). Moreover, intracellular factors, in particular, high-mobility group protein B1, were reported to upregulate the expression and release of IL-18 as well (He et al., 2012).

Multiple biological effects of IL-18 indicate an important role of this cytokine in cancer development. However, the impact of this cytokine on the formation of malignant tumors is controversial. On the one hand, many investigations have demonstrated strong antitumor activities of IL-18. Plenty in vitro and in vivo studies showed that transfer of *IL-18* gene decreased tumorigenicity and proliferation of various tumors (Fukumoto et al., 1997; Yoshimura et al., 2001; Nagai et al., 2002; Tanaka et al., 2002; Zhang and Wu, 2007; Agorio et al., 2007; Tse et al., 2011; Müller et al., 2011; Fan et al., 2012), and moreover, induced apoptosis (Ohtsuki et al., 1997; Liu et al., 2012) and inhibited angiogenesis within tumors (Zheng et al., 2009; Zheng et al., 2010).

Additionally, intratumoral and peritoneal administration of recombinant IL-18 demonstrated significant anticancer effect in series of in vivo experiments and in patients with malignant tumors (Micallef et al., 1997; Cao et al., 1999; Redlinger et al., 2003; Xia et al., 2003; Iwasaki et al., 2002; Subleski et al., 2006; Shiratori et al., 2007; Yamada et al., 2009). In addition, several research groups demonstrated that combination of IL-18 with other cytokines, such as IL-2, IL-12, IL-15, or IL-23 significantly reduces tumor growth and angiogenesis both in vitro and in vivo (Osaki et al., 1998; Coughlin et al., 1998; Redlinger et al., 2003; Smyth et al., 2004; Wang et al., 2004; Müller et al., 2011; Chen et al., 2012; Ni et al., 2012). Finally, it was found that simultaneous administration of IL-18 and monoclonal antibody rituximab promoted significant regression of human lymphoma xenografts in severe combined immunodeficiency mice (Srivastava et al., 2013).

Currently, the following mechanisms of IL-18-mediated anticancer immune response are known:

• Activation of immune cells.
• Production of IFN-γ and other anticancer cytokines.
• Expression of Fas ligand, thereby triggering Fas-mediated apoptosis in tumors.
• Downregulation of VEGF and other proangiogenic factors, such as CXCL2.

It is important to mention an interesting study by Du et al. (2012), who created IL-18-IL-12 fusion protein. The authors used polymerase chain reaction to obtain the fusion gene *IL-18-IL-12*, and then inserted it into viral vector to examine its antitumor activities in mice with LLC. Importantly, the authors observed IL-18-IL-12-induced increase in the secretion of IFN-γ and significant regression of tumor. Further in-depth investigations should be conducted to evaluate possible application of this fusion cytokine in cancer immunotherapy.

On the other hand, however, there are numerous findings reporting that IL-18 is involved in cancer development and progression. First, several studies provided an evidence of proangiogenic activities of IL-18. In particular, it was found that IL-18 is capable of upregulating a plethora of angiogenic factors, including VEGF, cell-derived factor 1 alpha, and monocyte chemotactic protein 1 via c-Jun, p38 MAPK, and NF-κB signaling pathways (Cho et al., 2006; Amin et al., 2007). In addition, VEGF has been reported to upregulate the expression of IL-18 as well (Kim et al., 2007). Furthermore, Park et al. (2001) revealed that IL-18 is able to promote angiogenesis both in vitro and in vivo. Importantly, these observations are in contrast with studies demonstrating antiangiogenic activities of IL-18 (Zheng et al., 2009; Zheng et al., 2010). Apparently, antiangiogenic effects in these findings may be caused due to IL-18-induced expression of other antiangiogenic cytokines, such as, for instance, IL-12. Second, IL-18 demonstrated significant prometastatic activities in series of experiments. Jiang et al. (2003a) observed significant upregulation of *IL-18* gene expression in highly metastatic cell line PLA801D. In their further investigations, the authors found that IL-18 is an important factor for the development of lung metastasis (Jiang et al., 2003b). Jung et al. (2006) found that IL-18 significantly increased migration and motility of cells in murine melanoma B16F10 cell lines, thereby contributing to prometastatic activity. Another study conducted by Zhang et al. (2011) demonstrated that IL-18 promotes metastasis in hepatoma cells due to upregulation of MMPs 2, 3, and 9, which modulate metastasis formation due to degradation of extracellular matrix (ECM) components. In accordance with previous findings, Cero et al. (2012) observed that administration of recombinant murine IL-18 in mice caused significant elevation of pulmonary mRNA levels of MMP. Furthermore, the authors observed that injection of IL-18 also increased mRNA levels of cathepsin S, a protein involved in the degradation of ECM and promotion of tumor growth (Fan et al., 2012; Burden et al., 2012).

Third, significantly elevated levels of IL-18 were observed in patients with various malignancies, including lung cancer (Naumnik et al., 2004; Okamoto et al., 2009), prostate cancer (Dwivedi et al., 2011), esophageal cancer (Tsuboi et al., 2004; Diakowska et al., 2006), ovarian cancer (Akahiro et al., 2004; Akgun et al., 2005; Le Page et al., 2006; Samsami Dehaghani et al., 2009), gastric carcinoma (Thong-Ngam et al., 2006; Ye et al., 2007; Haghshenas et al., 2009), breast cancer (Merendino et al., 2001; Günel et al., 2002; Eissa et al., 2005), colorectal carcinoma (Merendino et al., 2002; Haghshenas et al., 2009), hepatitis C virus-related hepatocellular carcinoma (Tangkijvanich et al., 2007; Perrella et al., 2009; Mohran and Ali-Eldin, 2011), oral cavity cancer (Jablonska et al., 2005), head and neck squamous cell carcinoma (Riedel et al., 2004), renal cell carcinoma (Sozen et al., 2004), bladder carcinoma (Bukan et al., 2003), different lymphomas (Takubo et al., 2001; Amo et al., 2001), and skin tumors (Park et al., 2001).

Fourth, it was found that the high serum levels of IL-18 were associated with disease severity and poor prognosis of patients with diffuse large B-cell lymphoma, multiple myeloma, gastric cancer, esophageal carcinoma, and pancreatic carcinoma (Kawabata et al., 2001; Alexandrakis et al., 2004; Carbone et al., 2009; Goto et al., 2011; Zhao et al., 2013).

Finally, there is evidence that IL-18 is able to stimulate tumor immune escape by upregulation of thrombospondin 1 (TSP-1) and regulating the expression of Fas ligand and reactive oxygen intermediates (Cho et al., 2000; Kim et al., 2006). TSP-1 is a major component of ECM; however, the impact of this molecule on carcinogenesis is controversial. Some researchers observed that TSP-1 acts as inhibitor of tumor growth and angiogenesis, whereas others reported totally opposite effects (reviewed by Sargiannidou et al., 2001; Lawler, 2002).

According to these contradictory data, the impact of IL-18 on cancer development seems ambiguous (Figure 2.2). It is clear that antitumor effects of IL-18 are offset by such carcinogenic activities as cathepsin- and MMP-induced degradation of ECM, stimulation of migration of cells, upregulation of numerous proangiogenic factors, enhancing tumor immune escape, and activation of NF-κB pathway, which plays a significant role in the suppression of apoptosis and induction of cell proliferation and inflammation (Karin et al., 2002). So far, therapeutic significance of this cytokine is questioned, and it is not yet clear if it brings more harm or benefit. Apparently, IL-18 is more conducive to tumor growth than to regression, and possibly, it would be helpful to examine the effect of IL-18 blockade in vivo in order to evaluate its possible application in clinical practice. In this regard, the most effective approach to conduct IL-18 blockade is the usage of the IL-18 binding protein (IL-18BP), a soluble glycoprotein performing high-affinity binding of IL-18, thereby neutralizing it (Dinarello and Fantuzzi, 2003). To date, knowledge about the impact of IL-18BP on cancer progression is limited, but it was found that neutralization of IL-18 by IL-18BP significantly decreased hepatic metastasis of melanoma cells in animal models (Carrascal et al., 2003). Perhaps, IL-18BP may become an effective anticancer agent, and therefore, further studies devoted to this issue are required.

To conclude, IL-18 has both pro- and anticarcinogenic activities, and many aspects in the relationship between this cytokine and formation of malignant tumors are unclear until now. A couple of informative review articles by Gracie et al. (2003), and Dinarello and Fantuzzi (2003) may be recommended for further reading regarding the biology of IL-18 and its role in disease.

2.3 INTERLEUKIN-33

Previously known as nuclear factor from high endothelial venules, IL-33 represents one of the newest members of the IL-1 superfamily. Although there is a high degree of homology between IL-33 and other representatives of the

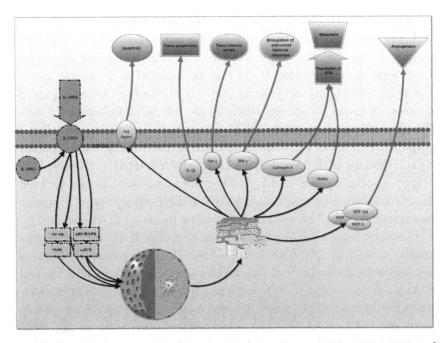

Figure 2.2 Schematic plan illustrates main pro- and anticarcinogenic activities of interleukin (IL)-18. MMP, matrix metalloproteinases; VEGF, vascular endothelial growth factor; MAPK, mitogen-activated protein kinase; SDF, stromal cell-derived factor; MCP, monocyte chemotactic protein. (For color version of this figure, the reader is referred to the online version of this book).

superfamily, the impact of IL-33 on the immune system is totally different. The main known function of this cytokine is to trigger antiinflammatory Th1-polarized immune response by expressing IL-4, IL-5, IL-6, and IL-13 in immune cells and increasing production of immunoglobulins (Liew et al., 2010; Anthony et al., 2011; Schmieder et al., 2012). Importantly, according to the recent reports it could be suggested that IL-33 is able to suppress the production and release of certain proinflammatory cytokines as well. In particular, Volarevic et al. (2012) demonstrated that *IL-33*-deficient mice with concanavalin A-induced liver injury had significantly elevated serum levels of IL-17, IFN-γ, and TNF-α as compared to wild-type animals. So, IL-33 is considered as an antiinflammatory mediator. Numerous agents have been reported to activate transcription and release of IL-33, including IL-1α, IL-1β, IL-3, TNF-α, IL-5, PDGF-BB, and IFN-γ (Xu et al., 2008; Masamune et al., 2010; Ikutani et al., 2012; Schmieder et al., 2012). Similar to other members of the IL-1 superfamily, the mature 18 kDa form of IL-33 is produced by the cleavage of a 30 kDa precursor molecule with an enzyme caspase-1. Importantly, not long ago it was discovered that the mature form of IL-33 may act as either an intracellular nuclear factor or a secreted agent, like IL-1α and IL-1β, respectively; therefore, IL-33 may be regarded as a "double agent" (Carriere, 2007; Gadina and Jefferies, 2007). IL-33 has been found expressed in almost all tissues and organs, especially in endothelial and epithelial cells. The natural ligand of IL-33 is the ST2 receptor, also known as interleukin 1 receptor-like 1. It can be found in two forms, soluble and transmembrane (ST2L). Binding of IL-33 to ST2L recruits MyD88, IRAK1, IRAK4, TNF receptor-associated factor 6, and possibly, other agents that have not yet been identified. Subsequent triggering of MAPK and NF-κB is thought to initiate the expression of the Th2-polarized phenotype (Gadina and Jefferies, 2007).

Currently, some evidence exists for the impact of IL-33 on cancer progression. Choi et al. (2009) demonstrated that IL-33 promotes angiogenesis and vasopermeability both in vivo and in vitro. The authors revealed that IL-33 is able to upregulate NO production in epithelial cells via PI3K/Akt-dependent activation of epithelial nitric oxide synthase. We have already noted that NO exerts procarcinogenic effects (Fukumura et al., 1997; Murohara et al., 1998), so the link between IL-33 and cancer progression seems to be established through NO-dependent synthesis of MMPs and bFGF. Furthermore, it was demonstrated that proangiogenic growth factors such as VEGF, IL-8, transforming growth factor beta (TGF-β), epidermal growth factor, and FGF are able to downregulate IL-33 in tumor endothelial cells and in highly metastatic human pancreatic carcinoma cells (Kuchler et al., 2008; Schmieder et al., 2012), suggesting the complicated cross talk between these agents. In addition, high serum levels of IL-33 were found increased in mice with expressed K-*ras*, an oncogene responsible for many cancers (Lee et al., 2009). Gao et al. (2013) reported that IL-33 triggers the proliferation, activation, and infiltration of CD8$^+$ T cells and NK cells via NF-κB signaling pathway, thereby inhibiting pulmonary metastasis in B16 melanoma and LLC mice. Masamune et al. (2010) reported that the expression of IL-33 mRNA was significantly elevated in culture-activated pancreatic stellate cells isolated from the pancreas of subjects with pancreatic cancer. Similarly, Schmieder et al. (2012) observed that mRNA expression and production of IL-33 and ST2 was increased in pancreatic adenocarcinoma cell line Colo35. In addition, Sun et al. (2011) reported that serum levels of IL-33 were significantly elevated in 68 Chinese patients with gastric carcinoma in comparison with 58 healthy blood donors. Furthermore, the authors indicated that IL-33 was associated with some poor prognostic factors, including depth of invasion, distant metastasis, and advanced stage. Finally, Jovanovic et al. (2011) revealed that ST2-deficient BALB/c mice with mammary carcinoma had higher cytotoxic activity of NK cells, as well as higher number of these cells as compared to wild-type animals. Additionally, the authors found that IL-17, IFN-γ, and TNF-α levels were increased in ST2-deficient mice, whereas the amount of IL-4 was decreased. In their further investigations, Jovanovic et al. (2012) suggested the hypothetical role of IL-33 in cancer development. The authors found that in the absence of ST2, particularly, in ST2-deficient mice, IL-33 does not trigger Th2 polarization and therefore prevents development of IL-4-, IL-10-, and IL-13-driven immunosuppressive response. Consequently, in the absence of the signal from IL-33, IL-12-mediated Th1 polarization of immune response does occur, thereby promoting tumor regression. Yet another possible mechanism of the influence of IL-33 on cancer cells may be related to the activation of eosinophils. In particular, several studies indicated that IL-33 is involved in the stimulation of the degranulation of eosinophils (Cherry et al., 2008), recruitment of eosinophils to tumor cells in vivo (Ikutani et al., 2012), development of the eosinophilia in the lung (Zhiguang et al., 2010), and exacerbation of eosinophil-mediated airway inflammation (Stolarski et al., 2010). However, it is not easy to determine whether this pathway contributes to cancer development or not, because the role of eosinophils in carcinogenesis is controversial. Eosinophils have been reported to have a different impact on different cancers (Looi, 1987; Nielsen et al., 1999; Dorta et al., 2002), and moreover, these immune cells are known to stimulate angiogenesis due to upregulation of VEGF expression in late stages of cancer development (Horiuchi and Weller, 1997). On the other hand, eosinophils are the essential part of proper and efficient immune response, and antitumor immune response is not an exception here.

To conclude, the precise role of IL-33 in cancer is unclear due to the lack of robust data supporting pro- or anticancer activities of this cytokine. However, we may currently speculate about the significance of several important carcinogenic pathways in which IL-33 and ST2 are involved; therefore, further in-depth studies should elaborate previous findings in order to clarify this issue.

2.4 NEXT AIMS AND FURTHER DIRECTIONS

In this final section, we discuss ILs that have been discovered recently. Not much is known about the biological effects and signaling pathways of these cytokines; moreover, there is virtually no research devoted to the investigation of the relationship between them and cancer. Due to the lack of information about these ILs, there are no substantial reviews below, only cursory description of known facts. Here, we can only propose potential directions of cancer-related investigations based on these known facts, and possibly, this may help researchers to choose promising areas of study.

2.4.1 Interleukin-36

In the early 2000s, the novel IL-1-like gene cluster was discovered by several research groups (Smith et al., 2000; Kumar et al., 2000). This cluster included genes that encode three agonists, IL-36α, IL-36β, and IL-36γ; one receptor IL-36Ra; one antagonist IL-36Ra; and one accessory protein. IL-36 exerts proinflammatory activity through MAPK and NF-κB (Towne et al., 2004; Chustz et al., 2011; Ramadas et al., 2012), and several reports indicate that IL-1 and TNF-α markedly upregulate the expression of IL-36 mRNA (Debets et al., 2001; Kumar et al., 2000; Lian et al., 2012). It is also known that the expression of IL-36 mRNA may be significantly enhanced in the presence of certain TLR receptor ligands, such as polyinosinic-polycytidylic acid and flagellin (Lian et al., 2012). It was found that IL-36β acts synergistically with IL-12 to promote polarization of Th1, and moreover, IL-36 signaling is involved in mediating Th1 immune responses to bacillus Calmette-Guérin infection in vivo (Vigne et al., 2012).

Currently, there is a lack of studies devoted to the investigation of the role of IL-36 in cancer; nevertheless, there is every reason to believe that this cytokine may be involved in occurrence and progression of cancer. In particular, it has been found to dramatically enhance various proinflammatory skin conditions (reviewed by Towne and Sims, 2012; Jensen, 2010). In brief, Debets et al. (2001) found that mRNA amounts of IL-36γ and IL-36Ra were significantly elevated in lesional psoriasis skin characterized by chronic cutaneous inflammation. Furthermore, a series of experiments by Blumberg et al. (2007) observed that mice injected with a plasmid containing the IL-37α gene demonstrated psoriasis-like skin changes affecting both the dermis and epidermis. In particular, these changes included parakeratosis, an increase in the number of neutrophils, dermal macrophages, and also an increase in epidermal thickness. In their further investigations, Blumberg et al. (2010) established a self-amplifying gene-expression loop between IL-36, IL-17, IL-22, and IL-23 in psoriatic-like skin, thereby suggesting a complex cross talk between these cytokines in the initiation of the inflammatory response. Carrier et al. (2011) found that all three IL-36 agonists stimulated the production of proinflammatory TNF-α, IL-6, and IL-8 in cultured primary human keratinocytes. In addition, the effect was more evident after addition of IL-17A or TNF-α to the cell culture. Lian et al. (2012) showed that IL-36 may act as alarmin, mediating pyroptosis (proinflammatory programmed cell death) in keratinocytes. Finally, IL-36 regulates the IL-23/IL-17/IL-22 axis in the development of psoriasiform dermatitis (Tortola et al., 2012). In addition, a series of experiments performed by Ramadas et al. (2006, 2011, 2012) revealed that IL-36α and IL-36γ exert proinflammatory activities in mice. In particular, it was demonstrated that IL-36α promoted CD4⁺4 cell proliferation and enhanced the production of cytokines IL-1α, IL-1β, TNF-α, IL-36γ, and chemokines CXCL1 and CXCL2 in a dose-dependent manner. Importantly, CXCL1 and CXCL2 were found associated with angiogenesis, tumor growth, migration, invasion, and survival of cancer cells (Burgess et al., 2012; Kuo et al., 2012; Sajadi et al., 2013; Sharma et al., 2013).

As seen, IL-36 may contribute to cancer progression through several pathways. Possibly, future research should be focused on the association between IL-36 and skin and lung cancers.

2.4.2 Interleukin-37

IL-37 was discovered in 2000 as a member of novel IL-1-like gene cluster; however, its functions and biological effects have long been unknown (Smith et al., 2000). During the experiments on the biological effects of IL-18BP, several research groups indicated that higher doses of this cytokine increased severity of plaque psoriasis and rheumatoid arthritis both in clinical studies and animal models (Tak et al., 2006; Banda et al., 2003). It was proposed that aside from ILBP, IL-18R may bind another orphan ligand, thereby activating proinflammatory immune response. Further research confirmed the existence of this orphan ligand, and it was IL-37. Furthermore, it was revealed that IL-37 may bind both IL-18R and IL-BP. There are five alternative splice variants of this cytokine, namely, IL-37a, IL-37b, IL-37c, IL-37d, and IL-37e. Of them, IL-37b is the most stable isoform, and therefore, it is the best studied one. Isoforms of IL-37 were found expressed in various tissues and organs, including lung, heart, brain, stomach, spleen, prostate, pancreas, liver, and kidney (Bufler et al., 2002). In addition, increased levels of different splice variants of IL-37 were indicated in tumors. In particular, IL-37 was expressed in stroma of colon carcinomas as well as in cells of lung carcinoma, melanoma, and ductal mammary carcinoma, but not in prostate cancer cells (Kumar et al., 2002).

According to the latest reports, IL-37 has multiple functions, playing a major role in the regulation of the immune system. Similar to IL-1α and IL-33, IL-37 is known to act as an intracellular nuclear factor affecting gene expression (Sharma et al., 2008; Ross et al., 2013). Nold et al. (2010) demonstrated that IL-4 downregulated the expression of IL-37, thereby inhibiting differentiation and activation of DCs and significantly suppressing the innate immunity. Moreover, the authors found that proinflammatory effects were significantly suppressed in IL-37 transgenic mice administered with several cytokines, such as IL-1β, TNF, IL-12, IL-18, and IL-12. In addition, the authors indicated that IL-37 expression was markedly upregulated by IL-1β, IFN-γ, IL-18, and TNF. Further research by Imaeda et al. (2013) revealed that TNF-α upregulates the expression of IL-37 via NF-κB and AP-1. Furthermore, glucocorticoids were reported to downregulate IL-37 in subjects with systemic lupus erythematosus (Song et al., 2013). It is known that IL-37 downregulates the expression of proinflammatory cytokines, including TNF-α, IL-1α, IL-6, MIP-2, and IL-10 (Sharma et al., 2008) but does not trigger the production of IFN-γ (Kumar et al., 2002) in macrophages and endothelial cells. McNamee et al. (2011) demonstrated that IL-37 activated the expression of antiinflammatory cytokine IL-10, thereby inhibiting inflammation in mice with dextran sulfate sodium-induced colitis. Finally, serum levels for IL-1α, IL-6, IL-5, and IL-9 were significantly decreased in IL-37 transgenic mice with concanavalin A-induced liver injury (Bulau et al., 2011).

There is evidence that antiinflammatory activities of IL-37 may be realized through the inhibition of decapentaplegic homolog 3 (Smad3) signaling pathway. Smad3 is a modulator of TGF-β activity, which is known to be associated with impaired local inflammatory response (Ashcroft et al., 1999), inhibition of cytotoxicity (Trotta et al., 2008), and suppression of activation of macrophages and DCs due to TGF-β-mediated downregulation of several cytokines (Musso et al., 1990; Werner et al., 2000). On the other hand, it was found that Smad3 mutant mice develop colorectal cancer (Zhu et al., 1998). The link between Smad3 and IL-37 was established by Nold et al. (2010), who found that silencing of Smad3 significantly inhibited the antiinflammatory activities of IL-37 in vivo. Moreover, Grimbsy et al. (2004) found that IL-37 is one of the agents that bind Smad3, and Nold et al. (2010) revealed that Smad3 and IL-37 form a functional complex. Other authors speculate that biological effects of IL-37 may be due to recruitment of one of the orphan accessory receptors of the IL-1 family, such as TIR8/SIGIRR (IL-1R8), TIGIRR-1 (IL-1R9), and TIGIRR-2 (IL-1R10); however, despite all these observations the precise signaling pathways of IL–37 still remain undiscovered (Boraschi et al., 2011).To conclude, all the above-mentioned observations show that IL–37 is a major suppressor of local and systemic inflammation. Other activities of IL–37 are obscure, and further in-depth research is necessary to determine possible disease-relevant properties of this cytokine. Comprehensive review articles by Boraschi et al. (2011) and Tete et al. (2012) may be recommended for further reading on the biology of IL–37.

2.4.3 Interleukin-38

In 2001, two research groups led by Lin and Bensen (Lin et al., 2001; Bensen et al., 2001), respectively, independently identified, cloned, and characterized a novel human cytokine, named IL–38. The new cytokine has a 41% homology with IL–1Ra and 43% homology with IL–36R. In addition, the *IL-38* gene was located adjacent to *IL-1Ra* and *IL-36Ra* genes within the *IL-1* gene cluster. The similarity between IL–38 and IL–36 seems to be obvious; IL–38 is able to bind to the IL–36R and its activity is very similar to IL–36 (Veerdonk et al., 2012). Although exact biological effects of IL–38 are unknown, the results obtained in several studies suggest that this cytokine may indirectly promote or inhibit tumor growth. Veerdonk et al. (2012) demonstrated that recombinant IL–38 inhibited the synthesis of IL–17A and IL–22 in human peripheral blood mononuclear cells (PBMCs) by 39% and 37%, respectively. Interestingly, the increase in the concentration of IL–38 resulted in the loss of inhibitory activity of this cytokine. In addition, the authors observed that recombinant IL–1Ra had a similar but more evident effect on PBMCs, suppressing IL–17A and IL–22 by 82% and 71%, respectively. Moreover, IL–38 was found to inhibit IL–36γ-induced production of IL–8 by 42%, but it did not affect the synthesis of IFN-γ (Veerdonk et al., 2012). Taking into account that IL–8 production correlates with the tumorigenicity, angiogenesis, and metastasis of tumors in numerous in vivo models (Waugh and Wilson, 2008), IL–38 may play a protective role against cancer progression. However, the authors demonstrated that both IL–36Ra and IL–38 are able to upregulate IL–6, which is known to be a key regulator of development and progression of esophageal cancer, colorectal carcinoma, melanoma, and gynecological malignancies (Groblewska et al., 2012; Coward and Kulbe, 2012; Hoejberg et al., 2012; Waldner et al., 2012). In particular, IL–6 concentrations in human DCs were increased by 100% in the presence of either IL–36Ra or IL–38 (Veerdonk et al., 2012). In addition, it is known that IL–38 possesses antiinflammatory properties, thereby exerting a protective role in the risk of cancer occurrence (Shaik et al., 2013).

Currently, there is a lack of studies investigating the role of IL-38 in the progression of malignant tumors, but the obtained findings indicate the need for research in this field. Taking into account that IL-38 is expressed generally in the skin, it would be feasible to focus further investigations precisely on skin cancers.

REFERENCES

Agorio, C., Schreiber, F., Sheppard, M., Mastroeni, P., Fernandez, M., Martinez, M.A., Chabalgoity, J.A., 2007. Live attenuated *Salmonella* as a vector for oral cytokine gene therapy in melanoma. J. Gene Med. 9 (5), 416–423.

Akahiro, J., Konno, R., Ito, K., Okamura, K., Yaegashi, N., 2004. Impact of serum interleukin-18 level as a prognostic indicator in patients with epithelial ovarian carcinoma. Int. J. Clin. Oncol. 9 (1), 42–46.

Akgun, M., Saglam, L., Kaynar, H., Yildirim, A.K., Mirici, A., Gorguner, M., Meral, M., Ozden, K., 2005. Serum IL-18 levels in tuberculosis: comparison with pneumonia, lung cancer and healthy controls. Respirology 10 (3), 295–299.

Alexandrakis, M.G., Passam, F.H., Sfiridaki, K., Moschandrea, J., Pappa, C., Liapi, D., Petreli, E., Roussou, P., Kyriakou, D.S., 2004. Interleukin-18 in multiple myeloma patients: serum levels in relation to response to treatment and survival. Leuk. Res. 28 (3), 259–266.

Amin, M.A., Mansfield, P.J., Pakozdi, A., Campbell, P.L., Ahmed, S., Martinez, R.J., Koch, A.E., 2007. Interleukin-18 induces angiogenic factors in rheumatoid arthritis synovial tissue fibroblasts via distinct signaling pathways. Arthritis Rheum. 56 (6), 1787–1797.

Amo, Y., Ohta, Y., Hamada, Y., Katsuoka, K., 2001. Serum levels of interleukin-18 are increased in patients with cutaneous T-cell lymphoma and cutaneous natural killer-cell lymphoma. Br. J. Dermatol. 145 (4), 674–676.

Anthony, R.M., Kobayashi, T., Wermeling, F., Ravetch, J.V., 2011. Intravenous gammaglobulin suppresses inflammation through a novel T(H)2 pathway. Nature 475 (7354), 110–113.

Apte, R.N., Voronov, E., 2002. Interleukin-1 – a major pleiotropic cytokine in tumor-host interactions. Semin. Cancer Biol. 12 (4), 277–290.

Arend, W.P., Dayer, J.M., 1990. Cytokines and cytokine inhibitors or antagonists in rheumatoid arthritis. Arthritis Rheum. 33 (3), 305–315.

Ashcroft, G.S., Yang, X., Glick, A.B., Weinstein, M., Letterio, J.L., Mizel, D.E., Anzano, M., Greenwell-Wild, T., Wahl, S.M., Deng, C., Roberts, A.B., 1999. Mice lacking Smad3 show accelerated wound healing and an impaired local inflammatory response. Nat. Cell Biol. 1 (5), 260–266.

Asumendi, A., Alvarez, A., MartMnez, I., Smedsrod, B., Vidal-Vanaclocha, F., 1995. Interleukin-1-dependent stimulation of mannose receptor activity in the hepatic sinusoidal endothelium. In: Knook, D., Wisse, E., Wake, K. (Eds.), Cells of the Hepatic Sinusoid. Kupffer Cell Foundation, Leiden, The Netherlands, pp. 209–211.

Banda, N.K., Vondracek, A., Kraus, D., Dinarello, C.A., Kim, S.H., Bendele, A., Senaldi, G., Arend, W.P., 2003. Mechanisms of inhibition of collagen-induced arthritis by murine IL-18 binding protein. J. Immunol. 170 (4), 2100–2105.

Bar, D., Apte, R.N., Voronov, E., Dinarello, C.A., Cohen, S., 2004. A continuous delivery system of IL-1 receptor antagonist reduces angiogenesis and inhibits tumor development. FASEB J. 18 (1), 161–163.

Barak, V., Nisman, B., Polliack, A., Vannier, E., Dinarello, C.A., 1998. Correlation of serum levels of interleukin-1 family members with disease activity and response to treatment in hairy cell leukemia. Eur. Cytokine Network 9 (1), 33–39.

Ben-Av, P., Crofford, L.J., Wilder, R.L., Hla, T., 1995. Induction of vascular endothelial growth factor expression in synovial fibroblasts by prostaglandin E and interleukin-1: a potential mechanism for inflammatory angiogenesis. FEBS Lett. 372 (1), 83–87.

Bensen, J.T., Dawson, P.A., Mychaleckyj, J.C., Bowden, D.W., 2001. Identification of a novel human cytokine gene in the interleukin gene cluster on chromosome 2q12-14. J. Interferon Cytokine Res. 2011 (21), 899–904.

Bernstein, S.H., Fay, J., Frankel, S., Christiansen, N., Baer, M.R., Jacobs, C., Blosch, C., Hanna, R., Herzig, G., 1999. A phase I study of recombinant human soluble interleukin-1 receptor (rhu IL-1R) in patients with relapsed and refractory acute myeloid leukemia. Cancer Chemother. Pharmacol. 43 (2), 141–144.

Bessis, N., Guery, L., Mantovani, A., Vecchi, A., Sims, J.E., Fradelizi, D., Boissier, M.C., 2000. The type II decoy receptor of IL-1 inhibits murine collagen-induced arthritis. Eur. J. Immunol. 30, 867–875.

Bloom, B.R., Bennett, B., 1966. Mechanism of a reaction in vitro associated with delayed-type hypersensitivity. Science 153 (3731), 80–82.

Blumberg, H., Dinh, H., Dean Jr, C., Trueblood, E.S., Bailey, K., Shows, D., Bhagavathula, N., Aslam, M.N., Varani, J., Towne, J.E., Sims, J.E., 2010. IL-1RL2 and its ligands contribute to the cytokine network in psoriasis. J. Immunol. 185 (7), 4354–4362.

Blumberg, H., Dinh, H., Trueblood, E.S., Pretorius, J., Kugler, D., Weng, N., Kanaly, S.T., Towne, J.E., Willis, C.R., Kuechle, M.K., Sims, J.E., Peschon, J.J., 2007. Opposing activities of two novel members of the IL-1 ligand family regulate skin inflammation. J. Exp. Med. 204 (11), 2603–2614.

Boraschi, D., Villa, L., Volpini, C., Boss'u, P., Censini, S., Chiara, P., Scapigliat, G., Nencioni, L., Bartalini, M., Matteucci, C., 1990. Differential activity of interleukin 1 alpha and interleukin 1 beta in the stimulation of the immune response in vivo. Eur. J. Immunol. 20, 317–321.

Boraschi, D., Lucchesi, D., Hainzl, S., Leitner, M., Maier, E., Mangelberger, D., Oostingh, G.J., Pfaller, T., Pixner, C., Posselt, G., Italiani, P., Nold, M.F., Nold-Petry, C.A., Bufler, P., Dinarello, C.A., 2011. IL-37: a new anti-inflammatory cytokine of the IL-1 family. Eur. Cytokine Network 22 (3), 127–147.

Born, T.L., Thomassen, E., Bird, T.A., Sims, J.E., 1998. Cloning of a novel receptor subunit, AcPL, required for interleukin-18 signaling. J. Biol. Chem. 273 (45), 29445–29450.

Botsios, C., Sfriso, P., Furlan, A., Punzi, L., Dinarello, C.A., 2008. Resistant Behçet disease responsive to anakinra. Ann. Intern. Med. 149, 284–286.

Bufler, P., Azam, T., Gamboni-Robertson, F., Reznikov, L.L., Kumar, S., Dinarello, C.A., Kim, S.H., 2002. A complex of the IL-1 homologue IL-1F7b and IL-18-binding protein reduces IL-18 activity. Proc. Natl. Acad. Sci. USA. 99 (21), 13723–13728.

Bukan, N., Sözen, S., Coskun, U., Sancak, B., Günel, N., Bozkirli, I., Senocak, C., 2003. Serum interleukin-18 and nitric oxide activity in bladder carcinoma. Eur. Cytokine Network 14 (3), 163–167.

Bulau, A.M., Fink, M., Maucksch, C., Kappler, R., Mayr, D., Wagner, K., Bufler, P., 2011. In vivo expression of interleukin-37 reduces local and systemic inflammation in concanavalin A-induced hepatitis. Sci. World J. 11, 2480–2490.

Burden, R.E., Gormley, J.A., Kuehn, D., Ward, C., Kwok, H.F., Gazdoiu, M., McClurg, A., Jaquin, T.J., Johnston, J.A., Scott, C.J., Olwill, S.A., 2012. Inhibition of Cathepsin S by Fsn0503 enhances the efficacy of chemotherapy in colorectal carcinomas. Biochimie 94 (2), 487–493.

Burgess, M., Cheung, C., Chambers, L., Ravindranath, K., Minhas, G., Knop, L., Mollee, P., McMillan, N.A., Gill, D., 2012. CCL2 and CXCL2 enhance survival of primary chronic lymphocytic leukemia cells in vitro. Leuk. Lymphoma 53 (10), 1988–1998.

Calligaris, L., Marchetti, F., Tommasini, A., Ventura, A., 2008. The efficacy of anakinra in an adolescent with colchicine-resistant familial Mediterranean fever. Eur. J. Pediatr. 167 (6), 695–696.

Camargo, M.C., Mera, R., Correa, P., Peek Jr, R.M., Fontham, E.T., Goodman, K.J., Piazuelo, M.B., Sicinschi, L., Zabaleta, J., Schneider, B.G., 2006. Interleukin-1beta and interleukin-1 receptor antagonist gene polymorphisms and gastric cancer: a meta-analysis. Cancer Epidemiol., Biomarkers Prev. 15 (9), 1674–1687.

Cao, R., Farnebo, J., Kurimoto, M., Cao, Y., 1999. Interleukin-18 acts as an angiogenesis and tumor suppressor. FASEB J. 13 (15), 2195–2202.

Carbone, A., Vizio, B., Novarino, A., Mauri, F.A., Geuna, M., Robino, C., Brondino, G., Prati, A., Giacobino, A., Campra, D., Chiarle, R., Fronda, G.R., Ciuffreda, L., Bellone, G., 2009. IL-18 paradox in pancreatic carcinoma: elevated serum levels of free IL-18 are correlated with poor survival. J. Immunother. 32 (9), 920–931.

Carmeliet, P., Dor, Y., Herbert, J.M., Fukumura, D., Brusselmans, K., Dewerchin, M., Neeman, M., Bono, F., Abramovitch, R., Maxwell, P., Koch, C.J., Ratcliffe, P., Moons, L., Jain, R.K., Collen, D., Keshert, E., 1998. Role of HIF-1alpha in hypoxia-mediated apoptosis, cell proliferation and tumour angiogenesis. Nature 394 (6692), 485–490.

Carmi, Y., Voronov, E., Dotan, S., Lahat, N., Rahat, M.A., Fogel, M., Huszar, M., White, M.R., Dinarello, C.A., Apte, R.N., 2009. The role of macrophage-derived IL-1 in induction and maintenance of angiogenesis. J. Immunol. 183 (7), 4705–4714.

Carrascal, M.T., Mendoza, L., Valcárcel, M., Salado, C., Egilegor, E., Tellería, N., Vidal-Vanaclocha, F., Dinarello, C.A., 2003. Interleukin-18 binding protein reduces b16 melanoma hepatic metastasis by neutralizing adhesiveness and growth factors of sinusoidal endothelium. Cancer Res. 63 (2), 491–497.

Carrier, Y., Ma, H.L., Ramon, H.E., Napierata, L., Small, C., O'Toole, M., Young, D.A., Fouser, L.A., Nickerson-Nutter, C., Collins, M., Dunussi-Joannopoulos, K., Medley, Q.G., 2011. Inter-regulation of Th17 cytokines and the IL-36 cytokines in vitro and in vivo: implications in psoriasis pathogenesis. J. Invest. Dermatol. 131 (12), 2428–2437.

Carriere, V., Roussel, L., Ortega, N., Lacorre, D.A., Americh, L., Aguilar, L., Bouche, G., Girard, J.P., 2007. IL-33, the IL-1-like cytokine ligand for ST2 receptor, is a chromatin-associated nuclear factor in vivo. Proc. Natl. Acad. Sci. USA. 104, 282–287.

Carter, D., Deibel Jr., M.R., Dunn, C.J., Tomich, C.S., Laborde, A.L., Slightom, J.L., Berger, A.E., Bienkowski, M.J., Sun, F.F., McEwan, R.N., 1990. Purification, cloning, expression and biological characterization of an interleukin-1 receptor antagonist protein. Nature 344 (6267), 633–638.

Cero, F.T., Hillestad, V., Løberg, E.M., Christensen, G., Larsen, K.O., Skjønsberg, O.H., 2012. IL-18 and IL-12 synergy induces matrix degrading enzymes in the lung. Exp. Lung Res. 38 (8), 406–419.

Chen, Z.F., Zhou, R., Xia, B., Deng, C.S., 2012. Interleukin-18 and -12 synergistically enhance cytotoxic functions of tumor-infiltrating lymphocytes. Chin. Med. J. (Engl.) 125 (23), 4245–4248.

Cherry, W.B., Yoon, J., Bartemes, K.R., Iijima, K., Kita, H., 2008. A novel IL-1 family cytokine, IL-33, potently activates human eosinophils. J. Allergy Clin. Immunol. 121, 1484–1490.

Chirivi, R.G., Chiodoni, C., Musiani, P., Garofalo, A., Bernasconi, S., Colombo, M.P., Giavazzi, R., 1996. IL-1alpha gene-transfected human melanoma cells increase tumor-cell adhesion to endothelial cells and their retention in the lung of nude mice. Int. J. Cancer 67 (6), 856–863.

Chirivi, R.G., Garofalo, A., Padura, I.M., Mantovani, A., Giavazzi, R., 1993. Interleukin 1 receptor antagonist inhibits the augmentation of metastasis induced by interleukin 1 or lipopolysaccharide in a human melanoma/nude mouse system. Cancer Res. 53 (20), 5051–5054.

Cho, D., Song, H., Kim, Y.M., Houh, D., Hur, D.Y., Park, H., Yoon, D., Pyun, K.H., Lee, W.J., Kurimoto, M., Kim, Y.B., Kim, Y.S., Choi, I., 2000. Endogenous interleukin18 modulates immune escape of murine melanoma cells by regulating the expression of Fas ligand and reactive oxygen intermediates. Cancer Res. 60 (10), 2703–2709.

Cho, M.L., Jung, Y.O., Moon, Y.M., Min, S.Y., Yoon, C.H., Lee, S.H., Park, S.H., Cho, C.S., Jue, D.M., Kim, H.Y., 2006. Interleukin-18 induces the production of vascular endothelial growth factor (VEGF) in rheumatoid arthritis synovial fibroblasts via AP-1-dependent pathways. Immunol. Lett. 103 (2), 159–166.

Choi, Y.S., Choi, H.J., Min, J.K., Pyun, B.J., Maeng, Y.S., Park, H., Kim, J., Kim, Y.M., Kwon, Y.G., Oct 1, 2009. Interleukin-33 induces angiogenesis and vascular permeability through ST2/TRAF6-mediated endothelial nitric oxide production. Blood 114 (14), 3117–3126.

Chustz, R.T., Nagarkar, D.R., Poposki, J.A., Favoreto Jr, S., Avila, P.C., Schleimer, R.P., Kato, A., 2011. Regulation and function of the IL-1 family cytokine IL-1F9 in human bronchial epithelial cells. Am. J. Respir. Cell Mol. Biol. 45 (1), 145–153.

Claesson-Welsh, L., Welsh, M., 2013. VEGFA and tumour angiogenesis. J. Intern. Med. 273 (2), 114–127.

Colotta, F., Re, F., Muzio, M., Bertini, R., Polentarutti, N., Sironi, M., Giri, J.G., Dower, S.K., Sims, J.E., Mantovani, A., 1993. Interleukin-1 type II receptor: a decoy target for IL-1 that is regulated by IL-4. Science 261, 472–475.

Conti, B., Park, L.C., Calingasan, N.Y., Kim, Y., Kim, H., Bae, Y., Gibson, G.E., Joh, T.H., 1999. Cultures of astrocytes and microglia express interleukin 18. Brain Res. Mol. Brain Res. 67 (1), 46–52.

Coughlin, C.M., Salhany, K.E., Wysocka, M., Aruga, E., Kurzawa, H., Chang, A.E., Hunter, C.A., Fox, J.C., Trinchieri, G., Lee, W.M., 1998. Interleukin-12 and interleukin-18 synergistically induce murine tumor regression which involves inhibition of angiogenesis. J. Clin. Invest. 101 (6), 1441–1452.

Coward, J.I., Kulbe, H., 2012. The role of interleukin-6 in gynaecological malignancies. Cytokine Growth Factor Rev. 23 (6), 333–342.

Daun, J.M., Ball, R.W., Burger, H.R., Cannon, J.G., 1999. Aspirin-induced increases in soluble IL-1 receptor type II concentrations in vitro and in vivo. J. Leukoc Biol. 65, 863–866.

David, J.R., Al-Askari, S., Lawrence, H.S., Thomas, L., 1964. Delayed hypersensitiviy in vitro. I. The specificity of inhibition of cell migration by antigens. J. Immunol. 93, 264–273.

Debets, R., Timans, J.C., Homey, B., Zurawski, S., Sana, T.R., Lo, S., Wagner, J., Edwards, G., Clifford, T., Menon, S., Bazan, J.F., Kastelein, R.A., 2001. Two novel IL-1 family members, IL-1 delta and IL-1 epsilon, function as an antagonist and agonist of NF-kappa B activation through the orphan IL-1 receptor-related protein 2. J. Immunol. 167 (3), 1440–1446.

Diakowska, D., Markocka-Maczka, K., Grabowski, K., Lewandowski, A., 2006. Serum interleukin-12 and interleukin-18 levels in patients with oesophageal squamous cell carcinoma. Exp. Oncol. 28 (4), 319–322.

Dinarello, C.A., 1994. The interleukin-1 family: 10 years of discovery. FASEB J. 8 (15), 1314–1325.

Dinarello, C.A., 1996. Biologic basis for interleukin-1 in disease. Blood 87 (6), 2095–2147.

Dinarello, C.A., Sep 2006. The paradox of pro-inflammatory cytokines in cancer. Cancer Metastasis Rev. 25 (3), 307–313. Review.

Dinarello, C.A., 2009. The Interleukin-1, the First Interleukin. The Crafoord Prize Lectures. Lund University, Sweden.

Dinarello, C.A., 2010. Why not treat human cancer with interleukin-1 blockade? Cancer Metastasis Rev. 29 (2), 317–329.

Dinarello, C.A., 2011. A clinical perspective of IL-1β as the gatekeeper of inflammation. Eur. J. Immunol. 41 (5), 1203–1217.

Dinarello, C.A., Fantuzzi, G., 2003. Interleukin-18 and host defense against infection. J. Infect. Dis. 187 (Suppl. 2), S370–S384.

Dinarello, C.A., Goldin, N.P., Wolff, S.M., 1974. Demonstration and characterization of two distinct human leukocytic pyrogens. J. Exp. Med. 139 (6), 1369–1381.

Dinarello, C.A., Wolff, S.M., 1978. Partial purification of human leukocytic pyrogen. Inflammation 2 (3), 179–189.

Dinarello, C.A., Wolff, S.M., 1978. Pathogenesis of fever in man. N. Engl. J. Med. 298 (11), 607–612.

Dorta, R.G., Landman, G., Kowalski, L.P., Lauris, J.R., Latorre, M.R., Oliveira, D.T., 2002. Tumour-associated tissue eosinophilia as a prognostic factor in oral squamous cell carcinomas. Histopathology 41, 152–157.

Du, G., Ye, L., Zhang, G., Dong, Q., Liu, K., Tian, J., 2012. Human IL18-IL2 fusion protein as a potential antitumor reagent by enhancing NK cell cytotoxicity and IFN-γ production. J. Cancer Res. Clin. Oncol. 138 (10), 1727–1736.

Dwivedi, S., Goel, A., Natu, S.M., Mandhani, A., Khattri, S., Pant, K.K., 2011. Diagnostic and prognostic significance of prostate specific antigen and serum interleukin 18 and 10 in patients with locally advanced prostate cancer: a prospective study. Asian Pac. J. Cancer Prev. 12 (7), 1843–1848.

Ebrahimi, B., Tucker, S.L., Li, D., Abbruzzese, J.L., Kurzrock, R., 2004. Cytokines in pancreatic carcinoma: correlation with phenotypic characteristics and prognosis. Cancer 101, 2727–2736.

Eisenberg, S.P., Evans, R.J., Arend, W.P., Verderber, E., Brewer, M.T., Hannum, C.H., Thompson, R.C., 1990. Primary structure and functional expression from complementary DNA of a human interleukin-1 receptor antagonist. Nature 343 (6256), 341–346.

Eissa, S.A., Zaki, S.A., El-Maghraby, S.M., Kadry, D.Y., 2005. Importance of serum IL-18 and RANTES as markers for breast carcinoma progression. J. Egypt. Natl. Cancer Inst. 17, 51–55.

Elaraj, D.M., Weinreich, D.M., Varghese, S., Puhlmann, M., Hewitt, S.M., Carroll, N.M., Feldman, E.D., Turner, E.M., Alexander, H.R., 2006. The role of interleukin 1 in growth and metastasis of human cancer xenografts. Clin. Cancer Res. 12 (4), 1088–1096.

El-Osta, II., Janku, F., Kurzrock, R., 2010. Successful treatment of Castleman's disease with interleukin-1 receptor antagonist (Anakinra). Mol. Cancer Ther. 9 (6), 1485–1488.

Fan, Q., Wang, X., Zhang, H., Li, C., Fan, J., Xu, J., 2012. Silencing cathepsin S gene expression inhibits growth, invasion and angiogenesis of human hepatocellular carcinoma in vitro. Biochem. Biophys. Res. Commun. 425 (4), 703–710.

Fan, X., Ye, M., Xue, B., Ke, Y., Wong, C.K., Xie, Y., 2012. Human dendritic cells engineered to secrete interleukin-18 activate MAGE-A3-specific cytotoxic T lymphocytes in vitro. Immunol. Invest. 41 (5), 469–483.

Farhat, F.S., Tfayli, A., Fakhruddin, N., Mahfouz, R., Otrock, Z.K., Alameddine, R.S., Awada, A.H., Shamseddine, A., 2012. Expression, prognostic and predictive impact of VEGF and bFGF in non-small cell lung cancer. Crit. Rev. Oncol. Hematol. 84 (2), 149–160.

Fleischmann, R.M., Tesser, J., Schiff, M.H., Schechtman, J., Burmester, G.R., Bennett, R., Modafferi, D., Zhou, L., Bell, D., Appleton, B., 2006. Safety of extended treatment with anakinra in patients with rheumatoid arthritis. Ann. Rheum. Dis. 65 (8), 1006–1012.

Fujiwaki, R.1, Iida, K., Nakayama, K., Kanasaki, H., Hata, K., Katabuchi, H., Okamura, H., Miyazaki, K., Apr 2003. Clinical significance of interleukin-1 receptor antagonist in patients with cervical carcinoma. Gynecol. Oncol. 89 (1), 77–83.

Fukumoto, H., Nishio, M., Nishio, K., Heike, Y., Arioka, H., Kurokawa, H., Ishida, T., Fukuoka, K., Nomoto, T., Ohe, Y., Saijo, N., 1997. Interferon-gamma-inducing factor gene transfection into Lewis lung carcinoma cells reduces tumorigenicity in vivo. Jpn. J. Cancer Res. 88 (5), 501–505.

Fukumura, D., Yuan, F., Endo, M., Jain, R.K., 1997. Role of nitric oxide in tumor microcirculation. Blood flow, vascular permeability, and leukocyte-endothelial interactions. Am. J. Pathol. 150 (2), 713–725.

Gadina, M., Jefferies, C.A., Jun 30, 2007. IL-33: a sheep in wolfs clothing? Sci. STKE. 2007(390):pe31.

Gao, K., Li, X., Zhang, L., Bai, L., Dong, W., Gao, K., Shi, G., Xia, X., Wu, L., Zhang, L., Jul 28, 2013. Transgenic expression of IL-33 activates CD8(+) T cells and NK cells and inhibits tumor growth and metastasis in mice. Cancer Lett. 335 (2), 463–471.

Garlind, A., Brauner, A., Hojeberg, B., Basun, H., Schultzberg, M., 1999. Soluble interleukin-1 receptor type II levels are elevated in cerebrospinal fluid in Alzheimer's disease patients. Brain Res. 826, 112–116.

Gery, I., Gershon, R.K., Waksman, B.H., 1971. Potentiation of cultured mouse thymocyte responses by factors released by peripheral leukocytes. J. Immunol. 107, 1778.

Gery, I., Gershon, R.K., Waksman, B.H., 1972. Potentiation of the T-lymphocyte response to mitogens. I. The responding cell. J. Exp. Med. 136 (1), 128–142.

Gherardi, R.K., Belec, L., Soubrier, M., Malapert, D., Zuber, M., Viard, J.P., Intrator, L., Degos, J.D., Authier, F.J., 1996. Overproduction of proinflammatory cytokines imbalanced by their antagonists in POEMS syndrome. Blood 87, 1458–1465.

Giri, J.G., Newton, R.C., Horuk, R., 1990. Identification of soluble interleukin-1 binding protein in cell-free supernatants. Evidence for soluble interleukin-1 receptor. J. Biol. Chem. 265 (29), 17416–17419.

Giri, J.G., Wells, J., Dower, S.K., McCall, C.E., Guzman, R.N., Slack, J., Bird, T.A., Shanebeck, K., Grabstein, K.H., Sims, J.E., 1994. Elevated levels of shed type II IL-1 receptor in sepsis. Potential role for type II receptor in regulation of IL-1 responses. J. Immunol. 153 (12), 5802–5809.

Goto, N., Tsurumi, H., Kasahara, S., Kanemura, N., Hara, T., Yasuda, I., Shimizu, M., Murakami, N., Sawada, M., Yamada, T., Takemura, M., Seishima, M., Kito, Y., Takami, T., Moriwaki, H., 2011. Serum interleukin-18 level is associated with the outcome of patients with diffuse large B-cell lymphoma treated with CHOP or R-CHOP regimens. Eur. J. Haematol. 87 (3), 217–227.

Gracie, J.A., Robertson, S.E., McInnes, I.B., 2003. Interleukin-18. J. Leukoc Biol. 73 (2), 213–224.

Grimsby, S., Jaensson, H., Dubrovska, A., Lomnytska, M., Hellman, U., Souchelnytskyi, S., Nov 5, 2004. Proteomics-based identification of proteins interacting with Smad3: SREBP-2 forms a complex with Smad3 and inhibits its transcriptional activity. FEBS Lett. 577 (1-2), 93–100.

Groblewska, M., Mroczko, B., Sosnowska, D., Szmitkowski, M., 2012. Interleukin 6 and C-reactive protein in esophageal cancer. Clin. Chim. Acta 413 (19–20), 1583–1590.

Günel, N., Coşkun, U., Sancak, B., Günel, U., Hasdemir, O., Bozkurt, S., 2002. Clinical importance of serum interleukin-18 and nitric oxide activities in breast carcinoma patients. Cancer 95 (3), 663–667.

Haddad, J.J., 2002. Recombinant human interleukin (IL)-1 beta-mediated regulation of hypoxia-inducible factor-1 alpha (HIF-1 alpha) stabilization, nuclear translocation and activation requires an antioxidant/reactive oxygen species (ROS)-sensitive mechanism. Eur. Cytokine Netw. 13 (2), 250–260.

Haghshenas, M.R., Hosseini, S.V., Mahmoudi, M., Saberi-Firozi, M., Farjadian, S., Ghaderi, A., 2009. IL-18 serum level and IL-18 promoter gene polymorphism in Iranian patients with gastrointestinal cancers. J Gastroenterol. Hepatol. 24 (6), 1119–1122.

Hamajima, N., Matsuo, K., Saito, T., Tajima, K., Okuma, K., Yamao, K., Tominaga, S., 2001. Interleukin 1 polymorphisms, lifestyle factors, and *Helicobacter pylori* infection. Jpn. J. Cancer Res. 92 (4), 383–389.

Harnack, U., Johnen, H., Pecher, G., 2011. IL-1 receptor antagonist anakinra enhances tumour growth inhibition in mice receiving peptide vaccination and beta-(1-3),(1-6)-D-glucan. Anticancer Res. 30 (10), 3959–3965.

He, Q.,You, H., Li, X.M., Liu,T.H.,Wang, P.,Wang, B.E., 2012. HMGB1 promotes the synthesis of pro-IL-1β and pro-IL-18 by activation of p38 MAPK and NF-κB through receptors for advanced glycation end-products in macrophages.Asian Pac.J. Cancer Prev. 13 (4), 1365–1370.

Hoejberg, L., Bastholt, L., Schmidt, H., 2012. Interleukin-6 and melanoma. Melanoma Res. 22 (5), 327–333.

Hoffmann, J., Junker, H., Schmieder, A.,Venz, S., Brandt, R., Multhoff, G., Falk,W., Radons, J., 2011. EGCG downregulates IL-1RI expression and suppresses IL-1-induced tumorigenic factors in human pancreatic adenocarcinoma cells. Biochem. Pharmacol. 82 (9), 1153–1162.

Horiuchi, T., Weller, P.F., 1997. Expression of vascular endothelial growth factor by human eosinophils: upregulation by granulocyte macrophage colony-stimulating factor and interleukin-5.Am.J. Respir. Cell Mol. Biol. 17, 70–77.

Hutchinson, N.I., Lark, M.W., MacNaul, K.L., Harper, C., Hoerrner, L.A., McDonnell, J., Donatelli, S., Moore,V., Bayne, E.K., 1992. In vivo expression of stromelysin in synovium and cartilage of rabbits injected intraarticularly with interleukin-1β. Arthritis Rheum. 35, 1227–1233.

Ikutani, M.,Yanagibashi,T., Ogasawara, M.,Tsuneyama, K.,Yamamoto, S., Hattori,Y., Kouro, T., Itakura, A., Nagai, Y., Takaki, S., Takatsu, K., 2012. Identification of innate IL-5-producing cells and their role in lung eosinophil regulation and antitumor immunity.J. Immunol. 188 (2), 703–713.

Imaeda, H.,Takahashi, K., Fujimoto,T., Kasumi, E., Ban, H., Bamba, S., Sonoda, H., Shimizu, T., Fujiyama,Y.,Andoh, A., 2013. Epithelial expression of interleukin-37b in inflammatory bowel disease. Clin. Exp. Immunol. 172 (3), 410–416.

Ito, H., Miki, C., Nov 1999. Profile of circulating levels of interleukin-1 receptor antagonist and interleukin-6 in colorectal cancer patients. Scand. J. Gastroenterol. 34 (11), 1139–1143.

Iwagaki, H., Hizuta,A.,Tanaka, N., 1997. Interleukin-1 receptor antagonists and other markers in colorectal cancer patients. Scand.J. Gastroenterol. 32, 577–581.

Iwasaki, T.,Yamashita, K., Tsujimura, T., Kashiwamura, S., Tsutsui, H., Kaisho, T., Sugihara, A., Yamada, N., Mukai, M.,Yoneda,T., Okamura, H.,Akedo, H.,Terada, N., 2002. Interleukin-18 inhibits osteolytic bone metastasis by human lung cancer cells possibly through suppression of osteoclastic bone-resorption in nude mice.J. Immunother. 25 (Suppl. 1), S52–S60.

Jablonska, E., Puzewska,W., Grabowska, Z., Jablonski, J.,Talarek, L., 2005.VEGF, IL-18 and NO production by neutrophils and their serum levels in patients with oral cavity cancer. Cytokine 30 (3), 93–99.

Jensen, L.E., 2010. Targeting the IL-1 family members in skin inflammation. Curr. Opin. Invest. Drugs 11 (11), 1211–1220.

Jiang, D.,Ying,W., Lu,Y., Wan, J., Zhai,Y., Liu,W., Zhu,Y., Qiu, Z., Qian, X., He, F., 2003a. Identification of metastasis-associated proteins by proteomic analysis and functional exploration of interleukin-18 in metastasis. Proteomics 3, 724–737.

Jiang, D.F., Liu,W.L., Lu,Y.L., Qiu, Z.Y., He, F.C., 2003b. Function of IL-18 in promoting metastasis of lung cancer. Zhonghua Zhongliu Zazhi 25, 348–352.

Jovanovic, I., Radosavljevic, G., Mitrovic, M., Juranic,V.L., McKenzie, A.N., Arsenijevic, N., Jonjic, S., Lukic, M.L., Jul 2011. ST2 deletion enhances innate and acquired immunity to murine mammary carcinoma. Eur. J. Immunol. 41 (7), 1902–1912.

Jovanovic, I.P., Pejnovic, N.N., Radosavljevic, G.D., Arsenijevic, N.N., Lukic, M.L., Mar 1, 2012. IL-33/ST2 axis in innate and acquired immunity to tumors. Oncoimmunology 1 (2), 229–231.

Jung, M.K., Song, H.K., Kim, K.E., Hur, D.Y., Kim,T., Bang, S., Park, H., Cho, D.H., 2006. IL-18 enhances the migration ability of murine melanoma cells through the generation of ROI and the MAPK pathway. Immunol. Lett. 107 (2), 125–130.

Kalliolias, G.D., Gordon, R.A., Ivashkiv, L.B., 2010. Suppression of TNF-alpha and IL-1 signaling identifies a mechanism of homeostatic regulation of macrophages by IL-27. J. Immunol. 185, 7047–7056.

Kamangar, F., Cheng, C., Abnet, C.C., Rabkin, C.S., 2006. Interleukin-1B polymorphisms and gastric cancer risk – a meta-analysis. Cancer Epidemiol. Biomarkers Prev. 15 (10), 1920–1928.

Kaminska, J., Kowalska, M.M., Nowacki, M.P., Chwalinski, M.G., Rysinska, A., Fuksiewicz, M., 2000. CRP, TNF-alpha, IL-1ra, IL-6, IL-8 and IL-10 in blood serum of colorectal cancer patients. Pathol. Oncol. Res. 6, 38–41.

Karin, M., Cao, Y., Greten, F.R., Li, Z.W., 2002. NF-kappaB in cancer: from innocent bystander to major culprit. Nat. Rev. Cancer 2 (4), 301–310.

Kawabata, T., Ichikura, T., Majima, T., Seki, S., Chochi, K., Takayama, E., Hiraide, H., Mochizuki, H., 2001. Preoperative serum interleukin-18 level as a postoperative prognostic marker in patients with gastric carcinoma. Cancer 92 (8), 2050–2055.

Keita, M., Ain Melk, Y., Pelmus, M., Bessette, P., Aris, A., 2011. Endometrioid ovarian cancer and endometriotic cells exhibit the same alteration in the expression of interleukin-1 receptor II: to a link between endometriosis and endometrioid ovarian cancer. J. Obstet. Gynaecol. Res. 37 (2), 99–107.

Kim, J., Kim, C., Kim, T.S., Bang, S.I., Yang, Y., Park, H., Cho, D., Jun 16, 2006. IL-18 enhances thrombospondin-1 production in human gastric cancer via JNK pathway. Biochem. Biophys. Res. Commun. 344 (4), 1284–1289.

Kim, K.E., Song, H., Kim, T.S., Yoon, D., Kim, C.W., Bang, S.I., Hur, D.Y., Park, H., Cho, D.H., 2007. Interleukin-18 is a critical factor for vascular endothelial growth factor-enhanced migration in human gastric cancer cell lines. Oncogene 26 (10), 1468–1476.

Konishi, N., Miki, C., Yoshida, T., Tanaka, K., Toiyama, Y., Kusunoki, M., 2005. Interleukin-1 receptor antagonist inhibits the expression of vascular endothelial growth factor in colorectal carcinoma. Oncology 68 (2–3), 138–145.

Korde Choudhari, S., Sridharan, G., Gadbail, A., Poornima, V., 2012. Nitric oxide and oral cancer: a review. Oral Oncol. 48 (6), 475–483.

Kos, M., Dabrowski, A., 2002. Tumour's angiogenesis–the function of VEGF and bFGF in colorectal cancer. Ann. Univ. Mariae Curie Sklodowska, Med. 57 (2), 556–561.

Krelin, Y., Voronov, E., Dotan, S., Elkabets, M., Reich, E., Fogel, M., Huszar, M., Iwakura, Y., Segal, S., Dinarello, C.A., Apte, R.N., 2007. Interleukin-1beta-driven inflammation promotes the development and invasiveness of chemical carcinogen-induced tumors. Cancer Res. 67 (3), 1062–1071.

Küchler, A.M., Pollheimer, J., Balogh, J., Sponheim, J., Manley, L., Sorensen, D.R., De Angelis, P.M., Scott, H., Haraldsen, G., Oct 2008. Nuclear interleukin-33 is generally expressed in resting endothelium but rapidly lost upon angiogenic or proinflammatory activation. Am. J. Pathol. 173 (4), 1229–1242.

Kujawaski, M., Kortylewski, M., Lee, H., Herrmann, A., Kay, H., Yu, H., 2008. Stat3 mediates myeloid cell-dependent tumor angiogenesis in mice. J. Clin. Invest. 118 (10), 3367–3377.

Kumar, S., Hanning, C.R., Brigham-Burke, M.R., Rieman, D.J., Lehr, R., Khandekar, S., Kirkpatrick, R.B., Scott, G.F., Lee, J.C., Lynch, F.J., Gao, W., Gambotto, A., Lotze, M.T., 2002. Interleukin-1F7B (IL-1H4/IL-1F7) is processed by caspase-1 and mature IL-1F7B binds to the IL-18 receptor but does not induce IFN-gamma production. Cytokine 18 (2), 61–71.

Kumar, S., McDonnell, P.C., Lehr, R., Tierney, L., Tzimas, M.N., Griswold, D.E., Capper, E.A., Tal-Singer, R., Wells, G.I., Doyle, M.L., Young, P.R., 2000. Identification and initial characterization of four novel members of the interleukin-1 family. J. Biol. Chem. 275, 10308–10314.

Kuo, P.L., Shen, K.H., Hung, S.H., Hsu,Y.L., 2012. CXCL1/GROα increases cell migration and invasion of prostate cancer by decreasing fibulin-1 expression through NF-κB/HDAC1 epigenetic regulation. Carcinogenesis 33 (12), 2477–2487.

Kutikhin, A.G.,Yuzhalin, A.E.,Volkov, A.N., Zhivotovskiy, A.S., Brusina, E.B., 2014. Correlation between genetic polymorphisms within IL-1B and TLR4 genes and cancer risk in a Russian population: a case-control study. Tumour Biol. 35 (5), 4821–4830.

Larsen, C.M., Faulenbach, M.,Vaag, A.,Volund, A., Ehses, J.A., Seifert, B., Mandrup-Poulsen, T., Donath, M.Y., 2007. Interleukin-1-receptor antagonist in type 2 diabetes mellitus. N. Engl. J. Med. 356, 1517–1526.

Lawler, J., 2002. Thrombospondin-1 as an endogenous inhibitor of angiogenesis and tumor growth. J. Cell Mol. Med. 6 (1), 1–12.

Le Page, C., Ouellet,V., Madore, J., Hudson, T.J., Tonin, P.N., Provencher, D.M., Mes-Masson, A.M., 2006. From gene profiling to diagnostic markers: IL-18 and FGF-2 complement CA125 as serum-based markers in epithelial ovarian cancer. Int. J. Cancer 118 (7), 1750–1758.

Lee, C.S., Jun, I.H., Kim, T.I., Byeon, S.H., Koh, H.J., Lee, S.C., 2012. Expression of 12 cytokines in aqueous humour of uveal melanoma before and after combined Ruthenium-106 brachytherapy and transpupillary thermotherapy. Acta Ophthalmol. 90 (4), e314–20.

Lee, K.A., Ki, C.S., Kim, H.J., Sohn, K.M., Kim, J.W., Kang, W.K., Rhee, J.C., Song, S.Y., Sohn, T.S., 2004. Novel interleukin 1beta polymorphism increased the risk of gastric cancer in a Korean population. J. Gastroenterol. 39 (5), 429–433.

Lee, S., Kang, J., Cho, M., Seo, E., Choi, H., Kim, E., Kim, J., Kim, H., Kang, G.Y., Kim, K.P., Park,Y.H.,Yu, D.Y.,Yum,Y.N., Park, S.N.,Yoon, D.Y., Jan 2009. Profiling of transcripts and proteins modulated by K-ras oncogene in the lung tissues of K-ras transgenic mice by omics approaches. Int. J. Oncol. 34 (1), 161–172.

Lefebvre,V., Peeters-Joris, C.,Vaes, G., 1991. Production of gelatin-degrading matrix metalloproteinases ('type IV collagenases') and inhibitors by articular chondrocytes during their dedifferentiation by serial subcultures and under stimulation by interleukin-1 and tumor necrosis factor a. Biochim. Biophys. Acta 1094, 8–18.

Lian, L.H., Milora, K.A., Manupipatpong, K.K., Jensen, L.E., 2012. The double-stranded RNA analogue polyinosinic-polycytidylic acid induces keratinocyte pyroptosis and release of IL-36γ. J. Invest. Dermatol. 132 (5), 1346–1353.

Librizzi, L., Noè, F.,Vezzani, A., de Curtis, M., Ravizza, T., 2012. Seizure-induced brainborne inflammation sustains seizure recurrence and blood-brain barrier damage. Ann. Neurol. 72 (1), 82–90.

Lie, P.P., Cheng, C.Y., Mruk, D.D., 2012. The biology of interleukin-1: emerging concepts in the regulation of the actin cytoskeleton and cell junction dynamics. Cell Mol. Life Sci. 69 (4), 487–500.

Liew, F.Y., Pitman, N.I., McInnes, I.B., 2010. Disease-associated functions of IL-33: the new kid in the IL-1 family. Nat. Rev. Immunol. 10 (2), 103–110.

Lin, H., Ho, A.S., Haley-Vicente, D., Zhang, J., Bernal-Fussell, J., Pace, A.M., Hansen, D., Schweighofer, K., Mize, N.K., Ford, J.E., 2001. Cloning and characterization of IL-1HY2, a novel interleukin-1 family member. J. Biol. Chem. 276, 20597–20602.

Liu, W., Han, B., Sun, B., Gao,Y., Huang,Y., Hu, M., 2012. Overexpression of interleukin-18 induces growth inhibition, apoptosis and gene expression changes in a human tongue squamous cell carcinoma cell line. J. Int. Med. Res. 40 (2), 537–544.

Looi, L.M., 1987. Tumor-associated tissue eosinophilia in nasopharyngeal carcinoma. A pathologic study of 422 primary and 138 metastatic tumors. Cancer 59, 466–470.

Lundström, W., Fewkes, N.M., Mackall, C.L., 2012. IL-7 in human health and disease. Semin. Immunol. 24 (3), 218–224.

Lv, M., Xiaoping, X., Cai, H., Li, D.,Wang, J., Fu, X.,Yu, F., Sun, M., Lv, Z., 2011. Cytokines as prognostic tool in breast carcinoma. Front Biosci. 16, 2515–2526.

Maier, J.A., Statuto, M., Ragnotti, G., 1994. Endogenous interleukin 1 alpha must be transported to the nucleus to exert its activity in human endothelial cells. Mol. Cell Biol. 14, 1845–1851.

March, C.J., Mosley, B., Larsen, A., Cerretti, D.P., Braedt, G., Price, V., Gillis, S., Henney, C.S., Kronheim, S.R., Grabstein, K., 1985. Cloning, sequence and expression of two distinct human interleukin-1 complementary DNAs. Nature 315 (6021), 641–647.

Marhaba, R., Nazarenko, I., Knöfler, D., Reich, E., Voronov, E., Vitacolonna, M., Hildebrand, D., Elter, E., Apte, R.N., Zöller, M., 2008. Opposing effects of fibrosarcoma cell-derived IL-1 alpha and IL-1 beta on immune response induction. Int. J. Cancer 123 (1), 134–145.

Masamune, A., Watanabe, T., Kikuta, K., Satoh, K., Kanno, A., Shimosegawa, T., Oct 2010. Nuclear expression of interleukin-33 in pancreatic stellate cells. Am. J. Physiol. Gastrointest. Liver Physiol. 299 (4), G821–G832.

McNamee, E.N., Masterson, J.C., Jedlicka, P., McManus, M., Grenz, A., Collins, C.B., Nold, M.F., Nold-Petry, C., Bufler, P., Dinarello, C.A., Rivera-Nieves, J., 2011. Interleukin 37 expression protects mice from colitis. Proc. Natl. Acad. Sci. USA. 108 (40), 16711–16716.

Merendino, R.A., Gangemi, S., Ruello, A., Bene, A., Losi, E., Lonbardo, G., Purello-Dambrosio, F., 2001. Serum levels of interleukin-18 and sICAM-1 in patients affected by breast cancer: preliminary considerations. Int. J. Biol. Markers 16, 126–129.

Merendino, R.A., Ruello, A., Cascinu, S., Ferlazzo, B., Bene, A., Bonanno, D., Quattrocchi, P., Caristi, N., Gangemi, S., 2002. Influence of 5-fluorouracil and folinic acid on interleukin-18 production in colorectal cancer patients. Int. J. Biol. Markers 17 (1), 63–66.

Micallef, M.J., Yoshida, K., Kawai, S., Hanaya, T., Kohno, K., Arai, S., Tanimoto, T., Torigoe, K., Fujii, M., Ikeda, M., Kurimoto, M., 1997. In vivo antitumor effects of murine interferon-gamma-inducing factor/interleukin-18 in mice bearing syngeneic Meth A sarcoma malignant ascites. Cancer Immunol. Immunother. 43 (6), 361–367.

Mo, C., Dai, Y., Kang, N., Cui, L., He, W., 2012. Ectopic expression of human MutS homologue 2 on renal carcinoma cells is induced by oxidative stress with interleukin-18 promotion via p38 mitogen-activated protein kinase (MAPK) and c-Jun N-terminal kinase (JNK) signaling pathways. J. Biol. Chem. 287 (23), 19242–19254.

Mohran, Z.Y., Ali-Eldin, F.A., 2011. Abdel Aal HA. Serum interleukin-18: does it have a role in the diagnosis of hepatitis C virus related hepatocellular carcinoma? Arab J. Gastroenterol. 12 (1), 29–33.

Müller, J., Feige, K., Wunderlin, P., Hödl, A., Meli, M.L., Seltenhammer, M., Grest, P., Nicolson, L., Schelling, C., Heinzerling, L.M., Jan 2011. Double-blind placebo-controlled study with interleukin-18 and interleukin-12-encoding plasmid DNA shows antitumor effect in metastatic melanoma in gray horses. J. Immunother. 34 (1), 58–64.

Murohara, T., Asahara, T., Silver, M., Bauters, C., Masuda, H., Kalka, C., Kearney, M., Chen, D., Symes, J.F., Fishman, M.C., Huang, P.L., Isner, J.M., 1998. Nitric oxide synthase modulates angiogenesis in response to tissue ischemia. J. Clin. Invest. 101 (11), 2567–2578.

Musso, T., Espinoza-Delgado, I., Pulkki, K., Gusella, G.L., Longo, D.L., Varesio, L., 1990. Transforming growth factor beta downregulates interleukin-1 (IL-1)-induced IL-6 production by human monocytes. Blood 76 (12), 2466–2469.

Mustea, A., Pirvulescu, C., Konsgen, D., Braicu, E.I., Yuan, S., Sun, P., Lichtenegger, W., Sehouli, J., 2008. Decreased IL-1 RA concentration in ascites is associated with a significant improvement in overall survival in ovarian cancer. Cytokine 42, 77–84.

Nagai, H., Hara, I., Horikawa, T., Oka, M., Kamidono, S., Ichihashi, M., 2002. Gene transfer of secreted-type modified interleukin-18 gene to B16F10 melanoma cells suppresses in vivo tumor growth through inhibition of tumor vessel formation. J. Invest. Dermatol. 119 (3), 541–548.

Nakao, S., Kuwano, T., Tsutsumi-Miyahara, C., Ueda, S., Kimura, Y.N., Hamano, S., Sonoda, K.H., Saijo, Y., Nukiwa, T., Strieter, R.M., Ishibashi, T., Kuwano, M., Ono, M., 2005. Infiltration of COX-2-expressing macrophages is a prerequisite for IL-1 beta induced neovascularization and tumor growth. J. Clin. Invest. 115 (11), 2979–2991.

Naumnik, W., Chyczewska, E., Kovalchuk, O., Tałałaj, J., Izycki, T., Panek, B., 2004. Serum levels of interleukin-18 (IL-18) and soluble interleukin-2 receptor (sIL-2R) in lung cancer. Rocz. Akad. Med. Bialymstoku 49, 246–251.

Ni, J., Miller, M., Stojanovic, A., Garbi, N., Cerwenka, A., 2012. Sustained effector function of IL-12/15/18-preactivated NK cells against established tumors. J. Exp. Med. 209 (13), 2351–2365.

Nicklin, M.J., Barton, J.L., Nguyen, M., FitzGerald, M.G., Duff, G.W., Kornman, K., 2002. A sequence-based map of the nine genes of the human interleukin-1 cluster. Genomics 79, 718–725.

Niedźwiecki, S., Stepień, T., Kuzdak, K., Stepień, H., Krupiński, R., Seehofer, D., Rayes, N., Ulrich, F., 2008. Serum levels of interleukin-1 receptor antagonist (IL-1ra) in thyroid cancer patients. Langenbecks Arch. Surg. 393 (3), 275–280.

Nielsen, H.J., Hansen, U., Christensen, I.J., Reimert, C.M., Brunner, N., Moesgaard, F., 1999. Independent prognostic value of eosinophil and mast cell infiltration in colorectal cancer tissue. J. Pathol. 189, 487–495.

Nold, M.F., Nold-Petry, C.A., Zepp, J.A., Palmer, B.E., Bufler, P., Dinarello, C.A., 2010. IL-37 is a fundamental inhibitor of innate immunity. Nat. Immunol. 11, 1014–1022.

Ohtsuki, T., Micallef, M.J., Kohno, K., Tanimoto, T., Ikeda, M., Kurimoto, M., 1997. Interleukin 18 enhances Fas ligand expression and induces apoptosis in Fas-expressing human myelomonocytic KG-1 cells. Anticancer Res. 17 (5A), 3253–3258.

Okamoto, M., Azuma, K., Hoshino, T., Imaoka, H., Ikeda, J., Kinoshita, T., Takamori, S., Ohshima, K., Edakuni, N., Kato, S., Iwanaga, T., Aizawa, H., 2009. Correlation of decreased survival and IL-18 in bone metastasis. Intern. Med. 48 (10), 763–773.

Okamoto, M., Liu, W., Luo, Y., Tanaka, A., Cai, X., Norris, D.A., Dinarello, C.A., Fujita, M., 2010. Constitutively active inflammasome in human melanoma cells mediating autoinflammation via caspase-1 processing and secretion of interleukin-1beta. J. Biol. Chem. 285 (9), 6477–6488.

Okamura, H., Tsutsi, H., Komatsu, T., Yutsudo, M., Hakura, A., Tanimoto, T., Torigoe, K., Okura, T., Nukada, Y., Hattori, K., Akita, K., Namba, M., Tanabe, F., Konishi, K., Fukuda, S., Kurimoto, M., 1995. Cloning of a new cytokine that induces IFN-gamma production by T cells. Nature 378 (6552), 88–91.

Oppenheim, J.J., Gery, I., 1993. From lymphodrek to interleukin 1 (IL-1). Immunol. Today 14 (5), 232–234.

Osaki, T., Péron, J.M., Cai, Q., Okamura, H., Robbins, P.D., Kurimoto, M., Lotze, M.T., Tahara, H., 1998. IFN-gamma-inducing factor/IL-18 administration mediates IFN-gamma- and IL-12-independent antitumor effects. J. Immunol. 160 (4), 1742–1749.

Pantschenko, A.G., Pushkar, I., Anderson, K.H., Wang, Y., Miller, L.J., Kurtzman, S.H., Barrows, G., Kreutzer, D.L., 2003. The interleukin-1 family of cytokines and receptors in human breast cancer: implications for tumor progression. Int. J. Oncol. 23 (2), 269–284.

Parekh, D.J., Ankerst, D.P., Baillargeon, J., Higgins, B., Platz, E.A., Troyer, D., Hernandez, J., Leach, R.J., Lokshin, A., Thompson, I.M., 2007. Assessment of 54 biomarkers for biopsy-detectable prostate cancer. Cancer Epidemiology. Biomarkers Prev. 16, 1966–1972.

Park, C.C., Morel, J.C., Amin, M.A., Connors, M.A., Harlow, L.A., Koch, A.E., 2001. Evidence of IL-18 as a novel angiogenic mediator. J. Immunol. 167 (3), 1644–1653.

Park, H., Byun, D., Kim, T.S., Kim, Y.I., Kang, J.S., Hahm, E.S., Kim, S.H., Lee, W.J., Song, H.K., Yoon, D.Y., Kang, C.J., Lee, C., Houh, D., Kim, H., Cho, B., Kim, Y., Yang, Y.H., Min, K.H., Cho, D.H., 2001. Enhanced IL-18 expression in common skin tumors. Immunol. Lett. 79 (3), 215–219.

Pascual, V., Allantaz, F., Arce, E., Punaro, M., Banchereau, J., 2005. Role of interleukin-1 (IL-1) in the pathogenesis of systemic onset juvenile idiopathic arthritis and clinical response to IL-1 blockade. J. Exp. Med. 201 (9), 1479–1486.

Perrella, O., Cuomo, O., Sbreglia, C., Monaco, A., Gnarini, M.R., Gentile, B., Perrella, M., Perrella, A., 2009. IL-18 and interferon-gamma in HCV-related hepatocellular carcinoma: a model of interplay between immune status and cancer. J. Biol. Regul. Homeostatic Agents 23 (4), 251–258.

Peters, V.A., Joesting, J.J., Freund, G.G., 2013. IL-1 receptor 2 (IL-1R2) and its role in immune regulation. Brain Behav. Immun. 32, 1–8.

Poch, B., Lotspeich, E., Ramadani, M., Gansauge, S., Beger, H.G., Gansauge, F., 2007. Systemic immune dysfunction in pancreatic cancer patients. Langenbeck's Arch. Surg. 392, 353–358.

Porta, C., Subhra Kumar, B., Larghi, P., Rubino, L., Mancino, A., Sica, A., 2007. Tumor promotion by tumor-associated macrophages. Adv. Exp. Med. Biol. 604, 67–86.

Pruitt, J.H., Welborn, M.B., Edwards, P.D., Harward, T.R., Seeger, J.W., Martin, T.D., Smith, C., Kenney, J.A., Wesdorp, R.I., Meijer, S., Cuesta, M.A., Abouhanze, A., Copeland 3rd, E.M., Giri, J., Sims, J.E., Moldawer, L.L., Oldenburg, H.S., 1996. Increased soluble interleukin-1 type II receptor concentrations in postoperative patients and in patients with sepsis syndrome. Blood 87 (8), 3282–3288.

Qian, L., Xiang, D., Zhang, J., Zhu, S., Gao, J., Wang, X., Gao, J., Zhang, Y., Shen, J., Yu, Y., Han, W., Wu, M., 2013. Recombinant human interleukin-1 receptor antagonist reduces acute lethal toxicity and protects hematopoiesis from chemotoxicity in vivo. Biomed. Pharmacother. 67 (2), 108–115.

Ramadas, R.A., Ewart, S.L., Iwakura, Y., Medoff, B.D., LeVine, A.M., 2012. IL-36a exerts pro-inflammatory effects in the lungs of mice. PLoS ONE 7 (9), e45784.

Ramadas, R.A., Ewart, S.L., Medoff, B.D., LeVine, A.M., 2011. Interleukin-1 family member 9 stimulates chemokine production and neutrophil influx in mouse lungs. Am. J. Respir. Cell Mol. Biol. 44, 134–145.

Ramadas, R.A., Li, X., Shubitowski, D.M., Samineni, S., Wills-Karp, M., Ewart, S.L., 2006. IL-1 Receptor antagonist as a positional candidate gene in a murine model of allergic asthma. Immunogenetics 58 (10), 851–855.

Rauschmayr, T., Groves, R.W., Kupper, T.S., 1997. Keratinocyte expression of the type 2 interleukin 1 receptor mediates local and specific inhibition of interleukin 1-mediated inflammation. Proc. Natl. Acad. Sci. USA. 94 (11), 5814–5819.

Re, F., Muzio, M., De Rossi, M., Polentarutti, N., Giri, J.G., Mantovani, A., Colotta, F., 1994. The type II "receptor" as a decoy target for interleukin 1 in polymorphonuclear leukocytes: characterization of induction by dexamethasone and ligand binding properties of the released decoy receptor. J. Exp. Med 179, 739–743.

Redlinger Jr, R.E., Mailliard, R.B., Lotze, M.T., Barksdale Jr, E.M., 2003. Synergistic interleukin-18 and low-dose interleukin-2 promote regression of established murine neuroblastoma in vivo. J. Pediatr. Surg. 38 (3), 301–307.

Ricote, M., Garcia-Tunon, I., Bethencourt, F.R., Fraile, B., Paniagua, R., Royuela, M., 2004. Interleukin-1 (IL-1alpha and IL-1beta) and its receptors (IL-1RI, IL-1RII, and IL-1Ra) in prostate carcinoma. Cancer 100, 1388–1396.

Riedel, F., Adam, S., Feick, P., Haas, S., Götte, K., Hörmann, K., 2004. Mannheim Alcohol Study Group. Expression of IL-18 in patients with head and neck squamous cell carcinoma. Int. J. Mol. Med. 13 (2), 267–272.

Robertson, M.J., Mier, J.W., Logan, T., Atkins, M., Koon, H., Koch, K.M., Kathman, S., Pandite, L.N., Oei, C., Kirby, L.C., Jewell, R.C., Bell, W.N., Thurmond, L.M., Weisenbach, J., Roberts, S., Dar, M.M., 2006. Clinical and biological effects of recombinant human interleukin-18 administered by intravenous infusion to patients with advanced cancer. Clin. Cancer Res. 12, 4265–4273.

Rosenwasser, L.J., Dinarello, C.A., Rosenthal, A.S., 1979. Adherent cell function in murine T-lymphocyte antigen recognition. IV. Enhancement of murine T-cell antigen recognition by human leukocytic pyrogen. J. Exp. Med. 150 (3), 709–714.

Ross, R., Grimmel, J., Goedicke, S., Möbus, A.M., Bulau, A.M., Bufler, P., Ali, S., Martin, M.U., 2013. Analysis of nuclear localization of interleukin-1 family cytokines by flow cytometry. J. Immunol. Methods 387 (1–2), 219–227.

Ruddle, N.H., Waksman, B.H., 1968. Cytotoxicity mediated by soluble antigen and lymphocytes in delayed hypersensitivity. I. Characterization of the phenomenon. J. Exp. Med. 128 (6), 1237–1254.

Saijo, Y., Tanaka, M., Miki, M., Usui, K., Suzuki, T., Maemondo, M., Hong, X., Tazawa, R., Kikuchi, T., Matsushima, K., Nukiwa, T., 2002. Proinflammatory cytokine IL-1 beta promotes tumor growth of Lewis lung carcinoma by induction of angiogenic factors: in vivo analysis of tumor-stromal interaction. J. Immunol. 169 (1), 469–475.

Sajadi, S.M., Khoramdelazad, H., Hassanshahi, G., Rafatpanah, H., Hosseini, J., Mahmoodi, M., Arababadi, M.K., Derakhshan, R., Hasheminasabzavareh, R., Hosseini-Zijoud, S.M., Ahmadi, Z., 2013. Plasma levels of CXCL1 (GRO-alpha) and CXCL10 (IP-10) are elevated in type 2 diabetic patients: evidence for the involvement of inflammation and angiogenesis/angiostasis in this disease state. Clin. Lab. 59 (1–2), 133–137.

Samsami Dehaghani, A., Shahriary, K., Kashef, M.A., Naeimi, S., Fattahi, M.J., Mojtahedi, Z., Ghaderi, A., 2009. Interleukin-18 gene promoter and serum level in women with ovarian cancer. Mol. Biol. Rep. 36 (8), 2393–2397.

Sargiannidou, I., Zhou, J., Tuszynski, G.P., 2001. The role of thrombospondin-1 in tumor progression. Exp. Biol. Med. (Maywood) 226 (8), 726–733.

Sasaki, K., Hattori, T., Fujisawa, T., Takahashi, K., Inoue, H., Takigawa, M., 1998. Nitric oxide mediates interleukin-1-induced gene expression of matrix metalloproteinases and basic fibroblast growth factor in cultured rabbit articular chondrocytes. J. Biochem 123 (3), 431–439.

Schmieder, A., Multhoff, G., Radons, J., Nov 2012. Interleukin-33 acts as a pro-inflammatory cytokine and modulates its receptor gene expression in highly metastatic human pancreatic carcinoma cells. Cytokine 60 (2), 514–521.

Semenza, G.L., 2007. Evaluation of HIF-1 inhibitors as anticancer agents. Drug Discovery Today 12 (19–20), 853–859.

Shaik, Y., Sabatino, G., Maccauro, G., Varvara, G., Murmura, G., Saggini, A., Rosati, M., Conti, F., Cianchetti, E., Caraffa, A., Antinolfi, P., Pandolfi, F., Potalivo, G., Galzio, R., Conti, P., Theoharides, T.C., 2013. IL-36 receptor antagonist with special emphasis on IL-38. Int. J. Immunopathol. Pharmacol. 26 (1), 27–36.

Sharma, B., Nawandar, D.M., Nannuru, K.C., Varney, M.L., Singh, R.K., 2013. Targeting CXCR2 enhances chemotherapeutic response, inhibits mammary tumor growth, angiogenesis, and lung metastasis. Mol. Cancer Ther. 12 (5), 799–808.

Sharma, S., Kulk, N., Nold, M.F., Gräf, R., Kim, S.H., Reinhardt, D., Dinarello, C.A., Bufler, P., 2008. The IL-1 family member 7b translocates to the nucleus and down-regulates proinflammatory cytokines. J. Immunol. 180 (8), 5477–5482.

Shiratori, I., Suzuki, Y., Oshiumi, H., Begum, N.A., Ebihara, T., Matsumoto, M., Hazeki, K., Kodama, K., Kashiwazaki, Y., Seya, T., 2007. Recombinant interleukin-12 and interleukin-18 antitumor therapy in a guinea-pig hepatoma cell implant model. Cancer Sci. 98 (12). 1936–42.

Simeoni, E., Dudler, J., Fleury, S., Li, J., Pagnotta, M., Pascual, M., von Segesser, L.K., Vassalli, G., 2007. Gene transfer of a soluble IL-1 type 2 receptor Ig fusion protein improves cardiac allograft survival in rats. Eur. J. Cardiothorac Surg. 31 (2), 222–228.

Sims, J.E., Dower, S.K., Nov-Dec 1994. Interleukin-1 receptors. Eur. Cytokine Netw. 5 (6), 539–546.

Smeets, R.L., Joosten, L.A., Arntz, O.J., Bennink, M.B., Takahashi, N., Carlsen, H., Martin, M.U., van den Berg, W.B., van de Loo, F.A., 2005. Soluble interleukin-1 receptor accessory protein ameliorates collagen-induced arthritis by a different mode of action from that of interleukin-1 receptor antagonist. Arthritis Rheum. 52 (7), 2202–2211.

Smith, D.E., Renshaw, B.R., Ketchem, R.R., Kubin, M., Garka, K.E., Sims, J.E., 2000. Four new members expand the interleukin-1 superfamily. J. Biol. Chem. 275 (2), 1169–1175.

Smith 2nd, J.W., Urba, W.J., Curti, B.D., Elwood, L.J., Steis, R.G., Janik, J.E., Sharfman, W.H., Miller, L.L., Fenton, R.G., Conlon, K.C., 1992. The toxic and hematologic effects of interleukin-1 alpha administered in a phase I trial to patients with advanced malignancies. J. Clin. Oncol. 10 (7), 1141–1152.

Smith Jr, M.F., Carl, V.S., Lodie, T., Fenton, M.J., 1998. Secretory interleukin-1 receptor antagonist gene expression requires both a PU.1 and a novel composite NF-kappaB/PU.1/GA-binding protein binding site. J. Biol. Chem. 273 (37), 24272–24279.

Smyth, M.J., Swann, J., Kelly, J.M., Cretney, E., Yokoyama, W.M., Diefenbach, A., Sayers, T.J., Hayakawa, Y., 2004. NKG2D recognition and perforin effector function mediate effective cytokine immunotherapy of cancer. J. Exp. Med. 200 (10), 1325–1335.

Song, J.K., Park, M.H., Choi, D.Y., Yoo, H.S., Han, S.B., Yoon do, Y., Hong, J.T., 2012. Deficiency of C-C chemokine receptor 5 suppresses tumor development via inactivation of NF-κB and upregulation of IL-1Ra in melanoma model. PLoS One 7 (5), e33747.

Song, L., Qiu, F., Fan, Y., Ding, F., Liu, H., Shu, Q., Liu, W., Li, X., 2013. Glucocorticoid regulates interleukin-37 in systemic lupus erythematosus. J. Clin. Immunol. 33 (1), 111–117.

Song, X., Voronov, E., Dvorkin, T., Fima, E., Cagnano, E., Benharroch, D., Shendler, Y., Bjorkdahl, O., Segal, S., Dinarello, C.A., Apte, R.N., 2003. Differential effects of IL-1 alpha and IL-1 beta on tumorigenicity patterns and invasiveness. J. Immunol. 171 (12), 6448–6456.

Sozen, S., Coskun, U., Sancak, B., Bukan, N., Gьnel, N., Tunc, L., Bozkirli, I., 2004. Serum levels of interleukin-18 and nitrite+nitrate in renal cell carcinoma patients with different tumor stage and grade. Neoplasma 51 (1), 25–29.

Spriggs, M.K., Nevens, P.J., Grabstein, K., Dower, S.K., Cosman, D., Armitage, R.J., McMahan, C.J., Sims, J.E., 1992. Molecular characterization of the interleukin-1 receptor (IL-1R) on monocytes and polymorphonuclear cells. Cytokine 4 (2), 90–95.

Srivastava, S., Pelloso, D., Feng, H., Voiles, L., Lewis, D., Haskova, Z., Whitacre, M., Trulli, S., Chen, Y.J., Toso, J., Jonak, Z.L., Chang, H.C., Robertson, M.J., Jun 2013. Effects of interleukin-18 on natural killer cells: costimulation of activation through Fc receptors for immunoglobulin. Cancer Immunol. Immunother. 62 (6), 1073–1082.

Stolarski, B., Kurowska-Stolarska, M., Kewin, P., Xu, D., Liew, F.Y., 2010. IL-33 exacerbates eosinophil-mediated airway inflammation. J. Immunol. 185 (6), 3472–3480.

Stoll, S., Jonuleit, H., Schmitt, E., Müller, G., Yamauchi, H., Kurimoto, M., Knop, J., Enk, A.H., 1998. Production of functional IL-18 by different subtypes of murine and human dendritic cells (DC): DC-derived IL-18 enhances IL-12-dependent Th1 development. Eur. J. Immunol. 28 (10), 3231–3239.

Subleski, J.J., Hall, V.L., Back, T.C., Ortaldo, J.R., Wiltrout, R.H., 2006. Enhanced antitumor response by divergent modulation of natural killer and natural killer T cells in the liver. Cancer Res. 66 (22), 11005–11012.

Sun, P., Ben, Q., Tu, S., Dong, W., Qi, X., Wu, Y., Dec 2011. Serum interleukin-33 levels in patients with gastric cancer. Dig. Dis. Sci. 56 (12), 3596–3601.

Symons, J.A., Eastgate, J.A., Duff, G.W., 1991. Purification and characterization of a novel soluble receptor for interleukin. J. Exp. Med. 174 (5), 1251–1254.

Tak, P.P., Bacchi, M., Bertolino, M., 2006. Pharmacokinetics of IL-18 binding protein in healthy volunteers and subjects with rheumatoid arthritis or plaque psoriasis. Eur. J. Drug Metab. Pharmacokinet. 31, 109–116.

Takeda, K., Tsutsui, H., Yoshimoto, T., Adachi, O., Yoshida, N., Kishimoto, T., Okamura, H., Nakanishi, K., Akira, S., 1998. Defective NK cell activity and Th1 response in IL-18-deficient mice. Immunity 8 (3), 383–390.

Takubo, T., Kumura, T., Kanashima, H., Nakao, T., Nakamae, H., Aoyama, Y., Yamamura, R., Ohta, T., Koh, K.R., Ohta, K., Yamane, T., Hino, M., Kamitani, T., Tatsumi, N., 2001. Analysis of IL-18 bioactivity and IL-18 mRNA in three patients with adult T-cell leukaemia, acute mixed lineage leukaemia, and acute lymphocytic leukaemia accompanied with high serum IL-18 levels. Haematologia (Budap) 31 (3), 231–235.

Tanaka, F., Hashimoto, W., Robbins, P.D., Lotze, M.T., Tahara, H., 2002. Therapeutic and specific antitumor immunity induced by co-administration of immature dendritic cells and adenoviral vector expressing biologically active IL-18. Gene Ther. 9 (21), 1480–1486.

Tangkijvanich, P., Thong-Ngam, D., Mahachai, V., Theamboonlers, A., Poovorawan, Y., 2007. Role of serum interleukin-18 as a prognostic factor in patients with hepatocellular carcinoma. World J. Gastroenterol. 13 (32), 4345–4349.

Tete, S., Tripodi, D., Rosati, M., Conti, F., Maccauro, G., Saggini, A., Cianchetti, E., Caraffa, A., Antinolfi, P., Toniato, E., Castellani, M.L., Conti, P., Theoharides, T.C., 2012. IL-37 (IL-1F7) the newest anti-inflammatory cytokine which suppresses immune responses and inflammation. Int. J. Immunopathol. Pharmacol. 25 (1), 31–38.

Thong-Ngam, D., Tangkijvanich, P., Lerknimitr, R., Mahachai, V., Theamboonlers, A., Poovorawan, Y., 2006. Diagnostic role of serum interleukin-18 in gastric cancer patients. World J. Gastroenterol. 12 (28), 4473–4477.

Tortola, L., Rosenwald, E., Abel, B., Blumberg, H., Schäfer, M., Coyle, A.J., Renauld, J.C., Werner, S., Kisielow, J., Kopf, M., 2012. Psoriasiform dermatitis is driven by IL-36-mediated DC-keratinocyte crosstalk. J. Clin. Invest. 122 (11), 3965–3976.

Towne, J.E., Garka, K.E., Renshaw, B.R., Virca, G.D., Sims, J.E., 2004. Interleukin (IL)-1F6, IL-1F8, and IL-1F9 signal through IL-1Rrp2 and IL-1RAcP to activate the pathway leading to NF-kappaB and MAPKs. J. Biol. Chem. 279 (14), 13677–13688.

Towne, J.E., Sims, J.E., 2012. IL-36 in psoriasis. Curr. Opin Pharmacol. 12 (4), 486–490.

Trotta, R., Dal Col, J., Yu, J., Ciarlariello, D., Thomas, B., Zhang, X., Allard 2nd, J., Wei, M., Mao, H., Byrd, J.C., Perrotti, D., Caligiuri, M.A., 2008. TGF-beta utilizes SMAD3 to inhibit CD16-mediated IFN-gamma production and antibody-dependent cellular cytotoxicity in human NK cells. J. Immunol. 181 (6), 3784–3792.

Tse, B.W., Russell, P.J., Lochner, M., Förster, I., Power, C.A., 2011. IL-18 inhibits growth of murine orthotopic prostate carcinomas via both adaptive and innate immune mechanisms. PLoS One 6 (9), e24241.

Tsuboi, K., Miyazaki, T., Nakajima, M., Fukai, Y., Masuda, N., Manda, R., Fukuchi, M., Kato, H., Kuwano, H., 2004. Serum interleukin-12 and interleukin-18 levels as a tumor marker in patients with esophageal carcinoma. Cancer Lett. 205 (2), 207–214.

Udagawa, N., Horwood, N.J., Elliott, J., Mackay, A., Owens, J., Okamura, H., Kurimoto, M., Chambers, T.J., Martin, T.J., Gillespie, M.T., 1997. Interleukin-18 (interferon-gamma-inducing factor) is produced by osteoblasts and acts via granulocyte/macrophage colony-stimulating factor and not via interferon-gamma to inhibit osteoclast formation. J. Exp. Med. 185 (6), 1005–1012.

Ushio, S., Namba, M., Okura, T., Hattori, K., Nukada, Y., Akita, K., Tanabe, F., Konishi, K., Micallef, M., Fujii, M., Torigoe, K., Tanimoto, T., Fukuda, S., Ikeda, M., Okamura, H., Kurimoto, M., 1996. Cloning of the cDNA for human IFN-gamma-inducing factor, expression in *Escherichia coli*, and studies on the biologic activities of the protein. J. Immunol. 156 (11), 4274–4279.

Vambutas, A., DeVoti, J., Goldofsky, E., Gordon, M., Lesser, M., Bonagura, V., 2009. Alternate splicing of interleukin-1 receptor type II (IL1R2) in vitro correlates with clinical glucocorticoid responsiveness in patients with AIED. PLoS One 4, e5293.

Vannier, E., Kaser, A., Atkins, M.B., Fantuzzi, G., Dinarello, C.A., Mier, J.W., Tilg, H., 1999. Elevated circulating levels of soluble interleukin-1 receptor type II during interleukin-2 immunotherapy. Eur. Cytokine Netw. 10 (1), 37–42.

Veerdonk, F.L., Stoeckman, A.K., Wu, G., Boeckermann, A.N., Azam, T., Netea, M.G., Joosten, L.A., van der Meer, J.W., Hao, R., Kalabokis, V., Dinarello, C.A., 2012. IL-38 binds to the IL-36 receptor and has biological effects on immune cells similar to IL-36 receptor antagonist. Proc. Natl. Acad. Sci. USA. 109 (8), 3001–3005.

Vidal-Vanaclocha, F., Amézaga, C., Asumendi, A., Kaplanski, G., Dinarello, C.A., 1994. Interleukin-1 receptor blockade reduces the number and size of murine B16 melanoma hepatic metastases. Cancer Res. 54 (10), 2667–2672.

Vidal-Vanaclocha, F., Asumendi, A., Rocha, M., Barbera-Guillem, E., 1993. Participation of endothelial cell mannose receptors in the B16 melanoma cell adhesion to the hepatic sinusoidal endothelium. In: Knook, D., Wisse, E. (Eds.), Cells of the hepatic sinusoid. Kupffer Cell Foundation, Leiden, The Netherlands, pp. 555–558.

Vidal-Vanaclocha, F., Alvarez, A., Asumendi, A., Urcelay, B., Tonino, P., Dinarello, C.A., 1996. Interleukin 1 (IL-1) dependent melanoma hepatic metastasis in vivo; increased endothelial adherence by IL-1-induced mannose receptors and growth factor production in vitro. J. Natl. Cancer Inst. 88 (3–4), 198–205.

Vidal-Vanaclocha, F., Fantuzzi, G., Mendoza, L., Fuentes, A.M., Anasagasti, M.J., Martín, J., Carrascal, T., Walsh, P., Reznikov, L.L., Kim, S.H., Novick, D., Rubinstein, M., Dinarello, C.A., 2000. IL-18 regulates IL-1beta-dependent hepatic melanoma metastasis via vascular cell adhesion molecule-1. Proc. Natl. Acad. Sci. USA 97 (2), 734–739.

Vigne, S., Palmer, G., Martin, P., Lamacchia, C., Strebel, D., Rodriguez, E., Olleros, M.L., Vesin, D., Garcia, I., Ronchi, F., Sallusto, F., Sims, J.E., Gabay, C., 2012. IL-36 signaling amplifies Th1 responses by enhancing proliferation and Th1 polarization of naive CD4[+] T cells. Blood 120 (17), 3478–3487.

Volarevic, V., Mitrovic, M., Milovanovic, M., Zelen, I., Nikolic, I., Mitrovic, S., Pejnovic, N., Arsenijevic, N., Lukic, M.L., 2012. Protective role of IL-33/ST2 axis in Con A-induced hepatitis. J. Hepatol. 56 (1), 26–33.

Voronov, E., Shouval, D.S., Krelin, Y., Cagnano, E., Benharroch, D., Iwakura, Y., Dinarello, C.A., Apte, R.N., 2003. IL-1 is required for tumor invasiveness and angiogenesis. Proc. Natl. Acad. Sci. USA. 100 (5), 2645–2650.

Waldner, M.J., Foersch, S., Neurath, M.F., 2012. Interleukin-6 – a key regulator of colorectal cancer development. Int. J. Biol. Sci. 8 (9), 1248–1253.

Wang, J., Kobayashi, Y., Sato, A., Kobayashi, E., Murakami, T., 2004. Synergistic anti-tumor effect by combinatorial gene-gun therapy using IL-23 and IL-18 cDNA. J. Dermatol. Sci. 36 (1), 66–68.

Wang, P., Xia, H.H., Zhang, J.Y., Dai, L.P., Xu, X.Q., Wang, K.J., 2006. Association of interleukin-1 gene polymorphisms with gastric cancer: a meta-analysis. Int. J. Cancer 120 (3), 552–562.

Waugh, D.J., Wilson, C., 2008. The interleukin-8 pathway in cancer. Clin. Cancer Res. 14 (21), 6735–6741.

Weinreich, D.M., Elaraj, D.M., Puhlmann, M., Hewitt, S.M., Carroll, N.M., Feldman, E.D., Turner, E.M., Spiess, P.J., Alexander, H.R., 2003. Effect of interleukin 1 receptor antagonist gene transduction on human melanoma xenografts in nude mice. Cancer Res. 63 (18), 5957–5961.

Weiss, T., Vitacolonna, M., Zöller, M., 2009. The efficacy of an IL-1alpha vaccine depends on IL-1RI availability and concomitant myeloid-derived suppressor cell reduction. J. Immunother. 32 (6), 552–564.

Werman, A., Werman-Venkert, R., White, R., Lee, J.K., Werman, B., Krelin, Y., Voronov, E., Dinarello, C.A., Apte, R.N., 2004. The precursor form of IL-1α is an intracrine proinflammatory activator of transcription. Proc Natl. Acad. Sci. USA. 101, 2434–2439.

Werner, F., Jain, M.K., Feinberg, M.W., Sibinga, N.E., Pellacani, A., Wiesel, P., Chin, M.T., Topper, J.N., Perrella, M.A., Lee, M.E., 2000. Transforming growth factor-beta 1 inhibition of macrophage activation is mediated via Smad3. J. Biol. Chem. 275 (47), 36653–36658.

Xia, D., Zheng, S., Zhang, W., He, L., Wang, Q., Pan, J., Zhang, L., Wang, J., Cao, X., 2003. Effective induction of therapeutic antitumor immunity by dendritic cells coexpressing interleukin-18 and tumor antigen. J. Mol. Med. (Berlin) 81 (9), 585–596.

Xu, D., Jiang, H.R., Kewin, P., Li, Y., Mu, R., Fraser, A.R., Pitman, N., Kurowska-Stolarska, M., McKenzie, A.N., McInnes, I.B., Liew, F.Y., 2008. IL-33 exacerbates antigen-induced arthritis by activating mast cells. Proc. Natl. Acad. Sci. USA 105 (31), 10913–10918.

Xu, J., Yin, Z., Cao, S., Gao, W., Liu, L., Yin, Y., Liu, P., Shu, Y., 2013. Systematic review and meta-analysis on the association between IL-1B polymorphisms and cancer risk. PLoS One 8 (5), e63654.

Xue, H., Lin, B., Ni, P., Xu, H., Huang, G., 2010. Interleukin-1B and interleukin-1 RN polymorphisms and gastric carcinoma risk: a meta-analysis. J. Gastroenterol. Hepatol. 25 (10), 1604–1617.

Yamada, N., Hata, M., Ohyama, H., Yamanegi, K., Kogoe, N., Nakasho, K., Futani, H., Okamura, H., Terada, N., 2009. Immunotherapy with interleukin-18 in combination with preoperative chemotherapy with ifosfamide effectively inhibits postoperative progression of pulmonary metastases in a mouse osteosarcoma model. Tumour Biol. 30 (4), 176–184.

Yao, J., Liu, L., Yang, M., 2014. Interleukin-23 receptor genetic variants contribute to susceptibility of multiple cancers. Gene 533 (1), 21–25.

Ye, Z.B., Ma, T., Li, H., Jin, X.L., Xu, H.M., 2007. Expression and significance of intratumoral interleukin-12 and interleukin-18 in human gastric carcinoma. World J. Gastroenterol. 13, 1747–1751.

Yoshimura, K., Hazama, S., Iizuka, N., Yoshino, S., Yamamoto, K., Muraguchi, M., Ohmoto, Y., Noma, T., Oka, M., 2001. Successful immunogene therapy using colon cancer cells (colon 26) transfected with plasmid vector containing mature interleukin-18 cDNA and the Igkappa leader sequence. Cancer Gene Ther. 8 (1), 9–16.

Yuzhalin, A.E., Kutikhin, A.G., 2012. Interleukin-12: clinical usage and molecular markers of cancer susceptibility. Growth Factors 30 (3), 176–191.

Yuzhalin, A., 2011. The role of interleukin DNA polymorphisms in gastric cancer. Hum. Immunol. 72 (11), 1128–1136.

Zhang, Y., Li, Y., Ma, Y., Liu, S., She, Y., Zhao, P., Jing, M., Han, T., Yan, C., Wu, Z., Gao, J., Ye, L., 2011. Dual effects of interleukin-18: inhibiting hepatitis B virus replication in HepG2.2.15 cells and promoting hepatoma cells metastasis. Am J. Physiol. Gastrointest Liver Physiol. 301 (3), G565–G573.

Zhang, Y.K., Huang, Z.J., Liu, S., Liu, Y.P., Song, A.A., Song, X.J., May 1, 2013. WNT signaling underlies the pathogenesis of neuropathic pain in rodents. J. Clin. Invest. 123 (5), 2268–2286.

Zhang, Z.Y., Wu, J.M., 2007. Anti-tumor effects induced by fusion of interleukin-18 gene transfected NCI-H460 lung cancer cell line with dendritic cells. Zhonghua Zhongliu Zazhi 29 (1), 17–20.

Zhao, Y., Schetter, A.J., Yang, G.B., Nguyen, G., Mathй, E.A., Li, P., Cai, H., Yu, L., Liu, F., Hang, D., Yang, H., Wang, X.W., Ke, Y., Harris, C.C., 2013. microRNA and inflammatory gene expression as prognostic marker for overall survival in esophageal squamous cell carcinoma. Int J. Cancer 132 (12), 2901–2909.

Zheng, J.N., Pei, D.S., Mao, L.J., Liu, X.Y., Sun, F.H., Zhang, B.F., Liu, Y.Q., Liu, J.J., Li, W., Han, D., 2010. Oncolytic adenovirus expressing interleukin-18 induces significant antitumor effects against melanoma in mice through inhibition of angiogenesis. Cancer Gene Ther. 17 (1), 28–36.

Zheng, J.N., Pei, D.S., Sun, F.H., Liu, X.Y., Mao, L.J., Zhang, B.F., Wen, R.M., Xu, W., Shi, Z., Liu, J.J., Li, W., 2009. Potent antitumor efficacy of interleukin-18 delivered by conditionally replicative adenovirus vector in renal cell carcinoma-bearing nude mice via inhibition of angiogenesis. Cancer Biol. Ther. 8 (7), 599–606.

Zhiguang, X., Wei, C., Steven, R., Wei, D., Wei, Z., Rong, M., Zhanguo, L., Lianfeng, Z., 2010. Over-expression of IL-33 leads to spontaneous pulmonary inflammation in mIL-33 transgenic mice. Immunol. Lett. 131, 159–165.

Zhu, Y., Richardson, J.A., Parada, L.F., Graff, J.M., 1998. Smad3 mutant mice develop metastatic colorectal cancer. Cell. 94 (6), 703–714.

CHAPTER 3

Interleukin-2 Superfamily and Cancer

There is grandeur in this view of life, with its several powers, having been originally breathed by the Creator into a few forms or into one; and that, whilst this planet has gone circling on according to the fixed law of gravity, from so simple a beginning endless forms most beautiful and most wonderful have been, and are being evolved.

Charles Darwin, English biologist (1809–1882)

3.1 INTERLEUKIN-2 AND CANCER

Interleukin (IL) 2 was originally described in the early 1980s as a growth factor for antigen-stimulated T cells and is one of the key molecules performing T-cell clonal expansion after antigen recognition. IL-2 is produced by activated CD4+ T cells, naive CD8+ T cells, and dendritic cells, and it enhances proliferation and differentiation of natural killer (NK) and regulatory T (Treg) cells (Nelson, 2004). In addition, it is a growth factor for cytotoxic T cells at late stages of the immune reaction (Nelson, 2004). In the absence of IL-2, T cells may suffer from the phenomenon of anergy (Nelson, 2004). The soluble IL-2 receptor (IL-2R) is considered as an antagonist of IL-2, and interferon-γ negatively affects the production of IL-2R (Nelson, 2004).

Disease progression or negative prognosis in cancer has been associated with decreased IL-2 concentrations or an elevation in soluble IL-2R level (Berghella et al., 1998; Shibata and Takekawa, 1999; Orditura et al., 2000; Niitsu et al., 2001; Naumnik and Chyczewska, 2001; Vuoristo et al., 2001; Neuner et al., 2002). IL-2 was approved for clinical use in 1992, and nowadays it is a current treatment option for patients with late-stage renal cell carcinoma and malignant melanoma, and complete clinical responses associated with long-term survival are reported relatively consistently in these cases (Grivas and Redman, 2011). The ability of IL-2 to promote both activation and tolerance has remained obscure since IL-2 may lead to a rapid T-cell expansion enhancing an immune response but may also stimulate Tregs in a similar manner (Atkins et al., 1999; Fisher et al., 2000; Sojka et al., 2005; Knoechel et al., 2005; Klapper et al., 2008; Coventry and Ashdown, 2012).

Interleukins in Cancer Biology
http://dx.doi.org/10.1016/B978-0-12-801121-8.00003-8

The aim of IL-2 treatment is to enhance effector T-cell immune response toward killing cancer cells (Grivas and Redman, 2011). In various trials carried out from 1992, IL-2 consistently showed complete clinical response rates at approximately 7% in two very different tumors, namely, renal cell carcinoma and malignant melanoma, although such favorable responses occurred randomly and unpredictably in trial populations (Atkins et al., 1999; Fisher et al., 2000; Klapper et al., 2008; Grivas and Redman, 2011; Prieto et al., 2012). Notably, 10-year-survival rates have been high in patients who consisted these 7% (Atkins et al., 1999; Fisher et al., 2000; Klapper et al., 2008; Grivas and Redman, 2011; Prieto et al., 2012). Interestingly, certain studies have reported effective clinical responses using intermittent short bolus IL-2 dosing rather than longer IL-2 infusions (Grivas and Redman, 2011; Quan et al., 2012). In certain situations, either IL-2 and/or IL-2R can be released or expressed by cancer cells themselves (Plaisance et al., 1993; Alileche et al., 1993; Coventry et al., 1996; Barbour and Coventry, 2003; Rangel-Corona et al., 2010). How this may affect cancer development and how it interacts with IL-2 treatment is currently unclear but an evaluation of IL-2 and IL-2R expression in tumor cells from biopsies prior to therapy might potentially be of clinical relevance (Coventry and Ashdown, 2012).

3.2 IL-4 AND CANCER

IL-4 is a multifunctional peptide, which may affect multiple cell types (Hallet et al., 2012). It is produced by macrophages, dendritic cells, mast cells, NK cells, natural killer T (NKT) cells, basophils, eosinophils, and T lymphocytes, and it is a well-characterized regulator of proliferation and immunoglobulin class switching in B cells (Wills-Karp and Finkelman, 2008; LaPorte et al., 2008; Ito et al., 2009; Koller et al., 2010). When IL-4 binds IL-4Rα with high affinity, resultant heterodimerization with either the gamma common chain (γc) forms the type I IL-4R, or with IL-13Rα1 forms the type II IL-4R (LaPorte et al., 2008; Ito et al., 2009). The type II IL-4R can also be generated by binding of IL-13 to IL-13Rα1 and further heterodimerization with IL-4Rα (Wills-Karp and Finkelman, 2008; LaPorte et al., 2008). The type I IL-4R complex is expressed on the surface of lymphoid T and NK cells, basophils, mast cells, and most mouse B cells, while type II IL-4R is detected on nonlymphoid and tumor cells (Wills-Karp and Finkelman, 2008; Koller et al., 2010).

Biological functions of IL-4 are diverse. It plays a pivotal role in adaptive and humoral immunity. Furthermore, it has been shown to trigger the differentiation of plasma cells from B cells and also the proliferation of activated T and B cells. Multiple studies have shown that IL-4 decreases the production of dentritic cells (DCs), macrophages, Th1 cells, and interferon (IFN)-gamma. Some studies indicated that IL-4 is involved in angiogenesis (Dehne et al., 2014) and allergy (Hershey et al., 1997). Certain studies implicate IL-4 as a suppressor of proinflammatory cytokines and an enhancer of the expression of antiinflammatory cytokine production (Opal and DePalo, 2000). Moreover, IL-4 has been found to contribute to the conversion of macrophages into tumor-associated macrophages. These cells are known to be key mediators of tumor angiogenesis. In particular, they were reported to enhance fibrin deposition via procoagulant activity and can promote the formation of new vessels (Wang and Joyce, 2010). Furthermore, tumor-associated macrophages are reported to have a considerable influence on metastatic processes as well (van Netten et al., 1993).

High IL-4 levels have been found in the tumor microenvironment and peripheral blood of patients with prostate, bladder, and breast cancers (Camp et al., 1996; Elsässer-Beile et al., 1998; Wise et al., 2000). Certain investigations found that type II IL-4R (IL-4Rα and IL-13Rα1 chains) is upregulated and activated in various epithelial tumor types including malignant glioma and ovarian, lung, breast, pancreatic, and colon cancers (Prokopchuk et al., 2005; Todaro et al., 2008). Nevertheless, expression of type I IL-4R (IL-4Rα and γC chains) remains to be examined in these malignant tumors. The IL-4/IL4-Rα complex on epithelial cancer cells increases resistance to apoptosis and may enhance tumor cell survival (Li et al., 2008; Hallett et al., 2012). Tumor-promoting macrophages can also be activated by IL-4 (Wang and Joyce, 2010). Additionally, IL-4 was found to induce mitogenesis, dedifferentiation, and metastasis in rhabdomyosarcoma model (Hosoyama et al., 2011). Treatment with the IL-4 neutralizing antibody alone has downregulated antiapoptotic proteins phosphoprotein enriched in diabetes (PED), cellular FLICE inhibitory protein (cFLIP) Bcl-xL, and Bcl-2, therefore decreasing the growth of breast and colon tumors (Todaro et al., 2008). Mice bearing colorectal tumors and treated with an anti–human IL-4 neutralizing antibody or with an antagonist of human IL-4Rα have demonstrated a modest decrease in tumor size in comparison with controls with either treatment alone (Todaro et al., 2007). However, efficacy of chemotherapy with oxaliplatin and/or 5-fluorouracil has been significantly improved when animals were cotreated with either of these modalities (Todaro et al., 2007). Importantly, these antitumor effects have been sustained after the cessation of treatment (Todaro et al., 2007). Thus, anti-IL-4/IL-4Rα treatment in combination with standard chemotherapy may have a synergistic effect in reducing tumor growth in patients (Todaro et al., 2007). In addition, IL-4 has been shown to directly enhance the proliferation of colon, breast, head and neck, ovarian, and prostate cancer cells, possibly via activation of downstream signal transducer and activator of transcription 6 (STAT6) signaling and upregulation of survivin (Zhang et al., 2008; Koller et al., 2010; Roca et al., 2012). It is worthy of note that clinical trials in which exogenous IL-4 has been tested as an antitumor agent have not been successful (Li et al., 2009). Results obtained from the implantation model have shown that tumor cell IL-4Rα is crucial for inducing proliferation but not survival in vivo (Koller et al., 2010). In the carcinogen model, IL-4Rα−/− mice have had significantly smaller tumors in comparison with wild-type mice (Koller et al., 2010). The reduction in tumor size has been due to decreased proliferation and a significant increase in apoptosis (Koller et al., 2010). This investigation has established a potential role for IL-4Rα in colon cancer, although it contradicts previous studies demonstrating a strong pro-survival effect of the IL-4/IL-4Rα complex in epithelial tumor cells (Todaro et al., 2007; Todaro et al., 2008; Li et al., 2008; Roca et al., 2012).

Much research has been done on evaluating the impact of inherited variations within the *IL-4* gene on tumor biology. In particular, genetic polymorphisms of *IL-4* gene can have considerable influence on gastric cancer etiology (reviewed by Yuzhalin, 2011). The mutant T allele for the promoter IL4-590C/T (rs2243250) polymorphism increases the expression of IL-4 dramatically, and therefore is of particular interest (Rosenwasser et al., 1995). Wu et al. (2003) identified that the carriage of the CT/CC genotype correlates with an increased risk of developing cardiac or diffuse-type gastric cancer (odds ratio (OR) = 1.64; 95% confidence interval (CI): 1.01–2.67 and OR = 2.44; 95% CI: 1.13–2.67, respectively) as compared to the TT genotype. However, in combined analyses using data from five previous studies, Sugimoto et al. (2010) found that this polymorphism was significantly associated with the decreased risk of noncardiac gastric cancer. Importantly, the protective effect was more evident in patients with the upregulated genotype, although this analysis included studies analyzing the Western population only, because the frequency of the TT genotype was too low among the Asian population. From these findings it could be concluded that carriers of the CC "down-IL-4" genotype are less protected against inflammation and therefore are more predisposed to cancer risk. Nevertheless, it is not easy to explain possible association between the angiogenic properties of IL-4 and cancer protection. On the one hand, angiogenesis can inhibit the source of inflammation at a precancerous stage, and the contribution of the IL-4 high-producing genotype is very clear. On the other hand, this genotype may provide a blood supply to the malignancy if the tumor has already been established, and hence it is possible to hypothesize that the TT genotype plays a protective role only in the occurrence, but not in the progression of gastric cancer. It is also important that the *IL4*-590T allele had the same effect in patients with colorectal (Yannopoulos et al., 2007) and prostate cancer (Tindall et al., 2010), which can also indicate a possible involvement of this genetic polymorphism in carcinogenesis and allows its possible use in the prediction of malignancies.

Another genetic polymorphism, *IL4*-168T/C (rs2070874), was examined by Wu et al. (2009), showing that the variant C allele correlates with a decreased gastric cancer risk in a Chinese population as compared to the wild-type TT genotype (OR = 0.81 for the TC genotype and OR = 0.83 for the TC/CC genotype, respectively). Moreover, the observed effect was more evident among individuals with cardiac gastric cancer (OR = 0.73 for the TC/CC vs TT genotype).

3.3 IL-7 AND CANCER

IL-7 was discovered as a human T-cell growth factor in 1987. IL-7 is mainly expressed in thymus and bone marrow, although small concentrations of this cytokine are produced by DCs, neurons, hepatocytes, and keratinocytes. Earlier studies have identified IL-7 as an essential cytokine for T-cell production, maturation and expansion (Goodwin and Namen, 1989–1990); therefore, it has been suggested as an ideal candidate for immune reconstitution (Morrissey et al., 1991; Alpdogan et al., 2001; Storek et al., 2003; Fry et al., 2003; Beq and Nugeyre, 2006; Leone et al., 2010; Parker et al., 2010). Importantly, IL-7 administration has not caused the acute inflammatory cytokine release in preclinical models unlike a number of other cytokines (Henriques et al., 2010). IL-7 administration induces massive and rapid T-cell migration from the blood into various organs including the lymph nodes, gut, and the skin (Beq et al., 2009) and leads to increase in both naive and memory T cells (Morre and Beq, 2012). Finally, the proliferative effects of IL-7 on the lymphocyte population are not limited to the αβ T cells since IL-7 also triggers the expansion of γδ T cells and invariant NKT cells (Morre and Beq, 2012). IL-7 can be produced by thymic epithelial cells, bone marrow stromal cells, liver and intestinal epithelial cells, keratinocytes, fibroblasts, dendritic cells, and macrophages (Fry and Mackall, 2002). In solid tissue, IL-7 is presented at the T-cell surface by fibronectin and heparin sulfate (Borghesi et al., 1999). The IL-7 receptor (IL-7R) is only present on the surface of hematopoietic lineage cells, including T cells, dendritic cells, macrophages, and NK subsets (Mackall et al., 2011). IL-7R is a heterodimer consisting of IL-7Rα (also known as CD127) and the common cytokine receptor γ-chain (γc; also known as CD132) (Pellegrini et al., 2009). However, when T cells become activated, the expression of IL-7Rα is downregulated, which prevents these cells from responding to IL-7 (Mackall et al., 2011). Conversely, when T-cell populations are decreased in size, circulating and tissue levels of IL-7 increase (Mackall et al., 2011). IL-7 mediates antiapoptotic and costimulatory proliferative signals through the activation of phosphatidylinositol 3-kinase (PI3K) and Janus kinase (JAK)–STAT pathway, downregulation of the cyclin-dependent kinase inhibitor p27 (also known as p27Kip1), and modulation of members of the Bcl-2 family (Pellegrini et al., 2009). In addition, IL-7 drives the clonal expansion and survival of immature B cells (Malin et al., 2010), and it has also been implicated as a mediator of survival and proliferation of malignant pre-B cells (Brown et al., 2003). IL-7 can also play a role in the development of some subsets of dendritic cells and thymic NK cells (Mackall et al., 2011).

It has been observed that IL-7 alone is not able to trigger antitumoral immune responses; however, any such response triggered by a vaccine, an adoptive T-cell therapy, or any therapy able to stimulate antigen-presenting cells may be amplified and prolonged by IL-7 treatment (Morre and Beq, 2012). For instance, combining IL-7 administration with a granulocyte-macrophage colony-stimulating factor (GM-CSF)-secreting tumor cell immunotherapy directed against colon cancer or malignant melanoma, Li et al. have observed an increased number of activated dendritic cells, T cells in lymphoid tissues, and an increase in activated effector T cells in the tumor microenvironment that has been associated with prolonged survival of tumor-bearing mice (Li et al., 2007). Short-term IL-7 therapy has enhanced vaccine-mediated immunity in a complex double-transgenic mouse model using lymphocytic choriomeningitis virus (LCMV) infection as a vaccine against a spontaneous SV40-driven tumor mouse model (Pellegrini et al., 2009).

3.4 IL-9 AND CANCER

IL-9 was first purified and characterized as a T-cell and mast-cell growth factor, respectively, termed p40, based on its molecular weight, or mast cell growth-enhancing activity (Uyttenhove et al., 1988; Hültner et al., 1990). The cloning and complete amino acid sequencing of p40 have detected it is structurally distinct from other T-cell growth factors (Van Snick et al., 1989; Yang et al., 1989), and this cytokine has been renamed IL-9 based on biological effects on both myeloid and lymphoid cells. IL-9 is mainly synthesized by T lymphocytes and mast cells (Schmitt et al., 1989; Hültner et al., 2000; Stassen et al., 2000). The relative amounts of IL-9 produced by mast cells and T cells in distinct situations have not been determined (Goswami and Kaplan, 2011). The IL-9R has two subunits: the α-chain (IL-9Rα) and the common γ-chain receptor shared by other cytokines such as IL-2, IL-4, and IL-7 (Renauld et al., 1992; Russell et al., 1994). IL-9-mediated signal transduction led to the activation of STAT1, STAT3, and STAT5 (Bauer et al., 1998); mitogen-activated protein kinase; and insulin receptor substrate–PI3K pathway (Yin et al., 1995; Demoulin et al., 1996; Demoulin et al., 2003). IL-9R is expressed on T cell lines and on effector T cells but not on naive T cells (Druez et al., 1990; Cosmi et al., 2004), and it is mainly expressed in Th2 and Th17 cells (Nowak et al., 2009). IL-9R can also be revealed on mast cells and polymorphonuclear cells in the lung (Abdelilah et al., 2001; Kearley et al., 2011). IL-9 may promote T-cell growth and Th17 development but has variable effects on Treg development (Elyaman et al., 2009; Nowak et al., 2009), affects B-cell development and functioning (Vink et al., 1999; Knoops et al., 2004; Fawaz et al., 2007), enhances growth and functioning of mast cells (Hültner et al., 1990; Townsend et al., 2000; Matsuzawa et al., 2003), enhances hematopoiesis (Donahue et al., 1990; Williams et al., 1990; Holbrook et al., 1991; Fujiki et al., 2002), potentiates allergic inflammation in the airway epithelial cells (Steenwinckel et al., 2007), and induces airway mucus production (Louahed et al., 2000). IL-9 shows proinflammatory activity in several mouse models of inflammation (Cheng et al., 2002), mediates allergic inflammation (Knoops et al., 2005), protects against intestinal parasites (Faulkner et al., 1997), and regulates immune response to infectious diseases (Dodd et al., 2009).

Ellmark et al. (2006) used antibody microarray analysis to examine the abundance of 127 proteins, among which are cytokines, chemokines, and complementary factors, among 35 malignant and normal stomach tissue samples. The authors found that tissue levels of IL-9 were significantly over-expressed in tumor tissues versus normal.

However, the role of IL-9 in cancer remains to be elusive. Further in-depth research is required to identify the role of this cytokine in carcinogenesis.

3.5 IL-13 AND CANCER

IL-13 is a multifunctional peptide structurally similar to IL-4, and it also affects multiple cell types, playing a role in hypersensitivity reactions via the influence on epithelial and smooth muscle cells (Wills-Karp and Finkelman,

2008; LaPorte et al., 2008; Ito et al., 2009; Koller et al., 2010; Hallett et al., 2012). As in the case with IL-4, it is produced by macrophages, dendritic cells, mast cells, NKT, NK cells, basophils, eosinophils, and T lymphocytes (Koller et al., 2010). IL-13 binds IL-13Rα2, which is distinct from IL-13Rα1 and present in two forms. A soluble form resulting from either alternative splicing or proteolytic cleavage has no signaling ability and has been coined the decoy receptor (Wills-Karp and Finkelman, 2008), while a larger membrane-spanning form leads to activation of downstream effectors. Importantly, IL-13 can act through type II IL-4R (IL-4Rα and IL-13Rα1) or through IL-13Rα2 (Hallett et al., 2012). The dominant signaling pathway activated by IL-13 binding to IL-13Rα1 is the STAT6 pathway (Wills-Karp and Finkelman, 2008), the same pathway activated by IL-4 binding to the type II IL-4R. After IL-13 binding to IL-13Rα2, ERK1/2 and AP-1-dependent induction of transforming growth factor beta (TGF-β) expression may occur (Fichtner-Feigl et al., 2006). Another mediator is 15-lipoxygenase-1 (15-LOX-1), which, in contrast, acts only in the absence of IL-13Rα2 (Hsi et al., 2011).

It is known that IL-13 is overexpressed in the tumor microenvironment and peripheral blood of patients with prostate, bladder, and breast cancers (Camp et al., 1996; Elsässer-Beile et al., 1998; Wise et al., 2000; Srabovici et al., 2011), while IL-13Rα2 is overexpressed in colon, pancreatic, ovarian tumors and malignant glioma (Fujisawa et al., 2009; Nguyen et al., 2011; Srabovici et al., 2011; Barderas et al., 2012). Increased levels of IL-13 have been observed in the peripheral blood of pancreatic, esophageal, and gastric cancer patients when compared to healthy controls (Gabitass et al., 2011). Possible role for IL-13 and its receptors IL-13Rα1 and IL-13Rα2 in colorectal cancer has been suggested (Barderas et al., 2012; Formentini et al., 2012). Unexpectedly, low IL-13 expression has been associated with declined overall survival compared to high IL-13 expression (Formentini et al., 2012). However, high expression of IL-13Rα2 in colon cancer patients may be considered as a predictor of poor outcome (Barderas et al., 2012). Targeting IL-13Rα2 with a specific immunotoxin in mice has led to decreased tumor burden and extended host survival (Fujisawa et al., 2012). A correlation between IL13-Rα2 expression and metastasis has been found in certain malignant tumors. In an orthotopic model of human ovarian cancer, IL-13Rα2-expressing tumors have metastasized to lymph nodes faster than IL-13Rα2-negative tumors and led to a higher rate of animal mortality (Fujisawa et al., 2012). Exogenous IL-13 treatment has been an additional cause of mortality in mice carrying IL-13Rα2-expressing tumors showing the role of IL-13/IL-13Rα2 in determining the aggressiveness of tumor cells (Fujisawa et al., 2012). Overexpression of IL-13Rα2 has been associated with increased invasion and metastasis, and decreased survival in a mouse model of human pancreatic cancer (Fujisawa et al., 2009). Genetic knockdown of IL-13Rα2 in tumor cells has reduced liver homing ability, resulting in increased survival of mice compared to those injected with IL-13Rα2-expressing cells (Barderas et al., 2012). In mouse models of glioblastoma multiforme, tumor cells that survive IL-13Rα2 targeted therapy have had less tumorigenic potential compared to untreated control cells (Nguyen et al., 2011).

Regarding apoptosis, IL-13 may be both pro- and antiapoptotic depending on receptor presence and/or signaling pathways activated. The IL-13-induced proapoptotic pathway is activated by 15-LOX-1, which catalyzes the oxidation of arachidonic and linoleic acids, leading to activation of Peroxisome proliferator-activated receptor gamma (PPARγ), whose ligands can further launch apoptosis (Hsi et al., 2011). Interestingly, IL-13-dependent production of 15-LOX-1 occurs only in the absence of IL-13Rα2 (Hsi et al., 2011). Decreased glioblastoma multiforme growth due to increased apoptosis has correlated with IL-13 (Hsi et al., 2011).

So, IL-13-dependent signaling can go via three routes (Hallett et al., 2012):

1. IL-13 can bind to IL-13Rα1, recruit IL-4Rα, and act through this heterodimer to phosphorylate STAT6 and promote proliferation and/or apoptotic resistance;
2. IL-13 can bind to soluble IL-13Rα2 decoy receptor and result in no signaling;
3. IL-13 can bind transmembrane monomeric IL-13Rα2 and induce TGF-β leading to increased metastasis.

In IL4Rα−/− mice, where any IL-13 signaling must be through IL13-Rα2, increased development of precancerous lesions has been demonstrated in an intestinal carcinogen mode, and these mice have had elevated TGF-β level (Ko et al., 2008). Activation of AP-1 by IL-13 signaling via IL-13Rα2 may also be a cause of production of other factors, including matrix metalloproteinases (MMPs), which are known to promote tumor growth, invasion, and metastasis (Fujisawa et al., 2012). On the contrary, when IL13-Rα2 expression is abrogated, IL-13 signaling through type II IL-4R can be possibly increased that may lead to the activation of IL13-induced apoptotic pathway (Hallett et al., 2012).

3.6 IL-15 AND CANCER

IL-15 was simultaneously codiscovered by two different laboratories in 1994 and characterized as a T-cell growth factor (Burton et al., 1994; Grabstein et al., 1994). The heterotrimeric IL-15 receptor consists of a beta subunit (IL-2R/15Rβ) that is shared with the IL-2R, a common gamma subunit (γc) shared with IL-2, IL-4, IL-7, IL-9, and IL-21, and a unique alpha subunit (IL-15Rα) that is a cause of receptor specificity to IL-15 (Giri et al., 1995). Due to the common receptor components and a sharing of the JAK1/JAK3/STAT5 signaling pathway, these two cytokines also share certain functions that include the stimulation of T-cell proliferation, the generation of cytotoxic T lymphocytes, stimulation of immunoglobulin production by B cells, and the generation and persistence of NK cells (Waldmann and Tagaya, 1999). IL-15 activates monocytes, macrophages, dendritic cells, and neutrophils, enhancing the release of cytokines and improving their participation in immunity against infectious agents (Badolato et al., 1997; Maeurer et al., 2000; D'Agostino et al., 2004). It stimulates NF-kB activation and production of IL-8 in neutrophils and enhances their phagocytic and antimicrobial activity (Girard et al., 1996; McDonald et al., 1998; Musso et al., 1998). Nevertheless, in contrast to IL-2, IL-15 is not required for the maintenance of Tregs (Berger et al., 2009). IL-2 has a key role in the elimination of self-reactive T cells while IL-15 is an antiapoptotic factor for T cells, B cells, neutrophils, eosinophils, and mast cells (Girard et al., 1996; Bulfone-Paus et al., 1997; Marks-Konczalik et al., 2000; Hoontrakoon et al., 2002; Bouchard et al., 2004). Toxicities of these interleukins are also different, with little vascular capillary leak observed with IL-15 in contrast to IL-2 (Munger et al., 1995). IL-15 mRNA is expressed by many cells including fibroblasts, keratinocytes, epithelial cells of various tissues, nerve cells, monocytes, macrophages, dendritic cells, and T cells (Anderson et al., 1995). However, detection of IL-15 protein is largely limited to monocytes/macrophages and dendritic cells (Steel et al., 2012). IL-15 also exerts various effects on nonhematological cells, having anabolic effect on muscle and supporting muscle cell differentiation (Quinn et al., 1995), potentiating angiogenesis (Angiolillo et al., 1997) and causing microglial growth and survival (Hanisch et al., 1997). Under normal circumstances, IL-15 acts as a cell-bound cytokine and is trans presented to responding cells together with costimulatory signals (Dubois et al., 2002). Soluble IL-15 mostly undergoes association with IL-15Rα before being presented efficiently to cells responding to this cytokine (Overwijk and Schluns, 2009).

It has been shown that proliferation of the murine T-cell lymphoma cell line LBC may be enhanced by IL-15 (Gravisaco et al., 2003). Moreover, spontaneous development of CD8+ T-cell leukemia has been demonstrated in IL-15 transgenic mice (Fehniger et al., 2001; Sato et al., 2011). In addition, it is known that IL-15 is able to inhibit apoptosis of primary human NK leukemia cells and NK tumor cell lines (Yamasaki et al., 2004), as well as to stimulate the growth of B-cell chronic lymphocytic leukemia (CLL) cells (Trentin et al., 1996). Human T-cell lymphotrophic virus (HTLV-1) Tax protein activates expression of IL-15 and IL-15Rα, so IL-15/IL-15Rα autocrine growth stimulation loop may influence the transformation and progression of HTLV-1-associated adult T-cell leukemia/lymphoma (ATLL) (Azimi et al., 1998; Kukita et al., 2002). In the case with acute lymphocytic leukemia (ALL), IL-15 expression has correlated with mediastinal and lymph node involvement, and IL-15 expression in precursor B-cell ALL has been associated with a lower 5-year relapse-free survival (Wu et al., 2010). In addition, higher IL-15 expression has correlated with a higher risk of central nervous system relapse (Cario et al., 2007). Regarding solid malignant tumors, no significant difference between cancer patients and healthy controls has been reported (Lissoni et al., 1998).

The direct administration of IL-15 has demonstrated antitumor effects in certain preclinical mouse tumor models (Munger et al., 1995; Kimura et al., 2000; Oh et al., 2003; Basak et al., 2008; Zhang et al., 2009; Yu et al., 2010), including increase in the survival of mice with metastatic CT26 colon cancer (Yu et al., 2010). Coadministration of anti-programmed cell death-1 ligand (PD-L1) and anti-cytotoxic lymphocyte antigen 4 monoclonal antibodies has been associated with declined expression of the immunosuppressive molecules PD-1 and IL-10 and has led to greater antitumor responses than IL-15 alone (Yu et al., 2010). Coadministration of anti-CD40 has increased IL-15Rα expression, whereas covalent binding of IL-15 to soluble IL-15Rα has elevated the biostability of IL-15 (Dubois et al., 2008; Zhang et al., 2009), providing greater antitumor response compared to IL-15 alone. Similarly, the coadministration of other cytokines such as IL-21 has augmented the antitumor efficacy of IL-15 in animal tumor models (Zeng et al., 2005). IL-15 may also be a promising vaccine adjuvant in preclinical models of cancer. Animals vaccinated with dendritic cells expressing IL-15, IL-15Rα, and truncated *neu* gene have remained tumor-free significantly longer than those vaccinated with *neu* alone (Steel et al., 2010). In addition, IL-15 is able to overcome defects in CD4-help to allow CD8+ immune responses and enhance antitumor antibody response (Oh et al., 2008). The IL-15/IL-21 combination enhanced cytotoxicity of NK cells and T cells toward tumor cells (Kishida et al., 2003; Pouw et al., 2010). Injection of IL-15 and IL-21 expression plasmids into mice has synergistically augmented antitumor immune response with complete regression of lymphomas in 80% of animals (Kishida et al., 2003). Therefore, IL-15 has been used in experimental tumor therapy in combination not only with IL-21 (Strengell et al., 2003; Zeng et al., 2005; Huarte et al., 2009; Pouw et al., 2010), but also with other interleukins, including IL-7 (Habibi et al., 2009) and IL-12 (Kimura et al., 2000). Combining radiofrequency thermal ablation of breast tumors with intralesional administration of IL-7 and IL-15 has induced tumor-specific immune response in breast carcinoma models in mice, and has inhibited tumor growth and formation of lung metastases (Habibi et al., 2009). In mice inoculated intraperitoneally with fibrosarcoma, combined treatment with IL-12 and IL-15 has led to synergistic antitumor effects (Kimura et al., 2000). In mouse melanoma model, subtherapeutic doses of IL-15 have enhanced antitumor effects of IL-12, accompanied by increased IFN-γ production (Lasek et al., 1999). Considering the fact that IL-12 has shown profound anticancer activities in a number of models (Yuzhalin and Kutikhin, 2012), the combination of IL-15 with this cytokine may be promising in the therapeutic context; therefore, further research on this issue is necessary. In addition, IL-15 has shown prolonged remission induced by cyclophosphamide in rhabdomyosarcoma-bearing mice (Evans et al., 1997; Chapoval et al., 1998). Moreover, IL-15 has raised antitumor activity of 5-fluorouracil in rats suffering from colorectal cancer (Cao et al., 1998). IL-15 combined with IL-21 has enhanced antitumor effects of T-cell receptor (TCR)-transduced tumor-specific T cells (Pouw et al., 2010), and T cells transduced with chimeric TCRs and IL-15 genes have shown improved antitumor effects in vivo (Hoyos et al., 2010). IL-15 has been demonstrated to potentiate rituximab-mediated antibody-dependent cellular cytotoxicity against B-cell lymphoma (Moga et al., 2008). Lung cancer cells engineered to express IL-15 have stopped their growth, and tumor cells transfected with both IL-15 and IL-12 genes have been completely rejected in all mice tested (Di Carlo et al., 2000).

Murine Meth A fibrosarcoma cells and human prostate cancer cells engineered to secrete IL-15 have also been completely rejected following injection into normal (Hazama et al., 1999; Kimura et al., 1999) or nude mice (Suzuki et al., 2001). IL-15 has significantly improved the therapeutic potency of the vaccine against malignant melanoma consisting of tumor cells transduced with genes for either tumor necrosis factor (TNF)-α, GM-CSF, or IL-12 (Lasek et al., 2004; Basak et al., 2008).

3.7 IL-21 AND CANCER

IL-21, the most recently identified member of the type I cytokine family, has been initially discovered by functional cloning (Parrish-Novak et al., 2000; Ma et al., 2011). This cytokine is predominantly produced by CD4+ T cells,

Th17 cells, and NKT cells (Parrish-Novak et al., 2000; Mehta et al., 2004; Spolski and Leonard, 2008). In addition, IL-21 mRNA expression has been found in stromal cells in lymph nodes (Parrish-Novak et al., 2000; Mehta et al., 2004; Spolski and Leonard, 2008). The IL-21 receptor (IL-21R) was first discovered by genomic and cDNA sequencing projects in 2000 as a putative type I family receptor bearing close resemblance to the IL-2R β chain (Parrish-Novak et al., 2000; Ozaki et al., 2000; Parrish-Novak et al., 2002). Expression of the IL-21R complex has been found in lymphoid tissues including spleen, thymus, and peripheral blood cells, on resting and activated B cells, T cells, NK cells, dendritic cells, macrophages, and keratinocytes (Spolski and Leonard, 2008). Like other type I cytokines, IL-21 signals via JAK/STAT pathway (Spolski and Leonard, 2008).

IL-21 therapy in mice has led to significant increase in the number of tumor-infiltrating and tumor-specific CD8+ T cells, protecting against the relapse (Skak et al., 2008). IL-21 therapy in humans has resulted in increased CD8+ T-cell expression of perforin and granzyme B, which may cause apoptosis of B-CLL cells (Jahrsdörfer et al., 2006; Davis et al., 2007). CLL B cells have undergone apoptosis following IL-21 stimulation (Jahrsdörfer et al., 2006), and IL-21 has been able to counteract the proliferative and antiapoptotic signals delivered by IL-15 to CLL B cells (de Totero et al., 2006; de Totero D et al., 2008). In addition, IL-21 treatment of CLL B cells along with fludarabine or rituximab has improved the direct cytotoxic effect of these drugs (Gowda et al., 2008). Normal plasma cells isolated from the spleen have lacked expression of IL-21R (Good et al., 2006), whereas its expression in primary myeloma cells has been observed (Ménoret et al., 2008). Constant expression of IL-21R on malignant plasma cells has allowed suggesting that IL-21 may be involved in the development of multiple myeloma either by increasing proliferation or by giving a survival advantage to the malignant cells (Brenne et al., 2002; Ménoret et al., 2008). Expression of IL-21R in both the primary human promyelocytic leukemia (HL) cells and HL cell lines has been identified using flow cytometry (Lamprecht et al., 2008; Scheeren et al., 2008). Expression of IL-21R has been positive on primary follicular lymphoma cells that underwent apoptosis in response to IL-21 stimulation (Akamatsu et al., 2007; de Totero et al., 2010). However, low IL-21R expression has been detected on cells from other follicular lymphomas that were resistant to IL-21-mediated apoptosis (de Totero et al., 2010), so lymphoma cells may become refractory to IL-21-mediated proapoptotic effects during progression. IL-21 has induced apoptosis in de novo diffuse large B-cell lymphoma primary tumors (Lamprecht et al., 2008). Moreover, IL-21 has promoted tumor regression and prolonged survival of mice harboring xenograft diffuse large B-cell lymphomas (Sarosiek et al., 2010). IL-21R is consistently expressed in mantle cell lymphoma cell lines and tumors (Gelebart et al., 2009). IL-21R has been highly expressed in HTLV-1-infected T cell lines, ATLL cell lines, and in primary ATL peripheral blood mononuclear cells (Ueda et al., 2005; Akamatsu et al., 2007). Although IL-21 has reported to have no demonstrable proliferative effects on cutaneous T cell lymphoma (CTCL) cells, IL-21 is able to protect these cells from apoptosis (Marzec et al., 2008; Yoon et al., 2008).

3.8 SUMMARY

To conclude, certain representatives of the IL-2 superfamily seem to have a considerable influence on cancer development. IL-2 has long been approved for clinical use and it is currently being used for patients with late-stage renal cell carcinoma and malignant melanoma. Importantly, the administration of this cytokine very often shows a complete clinical response and is associated with long-term survival. Multiple studies demonstrated that elevations in soluble IL-2R level or decreased IL-2 concentrations are associated with disease progression or negative prognosis in cancer. Considering IL-4, high levels of this cytokine have been detected in the peripheral blood and tumor microenvironment of patients with prostate cancer, bladder cancer, and breast cancer. Furthermore, several studies indicated that type II IL-4R (IL-4Rα and IL-13Rα1 chains) is upregulated and activated in various epithelial tumors, such as malignant glioma, ovarian, lung, breast, pancreas, and colon cancer. In addition, IL-4 has been shown to directly enhance the proliferation of colon, breast, head and neck, ovarian, and prostate cancer cells, possibly via activation of downstream STAT6 signaling and upregulation of surviving. Regarding IL-13, this interleukin has been found overexpressed in the tumor microenvironment and peripheral blood of patients with prostate, bladder, pancreatic, esophageal, gastric, and breast cancer, while IL-13Rα2 has been found overexpressed in colon, pancreatic, and ovarian tumors and in malignant glioma. Importantly, IL-13 may be both pro- and antiapoptotic depending on receptor presence and/or signaling pathways activated. Activation of AP-1 by IL-13 signaling via IL-13Rα2 may also be a cause of production of other factors including MMPs, which are known to promote tumor growth, invasion, and metastasis. The direct administration of IL-15 has shown antitumor effects in certain preclinical mouse tumor models. Also, it significantly improved the therapeutic potency of the vaccine against malignant melanoma consisting of tumor cells transduced with genes for either TNF-α, GM-CSF, or IL-12. IL-15 and

IL-21 seem to play a role in the development of hematological malignancies, whereas studies on the role of IL-7 and IL-9 in human cancer are still lacking.

REFERENCES

Abdelilah, S., Latifa, K., Esra, N., Cameron, L., Bouchaib, L., Nicolaides, N., Levitt, R., Hamid, Q., 2001. Functional expression of IL-9 receptor by human neutrophils from asthmatic donors: role in IL-8 release. J. Immunol. 166 (4), 2768–2774.

Akamatsu, N., Yamada, Y., Hasegawa, H., Makabe, K., Asano, R., Kumagai, I., Murata, K., Imaizumi, Y., Tsukasaki, K., Tsuruda, K., Sugahara, K., Atogami, S., 2007. High IL-21 receptor expression and apoptosis induction by IL-21 in follicular lymphoma. Cancer Lett. 256 (2), 196–206.

Alileche, A., Plaisance, S., Han, D.S., Rubinstein, E., Mingari, C., Bellomo, R., Jasmin, C., Azzarone, B., 1993. Human melanoma cell line M14 secretes a functional interleukin 2. Oncogene 8 (7), 1791–1796.

Alpdogan, O., Schmaltz, C., Muriglan, S.J., Kappel, B.J., Perales, M.A., Rotolo, J.A., Halm, J.A., Rich, B.E., van den Brink, M.R., 2001. Administration of interleukin-7 after allogeneic bone marrow transplantation improves immune reconstitution without aggravating graft-versus-host disease. Blood 98 (7), 2256–2265.

Anderson, D.M., Kumaki, S., Ahdieh, M., Bertles, J., Tometsko, M., Loomis, A., Giri, J., Copeland, N.G., Gilbert, D.J., Jenkins, N.A., et al., 1995. Functional characterization of the human interleukin-15 receptor alpha chain and close linkage of IL15RA and IL2RA genes. J. Biol. Chem. 270 (50), 29862–29869.

Angiolillo, A.L., Kanegane, H., Sgadari, C., Reaman, G.H., Tosato, G., 1997. Interleukin-15 promotes angiogenesis in vivo. Biochem. Biophys. Res. Commun. 233 (1), 231–237.

Atkins, M.B., Lotze, M.T., Dutcher, J.P., Fisher, R.I., Weiss, G., Margolin, K., Abrams, J., Sznol, M., Parkinson, D., Hawkins, M., Paradise, C., Kunkel, L., Rosenberg, S.A., 1999. High-dose recombinant interleukin 2 therapy for patients with metastatic melanoma: analysis of 270 patients treated between 1985 and 1993. J. Clin. Oncol. 17 (7), 2105–2116.

Azimi, N., Brown, K., Bamford, R.N., Tagaya, Y., Siebenlist, U., Waldmann, T.A., 1998. Human T cell lymphotropic virus type I Tax protein trans-activates interleukin 15 gene transcription through an NF-kappaB site. Proc. Natl. Acad. Sci. U S A 95 (5), 2452–2457.

Badolato, R., Ponzi, A.N., Millesimo, M., Notarangelo, L.D., Musso, T., 1997. Interleukin-15 (IL-15) induces IL-8 and monocyte chemotactic protein 1 production in human monocytes. Blood 90 (7), 2804–2809.

Barbour, A.H., Coventry, B.J., 2003. Dendritic cell density and activation status of tumour-infiltrating lymphocytes in metastatic human melanoma: possible implications for sentinel node metastases. Melanoma Res. 13 (3), 263–269.

Barderas, R., Bartolomé, R.A., Fernandez-Aceñero, M.J., Torres, S., Casal, J.I., 2012. High expression of IL-13 receptor α2 in colorectal cancer is associated with invasion, liver metastasis, and poor prognosis. Cancer Res. 72 (11), 2780–2790.

Basak, G.W., Zapala, L., Wysocki, P.J., Mackiewicz, A., Jakóbisiak, M., Lasek, W., 2008. Interleukin 15 augments antitumor activity of cytokine gene-modified melanoma cell vaccines in a murine model. Oncol. Rep. 19 (5), 1173–1179.

Bauer, J.H., Liu, K.D., You, Y., Lai, S.Y., Goldsmith, M.A., 1998. Heteromerization of the gammac chain with the interleukin-9 receptor alpha subunit leads to STAT activation and prevention of apoptosis. J. Biol. Chem. 273 (15), 9255–9260.

Beq, S., Nugeyre, M.T., Ho Tsong Fang, R., Gautier, D., Legrand, R., Schmitt, N., Estaquier, J., Barré-Sinoussi, F., Hurtrel, B., Cheynier, R., Israël, N., 2006. IL-7 induces immunological improvement in SIV-infected rhesus macaques under antiviral therapy. J. Immunol. 176 (2), 914–922.

Beq, S., Rozlan, S., Gautier, D., Parker, R., Mersseman, V., Schilte, C., Assouline, B., Rancé, I., Lavedan, P., Morre, M., Cheynier, R., 2009. Injection of glycosylated recombinant simian IL-7 provokes rapid and massive T-cell homing in rhesus macaques. Blood 114 (4), 816–825.

Berger, C., Berger, M., Hackman, R.C., Gough, M., Elliott, C., Jensen, M.C., Riddell, S.R., 2009. Safety and immunologic effects of IL-15 administration in nonhuman primates. Blood 114 (12), 2417–2426.

Berghella, A.M., Pellegrini, P., Del Beato, T., Marini, M., Tomei, E., Adorno, D., Casciani, C.U., 1998. The significance of an increase in soluble interleukin-2 receptor level in colorectal cancer and its biological regulating role in the physiological switching of the immune response cytokine network from TH1 to TH2 and back. Cancer Immunol. Immunother. 45 (5), 241–249.

Borghesi, L.A., Yamashita, Y., Kincade, P.W., 1999. Heparan sulfate proteoglycans mediate interleukin-7-dependent B lymphopoiesis. Blood 93 (1), 140–148.

Bouchard, A., Ratthé, C., Girard, D., 2004. Interleukin-15 delays human neutrophil apoptosis by intracellular events and not via extracellular factors: role of Mcl-1 and decreased activity of caspase-3 and caspase-8. J. Leukoc. Biol. 75 (5), 893–900.

Brenne, A.T., Ro, T.B., Waage, A., Sundan, A., Borset, M., Hjorth-Hansen, H., 2002. Interleukin-21 is a growth and survival factor for human myeloma cells. Blood 99 (10), 3756–3762.

Brown, V.I., Fang, J., Alcorn, K., Barr, R., Kim, J.M., Wasserman, R., Grupp, S.A., 2003. Rapamycin is active against B-precursor leukemia in vitro and in vivo, an effect that is modulated by IL-7-mediated signaling. Proc. Natl. Acad. Sci. U S A 100 (25), 15113–15118.

Bulfone-Paus, S., Ungureanu, D., Pohl, T., Lindner, G., Paus, R., Rückert, R., Krause, H., Kunzendorf, U., 1997. Interleukin-15 protects from lethal apoptosis in vivo. Nat. Med. 3 (10), 1124–1128.

Burton, J.D., Bamford, R.N., Peters, C., Grant, A.J., Kurys, G., Goldman, C.K., Brennan, J., Roessler, E., Waldmann, T.A., 1994. A lymphokine, provisionally designated interleukin T and produced by a human adult T-cell leukemia line, stimulates T-cell proliferation and the induction of lymphokine-activated killer cells. Proc. Natl. Acad. Sci. U S A 91 (11), 4935–4939.

Camp, B.J., Dyhrman, S.T., Memoli, V.A., Mott, L.A., Barth Jr, R.J., 1996. In situ cytokine production by breast cancer tumor-infiltrating lymphocytes. Ann. Surg. Oncol. 3 (2), 176–184.

Cao, S., Troutt, A.B., Rustum, Y.M., 1998. Interleukin 15 protects against toxicity and potentiates antitumor activity of 5-fluorouracil alone and in combination with leucovorin in rats bearing colorectal cancer. Cancer Res. 58 (8), 1695–1699.

Cario, G., Izraeli, S., Teichert, A., Rhein, P., Skokowa, J., Möricke, A., Zimmermann, M., Schrauder, A., Karawajew, L., Ludwig, W.D., Welte, K., 2007. High interleukin-15 expression characterizes childhood acute lymphoblastic leukemia with involvement of the CNS. J. Clin. Oncol. 25 (30), 4813–4820.

Chapoval, A.I., Fuller, J.A., Kremlev, S.G., Kamdar, S.J., Evans, R., 1998. Combination chemotherapy and IL-15 administration induce permanent tumor regression in a mouse lung tumor model: NK and T cell-mediated effects antagonized by B cells. J. Immunol. 161 (12), 6977–6984.

Cheng, G., Arima, M., Honda, K., Hirata, H., Eda, F., Yoshida, N., Fukushima, F., Ishii, Y., Fukuda, T., 2002. Anti-interleukin-9 antibody treatment inhibits airway inflammation and hyperreactivity in mouse asthma model. Am. J. Respir. Crit. Care Med. 166 (3), 409–416.

Cosmi, L., Liotta, F., Angeli, R., Mazzinghi, B., Santarlasci,V., Manetti, R., Lasagni, L.,Vanini, V., Romagnani, P., Maggi, E., Annunziato, F., Romagnani, S., 2004. Th2 cells are less susceptible than Th1 cells to the suppressive activity of CD25+ regulatory thymocytes because of their responsiveness to different cytokines. Blood 103 (8), 3117–3121.

Coventry, B.J.,Ashdown, M.L., 2012.The 20th anniversary of interleukin-2 therapy: bimodal role explaining longstanding random induction of complete clinical responses. Cancer Manage Res. 4, 215–221.

Coventry, B.J.,Weeks, S.C., Heckford, S.E., Sykes, P.J., Bradley, J., Skinner, J.M., 1996. Lack of IL-2 cytokine expression despite IL-2 messenger RNA transcription in tumor-infiltrating lymphocytes in primary human breast carcinoma: selective expression of early activation markers. J. Immunol. 156 (9), 3486–3492.

D'Agostino, P., Milano, S., Arcoleo, F., Di Bella, G., La Rosa, M., Ferlazzo,V., Caruso, R., Chifari, N., Vitale, G., Mansueto, S., Cillari, E., 2004. Interleukin-15, as interferon-gamma, induces the killing of Leishmania infantum in phorbol-myristate-acetate-activated macrophages increasing interleukin-12. Scand. J. Immunol. 60 (6), 609–614.

Davis, I.D., Skrumsager, B.K., Cebon, J., Nicholaou,T., Barlow, J.W., Moller, N.P., Skak, K., Lundsgaard, D., Frederiksen, K.S., Thygesen, P., McArthur, G.A., 2007. An open-label, two-arm, phase I trial of recombinant human interleukin-21 in patients with metastatic melanoma. Clin. Cancer Res. 13 (12), 3630–3636.

de Totero, D., Capaia, M., Fabbi, M., Croce, M., Meazza, R., Cutrona, G., Zupo, S., Loiacono, F.,Truini, M., Ferrarini, M., Ferrini, S., 2010. Heterogeneous expression and function of IL-21R and susceptibility to IL-21-mediated apoptosis in follicular lymphoma cells. Exp. Hematol. 38 (5), 373–383.

de Totero, D., Meazza, R., Capaia, M., Fabbi, M., Azzarone, B., Balleari, E., Gobbi, M., Cutrona, G., Ferrarini, M., Ferrini, S., 2008.The opposite effects of IL-15 and IL-21 on CLL B cells correlate with differential activation of the JAK/STAT and ERK1/2 pathways. Blood 111 (2), 517–524.

de Totero, D., Meazza, R., Zupo, S., Cutrona, G., Matis, S., Colombo, M., Balleari, E., Pierri, I., Fabbi, M., Capaia, M.,Azzarone, B., Gobbi, M., Ferrarini, M., Ferrini, S., 2006. Inter-leukin-21 receptor (IL-21R) is up-regulated by CD40 triggering and mediates pro-apoptotic signals in chronic lymphocytic leukemia B cells. Blood 107 (9), 3708–3715.

Dehne, N.,Tausendschön, M., Essler, S., Geis,T., Schmid,T., Brüne, B., 2014. IL-4 reduces the proangiogenic capacity of macrophages by down-regulating HIF-1α translation. J. Leukoc. Biol. 95 (1), 129–137.

Demoulin, J.B., Louahed, J., Dumoutier, L., Stevens, M., Renauld, J.C., 2003. MAP kinase activation by interleukin-9 in lymphoid and mast cell lines. Oncogene 22 (12), 1763–1770.

Demoulin, J.B., Uyttenhove, C., Van Roost, E., DeLestré, B., Donckers, D., Van Snick, J., Renauld, J.C., 1996.A single tyrosine of the interleukin-9 (IL-9) receptor is required for STAT activation, antiapoptotic activity, and growth regulation by IL-9. Mol. Cell. Biol. 16 (9), 4710–4716.

Di Carlo, E., Comes, A., Basso, S., De Ambrosis, A., Meazza, R., Musiani, P., Moelling, K., Albini,A., Ferrini, S., 2000.The combined action of IL-15 and IL-12 gene transfer can induce tumor cell rejection without T and NK cell involvement. J. Immunol. 165 (6), 3111–3118.

Dodd, J.S., Lum, E., Goulding, J., Muir, R.,Van Snick, J., Openshaw, P.J., 2009. IL-9 regulates pathology during primary and memory responses to respiratory syncytial virus infection. J. Immunol. 183 (11), 7006–7013.

Donahue, R.E.,Yang,Y.C., Clark, S.C., 1990. Human P40 T-cell growth factor (interleukin-9) supports erythroid colony formation. Blood 75 (12), 2271–2275.

Druez, C., Coulie, P., Uyttenhove, C.,Van Snick, J., 1990. Functional and biochemical characterization of mouse P40/IL-9 receptors. J. Immunol. 145 (8), 2494–2499.

Dubois, S., Mariner, J., Waldmann, T.A., Tagaya, Y., 2002. IL-15Ralpha recycles and presents IL-15 in trans to neighboring cells. Immunity 17 (5), 537–547.

Dubois, S., Patel, H.J., Zhang, M., Waldmann, T.A., Müller, J.R., 2008. Preassociation of IL-15 with IL-15R alpha-IgG1-Fc enhances its activity on proliferation of NK and CD8+/CD44highT cells and its antitumor action. J. Immunol. 180 (4), 2099–2106.

Ellmark, P., Ingvarsson, J., Carlsson, A., Lundin, B.S., Wingren, C., Borrebaeck, C.A., 2006 Sep. Identification of protein expression signatures associated with Helicobacter pylori infection and gastric adenocarcinoma using recombinant antibody microarrays. Mol. Cell Proteomics 5 (9), 1638–1646

Elsässer-Beile, U., Kölble, N., Grussenmeyer, T., Schultze-Seemann, W., Wetterauer, U., Gallati, H., Schulte, M.J., von Kleist, S., 1998. Th1 and Th2 cytokine response patterns in leukocyte cultures of patients with urinary bladder, renal cell and prostate carcinomas. Tumour Biol. 19 (6), 470–476.

Elyaman, W., Bradshaw, E.M., Uyttenhove, C., Dardalhon, V., Awasthi, A., Imitola, J., Bettelli, E., Oukka, M., van Snick, J., Renauld, J.C., Kuchroo, V.K., Khoury, S.J., 2009. IL-9 induces differentiation of TH17 cells and enhances function of FoxP3+ natural regulatory T cells. Proc. Natl. Acad. Sci. U S A 106 (31), 12885–12890.

Evans, R., Fuller, J.A., Christianson, G., Krupke, D.M., Troutt, A.B., 1997. IL-15 mediates anti-tumor effects after cyclophosphamide injection of tumor-bearing mice and enhances adoptive immunotherapy: the potential role of NK cell subpopulations. Cell Immunol. 179 (1), 66–73.

Faulkner, H., Humphreys, N., Renauld, J.C., Van Snick, J., Grencis, R., 1997. Interleukin-9 is involved in host protective immunity to intestinal nematode infection. Eur. J. Immunol. 27 (10), 2536–2540.

Fawaz, L.M., Sharif-Askari, E., Hajoui, O., Soussi-Gounni, A., Hamid, Q., Mazer, B.D., 2007. Expression of IL-9 receptor alpha chain on human germinal center B cells modulates IgE secretion. J. Allergy Clin. Immunol. 120 (5), 1208–1215.

Fehniger, T.A., Suzuki, K., Ponnappan, A., VanDeusen, J.B., Cooper, M.A., Florea, S.M., Freud, A.G., Robinson, M.L., Durbin, J., Caligiuri, M.A., 2001. Fatal leukemia in interleukin 15 transgenic mice follows early expansions in natural killer and memory phenotype CD8+ T cells. J. Exp. Med. 193 (2), 219–231.

Fichtner-Feigl, S., Strober, W., Kawakami, K., Puri, R.K., Kitani, A., 2006. IL-13 signaling through the IL-13alpha2 receptor is involved in induction of TGF-beta1 production and fibrosis. Nat. Med. 12 (1), 99–106.

Fisher, R.I., Rosenberg, S.A., Fyfe, G., 2000. Long-term survival update for high-dose recombinant interleukin-2 in patients with renal cell carcinoma. Cancer J. Sci. Am. 6 (Suppl. 1), S55–S57.

Formentini, A., Braun, P., Fricke, H., Link, K.H., Henne-Bruns, D., Kornmann, M., 2012. Expression of interleukin-4 and interleukin-13 and their receptors in colorectal cancer. Int. J. Colorectal Dis. 27 (10), 1369–1376.

Fry, T.J., Mackall, C.L., 2002. Interleukin-7: from bench to clinic. Blood 99 (11), 3892–3904.

Fry, T.J., Moniuszko, M., Creekmore, S., Donohue, S.J., Douek, D.C., Giardina, S., Hecht, T.T., Hill, B.J., Komschlies, K., Tomaszewski, J., Franchini, G., Mackall, C.L., 2003. IL-7 therapy dramatically alters peripheral T-cell homeostasis in normal and SIV-infected nonhuman primates. Blood 101 (6), 2294–2299.

Fujiki, H., Kimura, T., Minamiguchi, H., Harada, S., Wang, J., Nakao, M., Yokota, S., Urata, Y., Ueda, Y., Yamagishi, H., Sonoda, Y., 2002. Role of human interleukin-9 as a megakaryocyte potentiator in culture. Exp. Hematol. 30 (12), 1373–1380.

Fujisawa, T., Joshi, B., Nakajima, A., Puri, R.K., 2009. A novel role of interleukin-13 receptor alpha2 in pancreatic cancer invasion and metastasis. Cancer Res. 69 (22), 8678–8685.

Fujisawa, T., Joshi, B.H., Puri, R.K., 2012. IL-13 regulates cancer invasion and metastasis through IL-13Rα2 via ERK/AP-1 pathway in mouse model of human ovarian cancer. Int. J. Cancer 131 (2), 344–356.

Gabitass, R.F., Annels, N.E., Stocken, D.D., Pandha, H.A., Middleton, G.W., 2011. Elevated myeloid-derived suppressor cells in pancreatic, esophageal and gastric cancer are an independent prognostic factor and are associated with significant elevation of the Th2 cytokine interleukin-13. Cancer Immunol. Immunother. 60 (10), 1419–1430.

Gelebart, P., Zak, Z., Anand, M., Dien-Bard, J., Amin, H.M., Lai, R., 2009. Interleukin-21 effectively induces apoptosis in mantle cell lymphoma through a STAT1-dependent mechanism. Leukemia 23 (10), 1836–1846.

Girard, D., Paquet, M.E., Paquin, R., Beaulieu, A.D., 1996. Differential effects of interleukin-15 (IL-15) and IL-2 on human neutrophils: modulation of phagocytosis, cytoskeleton rearrangement, gene expression, and apoptosis by IL-15. Blood 88 (8), 3176–3184.

Giri, J.G., Kumaki, S., Ahdieh, M., Friend, D.J., Loomis, A., Shanebeck, K., DuBose, R., Cosman, D., Park, L.S., Anderson, D.M., 1995. Identification and cloning of a novel IL-15 binding protein that is structurally related to the alpha chain of the IL-2 receptor. EMBO J. 14 (15), 3654–3663.

Good, K.L., Bryant,V.L.,Tangye, S.G., 2006. Kinetics of human B cell behavior and amplification of proliferative responses following stimulation with IL-21. J. Immunol. 177 (8), 5236–5247.

Goodwin, R.G., Namen, A.E., 1989–1990. The cloning and characterization of interleukin-7.Year Immunol. 6, 127–139.

Goswami, R., Kaplan, M.H., 2011. A brief history of IL-9. J. Immunol. 186 (6), 3283–3288.

Gowda,A., Roda, J., Hussain, S.R., Ramanunni,A., Joshi,T., Schmidt, S., Zhang, X., Lehman, A., Jarjoura, D., Carson,W.E., Kindsvogel,W., Cheney, C., 2008. IL-21 mediates apoptosis through up-regulation of the BH3 family member BIM and enhances both direct and antibody-dependent cellular cytotoxicity in primary chronic lymphocytic leukemia cells in vitro. Blood 111 (9), 4723–4730.

Grabstein, K.H., Eisenman, J., Shanebeck, K., Rauch, C., Srinivasan, S., Fung,V., Beers, C., Richardson, J., Schoenborn, M.A.,Ahdieh, M., et al., 1994. Cloning of a T cell growth factor that interacts with the beta chain of the interleukin-2 receptor. Science 264 (5161), 965–968.

Gravisaco, M.J., Mongini, C., Alvarez, E., Ruybal, P., Escalada, A., Sanchez-Lockhart, M., Hajos, S.,Waldner, C., 2003. IL-2, IL-10, IL-15 and TNF are key regulators of murine T-cell lymphoma growth. Int. J. Mol. Med. 12 (4), 627–632.

Grivas, P.D., Redman, B.G., 2011. Immunotherapy of kidney cancer. Curr. Clin. Pharmacol. 6 (3), 151–163.

Habibi, M., Kmieciak, M., Graham, L., Morales, J.K., Bear, H.D., Manjili, M.H., 2009. Radiofrequency thermal ablation of breast tumors combined with intralesional administration of IL-7 and IL-15 augments anti-tumor immune responses and inhibits tumor development and metastasis. Breast Cancer Res.Treat. 114 (3), 423–431.

Hallett, M.A.,Venmar, K.T., Fingleton, B., 2012. Cytokine stimulation of epithelial cancer cells: the similar and divergent functions of IL-4 and IL-13. Cancer Res. 72 (24), 6338–6343.

Hanisch, U.K., Lyons, S.A., Prinz, M., Nolte, C.,Weber, J.R., Kettenmann, H., Kirchhoff, F., 1997. Mouse brain microglia express interleukin-15 and its multimeric receptor complex functionally coupled to Janus kinase activity. J. Biol. Chem. 272 (46), 28853–28860.

Hazama, S., Noma,T.,Wang, F., Iizuka, N., Ogura,Y.,Yoshimura, K., Inoguchi, E., Hakozaki, M., Hirose, K., Suzuki, T., Oka, M., 1999.Tumour cells engineered to secrete interleukin-15 augment anti-tumour immune responses in vivo. Br. J. Cancer 80 (9), 1420–1426.

Henriques, C.M., Rino, J., Nibbs, R.J., Graham, G.J., Barata, J.T., 2010. IL-7 induces rapid clathrin-mediated internalization and JAK3-dependent degradation of IL-7Ralpha in T cells. Blood 115 (16), 3269–3277.

Hershey, G.K., Friedrich, M.F., Esswein, L.A., Thomas, M.L., Chatila, T.A., 1997. The association of atopy with a gain-of-function mutation in the alpha subunit of the interleukin-4 receptor. N. Engl. J. Med. 337 (24), 1720–1725.

Holbrook, S.T., Ohls, R.K., Schibler, K.R., Yang, Y.C., Christensen, R.D., 1991. Effect of interleukin-9 on clonogenic maturation and cell-cycle status of fetal and adult hematopoietic progenitors. Blood 77 (10), 2129–2134.

Hoontrakoon, R., Chu, H.W., Gardai, S.J., Wenzel, S.E., McDonald, P., Fadok, V.A., Henson, P.M., Bratton, D.L., 2002. Interleukin-15 inhibits spontaneous apoptosis in human eosinophils via autocrine production of granulocyte macrophage-colony stimulating factor and nuclear factor-kappaB activation. Am. J. Respir. Cell. Mol. Biol. 26 (4), 404–412.

Hosoyama, T., Aslam, M.I., Abraham, J., Prajapati, S.I., Nishijo, K., Michalek, J.E., Zarzabal, L.A., Nelon, L.D., Guttridge, D.C., Rubin, B.P., Keller, C., 2011. IL-4R drives dedifferentiation, mitogenesis, and metastasis in rhabdomyosarcoma. Clin Cancer Res. 17 (9), 2757–2766.

Hoyos, V., Savoldo, B., Quintarelli, C., Mahendravada, A., Zhang, M., Vera, J., Heslop, H.E., Rooney, C.M., Brenner, M.K., Dotti, G., 2010. Engineering CD19-specific T lymphocytes with interleukin-15 and a suicide gene to enhance their anti-lymphoma/leukemia effects and safety. Leukemia 24 (6), 1160–1170.

Hsi, L.C., Kundu, S., Palomo, J., Xu, B., Ficco, R., Vogelbaum, M.A., Cathcart, M.K., 2011. Silencing IL-13Rα2 promotes glioblastoma cell death via endogenous signaling. Mol. Cancer Ther. 10 (7), 1149–1160.

Huarte, E., Fisher, J., Turk, M.J., Mellinger, D., Foster, C., Wolf, B., Meehan, K.R., Fadul, C.E., Ernstoff, M.S., 2009. Ex vivo expansion of tumor specific lymphocytes with IL-15 and IL-21 for adoptive immunotherapy in melanoma. Cancer Lett. 285 (1), 80–88.

Hültner, L., Druez, C., Moeller, J., Uyttenhove, C., Schmitt, E., Rüde, E., Dörmer, P., Van Snick, J., 1990. Mast cell growth-enhancing activity (MEA) is structurally related and functionally identical to the novel mouse T cell growth factor P40/TCGFIII (interleukin 9). Eur. J. Immunol. 20 (6), 1413–1416.

Hültner, L., Kölsch, S., Stassen, M., Kaspers, U., Kremer, J.P., Mailhammer, R., Moeller, J., Broszeit, H., Schmitt, E., 2000. In activated mast cells, IL-1 up-regulates the production of several Th2-related cytokines including IL-9. J. Immunol. 164 (11), 5556–5563.

Ito, T., Suzuki, S., Kanaji, S., Shiraishi, H., Ohta, S., Arima, K., Tanaka, G., Tamada, T., Honjo, E., Garcia, K.C., Kuroki, R., Izuhara, K., 2009. Distinct structural requirements for interleukin-4 (IL-4) and IL-13 binding to the shared IL-13 receptor facilitate cellular tuning of cytokine responsiveness. J. Biol. Chem. 284 (36), 24289–24296.

Jahrsdörfer, B., Blackwell, S.E., Wooldridge, J.E., Huang, J., Andreski, M.W., Jacobus, L.S., Taylor, C.M., Weiner, G.J., 2006. B-chronic lymphocytic leukemia cells and other B cells can produce granzyme B and gain cytotoxic potential after interleukin-21-based activation. Blood 108 (8), 2712–2719.

Kearley, J., Erjefalt, J.S., Andersson, C., Benjamin, E., Jones, C.P., Robichaud, A., Pegorier, S., Brewah, Y., Burwell, T.J., Bjermer, L., Kiener, P.A., Kolbeck, R., Lloyd, C.M., Coyle, A.J., Humbles, A.A., 2011. IL-9 governs allergen-induced mast cell numbers in the lung and chronic remodeling of the airways. Am. J. Respir. Crit. Care Med. 183 (7), 865–875.

Kimura, K., Nishimura, H., Hirose, K., Matsuguchi, T., Nimura, Y., Yoshikai, Y., 1999. Immunogene therapy of murine fibrosarcoma using IL-15 gene with high translation efficiency. Eur. J. Immunol. 29 (5), 1532–1542.

Kimura, K., Nishimura, H., Matsuzaki, T., Yokokura, T., Nimura, Y., Yoshikai, Y., 2000. Synergistic effect of interleukin-15 and interleukin-12 on antitumor activity in a murine malignant pleurisy model. Cancer Immunol. Immunother. 49 (2), 71–77.

Kishida, T., Asada, H., Itokawa, Y., Cui, F.D., Shin-Ya, M., Gojo, S., Yasutomi, K., Ueda, Y., Yamagishi, H., Imanishi, J., Mazda, O., 2003. Interleukin (IL)-21 and IL-15 genetic transfer synergistically augments therapeutic antitumor immunity and promotes regression of metastatic lymphoma. Mol. Ther. 8 (4), 552–558.

Klapper, J.A., Downey, S.G., Smith, F.O., Yang, J.C., Hughes, M.S., Kammula, U.S., Sherry, R.M., Royal, R.E., Steinberg, S.M., Rosenberg, S., 2008. High-dose interleukin-2 for the treatment of metastatic renal cell carcinoma: a retrospective analysis of response and survival in patients treated in the surgery branch at the National Cancer Institute between 1986 and 2006. Cancer 113 (2), 293–301.

Knoechel, B., Lohr, J., Kahn, E., Bluestone, J.A., Abbas, A.K., 2005. Sequential development of interleukin 2-dependent effector and regulatory T cells in response to endogenous systemic antigen. J. Exp. Med. 202 (10), 1375–1386.

Knoops, L., Louahed, J., Renauld, J.C., 2004. IL-9-induced expansion of B-1b cells restores numbers but not function of B-1 lymphocytes in xid mice. J. Immunol. 172 (10), 6101–6106.

Knoops, L., Louahed, J., Van Snick, J., Renauld, J.C., 2005. IL-9 promotes but is not necessary for systemic anaphylaxis. J. Immunol. 175 (1), 335–341.

Ko, C.W., Cuthbert, R.J., Orsi, N.M., Brooke, D.A., Perry, S.L., Markham, A.F., Coletta, P.L., Hull, M.A., 2008. Lack of interleukin-4 receptor alpha chain-dependent signalling promotes azoxymethane-induced colorectal aberrant crypt focus formation in Balb/c mice. J. Pathol. 214 (5), 603–609.

Koller, F.L., Hwang, D.G., Dozier, E.A., Fingleton, B., 2010. Epithelial interleukin-4 receptor expression promotes colon tumor growth. Carcinogenesis 31 (6), 1010–1017.

Kukita, T., Arima, N., Matsushita, K., Arimura, K., Ohtsubo, H., Sakaki, Y., Fujiwara, H., Ozaki, A., Matsumoto, T., Tei, C., 2002. Autocrine and/or paracrine growth of adult T-cell leukaemia tumour cells by interleukin 15. Br. J. Haematol. 119 (2), 467–474.

Lamprecht, B., Kreher, S., Anagnostopoulos, I., Jöhrens, K., Monteleone, G., Jundt, F., Stein, H., Janz, M., Dörken, B., Mathas, S., 2008. Aberrant expression of the Th2 cytokine IL-21 in Hodgkin lymphoma cells regulates STAT3 signaling and attracts Treg cells via regulation of MIP-3alpha. Blood 112 (8), 3339–3347.

LaPorte, S.L., Juo, Z.S., Vaclavikova, J., Colf, L.A., Qi, X., Heller, N.M., Keegan, A.D., Garcia, K.C., 2008. Molecular and structural basis of cytokine receptor pleiotropy in the interleukin-4/13 system. Cell. 132 (2), 259–272.

Lasek, W., Basak, G., Switaj, T., Jakubowska, A.B., Wysocki, P.J., Mackiewicz, A., Drela, N., Jalili, A., Kamiński, R., Kozar, K., Jakóbisiak, M., 2004. Complete tumour regressions induced by vaccination with IL-12 gene-transduced tumour cells in combination with IL-15 in a melanoma model in mice. Cancer Immunol. Immunother. 53 (4), 363–372.

Lasek, W., Golab, J., Maśliński, W., Switaj, T., Bałkowiec, E.Z., Stokłosa, T., Giermasz, A., Malejczyk, M., Jakóbisiak, M., 1999. Subtherapeutic doses of interleukin-15 augment the antitumor effect of interleukin-12 in a B16F10 melanoma model in mice. Eur. Cytokine Netw. 10 (3), 345–356.

Leone, A., Rohankhedkar, M., Okoye, A., Legasse, A., Axthelm, M.K., Villinger, F., Piatak Jr, M., Lifson, J.D., Assouline, B., Morre, M., Picker, L.J., Sodora, D.L., 2010. Increased CD4+ T cell levels during IL-7 administration of antiretroviral therapy-treated simian immunodeficiency virus-positive macaques are not dependent on strong proliferative responses. J. Immunol. 185 (3), 1650–1659.

Li, B., VanRoey, M.J., Jooss, K., 2007. Recombinant IL-7 enhances the potency of GM-CSF-secreting tumor cell immunotherapy. Clin. Immunol. 123 (2), 155–165.

Li, Z., Chen, L., Qin, Z., 2009. Paradoxical roles of IL-4 in tumor immunity. Cell. Mol. Immunol. 6 (6), 415–422.

Li, Z., Jiang, J., Wang, Z., Zhang, J., Xiao, M., Wang, C., Lu, Y., Qin, Z., 2008. Endogenous interleukin-4 promotes tumor development by increasing tumor cell resistance to apoptosis. Cancer Res. 68 (21), 8687–8694.

Lissoni, P., Rovelli, F., Mandalà, M., Barni, S., 1998. Blood concentrations of interleukin-15 in cancer patients and their variations during interleukin-2 immunotherapy: preliminary considerations. Int. J. Biol. Markers 13 (3), 169–171.

Louahed, J., Toda, M., Jen, J., Hamid, Q., Renauld, J.C., Levitt, R.C., Nicolaides, N.C., 2000. Interleukin-9 upregulates mucus expression in the airways. Am. J. Respir. Cell Mol. Biol. 22 (6), 649–656.

Ma, J., Ma, D., Ji, C., 2011. The role of IL-21 in hematological malignancies. Cytokine 56 (2), 133–139.

Mackall, C.L., Fry, T.J., Gress, R.E., 2011. Harnessing the biology of IL-7 for therapeutic application. Nat. Rev. Immunol. 11 (5), 330–342.

Maeurer, M.J., Trinder, P., Hommel, G., Walter, W., Freitag, K., Atkins, D., Störkel, S., 2000. Interleukin-7 or interleukin-15 enhances survival of *Mycobacterium tuberculosis*-infected mice. Infect. Immun. 68 (5), 2962–2970.

Malin, S., McManus, S., Cobaleda, C., Novatchkova, M., Delogu, A., Bouillet, P., Strasser, A., Busslinger, M., 2010. Role of STAT5 in controlling cell survival and immunoglobulin gene recombination during pro-B cell development. Nat. Immunol. 11 (2), 171–179.

Marks-Konczalik, J., Dubois, S., Losi, J.M., Sabzevari, H., Yamada, N., Feigenbaum, L., Waldmann, T.A., Tagaya, Y., 2000. IL-2-induced activation-induced cell death is inhibited in IL-15 transgenic mice. Proc. Natl. Acad. Sci. U S A 97 (21), 11445–11450.

Marzec, M., Halasa, K., Kasprzycka, M., Wysocka, M., Liu, X., Tobias, J.W., Baldwin, D., Zhang, Q., Odum, N., Rook, A.H., Wasik, M.A., 2008. Differential effects of interleukin-2 and interleukin-15 versus interleukin-21 on CD4+ cutaneous T-cell lymphoma cells. Cancer Res. 68 (4), 1083–1091.

Matsuzawa, S., Sakashita, K., Kinoshita, T., Ito, S., Yamashita, T., Koike, K., 2003. IL-9 enhances the growth of human mast cell progenitors under stimulation with stem cell factor. J. Immunol. 170 (7), 3461–3467.

McDonald, P.P., Russo, M.P., Ferrini, S., Cassatella, M.A., 1998. Interleukin-15 (IL-15) induces NF-kappaB activation and IL-8 production in human neutrophils. Blood 92 (12), 4828–4835.

Mehta, D.S., Wurster, A.L., Grusby, M.J., 2004. Biology of IL-21 and the IL-21 receptor. Immunol. Rev. 202, 84–95.

Ménoret, E., Maïga, S., Descamps, G., Pellat-Deceunynck, C., Fraslon, C., Cappellano, M., Moreau, P., Bataille, R., Amiot, M., 2008. IL-21 stimulates human myeloma cell growth through an autocrine IGF-1 loop. J. Immunol. 181 (10), 6837–6842.

Moga, E., Alvarez, E., Cantó, E., Vidal, S., Rodríguez-Sánchez, J.L., Sierra, J., Briones, J., 2008. NK cells stimulated with IL-15 or CpG ODN enhance rituximab-dependent cellular cytotoxicity against B-cell lymphoma. Exp. Hematol. 36 (1), 69–77.

Morre, M., Beq, S., 2012. Interleukin-7 and immune reconstitution in cancer patients: a new paradigm for dramatically increasing overall survival. Target. Oncol. 7 (1), 55–68.

Morrissey, P.J., Conlon, P., Braddy, S., Williams, D.E., Namen, A.E., Mochizuki, D.Y., 1991. Administration of IL-7 to mice with cyclophosphamide-induced lymphopenia accelerates lymphocyte repopulation. J. Immunol. 146 (5), 1547–1552.

Munger, W., DeJoy, S.Q., Jeyaseelan Sr, R., Torley, L.W., Grabstein, K.H., Eisenmann, J., Paxton, R., Cox, T., Wick, M.M., Kerwar, S.S., 1995. Studies evaluating the antitumor activity and toxicity of interleukin-15, a new T cell growth factor: comparison with interleukin-2. Cell Immunol 165 (2), 289–293.

Musso, T., Calosso, L., Zucca, M., Millesimo, M., Puliti, M., Bulfone-Paus, S., Merlino, C., Savoia, D., Cavallo, R., Ponzi, A.N., Badolato, R., 1998. Interleukin-15 activates proinflammatory and antimicrobial functions in polymorphonuclear cells. Infect. Immun. 66 (6), 2640–2647.

Naumnik, W., Chyczewska, E., 2001. The clinical significance of serum soluble interleukin 2 receptor (sIL-2R) concentration in lung cancer. Folia Histochem. Cytobiol. 39 (Suppl. 2), 185–186.

Nelson, B.H., 2004. IL-2, regulatory T cells, and tolerance. J. Immunol. 172 (7), 3983–3988.

Neuner, A., Schindel, M., Wildenberg, U., Muley, T., Lahm, H., Fischer, J.R., 2002. Prognostic significance of cytokine modulation in non-small cell lung cancer. Int. J. Cancer 101 (3), 287–292.

Nguyen, V., Conyers, J.M., Zhu, D., Gibo, D.M., Dorsey, J.F., Debinski, W., Mintz, A., 2011. IL-13Rα2-targeted therapy escapees: biologic and therapeutic implications. Transl. Oncol. 4 (6), 390–400.

Niitsu, N., Iijima, K., Chizuka, A., 2001. A high serum-soluble interleukin-2 receptor level is associated with a poor outcome of aggressive non-Hodgkin's lymphoma. Eur. J. Haematol. 66 (1), 24–30.

Nowak, E.C., Weaver, C.T., Turner, H., Begum-Haque, S., Becher, B., Schreiner, B., Coyle, A.J., Kasper, L.H., Noelle, R.J., 2009. IL-9 as a mediator of Th17-driven inflammatory disease. J. Exp. Med. 206 (8), 1653–1660.

Oh, S., Berzofsky, J.A., Burke, D.S., Waldmann, T.A., Perera, L.P., 2003. Coadministration of HIV vaccine vectors with vaccinia viruses expressing IL-15 but not IL-2 induces long-lasting cellular immunity. Proc. Natl. Acad. Sci. U S A 100 (6), 3392–3397.

Oh, S., Perera, L.P., Terabe, M., Ni, L., Waldmann, T.A., Berzofsky, J.A., 2008. IL-15 as a mediator of CD4+ help for CD8+ T cell longevity and avoidance of TRAIL-mediated apoptosis. Proc. Natl. Acad. Sci. U S A 105 (13), 5201–5206.

Opal, S.M., DePalo, V.A., 2000. Anti-inflammatory cytokines. Chest 117 (4), 1162–1172.

Orditura, M., Romano, C., De Vita, F., Galizia, G., Lieto, E., Infusino, S., De Cataldis, G., Catalano, G., 2000. Behaviour of interleukin-2 serum levels in advanced non-small-cell lung cancer patients: relationship with response to therapy and survival. Cancer Immunol. Immunother. 49 (10), 530–536.

Overwijk, W.W., Schluns, K.S., 2009. Functions of γC cytokines in immune homeostasis: current and potential clinical applications. Clin. Immunol. 132 (2), 153–165.

Ozaki, K., Kikly, K., Michalovich, D., Young, P.R., Leonard, W.J., 2000. Cloning of a type I cytokine receptor most related to the IL-2 receptor beta chain. Proc. Natl. Acad. Sci. U S A 97 (21), 11439–11444.

Parker, R., Dutrieux, J., Beq, S., Lemercier, B., Rozlan, S., Fabre-Mersseman, V., Rancez, M., Gommet, C., Assouline, B., Rancé, I., Lim, A., Morre, M., Cheynier, R., 2010. Interleukin-7 treatment counteracts IFN-α therapy-induced lymphopenia and stimulates SIV-specific cytotoxic T lymphocyte responses in SIV-infected rhesus macaques. Blood 116 (25), 5589–5599.

Parrish-Novak, J., Dillon, S.R., Nelson, A., Hammond, A., Sprecher, C., Gross, J.A., Johnston, J., Madden, K., Xu, W., West, J., Schrader, S., Burkhead, S., Heipel, M., Brandt, C., Kuijper, J.L., Kramer, J., Conklin, D., Presnell, S.R., Berry, J., Shiota, F., Bort, S., Hambly, K., Mudri, S., Clegg, C., Moore, M., Grant, F.J., Lofton-Day, C., Gilbert, T., Rayond, F., Ching, A., Yao, L., Smith, D., Webster, P., Whitmore, T., Maurer, M., Kaushansky, K., Holly, R.D., Foster, D., 2000. Interleukin 21 and its receptor are involved in NK cell expansion and regulation of lymphocyte function. Nature 408 (6808), 57–63.

Parrish-Novak, J., Foster, D.C., Holly, R.D., Clegg, C.H., 2002. Interleukin-21 and the IL-21 receptor: novel effectors of NK and T cell responses. J. Leukoc. Biol. 72 (5), 856–863.

Pellegrini, M., Calzascia, T., Elford, A.R., Shahinian, A., Lin, A.E., Dissanayake, D., et al., 2009. Adjuvant IL-7 antagonizes multiple cellular and molecular inhibitory networks to enhance immunotherapies. Nat. Med. 15 (5), 528–536.

Plaisance, S., Rubinstein, E., Alileche, A., Han, D.S., Sahraoui, Y., Mingari, M.C., Dhanji, S., Nguyen, L.T., Gronski, M.A., Morre, M., Assouline, B., Lahl, K., Sparwasser, T., Ohashi, P.S., Mak, T.W., 1993. Human melanoma cells express a functional interleukin-2 receptor. Int J. Cancer 55 (1), 164–170.

Pouw, N., Treffers-Westerlaken, E., Kraan, J., Wittink, F., ten Hagen, T., Verweij, J., Debets, R., 2010. Combination of IL-21 and IL-15 enhances tumour-specific cytotoxicity and cytokine production of TCR-transduced primary T cells. Cancer Immunol. Immunother. 59 (6), 921–931.

Prieto, P.A., Yang, J.C., Sherry, R.M., Hughes, M.S., Kammula, U.S., White, D.E., Levy, C.L., Rosenberg, S.A., Phan, G.Q., 2012. CTLA-4 blockade with ipilimumab: long-term follow-up of 177 patients with metastatic melanoma. Clin. Cancer Res. 18 (7), 2039–2047.

Prokopchuk, O., Liu, Y., Henne-Bruns, D., Kornmann, M., 2005. Interleukin-4 enhances proliferation of human pancreatic cancer cells: evidence for autocrine and paracrine actions. Br. J. Cancer 92 (5), 921–928.

Quan Jr, W.D., Quan, F.M., Perez, M., Johnson, E., 2012. Outpatient intravenous interleukin-2 with famotidine has activity in metastatic melanoma. Cancer Biother. Radiopharm. 27 (7), 442–445.

Quinn, L.S., Haugk, K.L., Grabstein, K.H., 1995. Interleukin-15: a novel anabolic cytokine for skeletal muscle. Endocrinology 136 (8), 3669–3672.

Rangel-Corona, R., Corona-Ortega, T., Soto-Cruz, I., López-Labra, A., Pablo-Arcos, T., Torres-Guarneros, C.F., Weiss-Steider, B., 2010. Evidence that cervical cancer cells secrete IL-2, which becomes an autocrine growth factor. Cytokine 50 (3), 273–277.

Renauld, J.C., Druez, C., Kermouni, A., Houssiau, F., Uyttenhove, C., Van Roost, E., Van Snick, J., 1992. Expression cloning of the murine and human interleukin 9 receptor cDNAs. Proc. Natl. Acad. Sci. U S A 89 (12), 5690–5694.

Roca, H., Craig, M.J., Ying, C., Varsos, Z.S., Czarnieski, P., Alva, A.S., Hernandez, J., Fuller, D., Daignault, S., Healy, P.N., Pienta, K.J., 2012. IL-4 induces proliferation in prostate cancer PC3 cells under nutrient-depletion stress through the activation of the JNK-pathway and survivin up-regulation. J. Cell Biochem. 113 (5), 1569–1580.

Rosenwasser, L.J., Klemm, D.J., Dresback, J.K., Inamura, H., Mascali, J.J., Klinnert, M., Borish, L., 1995. Promoter polymorphisms in the chromosome 5 gene cluster in asthma and atopy. Clin. Exp. Allergy 25 (Suppl. 2), 74–78. discussion 95–6.

Russell, S.M., Johnston, J.A., Noguchi, M., Kawamura, M., Bacon, C.M., Friedmann, M., Berg, M., McVicar, D.W., Witthuhn, B.A., Silvennoinen, O., et al., 1994. Interaction of IL-2R beta and gamma c chains with Jak1 and Jak3: implications for XSCID and XCID. Science 266 (5187), 1042–1045.

Sarosiek, K.A., Malumbres, R., Nechushtan, H., Gentles, A.J., Avisar, E., Lossos, I.S., 2010. Novel IL-21 signaling pathway up-regulates c-Myc and induces apoptosis of diffuse large B-cell lymphomas. Blood 115 (3), 570–580.

Sato, N., Sabzevari, H., Fu, S., Ju, W., Petrus, M.N., Bamford, R.N., Waldmann, T.A., Tagaya, Y., 2011. Development of an IL-15-autocrine CD8 T-cell leukemia in IL-15-transgenic mice requires the cis expression of IL-15Rα. Blood 117 (15), 4032–4040.

Scheeren, F.A., Diehl, S.A., Smit, L.A., Beaumont, T., Naspetti, M., Bende, R.J., Blom, B., Karube, K., Ohshima, K., van Noesel, C.J., Spits, H., 2008. IL-21 is expressed in Hodgkin lymphoma and activates STAT5: evidence that activated STAT5 is required for Hodgkin lymphomagenesis. Blood 111 (9), 4706–4715.

Schmitt, E., Van Brandwijk, R., Van Snick, J., Siebold, B., Rüde, E., 1989. TCGF III/P40 is produced by naive murine CD4+ T cells but is not a general T cell growth factor. Eur. J. Immunol. 19 (11), 2167–2170.

Shibata, M., Takekawa, M., 1999. Increased serum concentration of circulating soluble receptor for interleukin-2 and its effect as a prognostic indicator in cachectic patients with gastric and colorectal cancer. Oncology 56 (1), 54–58.

Skak, K., Kragh, M., Hausman, D., Smyth, M.J., Sivakumar, P.V., 2008. Interleukin 21: combination strategies for cancer therapy. Nat. Rev. Drug. Discov. 7 (3), 231–240.

Sojka, D.K., Hughson, A., Sukiennicki, T.L., Fowell, D.J., 2005. Early kinetic window of target T cell susceptibility to CD25+ regulatory T cell activity. J. Immunol. 175 (11), 7274–7280.

Spolski, R., Leonard, W.J., 2008. Interleukin-21: basic biology and implications for cancer and autoimmunity. Annu. Rev. Immunol. 26, 57–79.

Srabovici, N., Mujagic, Z., Mujanovic-Mustedanagic, J., Muminovic, Z., Softic, A., Begic, L., 2011. Interleukin 13 expression in the primary breast cancer tumour tissue. Biochem. Med. (Zagreb) 21 (2), 131–138.

Stassen, M., Arnold, M., Hültner, L., Müller, C., Neudörfl, C., Reineke, T., Schmitt, E., 2000. Murine bone marrow-derived mast cells as potent producers of IL-9: costimulatory function of IL-10 and kit ligand in the presence of IL-1. J. Immunol. 164 (11), 5549–5555.

Steel, J.C., Ramlogan, C.A., Yu, P., Sakai, Y., Forni, G., Waldmann, T.A., Morris, J.C., 2010. Interleukin-15 and its receptor augment dendritic cell vaccination against the neu oncogene through the induction of antibodies partially independent of CD4 help. Cancer Res. 70 (3), 1072–1081.

Steel, J.C., Waldmann, T.A., Morris, J.C., 2012. Interleukin-15 biology and its therapeutic implications in cancer. Trends Pharmacol. Sci. 33 (1), 35–41.

Steenwinckel, V., Louahed, J., Orabona, C., Huaux, F., Warnier, G., McKenzie, A., Lison, D., Levitt, R., Renauld, J.C., 2007. IL-13 mediates in vivo IL-9 activities on lung epithelial cells but not on hematopoietic cells. J. Immunol. 178 (5), 3244–3251.

Storek, J., Gillespy 3rd, T., Lu, H., Joseph, A., Dawson, M.A., Gough, M., Morris, J., Hackman, R.C., Horn, P.A., Sale, G.E., Andrews, R.G., Maloney, D.G., Kiem, H.P., 2003. Interleukin-7 improves CD4 T-cell reconstitution after autologous CD34 cell transplantation in monkeys. Blood 101 (10), 4209–4218.

Strengell, M., Matikainen, S., Sirén, J., Lehtonen, A., Foster, D., Julkunen, I., Sareneva, T., 2003. IL-21 in synergy with IL-15 or IL-18 enhances IFN-gamma production in human NK and T cells. J. Immunol. 170 (11), 5464–5469.

Sugimoto, M., Yamaoka, Y., Furuta, T., 2010. Influence of interleukin polymorphisms on development of gastric cancer and peptic ulcer. World. J. Gastroenterol. 16 (10), 1188–1200.

Suzuki, K., Nakazato, H., Matsui, H., Hasumi, M., Shibata, Y., Ito, K., Fukabori, Y., Kurokawa, K., Yamanaka, H., 2001. NK cell-mediated anti-tumor immune response to human prostate cancer cell, PC-3: immunogene therapy using a highly secretable form of interleukin-15 gene transfer. J. Leukoc. Biol. 69 (4), 531–537.

Tindall, E.A., Severi, G., Hoang, H.N., Ma, C.S., Fernandez, P., Southey, M.C., English, D.R., Hopper, J.L., Heyns, C.F., Tangye, S.G., Giles, G.G., Hayes, V.M., 2010. Australian Prostate Cancer BioResource. Comprehensive analysis of the cytokine-rich chromosome 5q31.1 region suggests a role for IL-4 gene variants in prostate cancer risk. Carcinogenesis 31 (10), 1748–1754.

Todaro, M., Alea, M.P., Di Stefano, A.B., Cammareri, P., Vermeulen, L., Iovino, F., Tripodo, C., Russo, A., Gulotta, G., Medema, J.P., Stassi, G., 2007. Colon cancer stem cells dictate tumor growth and resist cell death by production of interleukin-4. Cell Stem Cell 1 (4), 389–402.

Todaro, M., Lombardo, Y., Francipane, M.G., Alea, M.P., Cammareri, P., Iovino, F., Di Stefano, A.B., Di Bernardo, C., Agrusa, A., Condorelli, G., Walczak, H., Stassi, G., 2008. Apoptosis resistance in epithelial tumors is mediated by tumor-cell-derived interleukin-4. Cell Death Differ. 15 (4), 762–772.

Townsend, J.M., Fallon, G.P., Matthews, J.D., Smith, P., Jolin, E.H., McKenzie, N.A., 2000. IL-9-deficient mice establish fundamental roles for IL-9 in pulmonary mastocytosis and goblet cell hyperplasia but not T cell development. Immunity 13 (4), 573–583.

Trentin, L., Cerutti, A., Zambello, R., Sancretta, R., Tassinari, C., Facco, M., Adami, F., Rode-ghiero, F., Agostini, C., Semenzato, G., 1996. Interleukin-15 promotes the growth of leukemic cells of patients with B-cell chronic lymphoproliferative disorders. Blood 87 (8), 3327–3335.

Ueda, M., Imada, K., Imura, A., Koga, H., Hishizawa, M., Uchiyama, T., 2005. Expression of functional interleukin-21 receptor on adult T-cell leukaemia cells. Br. J. Haematol. 128 (2), 169–176.

Uyttenhove, C., Simpson, R.J., Van Snick, J., 1988. Functional and structural characterization of P40, a mouse glycoprotein with T-cell growth factor activity. Proc. Natl. Acad. Sci. U S A 85 (18), 6934–6938.

Van Snick, J., Goethals, A., Renauld, J.C., Van Roost, E., Uyttenhove, C., Rubira, M.R., Moritz, R.L., Simpson, R.J., 1989. Cloning and characterization of a cDNA for a new mouse T cell growth factor (P40). J. Exp. Med. 169 (1), 363–368.

van Netten, J.P., Ashmead, B.J., Parker, R.L., Thornton, I.G., Fletcher, C., Cavers, D., Coy, P., Brigden, M.L., 1993. Macrophage-tumor cell associations: a factor in metastasis of breast cancer? J. Leukocyte Biol. 54 (4), 360–362.

Vink, A., Warnier, G., Brombacher, F., Renauld, J.C., 1999. Interleukin 9-induced in vivo expansion of the B-1 lymphocyte population. J. Exp. Med. 189 (9), 1413–1423.

Vuoristo, M.S., Laine, S., Huhtala, H., Parvinen, L.M., Hahka-Kemppinen, M., Korpela, M., Kumpulainen, E., Kellokumpu-Lehtinen, P., 2001. Serum adhesion molecules and inter-leukin-2 receptor as markers of tumour load and prognosis in advanced cutaneous mel-anoma. Eur. J. Cancer 37 (13), 1629–1634.

Waldmann, T.A., Tagaya, Y., 1999. The multifaceted regulation of interleukin-15 expression and the role of this cytokine in NK cell differentiation and host response to intracellular pathogens. Annu. Rev. Immunol. 17, 19–49.

Wang, H.W., Joyce, J.A., 2010. Alternative activation of tumor-associated macrophages by IL-4: priming for protumoral functions. Cell Cycle 9 (24), 4824–4835.

Wu, J., Lu, Y., Ding, Y.B., Ke, Q., Hu, Z.B., Yan, Z.G., Xue, Y., Zhou, Y., Hua, Z.L., Shu, Y.Q., Liu, P., Shen, J., Xu, Y.C., Shen, H.B., 2009. Promoter polymorphisms of IL2, IL4, and risk of gastric cancer in a high-risk Chinese population. Mol. Carcinog. 48 (7), 626–632.

Williams, D.E., Morrissey, P.J., Mochizuki, D.Y., de Vries, P., Anderson, D., Cosman, D., Boswell, H.S., Cooper, S., Grabstein, K.H., Broxmeyer, H.E., 1990. T-cell growth factor P40 promotes the proliferation of myeloid cell lines and enhances erythroid burst for-mation by normal murine bone marrow cells in vitro. Blood 76 (5), 906–911.

Wills-Karp, M., Finkelman, F.D., 2008. Untangling the complex web of IL-4- and IL-13-mediated signaling pathways. Sci. Signal 1 (51), pe55.

Wise, G.J., Marella, V.K., Talluri, G., Shirazian, D., 2000. Cytokine variations in patients with hormone treated prostate cancer. J. Urol. 164 (3 Pt 1), 722–725.

Wu, M.S., Wu, C.Y., Chen, C.J., Lin, M.T., Shun, C.T., Lin, J.T., 2003. Interleukin-10 geno-types associate with the risk of gastric carcinoma in Taiwanese Chinese. Int. J. Cancer 104 (5), 617–623.

Wu, S., Fischer, L., Gökbuget, N., Schwartz, S., Burmeister, T., Notter, M., Hoelzer, D., Fuchs, H., Blau, I.W., Hofmann, W.K., Thiel, E., 2010. Expression of interleukin 15 in primary adult acute lymphoblastic leukemia. Cancer 116 (2), 387–392.

Yamasaki, S., Maeda, M., Ohshima, K., Kikuchi, M., Otsuka, T., Harada, M., 2004. Growth and apoptosis of human natural killer cell neoplasms: role of interleukin-2/15 signaling. Leuk. Res. 28 (10), 1023–1031.

Yang, Y.C., Ricciardi, S., Ciarletta, A., Calvetti, J., Kelleher, K., Clark, S.C., 1989. Expression cloning of cDNA encoding a novel human hematopoietic growth factor: human homo-logue of murine T-cell growth factor P40. Blood 74 (6), 1880–1884.

Yannopoulos, A., Nikiteas, N., Chatzitheofylaktou, A., Tsigris, C., 2007. The (-590 C/T) polymorphism in the interleukin-4 gene is associated with increased risk for early stages of colorectal adenocarcinoma. In Vivo 21 (6), 1031–1035.

Yin, T., Keller, S.R., Quelle, F.W., Witthuhn, B.A., Tsang, M.L., Lienhard, G.E., Ihle, J.N., Yang, Y.C., 1995. Interleukin-9 induces tyrosine phosphorylation of insulin receptor substrate-1 via JAK tyrosine kinases. J. Biol. Chem. 270 (35), 20497–20502.

Yoon, J.S., Newton, S.M., Wysocka, M., Troxel, A.B., Hess, S.D., Richardson, S.K., Lin, J.H., Benoit, B.M., Kasprzycka, M., Wasik, M.A., Rook, A.H., 2008. IL-21 enhances antitumor responses without stimulating proliferation of malignant T cells of patients with Sézary syndrome. J. Invest. Dermatol. 128 (2), 473–480.

Yu, P., Steel, J.C., Zhang, M., Morris, J.C., Waldmann, T.A., 2010. Simultaneous blockade of multiple immune system inhibitory checkpoints enhances antitumor activity mediated by interleukin-15 in a murine metastatic colon carcinoma model. Clin. Cancer Res. 16 (24), 6019–6028.

Yuzhalin, A.E., Kutikhin, A.G., 2012. Interleukin-12: clinical usage and molecular markers of cancer susceptibility. Growth Factors 30 (3), 176–191.

Yuzhalin, A., 2011. The role of interleukin DNA polymorphisms in gastric cancer. Hum. Immunol. 72 (11), 1128–1136.

Zeng, R., Spolski, R., Finkelstein, S.E., Oh, S., Kovanen, P.E., Hinrichs, C.S., Pise-Masison, C.A., Radonovich, M.F., Brady, J.N., Restifo, N.P., Berzofsky, J.A., Leonard, W.J., 2005. Synergy of IL-21 and IL-15 in regulating CD8+ T cell expansion and function. J. Exp. Med. 201 (1), 139–148.

Zhang, M., Yao, Z., Dubois, S., Ju, W., Müller, J.R., Waldmann, T.A., 2009. Interleukin-15 combined with an anti-CD40 antibody provides enhanced therapeutic efficacy for murine models of colon cancer. Proc. Natl. Acad. Sci. U S A 106 (18), 7513–7518.

Zhang, W.J., Li, B.H., Yang, X.Z., Li, P.D., Yuan, Q., Liu, X.H., Xu, S.B., Zhang, Y., Yuan, J., Gerhard, G.S., Masker, K.K., Dong, C., Koltun, W.A., Chorney, M.J., 2008. IL-4-induced Stat6 activities affect apoptosis and gene expression in breast cancer cells. Cytokine 42 (1), 39–47.

CHAPTER 4

Interleukin-3, Interleukin-5, and Cancer

This is the highest wisdom that I own; freedom and life are earned by those alone who conquer them each day anew.
Johann Wolfgang von Goethe, German writer (1749–1832)

4.1 INTRODUCTION INTO THE HEMATOPOIETIC FAMILY OF CYTOKINES

Hematopoietic cytokines tightly control the production and differentiation of myeloid hematopoietic cells and their precursors (Ariai et al., 1990). The family of hematopoietic growth factors includes three main representatives, namely, interleukin (IL)-3, IL-5, and granulocyte-macrophage colony-stimulating factor (GM-CSF). Taking into account their main role in the body, we should bear in mind that these ILs may be considered as agents related with hematopoietic malignancies only. That is, we shall not discuss any other cancer types in this chapter simply because neither IL-3 nor IL-5 has ever been studied in relation to malignancies other than hematopoietic.

At first glance, IL-3 and IL-5 are quite similar in their set of biological activities. Their main distinction from other ILs is the fact that both IL-3 and IL-5 share the same type of receptors called "the gp140 family". In other words, the gp140 receptor is a distinctive feature of the hematopoietic ILs. It comprises two subunits, the common β-chain (gp140) and the α-chain, which is unique for IL-3, IL-5, and GM-CSF. However, in fact, IL-3 and IL-5 have a number of differences. It is important that they interact with cancer cells through different mechanisms, which will be considered in this chapter.

4.2 INTERLEUKIN-3

4.2.1 Brief Description of IL-3

The human IL-3 is characterized as a 32 kDa monomeric cytokine regulating the production and differentiation of multilineage hematopoietic progenitors from the bone marrow. IL-3 was first discovered in 1981 by Ihle et al. (1981)

Interleukins in Cancer Biology
http://dx.doi.org/10.1016/B978-0-12-801121-8.00004-X

who purified this cytokine from concanavalin A-stimulated lymphocytes. At that date the only known ability of the new molecule was the capability to induce production of 20α-hydroxysteroid dehydrogenase in splenic lymphocytes from athymic mice. However, further research revealed that IL-3 has a large number of other significant effects on the body. First of all, it was revealed that this cytokine is able to govern generation and maintenance of multipotent hematopoietic stem cells as well as their differentiation to myeloid progenitor cells (Aldinucci et al., 2005). In addition, it was discovered that IL-3 also modulates activation, proliferation, self-renewal, and survival of multiple cell lineages, including monocytes (Suzuki et al., 2004), eosinophils (Lampinen et al., 2004), stromal cells (Yamada et al., 2000), B cells (Kinashi et al., 1988), erythroid cells (Sieff et al., 1987), neutrophils (Lindemann and Mertelsmann, 1993), monocytes (Sieff et al., 1987), multipotent progenitors (Lindemann and Mertelsmann, 1993), megakaryocytes (Sieff et al., 1987), and mast cells (Itakura et al., 2001). It is interesting that IL-3 was reported to stimulate proliferation of plasmacytoid dendritic cells as well (Demoulin et al., 2012). Furthermore, a couple of studies revealed that IL-3 is able to promote migration and proliferation of endothelial cells and vascular smooth muscle cells, suggesting its direct involvement in angio- and atherogenesis (Dentelli et al., 1999; Brizzi et al., 2001). Finally, there is increasing evidence that IL-3 may also inhibit osteoclast and osteoblast formation (Ehrlich et al., 2005; Gupta et al., 2010).

IL-3 is primarily secreted by activated T cells, mast cells, basophils, and eosinophils (Aldinucci et al., 2005). Biological activities of this cytokine are exerted through IL-3 receptor (IL-3R), which is composed of two chains (Reddy et al., 2000). The first chain is a ligand-specific α subunit, which directly binds the ligand. The second chain represents a β subunit, which is shared with IL-5 and granulocyte colony-stimulating factor (G-CSF) as mentioned above. The β subunit does not bind IL-3 per se but it is necessary for high-affinity binding between the α chain and the ligand (Hayashida et al., 1990; Kitamura et al., 1991; Korpelainen et al., 1996). Although it is generally known that IL-3R is expressed exclusively on the surface of various hematopoietic cells (Korpelainen et al., 1996), some studies showed that it may also be expressed by fibroblasts, endothelial cells, and smooth muscle cells (Brizzi et al., 1993; Colotta et al., 1993; Korpelainen et al., 1993).

There is strong evidence to suggest that IL-3 has a major regulatory function within the body. First of all, numerous studies showed that this IL participates in the stimulation of growth and differentiation processes synergistically with other cytokines, such as thrombopoietin, G-CSF, GM-CSF, or IL-6 (McNiece et al., 1988; Paquette et al., 1988; Geissler et al., 1990, 1996; Ulich et al., 1990; Farese et al., 1993; Winton et al., 1994; Lemoli et al., 1996). In particular, IL-3 was reported to expand the pool of circulating hematopoietic progenitor cells, induce neutrophil recovery (Lemoli et al., 1996), augment megakaryocyte colony formation (McNiece et al., 1988), promote hematopoietic regeneration (Winton et al., 1994), and stimulate the mobilization of hematopoietic progenitor cells (Geissler et al., 1996). In addition, IL-3 was found associated with transmigration of neutrophils across endothelial monolayers and upregulated production of numerous regulatory agents such as G-CSF, IL-6, IL-8, and E-selectin (Korpelainen et al., 1993, 1996). Regarding the regulation of IL-3 expression, this cytokine is known to be profoundly upregulated by tumor necrosis factor alpha and interferon gamma (Korpelainen et al., 1995, 1996).

4.2.2 Overview of IL-3 Signaling Pathways in Cancer

It has long been known that IL-3 possesses a complex tumor-promoting effect. In particular, this cytokine is responsible for preventing apoptosis, promoting angiogenesis, and stimulating proliferation and survival in malignant hematopoietic cells (Guthridge et al., 1998; Schrader, 1998; Blalock et al., 1999). It is important to note that all these protumorigenic activities are implemented through different signaling pathways triggered by the IL-3/IL-3R complex. We shall describe them briefly to show the overall picture of the effects of IL-3 on tumor cells.

First of all, binding of IL-3 to IL-3R triggers the autophosphorylation of Jak2, enabling it to further phosphorylate and activate Signal transducer and activator of transcription 5 (STAT5), a transcription factor constitutively phosphorylated in tumor cells (reviewed by Van Etten, 2007). Several research groups showed that patients with different hematopoietical malignancies exhibited a dose-dependent activation of STAT5 in response to IL-3 and other hematopoietic growth factors (Mui et al., 1995; Du et al., 2011; Padron et al., 2013). Importantly, impaired STAT5 signaling has long been known to underlie the pathogenesis of various hematological malignancies as well as myeloproliferative disorders (reviewed by Hennighausen and Robinson, 2008). In cancer, activated STAT5 is responsible for modulation of the evasion of the immune response, stimulation of angiogenesis, cell survival, proliferation, migration, and invasion (Nosaka et al., 1999; Yu and Jove, 2004; Hennighausen and Robinson, 2008). In particular, IL-3 is well known to regulate the expression of a prosurvival antiapoptotic protein Bcl-xl through the activation of STAT5 (Shinjyo et al., 2001). It is interesting to note that it was found that hematopoietic GTPase RhoH is able to significantly regulate IL-3-driven activation of STAT5. In particular, decreased RhoH levels resulted in a marked upregulation of IL-3-dependent cell growth, STAT5 activity, and an upregulation of IL-3R surface expression (Gündogdu et al., 2010). It should also be noted that finally, STAT5 is involved in endothelial and smooth muscle cell migration and regulation, thereby suggesting its role in angiogenesis (Brizzi et al., 1999, 2002). Together, these observations suggest a strong cross talk between IL-3 and STAT5 as well as their profound impact on hematopoietic cancer development.

The second consequence of the mediation of the IL/IL-R complex is the activation of the adaptor protein Shc. In turn, this leads to the formation of a complex of Shc with two other adaptor proteins, Grb2 and Sos-1. This complex is able to trigger Ras protein, which consequently leads to two different actions. The first action is the activation of mitogenic signals through subsequent phosphorylation of Raf, MEK1, ERK1, and ERK2 (Berra et al., 1995; Blaikie et al., 1994). The second consequence of the IL-3-driven activation of Ras is prevention of apoptosis via phosphoinositide 3-kinase (PI3K)/Akt-modulated pathway. In short, IL-3-mediated triggering of Akt leads to the phosphorylation of the proapoptotic protein Bad, which is also known as bcl-2 antagonist of cell death. The phosphorylation of Bad then promotes its association with adaptor protein 14-3-3, thereby preventing it from transportation to the mitochondrion where it may exert its proapoptotic activities through forming complex with bcl-2 and bcl-xL. Furthermore, the activation of Akt leads to upregulation of nuclear factor kappaB (NF-κB) through the phosphorylation of IκB kinase. It is believed that NF-κB is able to inhibit c-Myc-induced apoptosis and hence regarded as an antiapoptotic molecule (Romashkova and Makarov, 1999; Chang et al., 2003).

Finally, the relationship between IL-3 signaling pathways and an oncoprotein Bcr-Abl has been demonstrated not long ago. The Bcr-Abl oncoprotein is activated by the STAT5 pathway regardless of Jak2 triggering (Ilaria and Van Etten, 1996), and it was found that the presence of IL-3R is critical for Bcr-Abl-modulated oncogenic transformation of myeloid progenitors in Philadelphia chromosome-positive chronic myeloid leukemia and lymphoid progenitors in Philadelphia chromosome-positive lymphoid leukemia in vitro (Tao et al., 2008).

To sum up, Figure 4.1 briefly represents the main signaling pathways of IL-3 involved in hematopoietic carcinogenesis.

4.2.3 IL-3 in Tumor Models

Numerous studies provided the evidence for IL-3-mediated prevention of apoptosis and other protumorigenic activities of this cytokine. To be concise, we will only mention the major achievements that have been made

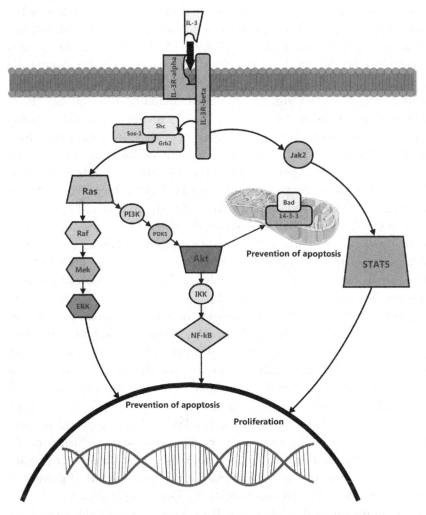

Figure 4.1 Known molecular mechanisms of IL-3-mediated cell proliferation and prevention of apoptosis. (For color version of this figure, the reader is referred to the online version of this book.)

on this issue. One of the first reports on this problem was provided by Lotem and Sachs (1992), who showed the inhibitory effect of IL-3 on apoptosis triggered by transforming growth factor beta1 in myeloid leukemic cells. Furthermore, Collins et al. (1992), showed that IL-3 is able to protect IL-3-dependent murine bone marrow cells from programmed cell death triggered either by etoposide treatment or ionizing radiation. In addition, Clayberger et al. (1992) demonstrated that recombinant IL-3 is able to stimulate growth of primary follicular lymphoma in vitro. Further research by Kinoshita et al. (1995) revealed an essential mechanism of IL-3-mediated suppression of apoptosis, which involves Shc, Ras, Raf-1, and mitogen-activated protein kinase (MAPK). Additionally, similar findings were obtained by Gotoh et al. (1996) who demonstrated antiapoptotic activities of IL-3 on the Ba/F3 proB cell line. In their study, the authors found out that IL-3 directly inhibited apoptosis through Shc/Ras/MAPK/c-fos-pathway. In addition, the researchers indicated a novel mechanism based on IL-3-driven triggering of Shc/c-myc pathway, which might independently inhibit apoptosis as well. Nishii et al. (1999) found that IL-3 efficiently augmented the survival of pre-B acute lymphoblastic leukemia cell line in the presence of stromal cells. Consistent with previous findings, the authors indicated that IL-3 directly upregulated the expression of Bcl-2, thereby confirming that the observed survival is associated with Bad/bcl-2-mediated inhibition of apoptosis. Aldinucci et al. (2002) demonstrated that exposure of Hodgkin disease cell lines HDLM2 and L1236 to recombinant IL-3 rescued cells from apoptosis in a dose-dependent manner. Interestingly, the authors also indicated that the overwhelming majority (>90%) of 19 tissue samples of Hodgkin disease constantly expressed IL-3Rα regardless of the histological subtype and their antigenic phenotype. However, these samples did not constitutively express IL-3 transcripts at all. Additionally, the authors revealed that the addition of recombinant IL-3 promoted growth and survival of Hodgkin disease cell lines either in combination with IL-9 and stem cell factor or alone (Aldinucci et al., 2002). As mentioned earlier, IL-3 was suspected in contributing to cell proliferation and proangiogenic activity (Brizzi et al., 1993, 2001; Korpelainen et al., 1995), thereby suggesting another procarcinogenic pathway of this cytokine. Also, it was found that IL-3 promoted survival of tumor-derived endothelial cells (Deregibus et al., 2002). Finally, direct tumor-promoting effects of IL-3 were shown in the studies by Bergui et al. (1989), Berdel et al. (1989), Dippold et al. (1991), Block et al. (1992) and Pedrazzoli et al. (1994).

However, it is worth noting that there are a large number of findings that may cast a doubt on the claim IL-3 is a procarcinogenic cytokine. Hsu and Hsu (1990) showed that IL-3 was not able to modulate the proliferation and differentiation of cultured Hodgkin disease cell lines HDLM-1 and KM-H2 alone or in combination with various colony-stimulating factors. Furthermore, the authors indicated that IL-3 did not change the expression profile of other cytokines synthesized by cancer cells. According to the study by Vellenga et al. (1991), IL-3 enhanced the tumor growth only in 1 out of 11 small cell lung cancer cell lines. Similarly, Guillaume et al. (1993) found no stimulatory effect of IL-3 on 34 different cancer cell lines derived from seven histological cell types. In addition, it is necessary to mention a study by Izquierdo et al. (1995), who failed to trace an association between IL-3 and stimulation of cancer progression. In particular, the investigators found minimal effects of this cytokine on tumor growth with only 4% (3 out of 72) of the tumors showing proliferation at 100 ng/ml of IL-3. Some researchers show that IL-3 can hardly promote tumor growth, whereas other authors indicate that it may exert anticancer activities. Particularly, Brach et al. (1990) demonstrated that IL-3 dramatically increased the efficacy of cytosine arabinoside for the elimination of leukemic stem cells, thereby suggesting possible anticancer effect of this cytokine. On the other hand, the authors noticed that IL-3 directly affected expression patterns of the proto-oncogenes *c-myc*, *c-fms*, and *c-fos*. Moreover, Younes et al. (1994) showed that IL-3 profoundly inhibited the growth of follicular small cleaved cell lymphoma cells in a dose-dependent manner. Additionally, the authors observed that IL-3 killed all the malignant but not normal lymphocytes in a dose-dependent manner as well. Finally, Sasaki et al. (1992) showed that 1500 U/kg dose of recombinant IL-3 injected intralesionally into BALB/c mice bearing Meth-A solid tumors resulted in tumor growth inhibition by 34% at 24 days after tumor inoculation. More interestingly, the observed effect gradually declined and vanished after pretreatment with anti-IL-3 monoclonal antibodies.

4.2.4 IL-3 Serum Levels and Cancer

For several years, little effort has been devoted to the study of prognostic role of serum IL-3 in the context of cancer. It should be useful to briefly mention these scarce studies. The levels of IL-3 were significantly lower in 40 patients with pancreatic and ampullary cancer as compared to 40 healthy volunteers (Vasiliades et al., 2012). A similar correlation was found in 48 patients with pancreatic cancer in comparison with 40 healthy subjects

(Mroczko et al., 2005a). On the other hand, the expression of IL-3 was markedly elevated in prostate cancer patients as well as in subjects with benign prostatic hyperplasia (Zhang et al., 2010). Similarly, Teruya-Feldstein et al. (2000) demonstrated high expression levels of IL-3 in tissue samples collected from patients with Hodgkin disease. In addition, some studies have demonstrated inconsistent findings. In particular, the analysis of serum IL-3 levels among 95 colorectal cancer patients and 65 healthy blood donors showed no statistically significant differences (Mroczko et al., 2007), whereas the previous results revealed a positive association in the samples of 75 cases and 40 controls and 30 cases and 20 controls (Mroczko et al., 2003, 2005b). Finally, no differences in IL-3 serum levels were found between 60 nasopharyngeal carcinoma patients and 40 normal healthy subjects (Liu et al., 2001).

4.2.5 IL-3R and Cancer: Dangerous Liaisons?

Having considered IL-3 itself, we shall now focus our attention on IL-3R because it seems to be very interesting in the context of cancer. As mentioned earlier, IL-3R belongs to the gp140 family of IL receptors. It is composed of two subunits, namely, an α subunit of 60–70 kDa and a β subunit of 130–140 kDa (Miyajima et al., 1992). The β subunit of the IL-3R is also shared by the receptors for IL-5 and GM-CSF (Miyajima et al., 1992). So far, the relationship between IL-3R and cancer has been widely investigated in two aspects: the expression patterns of IL-3R in cancer patients and use of IL-3R as a therapeutic agent for cancer treatment.

There is a large number of studies assessing the serum levels of IL-3 in patients with cancer (Table 4.1). In particular, overexpression of IL-3R has been found in various hematopoietic cancers, including B-cell chronic lymphocytic leukemia (Trentin et al., 1994), B-lineage acute lymphoblastic leukemia (Uckun et al., 1989; Testa et al., 2002; Nakase et al., 2007), pre-B lymphoma (Park et al., 1989), acute myeloid leukemia (Muñoz et al., 2001; Jordan et al., 2000; Testa et al., 2002; Du et al., 2011), follicular lymphoma (Clayberger et al., 1992; Younes et al., 1994), large cell lymphoma (Clayberger et al., 1992), Hodgkin disease (Aldinucci et al., 2002; Bosshart, 2003), hairy cell leukemia (Muñoz et al., 2001), and malignant plasma cell precursors (Bergui et al., 1989).

According to these observations, it is possible to suggest that IL-3R may be used as a diagnostic marker for hematological malignancies. Furthermore, several authors even proposed that flow cytometry analysis of IL-3R expression may be useful for diagnosing classical Hodgkin lymphoma (Fromm et al., 2006, 2009; Fromm 2011).

Table 4.1 Summary of Studies Investigating the Expression Patterns of IL-3R in Patients with Hematologic Malignancies

Author	Cancer Type	Patients	Cell Lines	Expression Pattern (Molecules per Cell), If Provided	Additional Information
Park et al. (1989)	Myelogenous leukemia, pre–B lymphoma	N/A	KG-1, JM-1, BMB, Nalm-6, RW	KG-1: 275 ± 60; JM-1: 90 ± 45; BMB: 120 ± 30;	
Bergui et al. (1989)	Multiple myeloma	5 men and 6 women	N/A	N/A	All multiple myeloma plasma cell precursors had IL-3R expressed
Uckun et al. (1989)	B-cell precursor lympho-blastic leukemia	12	N/A	146–1433 (mean 627 ± 250)	
Clayberger et al. (1992)	Large cell lymphoma, follicular lymphoma	1 LCL, 3 FL	N/A	N/A	All samples showed high levels of IL-3R
Trentin et al. (1994)	B-cell chronic lymphocytic leukemia	8 men and 4 women aged from 48 to 66 years	N/A	N/A	
Jordan et al. (2000)	Acute myeloid leukemia	18	N/A	N/A	16 of 18 specimens had strongly expressed IL-3R
Muñoz et al., (2001)	Acute myeloid leukemia, chronic lymphocytic leukemia, Burkitt's lymphoma, follicular lymphoma, hairy cell leukemia, mantle-cell lymphoma	45 patients with AML (19 ALL, 13 B-ALL, 6T-ALL); 77 (CLL), 12 MCL, 5 FL, 7 HCL, 2 Burkitt's lymphoma	N/A	N/A	High expression of IL-3R was found in 95% acute leukemia samples and 100% of B-lymphoid lineage samples
Testa et al. (2002)	Acute myeloid leukemia, B-acute lymphoid leukemia, T-acute lymphoid leukemia	79 patients with AML, 25 patients with (B-ALL), and 7 patients with (T-ALL)	N/A	N/A	Overexpression of IL-3R was found in 60% of AML cases, 100% of B-ALL cases and less than 10% of T-ALL cases

Continued

Table 4.1 Summary of Studies Investigating the Expression Patterns of IL-3R in Patients with Hematologic Malignancies—Cont'd

Author	Cancer Type	Patients	Cell Lines	Expression Pattern (Molecules per Cell), If Provided	Additional Information
Aldinucci et al. (2002)	Hodgkin disease	19	L428, KMH2, HDLM2, L540	N/A	All cell lines and tissues expressed IL-3R; L428 and HDLM2 cells showed the highest surface density
Bosshart (2003)	Multiple myeloma	11			
Nakase et al. (2007)	Acute lymphoblastic leukemia (ALL)	138	N/A	Median: 117; Max: 6155; mean: 469	No association between IL-3R expression and clinical outcome
Du et al. (2011)	Acute myeloid leukemia	13	N/A	N/A	IL-3Rα was overexpressed on CD34+ CD38– cells from FA patients with AML, but not in the total CD34+ population or in more primitive CD34+ CD38– cells of normal bone marrow
Fromm et al. (2011)	Various hematopoietic malignancies	274	N/A	N/A	IL-3R was highly expressed in patients with classical HD

CLL, Chronic lymphocytic leukemia; MCL, Mantle cell lymphoma; FL, Follicular lymphoma; HCL, Hairy cell leukemia; HD, Hodgkin's disease; FA, Fanconi anemia.

Intriguingly enough, there is accumulating evidence that IL-3R may be used for modern targeted cancer therapies. First of all, we should mention an interesting study performed by Du et al. (2007), who developed an immunotoxin against hematological malignancies. The immunotoxin targeting IL-3R was based on *Pseudomonas* exotoxin A and named 26292(Fv)-PE38-KDEL. During the study, it demonstrated profound cytotoxic activity against IL-3R-expressing cell lines TF-1, Molm-13, and Molm-14, thereby suggesting its further development for the possible treatment of IL-3R-expressing malignancies. Another study was performed by Stein et al. (2010), who created an IL3-R-specific immunotoxin of a similar design, called CD123-ETA'. The authors showed that CD123-ETA' was able to effectively eliminate cultured acute myeloid leukemia (AML)-derived cells. However, these immunotoxins have a serious limitation, namely, elicitation of an immune response resulting in the production of neutralizing antibodies, which does not allow repeated application of the agent within the framework of a therapeutic setting.

Another promising therapeutic agent on the basis of IL-3R targeting is $DT_{388}IL3$, which is supposed to kill all the IL-3-expressing cells within the body. $DT_{388}IL3$ was engineered by Frankel et al. (2000) and it represents a fusion protein comprising the human IL-3 linked to the truncated form of diphtheria toxin (DT_{388}). So far, a series of preclinical studies demonstrated the effectiveness of this agent in vivo with no adverse side effects or toxicity against normal bone marrow progenitors (Frankel et al. 2000, 2001; Feuring-Buske et al. 2002). What is more interesting is that $DT_{388}IL3$ has also been reported to synergize with chemotherapy agent cytarabine (Hogge et al., 2004) and tyrosine kinase inhibitors (Kim et al., 2010) in eliminating leukemic progenitors.

It is clear that $DT_{388}IL3$ may be used as a powerful drug for hematopoietic malignancies. Currently, $DT_{388}IL3$ is undergoing phase 1 clinical study in 40 patients with AML (Frankel et al., 2008). Finally, studies by Jin et al. (2009) and Du et al. (2011) showed that IL-3R-neutralizing monoclonal antibody 7G3 effectively activated innate immunity, reduced survival of malignant cells, and inhibited cancer progression in immunodeficient mice with AML.

4.2.6 Summary

From the research that has been carried out in past decades, it becomes increasingly clear that IL-3 is an essential factor for the regulation of proliferation, apoptosis inhibition, and survival of hematopoietic cells. Although many peculiarities of IL-3 singling remain poorly understood, it is clearly evident that this cytokine plays a leading role in the development of hematopoietic malignancies. So far, there are several recognized molecular mechanisms that indicate that IL-3 may contribute to hematopoietic cancer development. First, IL-3 seems to protect malignant cells from apoptosis thereby contributing to their survival. Second, it was repeatedly shown that IL-3 has a great impact on cell proliferation. Third, there is an established molecular pathway that links IL-3 with angiogenesis and endothelial cell survival. However, continued research on this issue appears fully justified because studies on animal models and cell cultures are inconsistent and conflicting. Furthermore, there still is a lack of large-scale prospective studies assessing the prognostic role of serum IL-3. Therefore, further study of the issue is still required. Another important conclusion is that IL-3R is likely to become a diagnostic marker for hematopoietic malignancies, since numerous studies have demonstrated overexpression of IL-3R in this group of diseases. What is more interesting is that IL-3R is currently being tested as an aim for targeted therapy. To date, several potential drugs have been developed; among them, $DT_{388}IL3$ has demonstrated the best results. Currently, there is substantial reason to believe that this approach could be useful for the treatment of various hematopoietic malignancies without serious toxicities. From the outcome of the clinical trials on $DT_{388}IL3$, it would be possible to conclude whether or not this drug is suitable for proper cancer treatment.

4.3 INTERLEUKIN-5

4.3.1 Brief Overview of IL-5

IL-5 was discovered during the experiments by Schimpl and Wecker (1972), who were investigating concanavalin A-treated lymphocyte cultures. Initially, IL-5 was designated as T-cell replacing factor (TRF) because it was demonstrated to activate B-cell differentiation in the absence of T cells. Further research revealed that TRF has plenty of other functions, such as regulation of immunoglobulin synthesis as well as influence on T cells, eosinophils, and basophils. Due to the similarity to other ILs, it was eventually renamed as "interleukin 5" (Takatsu et al., 1988).

IL-5 represents a 15 kDa homodimeric protein comprising two helical bundle motifs. A 30 kDa primary transcript of IL-5 requires further proteolytic cleavage to form a 134 amino acid mature protein. IL-5 is generally known to be produced by eosinophils, basophils, CD4+ Th2 lymphocytes, CD34+ progenitor cells, mast cells, invariant natural killer T cells, and Reed

Sternberg cells (Sehmi et al., 1997; Phillips et al., 2003; Sakuishi et al., 2007; Takatsu, 2011). Production of IL-5 may be triggered by either various allergens or bacteria (e.g., *Mycobacterium tuberculosis* or *Toxocara canis*).The biological effect of IL-5 is exerted through IL-5 receptor, which is expressed ubiquitously in the human body (Takaki et al., 1990). As it was mentioned earlier, the receptor is composed of a common βc subunit and a unique IL-5α subunit.The cytokine binds specifically to the latter subunit, but further transition of a signal is impossible without a former one. Interestingly enough, different signaling pathways are found to be triggered by IL-5 in different cells. It is known that in B cells, IL-5 acts through PI3K, Jak2, Btk tyrosine kinases,Vav, Shc, and HS1 (Sato et al., 1994; Adachi and Alam, 1998), whereas in eosinophils it has been reported to activate Jak2/Stat1, Lyn, MAPK, PI3K, and Syk pathways (Pazdrak et al., 1995;Yousefi et al., 1996;Adachi and Alam, 1998).The gene encoding IL-5 share the same cluster with *IL-3, IL-4, IL-13*, and *GM-CSF* genes in mice and humans (Le Beau et al., 1989).

Biological functions of IL-5 are highly diverse, and hence we will briefly mention only the basic ones. First, IL-5 is regarded as a major factor for growth and differentiation of activated T cells and B cells. Second, it has a profound impact on differentiation, activation, survival, and proliferation of eosinophils (Takatsu et al., 1994; Takatsu and Nakajima, 2008). It has been showed that *IL-5*-deficient mice have decreased numbers of circulating eosinophils and cannot implement eosinophilic response to infections (Foster et al., 1996; Kopf et al., 1996).Third, this cytokine is widely known to attract eosinophils as well as prevent them from apoptosis (Ochiai et al., 1997; Hamelmann et al., 1999;Tomaki et al., 2000). Fourth, the production of IL-5 was found to be significantly increased by IL-2. In particular, stimulation with IL-2 profoundly contributed to IL-5 synthesis in a specific subset of Peyer's patch cells both in vitro and in vivo (Kuraoka et al., 2004). Furthermore, IL-5 in turn is able to augment the IL-2-mediated production of cytotoxic T cells and stimulate mediator release from basophils (Huston et al., 1996). Fifth, overexpression of IL-5 was found associated with markedly increased circulating levels of IgM, IgA, and IgE, which suggests that this cytokine contributes to a major alteration in the immune profile (Tominaga et al., 1991). As seen from the above-mentioned data, IL-5 is of great biological significance. Finally, it should be noted that the review by Takatsu (2011) summarizes the knowledge of the structure, functions, and signaling of IL-5 and hence may be recommended for further reading.

Nowadays, IL-5 is believed to play a role in a broad range of diseases. The use of anti-IL5 antibody therapy has demonstrated a potential efficacy in patients with asthma, atopic dermatitis, nasal polyposis, hypereosino-philic syndrome, eosinophilic esophagitis, and Churg–Strauss syndrome (reviewed by Corren, 2012). With regards to malignant disease, the studies are scarce and limited. We shall briefly summarize and discuss them.

4.3.2 Potential Impact of IL-5 on Cancer Development

4.3.2.1 IL-5, Eosinophilia, and Cancer

Since it is clear that IL-5 exerts its biological effects mainly on eosinophils, the simplest way to analyze the impact of IL-5 on features of cancer development is to take a look at tumor-associated eosinophilia. Although the precise impact of eosinophils on malignant disease is unclear, there is a large amount of evidence that they may exert both pro- and anticancer activities (Gatault et al., 2012). So far, plenty of studies indicated a possible correlation between high IL-5 levels and cancer development. A remarkable example demonstrating the involvement of IL-5 in the development of eosinophilia in cancer was provided by Walter et al. (2002), who first reported a case of metastatic head and neck squamous cell carcinoma with marked blood eosinophilia and increased serum levels of IL-5. Similar associations were also found among patients with colon cancer (Anagnostopoulos et al., 2005; Kato et al., 2010), lung cancer (Pandit et al., 2007), nasopharyngeal carcinoma (Liu et al., 2001), hemangioendothelioma (Kimura et al., 2006), and peripheral T-cell lymphoma (Matsunaga et al., 2006; Thielen et al., 2008). According to these findings, the evidence of the link between IL-5 and tumor-associated eosinophilia seems to be clearly established. Nevertheless, almost all the existing reports on this issue are sporadic case reports, and further research should be performed to investigate the problem more profoundly.

In contrast to the results of the above-mentioned studies, it is necessary to mention an interesting study by Ikutani et al. (2012), who revealed that IL-5-driven activation of eosinophils may prevent metastasis formation and provoke antitumor immunity. In particular, the authors showed that IL-5-deficient mice or mice treated with anti-IL-5 monoclonal antibodies exhibited impaired eosinophil regulation and increased lung tumor metastasis. Moreover, the authors indicated that administration of recombinant IL-5 resulted in suppressed progression of metastasis. Another study performed by Yamazaki et al. (2005) showed that IL-5-mediated eosinophilia correlated with a good prognosis of cervical cancer: the 5-year cause-specific survival rate was 76% for patients with eosinophilia and 53% for patients without eosinophilia.

4.3.2.2 Prognostic Role of IL-5 in Cancer

According to a study by Eiró et al. (2013), high levels of IL-5 were associated with breast cancer metastasis through a significant increase in CD68$^+$/(CD3$^+$CD20$^+$) cell ratio. Furthermore, elevated amounts of IL-5 were found in 28 patients with chronic lymphocytic leukemia/small lymphocytic lymphoma (Karmali et al., 2013). Similarly, increased circulating levels of IL-5 were observed in 51 patients with advanced serous ovarian cancer as compared to 46 healthy controls (Zhu et al., 2010). Additionally, elevated levels of IL-5 were found in patients with colorectal cancer treated with a cancer vaccine based on dendritic cells pulsed with an allogeneic melanoma cell lysate (Burgdorf et al., 2009). Moreover, IL-5 levels correlated with the grade and severity of urothelial carcinoma of bladder among 72 patients (Satyam et al., 2011).

In contrast to the above-mentioned findings, there was no correlation obtained between higher IL-5 serum levels and survival in patients with lung cancer (Enewold et al., 2009, 359 cases) as well as non–Hodgkin lymphoma risk (Conroy et al., 2013, 272 cases and 541 controls). Moreover, levels of IL-5 were not established as a prognostic factor either for 80 patients with nasopharyngeal carcinoma (Lu et al., 2012) or for 94 subjects with adult T-cell leukemia/lymphoma (Inagaki et al., 2006). Furthermore, there was no association between IL-5 expression patterns in serum of 20 patients with adenoid cystic carcinoma, 20 subjects with squamous cell carcinoma of the head and neck, and 20 healthy blood donors (Hoffmann et al., 2007). Finally, IL-5 levels did not correlate with survival in 86 subjects with advanced non-small cell lung cancer (Su et al., 2011).

Several recent studies have analyzed the effect of cancer chemotherapy on the concentration of IL-5 in circulating blood. First, significant changes in the levels of IL-5 were observed in 60 subjects with recurrent prostate cancer after treatment with lenalidomide (Zabransky et al., 2012). Similarly, Argiris et al. (2011) detected altered IL-5 levels in 31 patients with head and neck cancer treated with therapy containing cetuximab. According to the study by Wang et al. (2012), serum levels of IL-5 were found decreased in patients with esophageal carcinoma who underwent two courses of chemotherapy treatment with tegafur and lentinan. Regarding radiotherapy, some research claims that it is unlikely to have an impact on IL-5 levels. Lopes and Callera (2012) revealed that 45 patients with prostate cancer who received three-dimensional conformal blocking radiation therapy had a stable concentration of IL-5 during the course.

An intriguing cross talk between IL-5 and IL-2 was discovered by Tomova et al. (2006), who used IL-2 for the treatment of 13 patients with primary or metastatic gastrointestinal malignancies. The authors found out that local IL-2 therapy caused significant increase in serum IL-5 levels. The first IL-2 injection boosted the expression by three times, the subsequent injection resulted in more than ninefold increase in IL-5 levels, showing that repeated administration of IL-2 profoundly affects IL-5 production. Furthermore, similar findings were obtained by Cragun et al. (2005). The authors indicated that circulating levels of IL-5 peaked 1 week after starting IL-2 therapy in 22 melanoma patients. Moreover, all the patients developed a marked eosinophilia correlating in magnitude with peak IL-5 serum levels (Cragun et al., 2005). In addition, it is interesting to mention a study by Rivoltini et al. (1993), who discovered that in vivo administration of IL-5 caused activation of IL-2 and eosinophils with subsequent cytotoxicity against malignant cells.

4.3.2.3 Summary

To date, the peculiarities of the structure, functioning, and regulation of IL-5 have been studied well enough to trace the relationship between this IL and various diseases. Nevertheless, the precise role of this cytokine in cancer is currently a subject of debates. The existing data on the impact of IL-5 on cancer risk and prognosis are conflicting. Furthermore, there is only one study devoted to the impact of IL-5 on survival of cancer patients. Further research is needed to elaborate this issue. Considering the impact of IL-5 on cancer development, two major mechanisms may be emphasized. The first pathway is based on a strong link between IL-5 and eosinophils, which is due to the IL-5-mediated regulation of eosinophils. It is certainly accepted that IL-5 is involved in the recruitment of eosinophils into the tumor. However, their exact impact on cancer development is difficult to evaluate due to the fact that in different stages of tumor development eosinophils may play different roles. For instance, it is well known that eosinophils synthesize vascular endothelial growth factor; hence, they may support tumors at late stages by contributing to angiogenesis. On the other hand, they may exert antitumor activity at early stages of tumor development. Therefore, in different cases the impact of IL-5 can be either advantageous or disadvantageous. So, in this regard, the impact of IL-5 may be variously interpreted. The second pathway lies in the ambivalent interaction between IL-2 and IL-5, which should be investigated more thoroughly. Possibly, IL-2 may synergize with IL-5 to promote antitumor activities or act as a downstream mediator of anticancer immune response.

To conclude, more research is desirable to extend our knowledge of the relationship between IL-5 and malignant disease.

REFERENCES

Adachi, T., Alam, R., 1998. The mechanism of IL-5 signal transduction. Am. J. Physiol. 275 (3 Pt 1), C623–C633.

Aldinucci, D., Olivo, K., Lorenzon, D., Poletto, D., Gloghini, A., Carbone, A., Pinto, A., 2005. The role of interleukin-3 in classical Hodgkin's disease. Leuk. Lymphoma 46 (3), 303–311.

Aldinucci, D., Poletto, D., Gloghini, A., Nanni, P., Degan, M., Perin, T., Ceolin, P., Rossi, F.M., Gattei, V., Carbone, A., Pinto, A., 2002. Expression of functional interleukin-3 receptors on Hodgkin and Reed-Sternberg cells. Am. J. Pathol. 160 (2), 585–596.

Anagnostopoulos, G., Sakorafas, G., Kostopoulos, P., Margantinis, G., Tsiakos, S., Terpos, E., Pavlakis, G., Fortun, P., Arvanitidis, D., 2005. Disseminated colon cancer with severe peripheral blood eosinophilia and elevated serum levels of interleukine-2, interleukine-3, interleukine-5, and GM-CSF. J. Surg. Oncol. 89, 273–275.

Arai, K.I., Lee, F., Miyajima, A., Miyatake, S., Arai, N., 1990. Yokota T. Cytokines: coordinators of immune and inflammatory responses. Annu. Rev. Biochem. 59, 783–836.

Argiris, A., Lee, S.C., Feinstein, T., Thomas, S., Branstetter 4th, B.F., Seethala, R., Wang, L., Gooding, W., Grandis, J.R., Ferris, R.L., 2011. Serum biomarkers as potential predictors of antitumor activity of cetuximab-containing therapy for locally advanced head and neck cancer. Oral Oncol. 47 (10), 961–966.

Berdel, W.E., Danhauser-Riedl, S., Steinhauser, G., Winton, E.F., 1989. Various human hematopoietic growth factors (interleukin-3, GM-CSF, G-CSF) stimulate clonal growth of nonhematopoietic tumor cells. Blood 73 (1), 80–83.

Bergui, L., Schena, M., Gaidano, G., Riva, M., Calligaris-Cappio, F., 1989. Interleukin 3 and interleukin 6 synergistically promote the proliferation and differentiation of malignant plasma cell precursors in multiple myeloma. J. Exp. Med. 170, 613–618.

Berra, E., Diaz-Meco, M.T., Lozano, J., Frutos, S., Municio, M.M., Sanchez, P., Sanz, L., Moscat, J., 1995. Evidence for a role of MEK and MAPK during signal transduction by protein kinase C zeta. EMBO J. 14, 6157–6163.

Blaikie, P., Immanuel, D., Wu, J., Li, N., Yajnik, V., Margolis, B., 1994. A region in Shc distinct from the SH2 domain can bind tyrosine-phosphorylated growth factor receptors. J. Biol. Chem. 269, 32031–32034.

Blalock, W.L., Weinstein-Oppenheimer, C., Chang, F., Hoyle, P.E., Wang, X.Y., Algate, P.A., Franklin, R.A., Oberhaus, S.M., Stilman, L.S., McCubrey, J.A., 1999. Signal transduction, cell cycle regulatory, and anti-apoptotic pathways regulated by IL-3 in hematopoietic cells: possible sites for intervention with anti-neoplastic drugs. Leukemia 13, 1109–1166.

Block, T., Schmid, F., Geffken, B., Treiber, U., Busch, R., Hartung, R., 1992. Modulation of in vitro cell growth of human and murine urothelial tumor cell lines under the influence of interleukin-3, granulocyte-, macrophage- and granulocyte-colony-stimulating factor. Urol. Res. 20 (4), 289–292.

Bosshart, H., 2003. Interleukin-3 receptors in Hodgkin's disease. Am. J. Pathol. 162 (1), 355–356.

Brach, M., Klein, H., Platzer, E., Mertelsmann, R., Herrmann, F., 1990. Effect of interleukin 3 on cytosine arabinoside-mediated cytotoxicity of leukemic myeloblasts. Exp. Hematol. 18 (7), 748–753.

Brizzi, M.F., Formato, L., Dentelli, P., Rosso, A., Pavan, M., Garbarino, G., Pegoraro, M., Camussi, G., Pegoraro, L., 2001. Interleukin-3 stimulates migration and proliferation of vascular smooth muscle cells: a potential role in atherogenesis. Circulation 103 (4), 549–554.

Brizzi, M.F., Garbarino, G., Rossi, P.R., Pagliardi, G.L., Arduino, C., Avanzi, G.C., Pegoraro, L., 1993. Interleukin 3 stimulates proliferation and triggers endothelial-leukocyte adhesion molecule 1 gene activation of human endothelial cells. J. Clin. Invest. 91 (6), 2887–2892.

Burgdorf, S.K., Claesson, M.H., Nielsen, H.J., Rosenberg, J., 2009. Changes in cytokine and biomarker blood levels in patients with colorectal cancer during dendritic cell-based vaccination. Acta Oncol. 48 (8), 1157–1164.

Chang, F., Lee, J.T., Navolanic, P.M., Steelman, L.S., Shelton, J.G., Blalock, W.L., Franklin, R.A., McCubrey, J.A., 2003. Involvement of PI3K/Akt pathway in cell cycle progression, apoptosis, and neoplastic transformation: a target for cancer chemotherapy. Leukemia 17 (3), 590–603.

Clayberger, C., Luna-Fineman, S., Lee, J.E., Pillai, A., Campbell, M., Levy, R., Krensky, A.M., 1992. Interleukin 3 is a growth factor for human follicular B cell lymphoma. J. Exp. Med. 175, 371–376.

Collins, M.K., Marvel, J., Malde, P., Lopez-Rivas, A., 1992. Interleukin 3 protects murine bone marrow cells from apoptosis induced by DNA damaging agents. J. Exp. Med. 176 (4), 1043–1051.

Colotta, F., Bussolino, F., Polentarutti, N., Guglielmetti, A., Sironi, M., Bocchietto, E., De Rossi, M., Mantovani, A., 1993. Differential expression of the common beta and specific alpha chains of the receptors for GM-CSF, IL-3, and IL-5 in endothelial cells. Exp. Cell Res. 206 (2), 311–317.

Conroy, S.M., Maskarinec, G., Morimoto, Y., Franke, A.A., Cooney, R.V., Wilkens, L.R., Goodman, M.T., Hernadez, B.Y., Le Marchand, L., Henderson, B.E., Kolonel, L.N., 2013. Non-Hodgkin lymphoma and circulating markers of inflammation and adiposity in a nested case-control study: the multiethnic cohort. Cancer Epidemiol. Biomarkers Prev. 22 (3), 337–347.

Corren, J., 2012. Inhibition of interleukin-5 for the treatment of eosinophilic diseases. Discov. Med. 13 (71), 305–312.

Cragun, W.C., Yamshchikov, G.V., Bissonette, E.A., Smolkin, M.E., Eastham, S., Petroni, G.R., Schrecengost, R.S., Woodson, E.M., Slingluff Jr, C.L., 2005. Low-dose IL-2 induces cytokine cascade, eosinophilia, and a transient Th2 shift in melanoma patients. Cancer Immunol. Immunother. 54 (11), 1095–1105.

Demoulin, S., Roncarati, P., Delvenne, P., Hubert, P., 2012. Production of large numbers of plasmacytoid dendritic cells with functional activities from CD34(+) hematopoietic progenitor cells: use of interleukin-3. Exp. Hematol. 40 (4), 268–278.

Dentelli, P., Del Sorbo, L., Rosso, A., Molinar, A., Garbarino, G., Camussi, G., Pegoraro, L., Brizzi, M.F., 1999. Human IL-3 stimulates endothelial cell motility and promotes in vivo new vessel formation. J. Immunol. 163 (4), 2151–2159.

Deregibus, M.C., Cantaluppi, V., Doublier, S., Brizzi, M.F., Deambrosis, I., Albini, A., Camussi, G., 2002. HIV-1-Tat protein activates phosphatidylinositol 3-kinase/AKT-dependent survival pathways in Kaposi's sarcoma cells. J. Biol. Chem. 277 (28), 25195–25202.

Dippold, W.G., Klingel, R., Kerlin, M., Schwaeble, W., Meyer zum Büschenfelde, K.H., 1991. Stimulation of pancreas and gastric carcinoma cell growth by interleukin 3 and granulocyte-macrophage colony-stimulating factor. Gastroenterology 100 (5 Pt 1), 1338–1344.

Du, W., Li, X.E., Sipple, J., Pang, Q., 2011. Overexpression of IL-3Rα on CD34+CD38- stem cells defines leukemia-initiating cells in Fanconi anemia AML. Blood 117 (16), 4243–4252.

Du, X., Ho, M., Pastan, I., 2007. New immunotoxins targeting CD123, a stem cell antigen on acute myeloid leukemia cells. J. Immunother. 30 (6), 607–613.

Ehrlich, L.A., Chung, H.Y., Ghobrial, I., Choi, S.J., Morandi, F., Colla, S., Rizzoli, V., Roodman, G.D., Giuliani, N., 2005. IL-3 is a potential inhibitor of osteoblast differentiation in multiple myeloma. Blood 106 (4), 1407–1414.

Eiró, N., Fernandez-Garcia, B., González, L.O.,Vizoso, F.J., 2013. Cytokines related to MMP-11 expression by inflammatory cells and breast cancer metastasis. Oncoimmunology 2 (5), e24010.

Enewold, L., Mechanic, L.E., Bowman, E.D., Zheng,Y.L.,Yu, Z.,Trivers, G.,Alberg,A.J., Harris, C.C., 2009. Serum concentrations of cytokines and lung cancer survival in African Americans and Caucasians. Cancer Epidemiol. Biomarkers Prev. 18 (1), 215–222.

Farese,A.M.,Williams, D.E., Seiler, F.R., MacVittie,T.J., 1993. Combination protocols of cytokine therapy with interleukin-3 and granulocyte-macrophage colony-stimulating factor in a primate model of radiation-induced marrow aplasia. Blood 82 (10), 3012–3018.

Feuring-Buske, M., Frankel, A.E., Alexander, R.L., Gerhard, B., Hogge, D.E., 2002. A diphtheria toxin-interleukin 3 fusion protein is cytotoxic to primitive acute myeloid leukemia progenitors but spares normal progenitors. Cancer Res. 62 (6), 1730–1736.

Foster, P.S., Hogan, S.P., Ramsay, A.J., Matthaei, K.I.,Young, I.G., 1996. Interleukin 5 deficiency abolishes eosinophilia, airways hyperreactivity, and lung damage in a mouse asthma model. J. Exp. Med. 183, 195–201.

Frankel, A., Liu, J.S., Rizzieri, D., Hogge, D., 2008. Phase I clinical study of diphtheria toxin-interleukin 3 fusion protein in patients with acute myeloid leukemia and myelodysplasia. Leuk. Lymphoma 49 (3), 543–553.

Frankel,A.E., Baer, M.R., Hogge, D.E., Stuart, R.K., 2001. Immunotherapy of acute myeloid leukemia. Curr. Pharm. Biotechnol. 2 (3), 209–215.

Frankel, A.E., McCubrey, J.A., Miller, M.S., Delatte, S., Ramage, J., Kiser, M., Kucera, G.L., Alexander, R.L., Beran, M.,Tagge, E.P., Kreitman, R.J., Hogge, D.E., 2000. Diphtheria toxin fused to human interleukin-3 is toxic to blasts from patients with myeloid leukemias. Leukemia 14 (4), 576–585.

Fromm, J.R., Kussick, S.J., Wood, B.L., 2006. Identification and purification of classical Hodgkin cells from lymph nodes by flow cytometry and flow cytometric cell sorting. Am. J. Clin. Pathol. 126 (5), 764–780.

Fromm, J.R., Thomas, A., Wood, B.L., 2009. Flow cytometry can diagnose classical Hodgkin lymphoma in lymph nodes with high sensitivity and specificity.Am. J. Clin. Pathol. 131 (3), 322–332.

Fromm, J.R., 2011. Flow cytometric analysis of CD123 is useful for immunophenotyping classical Hodgkin lymphoma. Cytometry B Clin. Cytom. 80 (2), 91–99.

Gatault, S., Legrand, F., Delbeke, M., Loiseau, S., Capron, M., 2012. Involvement of eosinophils in the anti-tumor response. Cancer Immunol. Immunother. 61 (9), 1527–1534.

Geissler, K., Peschel, C., Niederwieser, D., Strobl, H., Goldschmitt, J., Ohler, L., Bettelheim, P., Kahls, P., Huber, C., Lechner, K., Höcker, P., Kolbe, K., 1996. Potentiation of granulocyte colony-stimulating factor-induced mobilization of circulating progenitor cells by seven-day pretreatment with interleukin-3. Blood 87 (7), 2732–2739.

Geissler, K.,Valent, P., Mayer, P., Liehl, E., Hinterberger,W., Lechner, K., Bettelheim, P., 1990. Recombinant human interleukin-3 expands the pool of circulating hematopoietic progenitor cells in primates–synergism with recombinant human granulocyte/macrophage colony-stimulating factor. Blood 75 (12), 2305–2310.

Gotoh, N.,Tojo,A., Shibuya, M., 1996.A novel pathway from phosphorylation of tyrosine residues 239/240 of Shc, contributing to suppress apoptosis by IL-3. EMBO J. 15 (22), 6197–6204.

Guillaume,T., Sekhavat, M., Rubinstein, D.B., Hamdan, O., Symann, M.L., 1993.Transcription of genes encoding granulocyte-macrophage colony-stimulating factor, interleukin 3, and interleukin 6 receptors and lack of proliferative response to exogenous cytokines in nonhematopoietic human malignant cell lines. Cancer Res. 53 (13), 3139–3144.

Gündogdu, M.S., Liu, H., Metzdorf, D., Hildebrand, D., Aigner, M., Aktories, K., Heeg, K., Kubatzky, K.F., 2010. The haematopoietic GTPase RhoH modulates IL3 signalling through regulation of STAT activity and IL3 receptor expression. Mol. Cancer 9, 225.

Gupta, N., Barhanpurkar, A.P., Tomar, G.B., Srivastava, R.K., Kour, S., Pote, S.T., Mishra, G.C., Wani, M.R., 2010. IL-3 inhibits human osteoclastogenesis and bone resorption through downregulation of c-Fms and diverts the cells to dendritic cell lineage. J. Immunol. 185 (4), 2261–2272.

Guthridge, M.A., Stomski, F.C., Thomas, D., 1998. Mechanism of activation of the GM-CSF-IL-3, and IL-5 family of receptors. Stem Cells 16, 301–313.

Hamelmann, E., Takeda, K., Schwarze, J., Vella, A.T., Irvin, C.G., Gelfand, E.W., 1999. Development of eosinophilic airway inflammation and airway hyperresponsiveness requires interleukin-5 but not immunoglobulin E or B lymphocytes. Am. J. Respir. Cell Mol. Biol. 21 (4), 480–489.

Hayashida, K., Kitamura, T., Gorman, D.M., Arai, K.-I., Yokota, T., Miyajima, A., 1990. Molecular cloning of a second subunit of the receptor for human granulocyte-macrophage colony-stimulating factor (GM-CSF): reconstitution of a high-affinity GM-CSF receptor. Proc. Natl. Acad. Sci. USA 87, 9655–9659.

Hennighausen, L., Robinson, G.W., 2008. Interpretation of cytokine signaling through the transcription factors STAT5A and STAT5B. Genes Dev. 22 (6), 711–721.

Hoffmann, T.K., Sonkoly, E., Homey, B., Scheckenbach, K., Gwosdz, C., Bas, M., Chaker, A., Schirlau, K., Whiteside, T.L., 2007. Aberrant cytokine expression in serum of patients with adenoid cystic carcinoma and squamous cell carcinoma of the head and neck. Head Neck 29 (5), 472–478.

Hogge, D.E., Feuring-Buske, M., Gerhard, B., Frankel, A.E., 2004. The efficacy of diphtheria-growth factor fusion proteins is enhanced by co-administration of cytosine arabinoside in an immunodeficient mouse model of human acute myeloid leukemia. Leuk. Res. 28 (11), 1221–1226.

Huston, M.M., Moore, J.P., Mettes, H.L., Tavana, G., Huston, D.P., 1996. Human B Cells express IL-5 receptor messenger ribonucleic acid and respond to IL-5 with enhanced IgM production after mitogenic stimulation with Moraxella catarrhalis. J. Immunol. 156, 1392–1401.

Ihle, J.N., Pepersack, L., Rebar, L., 1981. Regulation of T cell differentiation: in vitro induction of 20 alpha-hydroxysteroid dehydrogenase in splenic lymphocytes from athymic mice by a unique lymphokine. J. Immunol. 126 (6), 2184–2189.

Ikutani, M., Yanagibashi, T., Ogasawara, M., Tsuneyama, K., Yamamoto, S., Hattori, Y., Kouro, T., Itakura, A., Nagai, Y., Takaki, S., Takatsu, K., 2012. Identification of innate IL-5-producing cells and their role in lung eosinophil regulation and antitumor immunity. J. Immunol. 188 (2), 703–713.

Ilaria Jr, R.L., Van Etten, R.A., 1996. P210 and P190(BCR/ABL) induce the tyrosine phosphorylation and DNA binding activity of multiple specific STAT family members. J. Biol. Chem. 271 (49), 31704–31710.

Inagaki, A., Ishida, T., Ishii, T., Komatsu, H., Iida, S., Ding, J., Yonekura, K., Takeuchi, S., Takatsuka, Y., Utsunomiya, A., Ueda, R., 2006. Clinical significance of serum Th1-, Th2- and regulatory T cells-associated cytokines in adult T-cell leukemia/lymphoma: high interleukin-5 and -10 levels are significant unfavorable prognostic factors. Int. J. Cancer 118 (12), 3054–3061.

Itakura, A., Miura, Y., Hikasa, Y., Kiso, Y., Matsuda, H., 2001. Interleukin-3 and stem cell factor modulate cell cycle regulatory factors in mast cells: negative regulation of p27Kip1 in proliferation of mast cells induced by interleukin-3 but not stem cell factor. Exp. Hematol. 29, 803–811.

Izquierdo, M.A., Degen, D., Myers, L., Levitt, D.J., Von Hoff, D.D., 1995. Effects of the hematopoietic growth factors GM-CSF, IL-3, and IL-6 on human tumor colony-forming units taken directly from patients. Ann. Oncol. 6 (9), 927–932.

IL-3, IL-5, and Cancer **111**

Jin, L., Lee, E.M., Ramshaw, H.S., Busfield, S.J., Peoppl, A.G., Wilkinson, L., Guthridge, M.A., Thomas, D., Barry, E.F., Boyd, A., Gearing, D.P., Vairo, G., Lopez, A.F., Dick, J.E., Lock, R.B., 2009. Monoclonal antibody-mediated targeting of CD123, IL-3 receptor alpha chain, eliminates human acute myeloid leukemic stem cells. Cell Stem Cell. 5 (1), 31–42.

Jordan, C.T., Upchurch, D., Szilvassy, S.J., Guzman, M.L., Howard, D.S., Pettigrew, A.L., Meyerrose, T., Rossi, R., Grimes, B., Rizzieri, D.A., Luger, S.M., Phillips, G.L., 2000. The interleukin-3 receptor alpha chain is a unique marker for human acute myelogenous leukemia stem cells. Leukemia 14 (10), 1777–1784.

Karmali, R., Paganessi, L.A., Frank, R.R., Jagan, S., Larson, M.L., Venugopal, P., Gregory, S.A., Christopherson 2nd, K.W., 2013. Aggressive disease defined by cytogenetics is associated with cytokine dysregulation in CLL/SLL patients. J. Leukoc. Biol. 93 (1), 161–170.

Kato, H., Kohata, K., Yamamoto, J., Ichikawa, S., Watanabe, M., Ishizawa, K., Ichinohasama, R., Harigae, H., 2010. Extreme eosinophilia caused by interleukin-5-producing disseminated colon cancer. Int. J. Hematol. 91 (2), 328–330.

Kim, H.P., Frankel, A.E., Hogge, D.E., 2010. A diphtheria toxin interleukin-3 fusion protein synergizes with tyrosine kinase inhibitors in killing leukemic progenitors from BCR/ABL positive acute leukemia. Leuk. Res. 34 (8), 1035–1042.

Kimura, T., Mukai, M., Kaneko, Y., Hirakata, M., Okamoto, S., Sakamoto, M., Okada, Y., Ikeda, Y., 2006. Unusual hemangioendothelioma of the liver with epithelioid morphology associated with marked eosinophilia: autopsy case. Pathol Int. 56 (11), 694–701.

Kinashi, T., Inaba, K., Tsubata, T., Tashiro, K., Palacios, R., Honjo, T., 1988. Differentiation of an interleukin 3-dependent precursor B-cell clone into immunoglobulin-producing cells in vitro. Proc. Natl. Acad. Sci. USA 85, 4473–4477.

Kinoshita, T., Yokota, T., Arai, K., Miyajima, A., 1995. Suppression of apoptotic death in hematopoietic cells by signalling through the IL-3/GM-CSF receptors. EMBO J. 14 (2), 266–275.

Kitamura, T., Sato, N., Arai K-, I., Miyajima, A., 1991. Expression cloning of the human IL-3 receptor cDNA reveals a shared β subunit for the human IL-3 and GM-CSF receptors. Cell 66, 1165–1174.

Kopf, M., Brombacher, F., Hodgkin, P.D., Ramsay, A.J., Milbourne, E.A., Dai, W.J., Ovington, K.S., Behm, C.A., Kohler, G., Young, I.G., Matthaei, K.I., 1996. IL-5 deficient mice have a developmental defect in CD5z B-1 cells and lack eosinophilia but have normal antibody and cytotoxic T cell responses. Immunity 4, 15–24.

Korpelainen, E.I., Gamble, J.R., Smith, W.B., Dottore, M., Vadas, M.A., Lopez, A.F., 1995. Interferon-gamma upregulates interleukin-3 (IL-3) receptor expression in human endothelial cells and synergizes with IL-3 in stimulating major histocompatibility complex class II expression and cytokine production. Blood 86 (1), 176–182.

Korpelainen, E.I., Gamble, J.R., Smith, W.B., Goodall, G.J., Qiyu, S., Woodcock, J.M., Dottore, M., Vadas, M.A., Lopez, A.F., 1993. The receptor for interleukin 3 is selectively induced in human endothelial cells by tumor necrosis factor alpha and potentiates interleukin 8 secretion and neutrophil transmigration. Proc. Natl. Acad. Sci. USA 90 (23), 11137–11141.

Korpelainen, E.I., Gamble, J.R., Vadas, M.A., Lopez, A.F., 1996. IL-3 receptor expression, regulation and function in cells of the vasculature. Immunol. Cell Biol. 74 (1), 1–7.

Kuraoka, M., Hashiguchi, M., Hachimura, S., Kaminogawa, S., 2004. CD4(-)c-kit(-)CD3epsilon(-)IL-2Ralpha(+) Peyer's patch cells are a novel cell subset which secrete IL-5 in response to IL-2: implications for their role in IgA production. Eur. J. Immunol. 34 (7), 1920–1929.

Lampinen, M., Carlson, M., Hakansson, L.D., Venge, P., 2004. Cytokine-regulated accumulation of eosinophils in inflammatory disease. Allergy 59, 793–805.

Le Beau, M.M., Lemons, R.S., Espinosa 3rd, R., Larson, R.A., Arai, N., Rowley, J.D., 1989. Interleukin-4 and interleukin-5 map to human chromosome 5 in a region encoding growth factors and receptors and are deleted in myeloid leukemias with a del(5q). Blood 73 (3), 647–650.

Lemoli, R.M., Rosti, G., Visani, G., Gherlinzoni, F., Miggiano, M.C., Fortuna, A., Zinzani, P., Tura, S., 1996. Concomitant and sequential administration of recombinant human granulocyte colony-stimulating factor and recombinant human interleukin-3 to accelerate hematopoietic recovery after autologous bone marrow transplantation for malignant lymphoma. J. Clin. Oncol. 14 (11), 3018–3025.

Lindemann, A., Mertelsmann, R., 1993. Interleukin-3: structure and function. Cancer Invest. 11 (5), 609–623.

Liu, C.M., Ko, J.J., Shun, C.T., Hsiao, T.Y., Sheen, T.S., 2001. Soluble adhesion molecules and cytokines in tumor-associated tissue eosinophilia of nasopharyngeal carcinoma. Acta Otolaryngol. 121 (4), 534–538.

Lopes, C.O., Callera, F., 2012. Three-dimensional conformal radiotherapy in prostate cancer patients: rise in interleukin 6 (IL-6) but not IL-2, IL-4, IL-5, tumor necrosis factor-α, MIP-1-α, and LIF levels. Int. J. Radiat. Oncol. Biol. Phys. 82 (4), 1385–1388.

Lotem, J., Sachs, L., 1992. Hematopoietic cytokines inhibit apoptosis induced by transforming growth factor beta 1 and cancer chemotherapy compounds in myeloid leukemic cells. Blood 80 (7), 1750–1757.

Lu, K., Feng, X., Deng, Q., Sheng, L., Liu, P., Xu, S., Su, D., 2012. Prognostic role of serum cytokines in patients with nasopharyngeal carcinoma. Onkologie 35 (9), 494–498.

Matsunaga, T., Sato, T., Iyama, S., Tanaka, S., Murase, K., Sato, Y., Kobune, M., Takimoto, R., Kato, J., Kuroda, H., Niitsu, Y., 2006. Peripheral T-cell lymphoma presenting with eosinophilia due to interleukin-5 produced by lymphoma cells. Rinsho Ketsueki 47 (11), 1457–1462.

McNiece, I.K., McGrath, H.E., Quesenberry, P.J., 1988. Granulocyte colony-stimulating factor augments in vitro megakaryocyte colony formation by interleukin-3. Exp. Hematol. 16 (9), 807–810.

Miyajima, A., Kitamura, T., Harada, N., Yokota, T., Arai, K., 1992. Cytokine receptors and signal transduction. Annu. Rev. Immunol. 10, 295–331.

Mroczko, B., Ławicki, S., Szmitkowski, M., Czygier, M., Okulczyk, B., Piotrowski, Z., 2003. Selected hematopoietic cytokines in patients with colorectal cancer. Pol. Merkuriuzs Lek. 15 (89), 416–419.

Mroczko, B., Szmitkowski, M., Wereszczyńska-Siemiatkowska, U., Jurkowska, G., 2005a. Hematopoietic cytokines in the sera of patients with pancreatic cancer. Clin. Chem. Lab. Med. 43 (2), 146–150.

Mroczko, B., Szmitkowski, M., Wereszczyńska-Siemiatkowska, U., Okulczyk, B., 2005b. Stem cell factor (SCF) and interleukin 3 (IL-3) in the sera of patients with colorectal cancer. Dig. Dis. Sci. 50 (6), 1019–1024.

Mroczko, B., Szmitkowski, M., Wereszczyńska-Siemiatkowska, U., Okulczyk, B., Kedra, B., 2007. Pretreatment serum levels of hematopoietic cytokines in patients with colorectal adenomas and cancer. Int. J. Colorectal Dis. 22 (1), 33–38.

Mui, A.L., Wakao, H., O'Farrell, A.M., Harada, N., Miyajima, A., 1995. Interleukin-3, granulocyte-macrophage colony stimulating factor and interleukin-5 transduce signals through two STAT5 homologs. EMBO J. 14 (6), 1166–1175.

Muñoz, L., Nomdedéu, J.F., López, O., Carnicer, M.J., Bellido, M., Aventín, A., Brunet, S., Sierra, J., 2001. Interleukin-3 receptor alpha chain (CD123) is widely expressed in hematologic malignancies. Haematologica 86 (12), 1261–1269.

Nakase, K., Kita, K., Miwa, H., Nishii, K., Shikami, M., Tanaka, I., Tsutani, H., Ueda, T., Nasu, K., Kyo, T., Dohy, H., Shiku, H., Katayama, N., 2007. Clinical and prognostic significance of cytokine receptor expression in adult acute lymphoblastic leukemia: interleukin-2 receptor alpha-chain predicts a poor prognosis. Leukemia 21 (2), 326–332.

Nishii, K., Katayama, N., Miwa, H., Shikami, M., Masuya, M., Shiku, H., Kita, K., 1999. Survival of human leukemic B-cell precursors is supported by stromal cells and cytokines: association with the expression of bcl-2 protein. Br. J. Haematol. 105, 701–710.

Nosaka, T., Kawashima, T., Misawa, K., Ikuta, K., Mui, A.L., Kitamura, T., 1999. STAT5 as a molecular regulator of proliferation, differentiation and apoptosis in hematopoietic cells. EMBO J. 18 (17), 4754–4765.

Ochiai, K., Kagami, M., Matsumura, R., Romioka, H., 1997. IL-5 but not interferon-gamma (IFN-gamma) inhibits eosinophil apoptosis by up-regulation of bcl-2 expression. Clin. Exp. Immunol. 107, 198–204.

Padron, E., Painter, J.S., Kunigal, S., Mailloux, A.W., McGraw, K., McDaniel, J.M., Kim, E., Bebbington, C., Baer, M., Yarranton, G., Lancet, J., Komrokji, R.S., Abdel-Wahab, O., List, A.F., Epling-Burnette, P.K., 2013. GM-CSF-dependent pSTAT5 sensitivity is a feature with therapeutic potential in chronic myelomonocytic leukemia. Blood 121 (25), 5068–5077.

Pandit, R., Scholnik, A., Wulfekuhler, L., Dimitrov, N., 2007. Non-small cell lung cancer associated with excessive eosinophilia and secretion of interleukin-5 as a paraneoplastic syndrome. Am. J. Hematol. 82, 234–237.

Paquette, R.L., Zhou, J.Y., Yang, Y.C., Clark, S.C., Koeffler, H.P., 1988. Recombinant gibbon interleukin-3 acts synergistically with recombinant human G-CSF and GM-CSF in vitro. Blood 71 (6), 1596–1600.

Park, L., Waldron, P.E., Friend, D., Sassenfeld, H.M., Price, V., Anderson, D., Cosman, D., Andrews, R.G., Bernstein, I.D., Urdal, D.L., 1989. Interleukin-3, GMCSF and G-CSF receptor expression on cell lines and primary leukemia cells: receptor heterogeneity and relationship to growth factor responsiveness. Blood 74, 56–65.

Pazdrak, K., Schreiber, D., Forsythe, P., Justement, L., Alam, R., 1995. The intracellular signal transduction mechanism of interleukin 5 in eosinophils: the involvement of lyn tyrosine kinase and the Ras-Raf-1-MEK-microtubule-associated protein kinase pathway. J. Exp. Med. 181 (5), 1827–1834.

Pedrazzoli, P., Bacciocchi, G., Bergamaschi, G., Cazzola, M., Danova, M., Gibelli, N., Giordano, M., Lazzaro, A., Locatelli, F., Pavesi, L., 1994. Effects of granulocyte-macrophage colony-stimulating factor and interleukin-3 on small cell lung cancer cells. Cancer Invest. 12 (3), 283–288.

Phillips, C., Coward, W.R., Pritchard, D.I., Hewitt, C.R., 2003. Basophils express a type 2 cytokine profile on exposure to proteases from helminthes and house dust mites. J. Leukoc. Biol. 73, 165–171.

Reddy, E.P., Korapati, A., Chaturvedi, P., Rane, S., 2000. IL-3 signaling and the role of Src kinases, JAKs and STATs: a covert liaison unveiled. Oncogene 19 (21), 2532–2547.

Rivoltini, L., Viggiano, V., Spinazzè, S., Santoro, A., Colombo, M.P., Takatsu, K., Parmiani, G., 1993. In vitro anti-tumor activity of eosinophils from cancer patients treated with subcutaneous administration of interleukin 2. Role of interleukin 5. Int. J. Cancer 54 (1), 8–15.

Romashkova, J.A., Makarov, S.S., 1999. NF-kappaB is a target of AKT in anti-apoptotic PDGF signalling. Nature 401 (6748), 86–90.

Sakuishi, K., Oki, S., Araki, M., Porcelli, S.A., Miyake, S., Yamamura, T., 2007. Invariant NKT cells biased for IL-5 production act as crucial regulators of inflammation. J. Immunol. 179, 3452–3462.

Sasaki, H., Schmitt, D.A., Hayashi, Y., Pollard, R.B., Suzuki, F., 1992. Inhibition of tumor growth by the intralesional administration of interleukin-3 into mice implanted with solid tumors. Anticancer Res. 12 (2), 313–315.

Sato, S., Katagiri, T., Takaki, S., Kikuchi, Y., Hitoshi, Y., Yonehara, S., Tsukada, S., Kitamura, D., Watanabe, T., Witte, O., Takatsu, K., 1994. IL-5 receptor-mediated tyrosine phosphorylation of SH2/SH3-containing proteins and activation of Bruton's tyrosine and Janus 2 kinases. J. Exp. Med. 180 (6), 2101–2111.

Satyam, A., Singh, P., Badjatia, N., Seth, A., Sharma, A., 2011. A disproportion of TH1/TH2 cytokines with predominance of TH2, in urothelial carcinoma of bladder. Urol. Oncol. 29 (1), 58–65.

Schimpl, A., Wecker, E., 1972. Replacement of T-cell function by a T-cell product. Nat. New Biol. 237 (70), 15–17.

Schrader, J.W., 1998. Interleukin-3. In: Thomson, A. (Ed.), The Cytokine Handbook, third ed. Academic Press, San Diego, pp. 105–132.

Sehmi, R., Wood, L.J., Watson, R., Foley, R., Hamid, Q., O'Byrne, P.M., Denburg, J.A., 1997. Allergen-induced increases in IL-5 receptor alpha-subunit expression on bone marrow-derived CD34+ cells from asthmatic subjects. A novel marker of progenitor cell commitment towards eosinophilic differentiation. J. Clin. Invest. 100, 2466–2475.

Shinjyo, T., Kuribara, R., Inukai, T., Hosoi, H., Kinoshita, T., Miyajima, A., Houghton, P.J., Look, A.T., Ozawa, K., Inaba, T., 2001. Downregulation of Bim, a proapoptotic relative of Bcl-2, is a pivotal step in cytokine-initiated survival signaling in murine hematopoietic progenitors. Mol. Cell Biol. 21 (3), 854–864.

Sieff, C.A., Niemeyer, C.M., Nathan, D.G., Ekern, S.C., Bieber, F.R., Yang, Y.C., Wong, G., Clark, S.C., 1987. Stimulation of human hematopoietic colony formation by recombinant gibbon multi-colony-stimulating factor or interleukin 3. J. Clin. Invest. 80 (3), 818–823.

Stein, C., Kellner, C., Kügler, M., Reiff, N., Mentz, K., Schwenkert, M., Stockmeyer, B., Mackensen, A., Fey, G.H., 2010. Novel conjugates of single-chain Fv antibody fragments specific for stem cell antigen CD123 mediate potent death of acute myeloid leukaemia cells. Br. J. Haematol. 148 (6), 879–889.

Su, C., Zhou, C., Zhou, S., Xu, J., 2011. Serum cytokine levels in patients with advanced non-small cell lung cancer: correlation with treatment response and survival. Med. Oncol. 28 (4), 1453–1457.

Suzuki, H., Katayama, N., Ikuta, Y., Mukai, K., Fujieda, A., Mitani, H., Araki, H., Miyashita, H., Hoshino, N., Nishikawa, H., Nishii, K., Minami, N., Shiku, H., 2004. Activities of granulocyte-macrophage colony-stimulating factor and interleukin-3 on monocytes. Am. J. Hematol. 75, 179–189.

Takaki, S., Tominaga, A., Hitoshi, Y., Mita, S., Sonoda, E., Yamaguchi, N., Takatsu, K., 1990. Molecular cloning and expression of the murine interleukin-5 receptor. EMBO J. 9 (13), 4367–4374.

Takatsu, K., Nakajima, H., 2008. IL-5 and eosinophilia. Curr. Opin. Immunol. 20 (3), 288–294.

Takatsu, K., Takaki, S., Hitoshi, Y., 1994. Interleukin-5 and its receptor system: implications in the immune system and inflammation. Adv. Immunol. 57, 145–190.

Takatsu, K., Tominaga, A., Harada, N., Mita, S., Matsumoto, M., Takahashi, T., Kikuchi, Y., Yamaguchi, N., 1988. T cell-replacing factor (TRF)/interleukin 5 (IL-5): molecular and functional properties. Immunol. Rev. 102, 107–135.

Takatsu, K., 2011. Interleukin-5 and IL-5 receptor in health and diseases. Proc. Jpn. Acad. Ser. B Phys. Biol. Sci. 87 (8), 463–485.

Tao, W.J., Lin, H., Sun, T., Samanta, A.K., Arlinghaus, R., 2008. BCR-ABL oncogenic transformation of NIH 3T3 fibroblasts requires the IL-3 receptor. Oncogene 27 (22), 3194–3200.

Teruya-Feldstein, J., Tosato, G., Jaffe, E.S., 2000. The role of chemokines in Hodgkin's disease. Leuk. Lymphoma 38 (3–4), 363–371.

Testa, U., Riccioni, R., Militi, S., Coccia, E., Stellacci, E., Samoggia, P., Latagliata, R., Mariani, G., Rossini, A., Battistini, A., Lo-Coco, F., Peschle, C., 2002. Elevated expression of IL-3Ralpha in acute myelogenous leukemia is associated with enhanced blast proliferation, increased cellularity, and poor prognosis. Blood 100 (8), 2980–2988.

Thielen, C., Radermacher, V., Trimeche, M., Roufosse, F., Goldman, M., Boniver, J., de Leval, L., 2008. TARC and IL-5 expression correlates with tissue eosinophilia in peripheral T-cell lymphomas. Leuk. Res. 32 (9), 1431–1438.

Tomaki, M., Zhao, L.L., Lundahl, J., Sjöstrand, M., Jordana, M., Lindén, A., O'Byrne, P., Lötvall, J., 2000. Eosinophilopoiesis in a murine model of allergic airway eosinophilia: involvement of bone marrow IL-5 and IL-5 receptor alpha. J. Immunol. 165 (7), 4040–4050.

Tominaga, A., Takaki, S., Koyama, N., Katoh, S., Matsumoto, R., Migita, M., Hitoshi, Y., Hosoya, Y., Yamauchi, S., Kanai, Y., Miyazaki, J.I., Usuku, G., Yamamura, K.I., Takatsu, K., 1991. Transgenic mice expressing a B cell growth and differentiation factor gene (interleukin 5) develop eosinophilia and autoantibody production. J. Exp. Med. 173 (2), 429–437.

Tomova, R., Pomakov, J., Jacobs, J.J., Adjarov, D., Popova, S., Altankova, I., Den Otter, W., Krastev, Z., 2006. Changes in cytokine profile during local IL-2 therapy in cancer patients. Anticancer Res. 26 (3A), 2037–2047.

Trentin, L., Zambello, R., Agostini, C., Enthammer, C., Cerruti, A., Adami, F., Zamboni, S., Semenzato, G., 1994. Expression and regulation of tumor necrosis factor, interleukin-2, and hematopoietic growth factor receptors in B-cell chronic lymphocytic leukemia. Blood 84, 4249–4256.

Uckun, F.M., Gesner, T.G., Song, C.W., Mayers, D.E., Mufson, A., 1989. Leukemic B-cell precursors express functional receptors for human interleukin-3. Blood 73, 533–542.

Ulich, T.R., del Castillo, J., McNiece, I.K., Yin, S.M., Irwin, B., Busser, K., Guo, K.Z., 1990. Acute and subacute hematologic effects of multi-colony stimulating factor in combination with granulocyte colony-stimulating factor in vivo. Blood 75 (1), 48–53.

Van Etten, R.A., 2007. Aberrant cytokine signaling in leukemia. Oncogene 26 (47), 6738–6749.

Vasiliades, G., Kopanakis, N., Vasiloglou, M., Zografos, G., Margaris, H., Masselou, K., Kokosi, E., Liakakos, T., 2012. Role of the hematopoietic cytokines SCF, IL-3, GM-CSF and M-CSF in the diagnosis of pancreatic and ampullary cancer. Int. J. Biol. Markers 27 (3), e186–e194.

Vellenga, E., Biesma, B., Meyer, C., Wagteveld, L., Esselink, M., de Vries, E.G., 1991. The effects of five hematopoietic growth factors on human small cell lung carcinoma cell lines: interleukin 3 enhances the proliferation in one of the eleven cell lines. Cancer Res. 51 (1), 73–76.

Walter, R., Joller-Jemelka, H.I., Salomon, F., 2002. Metastatic squamous cell carcinoma with marked blood eosinophilia and elevated serum interleukin-5 levels. Exp. Hematol. 30 (1), 1–2.

Wang, J.L., Bi, Z., Zou, J.W., Gu, X.M., 2012. Combination therapy with lentinan improves outcomes in patients with esophageal carcinoma. Mol. Med. Rep. 5 (3), 745–748.

Winton, E.F., Srinivasiah, J., Kim, B.K., Hillyer, C.D., Strobert, E.A., Orkin, J.L., Swenson, R.B., McClure, H.M., Myers, L.A., Saral, R., 1994. Effect of recombinant human interleukin-6 (rhIL-6) and rhIL-3 on hematopoietic regeneration as demonstrated in a non-human primate chemotherapy model. Blood 84 (1), 65–73.

Yamada, M., Suzu, S., Tanaka-Douzono, M., Wakimoto, N., Hatake, K., Hayasawa, H., Motoyoshi, K., 2000. Effect of cytokines on the proliferation/differentiation of stroma-initiating cells. J. Cell. Physiol. 184, 351–355.

Yamazaki, H., Inoue, T., Tanaka, E., Isohashi, F., Koizumi, M., Shuo, X., Nakamura, H., Inoue, T., Aug 2005. Pelvic irradiation-induced eosinophilia is correlated to prognosis of cervical cancer patients and transient elevation of serum interleukin 5 level. Radiat. Med. 23 (5), 317–321.

Younes, A., Drach, J., Katz, R., Jendiroba, D., Sabourian, M.H., Sarris, A.H., Swan Jr, F., Hill, D., Cabanillas, F., Ford, R., 1994. Growth inhibition of follicular small-cleaved-cell lymphoma cells in short-term culture by interleukin-3. Ann. Oncol. 5, 265–268.

Yousefi, S., Hoessli, D.C., Blaser, K., Mills, G.B., Simon, H.U., 1996. Requirement of Lyn and Syk tyrosine kinases for the prevention of apoptosis by cytokines in human eosinophils. J. Exp. Med. 183 (4), 1407–1414.

Yu, H., Jove, R., 2004. The STATs of cancer–new molecular targets come of age. Nat. Rev. Cancer 4 (2), 97–105.

Zabransky, D.J., Smith, H.A., Thoburn, C.J., Zahurak, M., Keizman, D., Carducci, M., Eisenberger, M.A., McNeel, D.G., Drake, C.G., Antonarakis, E.S., 2012. Lenalidomide modulates IL-8 and anti-prostate antibody levels in men with biochemically recurrent prostate cancer. Prostate 72 (5), 487–498.

Zhang, L., Sun, S.K., Shi, L.X., Zhang, X., 2010. Serum cytokine profiling of prostate cancer and benign prostatic hyperplasia using recombinant antibody microarray. Zhonghua Nan Ke Xue 16 (7), 584–588.

Zhu, X., Ying, L.S., Xu, S.H., Zhu, C.H., Xie, J.B., 2010. Clinicopathologic and prognostic significance of serum levels of cytokines in patients with advanced serous ovarian cancer prior to surgery. Zhonghua Bing Li Xue Za Zhi 39 (10), 666–670.

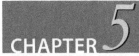

CHAPTER 5

IL-6 Family and Cancer

Medicine is not only a science; it is also an art. It does not consist of compounding pills and plasters; it deals with the very processes of life, which must be understood before they may be guided.

Paracelsus, Swiss German Physician (1493–1541)

5.1 INTERLEUKIN-6

5.1.1 Overview

Interleukin (IL)-6 is a 28 kDa glycoprotein with a molecular weight of 184 amino acids, composed of four α-helices arranged in an up–up–down–down topology. It was first cloned by Hiran et al. (1986) and initially designated B-cell differentiation factor because of the ability to stimulate the final maturation of B cells into immunoglobulin-secreting cells.

IL-6 is produced by T cells, B cells, macrophages, neutrophils, monocytes, keratinocytes, fibroblasts, endothelial cells, epithelial cells, osteoblasts, chondrocytes, adipocytes, and mesangial cells. The expression of the *IL-6* gene is driven by inflammatory response, which in turn is triggered by interferons (IFNs), tumor necrosis factor (TNF), IL-1, and bacterial lipopolysaccharide (LPS) and endotoxin.

IL-6 is a pleiotropic cytokine, possessing a wide range of functions depending on the expressing tissue and condition. In general, IL-6 promotes the differentiation of Th2 and Th17 cells, while it suppresses the generation of Treg cells. This cytokine is involved in the development of chronic inflammation, antigen-specific immune responses, and regulation of host defense mechanisms. In particular, IL-6 has strong pyrogenic activity and is involved in the expression and release of acute phase proteins in liver tissue. In addition, it also plays a role in hematopoiesis through the upregulation of VEGF and IL-3-mediated formation of blast cell colonies.

Multiple studies demonstrated a relationship between IL-6 and angiogenesis through the upregulation of vascular endothelial growth factor (VEGF) in various solid malignancies (reviewed by Middleton et al. (2014)). Differentiation of myeloid cells, macrophages, T lymphocytes, and megakaryocytes is also under control of IL-6 (Hassan and Drexler, 1995; Heike and Nakahate, 2002; Neurath and Finotto, 2011).

Interleukins in Cancer Biology
http://dx.doi.org/10.1016/B978-0-12-801121-8.00005-1

In epithelial cells, IL-6 promotes cell proliferation, whereas in endothelial cells it activates molecules of cell adhesion. In bone, IL-6 was reported to promote osteoclast formation and contribute to bone resorption. Finally, IL-6 is a maturing agent and stimulatory factor for many cells, including lymphocytes and hepatocytes. Differentiation of B cells into antibody-secreting plasma cells is also affected by this cytokine (reviewed by Neurath and Finotto (2011)).

It is also necessary to mention the role of IL-6 in skeletal muscle, which is the major source of this cytokine. Recent studies showed that IL-6 is involved in the regulation of adult skeletal muscle growth and regeneration; moreover, it acts as antiinflammatory myokine in contrast to its proinflammatory functions in other tissues. Functional studies have revealed that IL-6 triggers the proliferation of muscle stem cells; on the other hand, it can also modulate muscle atrophy under certain conditions as well (reviewed by Muñoz-Cánoves et al. (2013)).

Considering the influence of IL-6 on diseases, this cytokine has been associated with arthritis (Swaak et al., 1988), hepatic lipid metabolic disorders (Hassan et al., 2014), systemic sclerosis (Muangchan and Pope, 2012), coronary heart disease (Hingorani et al., 2012), asthma (DiCosmo et al., 1994; Tsuchiya et al., 2010), inflammatory bowel disease (Mitsuyama et al., 2006; Mudter and Neurath, 2007), acquired immune deficiency syndrome (Breen et al., 1990), and neurodegenerative diseases (Spooren et al., 2011; Koziorowski et al., 2012).

5.1.2 Role of IL-6 in Tumorigenesis

Aberrant IL-6 pathways were observed in numerous cancers. Overexpression of IL-6 serum levels as well as mRNA and protein levels were found increased in patients with Burkitt lymphoma (Aka et al., 2014), multiple myeloma (Alexandrakis et al., 2004), ovarian cancer (Berek et al., 1991), endometrial cancer (Bellone et al., 2005), lung cancer (Songür et al., 2004), and esophageal carcinoma (Oka et al., 1996; Wang et al., 1999; Krzystek-Korpacka et al., 2008; Fujiwara et al., 2011).

High IL-6 levels have been repeatedly associated with poor prognosis in patients with breast cancer (Bachelot et al., 2003; Cho et al., 2013), gastric cancer (Ashizawa et al., 2005; Liao et al., 2008; Ikeguchi et al., 2009; Necula et al., 2012), advanced esophageal squamous cell carcinoma (Chen et al., 2013a; Yoneda et al., 2013), renal cell carcinoma (Ljungberg et al., 1997), colorectal cancer (Belluco et al., 2000; Shimazaki et al., 2013), bladder cancer (Chen et al., 2013b), oral squamous cell carcinoma (Chen et al., 2012), lung cancer (Ujiie et al., 2012), chronic lymphocytic leukemia (Yoon et al., 2012), advanced pancreatic cancer (Mitsunaga et al., 2013) and hepatocellular carcinoma (Porta et al., 2008; Pang et al., 2011; Jang et al., 2012; Aleksandrova et al., 2014).

Several groups reported that the reduction in IL-6 levels correlated with better response to anticancer therapy (Plante et al., 1994; Zhang and Adachi, 1999).

Multiple studies demonstrated direct effect of IL-6 on tumorigenesis. The involvement of this cytokine in cancer development has been shown in vitro and in vivo, in models of colon cancer (Foran et al., 2010), multiple myeloma (Ishikawa et al., 2005; Rutsch et al., 2010), ovarian cancer (Huang et al., 2000; Rosen et al., 2006), prostate cancer (Qiu et al., 1998; Rojas et al., 2011), lung cancer (Gao et al., 2007), breast cancer (Sansone et al., 2007; Lesile et al., 2010), bladder cancer (Okamoto et al., 1995; Neiva et al., 2014), oral squamous cell carcinoma (Chuang et al., 2014), glioma (Cui et al., 2014), hepatocellular carcinoma (He et al., 2013), melanoma (Valles et al., 2013), pancreatic cancer (Zhang et al., 2013a), nasopharyngeal cancer (Zhang et al., 2013b), and head and neck cancers (Yadav et al., 2011).

Several molecular mechanisms are proposed to be culprits for IL-6-driven carcinogenesis (Figure 5.1). It is known that this cytokine triggers Janus kinase (JAK)/Signal transducer and activator of transcription (STAT3), Phosphoinositide 3-kinase (PI3K)/Akt, and Ras, three main signaling pathways

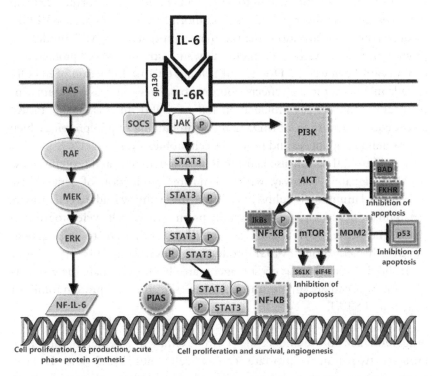

Figure 5.1 IL-6 signaling pathways. (For color version of this figure, the reader is referred to the online version of this book.)

involved in tumor development. Activation of these pathways by IL-6 leads to the promotion of invasion and migration of tumor cells, angiogenesis, antiapoptotic activity, and increased cell proliferation (reviewed by Ataie-Kachoie et al. (2013a)).

It is widely known that STAT3 is involved in tumorigenesis, as this transcription factor has been found activated in a variety of human cancers and human tumor cell lines. In particular, STAT3 has been repeatedly associated with inflammation, cell proliferation and survival, prometastatic activities, and angiogenesis (reviewed by Siveen et al. (2014)).

Aberrant activation of PI3K/Akt pathway occurs more frequently than any other pathway in patients with cancer (Bellacosa et al., 2005). Through the activation of the PI3K/Akt pathway, IL-6 promotes inhibition of apoptosis, angiogenesis, and cell proliferation and survival. These effects are due to IL-6-driven activation of mammalian target of rapamycin (mTOR), nuclear factor kappaB (NF-κB), and Mouse double minute 2 homolog (MDM2), and suppression of proapoptotic proteins Bcl-2-associated death promoter (BAD) and FKHR. NF-κB has an essential role in tumor biology. On the one hand, it stimulates the immune system to target and eliminate transformed cells; on the other hand, however, it exhibits protumorigenic activities, such as VEGF-mediated neovascularization, matrix metalloproteinase (MMP)-modulated promotion of cell invasiveness and motility, and activation of cell proliferation and survival (reviewed by Hoesel and Schmid (2013)). Induction of mTOR cascade inhibits autophagy, affects ribosome biogenesis, increases protein synthesis, and stimulates cell proliferation and survival (Kim et al., 2002). PI3K/Akt-mediated activation of MDM2 results in binding of p53 protein, which in turn inhibits apoptosis and promotes cell proliferation.

In addition, IL-6 can also activate Ras/mitogen-activated protein kinase (MAPK) signaling pathway, which stimulates production of acute phase proteins and immunoglobulins. In addition, this pathway leads to cell growth, differentiation, and survival through the promotion of cell cycle progression (Shaul and Seger, 2007). Also, Ras/MAPK pathway leads to angiogenesis through the activation of VEGF production (Slevin et al., 2000).

It should be noted that certain agents are able to terminate these signaling pathways, namely, suppressor of cytokine signaling and protein inhibitor of activated STAT.

Substantial evidence has been obtained that IL-6 may have an impact on drug resistance. Borsellino et al. (1995) examined whether or not IL-6 protects two human prostate cancer cell lines PC-3 and DU145 from programmed death induced by chemotherapy drugs *cis*-diamminedichloroplatinum, etoposide, and adriamycin. The authors found that the presence of IL-6 in cell line markedly restricts the cytotoxic effect of *cis*-diamminedichloroplatinum and etoposide; in addition, the neutralization of IL-6 sensitized the cells to cytotoxicity. In accordance with previous report, Mizutani et al. (1995) showed that either anti-IL-6 monoclonal antibody or anti-IL-6 receptor (IL-6R) monoclonal antibody enhances the sensitization of human renal cell carcinoma cell line to *cis*-diamminedichloroplatinum. A series of studies by Seiden group showed that the production of IL-6 in ovarian cancer cell lines plays a pivotal role against chemotherapy drug paclitaxel (Duan et al., 1999; Penson et al., 2000). Similarly, Conze et al. (2001) demonstrated that multidrug-resistant breast cancer cell line MCF7/ADR produces high levels of IL-6 as compared to conventional breast cancer cell line MCF7. It was also observed that pretreatment of MCF7 cells with IL-6 resulted in 8- to 10-fold increase in resistance to doxorubicin, clearly showing that IL-6 confers drug resistance. Additionally, the authors showed that the observed drug resistance correlates with IL-6-driven activation of C/EBP family of transcription factors. Finally, Pu et al. (2004) showed that IL-6 acts as a survival factor against β-lapachone-induced apoptosis in PC-3 prostate cancer cell line.

A study by Kottke et al. (2013) contains a new and important insight on the role of IL-6 in cancer immunity. The authors aimed to examine whether or not certain proinflammatory cytokines are associated with development of tumor recurrence from dormancy. The production of cytokines was analyzed in mice inoculated with B-16 Ova melanoma cell lines, apparently cured by various therapies, including chemotherapy, virotherapy, immunotherapy, or T cell therapy. All mice were divided into three groups, namely, those in which recurrences were not observant, those that were just developing recurrences, and those that had fully established recurrences. Strikingly, IL-6 serum levels were only present in mice with palpable recurrences at an early stage (<0.2 cm), but neither at later stages (>0.5 cm) nor in mice with tumor recurrence at all. These findings suggest that IL-6 may be used as a valuable marker of a stage at which a dormant tumor is starting to expand and recur. The authors hypothesized that this observation can promote the development of newer screening methods for minimal residual disease diagnosis and evaluating the risk of cancer recurrence.

Another interesting study was performed by Brighenti et al. (2014), who revealed that IL-6 markedly downregulated the expression and activity of p53 in human hepatocellular carcinoma cell line HepG2. The authors showed that the observed effect was due to IL-6-driven stimulation of rRNA transcription, which resulted in a significant reduction in the availability of ribosomal proteins for the binding to MDM2, thereby enhancing the MDM2-dependent proteasomal digestion of p53; hence, IL-6 exhibited a marked reduction of apoptosis, thereby favoring cancer development. Furthermore, the authors identified that IL-6-driven p53 downregulation leads to the epithelial–mesenchymal transition, a process by which epithelial cells lose their cell polarity and cell–cell adhesion, and obtain invasive properties. The authors also observed a marked downregulation of E-cadherin levels through the upregulation of a transcriptional repressor Slug in HepG2 as well as in normal colon cancer cell line NCM460. Altogether, these findings provide strong support for the direct involvement of IL-6 in tumorigenesis.

5.1.3 Anti-IL-6 Receptor Therapy in Patients with Cancer

A humanized anti-IL-6R monoclonal antibody tocilizumab was developed over a decade ago and has been extensively used for the treatment of moderate to severe rheumatoid arthritis and systemic juvenile idiopathic arthritis (Venkiteshwaran, 2009). It is also therapeutically effective against Castleman's disease and Crohn's disease (Ito et al., 2004; Nishimoto et al., 2005). In recent years, considerable attention has been paid to investigate anticancer potential of tocilizumab.

In the study by Shinriki et al. (2009), a xenograft mouse model inoculated with SAS human oral cancer cell line has shown drastic suppression of tumor growth after 20-day-long course of tocilizumab. The authors demonstrated that antitumorigenic effect of tocilizumab was due to the inhibition of VEGF expression and suppression of angiogenesis. Also, it was found that STAT3 phosphorylation was markedly reduced during the treatment. Importantly, the antitumor activity has continued after cessation of drug administration. Further investigations by Shinriki et al. (2011) revealed that tocilizumab is also involved in the blockade of Akt phosphorylation in oral squamous cell carcinoma cell line. The authors have replicated their findings in vitro, showing that tocilizumab prevents lymphangiogenesis in oral squamous cell carcinoma cell line.

Recent findings by Oguro et al. (2013) implicate tocilizumab as an important antitumorigenic agent against renal cell carcinoma. The authors showed that combination therapy with tocilizumab and IFN-α resulted in a profound decrease in 786-O renal cell carcinoma xenografts in nude mice. However, the use of either IFN-α or tocilizumab alone did not lead to tumor regression. Investigating molecular mechanisms of tocilizumab action in 786-O cells, the authors found a strong decrease in STAT3 and ERK phosphorylation and an increase in STAT1 phosphorylation, which is consistent with previous reports. Considering the fact that IL-6 is associated with poor prognosis in patients with renal cell carcinoma, further research devoted to use of tocilizumab in the treatment of this malignancy seems fully justified.

Finally, several recent studies reported beneficial effects of tocilizumab for the treatment of severe cancer-related cachexia (Ando et al., 2013; Hirata et al., 2013). The administration of the drug resulted in physical condition recovery, body weight increase, prompt recovery of appetite, improved anemia, increased dietary intake, and improved inflammatory and nutritional parameters.

It should also be noted that there are several other anti-IL-6 antibodies that have been developed recently. These are BE-8 and Siltuximab (CNTO 328), developed by Diaclone and Centocor, respectively (Fulciniti et al., 2009; Puchalski et al., 2010). Siltuximab is currently being involved in a number of clinical trials to treat ovarian cancer (Coward et al., 2011), renal cell carcinoma (Rossi et al., 2010), and prostate cancer (Dorff et al., 2010; Karkera et al., 2011; Fizazi et al., 2012), whereas the impact of BE-8 is being investigated in patients with lymphoma (Emilie et al., 1994) and multiple myeloma (Moreau et al., 2010).

Siltuximab showed good safety results across the trials, as no adverse events related to this drug were indicated. However, despite the fact that one group revealed a significant decrease in phosphorylation of STAT3 and p44/p42 MAPKs during the treatment of 20 patients with early prostate cancer (Fizazi et al., 2012), another trial failed to demonstrate an improvement in outcomes of 48 patients with metastatic castration-resistant prostate cancer (Karkera et al., 2011). Similarly, the drug did not demonstrate profound effect as monotherapy in the treatment of castration-resistant prostate cancer in a phase II trial involving 40 patients after progression on taxane chemotherapy (Dorf et al., 2010).

In the clinical trial involving 18 patients with ovarian cancer, only one had a partial response and seven had periods of disease stabilization. A decrease in IL-6-mediated factors, such as CCL2, CXCL12, and VEGF has been observed in serum of the patients (Coward et al., 2011).

Finally, the administration of siltuximab to 68 patients with progressive metastatic renal cell carcinoma stabilized disease in more than a half of subjects. However, only one partial response was observed (Rossi et al., 2010).

Considering the results from BE-8 trials, it was found that combination therapy of BE-8, dexamethasone, and high-dose melphalan, followed by autologous stem cell transplantation, markedly suppressed the activity of IL-6 in 16 patients with advanced multiple myeloma (Moreau et al., 2000). Six patients (37.5%) had a complete response that was confirmed by immunofixation and seven (43.7%) achieved a partial response. No adverse side effects, toxic or allergic reactions were observed during the trial. Also, the administration of BE-8 to 11 patients with lymphoma resulted in an improvement of clinical conditions, such as increased appetite and improved well-being, in seven patients (Emilie et al., 1994). Importantly, the progression of the disease as well as clinical symptoms was stopped in six and four patients, respectively. However, in this trial, BE-8 caused mild side effects, including moderate thrombocytopenia, and an occasional decrease in neutrophil counts.

In recent years, the use of JAK inhibitors is considered to be an attractive way to suppress IL-6 signaling in cancers. In particular, the administration of JAK/2 inhibitor AZD148 has shown tumor regression in preclinical models of IL-6-modulated breast, ovarian, and prostate cancers. Another JAK/2 inhibitor INCB018424 has demonstrated clinical improvements in phase III clinical trials so far (reviewed by Sansone and Bromberg (2012)).

It is also important to briefly mention several agents that are known as natural inhibitors of IL-6 signaling, production, and release. First, nonsteroidal antiinflammatory drugs (NSAIDs) have been reported to downregulate the bioactivity and expression of IL-6 through the inhibition of NF-κB (Tsuboi et al., 1995; Kang et al., 2001). Anticancer effects of NSAIDs have been observed in human hepatocellular carcinoma cell lines Hep3B, HepG2, Huh-7, SNU-387, and SNU-449 (Liu et al., 2011). Similar effects of NSAIDs were indicated in four human oral squamous cell carcinoma cell lines (Nikitakis et al., 2002).

Tetracyclines are broad-spectrum polyketide antibiotics extensively used for the treatment of infection. Apart from antibiotic activity, tetracyclines possess antiinflammatory and immunomodulatory properties. Recent studies revealed that tetracycline exerts antiinflammatory activities through the inhibition of mRNA and protein levels of TNF-α and IL-6 (Jiang et al., 2012). Antitumor effects of tetracyclines have been demonstrated in various cancers. A chemically modified tetracycline chemically modified tetracycline (CMT) was reported to suppress bone metastases and delay the development of paraplegia in a rat model of prostate cancer (Selzer et al., 1999). In another study, administration of doxycycline to MDA-MB-231 human breast cancer cell line resulted in significant tumor growth inhibition through the expression of osteonectin, a glycoprotein involved in extracellular matrix remodeling (Dhanesuan et al., 2002). Recent study by Pourgholami et al. (2012) demonstrated that minocycline markedly suppressed cell proliferation and colony formation in human ovarian cancer cell lines A2780, OVCAR-3, and SKOV-3. In addition, it was found that minocycline induced cell cycle arrest in these cell lines through the downregulation of cyclins A, B, and E. Further studies by this group showed that minocycline drives multiple pathways in cancer cells, leading to apoptosis, and downregulation of angiogenesis and metastasis (Ataie-Kachoie et al., 2013b; Pourgholami et al., 2013).

Finally, corticosteroids have been repeatedly reported to have antiinflammatory and immunomodulatory effects through the inhibition of IL-6 (Waage et al., 1990). Despite severe side effects caused by corticosteroids, they are extensively used for the treatment of autoimmune disorders and several cancers, such as multiple myeloma and prostate cancer (Nonomura et al., 2008; Morgan, 2010).

5.1.4 Summary

There is strong evidence that IL-6 has an impact on the development of chronic inflammation and associated diseases, including malignant tumors. This cytokine was shown to be involved in multiple cancer pathways, including stimulation of tumor proliferation, angiogenesis, and proapoptotic and prometastatic activities. In addition, increased IL-6 mRNA and protein levels were detected in patients with various cancers and correlated with poor prognosis in many studies. Recent studies have also highlighted the role of this cytokine in tumor recurrence. The impact of IL-6 on the resistance to chemotherapy drugs is certainly of great interest as well. It is very likely that certain IL-6 signaling inhibitors will soon be used in cancer therapy.

5.2 INTERLEUKIN-11

5.2.1 Overview

IL-11 is a 178-amino acid four-helical cytokine first identified in bone marrow-derived stromal cells by Paul et al. (1990). It shares a 22% homology with IL-6 and is also known as adipogenesis inhibitory factor and oprelvekin. Earlier studies demonstrated that IL-11 is involved in hematopoiesis; in particular, it was reported to promote the T-cell-dependent development of immunoglobulin-producing B cells and also synergize with IL-3 in supporting murine megakaryocyte colony formation (Paul et al., 1990).

Further studies, however, implicated IL-11 as a diverse cytokine with numerous immune functions.

In culture, IL-11 is secreted by multiple cells, including lymphocytes, B cells, macrophages, endothelial cells, hematopoietic cells, chondrocytes, osteoclasts, synoviocytes, trophoblasts, and fibroblasts (reviewed by Putoczki and Ernst (2010)). The sources of IL-11 in vivo are less investigated and require further studies. Considering IL-11 receptor α (IL-11Rα), it has two transmembrane isoforms, one of which, namely, IL-11Rα1, is expressed in small amounts in the kidney, muscle, thymus, bone marrow, testis, spleen, heart, uterus, brain, lung, intestines, salivary glands, ovary, and bladder, whereas IL-11Rα2 can only be found in lymph nodes, testis, and thymus (Davidson et al., 1997; Robb et al., 1997; Romas et al., 1996).

IL-11 exerts its biological activities through forming a high-affinity hexameric complex comprising IL-11 itself, IL-11R, and gp130. This leads to the initiation of the JAK/STAT pathway, involving JAK1, STAT3, and, to a lesser extent, STAT1 (Barton et al., 2000).

Biological effects of IL-11 are diverse and focused primarily on hematopoietic cells. In particular, IL-11 is involved in B-cell IgG production, activation of certain lymphocytes, and stimulation of erythropoiesis (reviewed by Putoczki and Ernst (2010)). Multiple experiments on animal models revealed profound antiinflammatory activities of this cytokine (Trepicchio and Dorner, 1998). IL-11 is responsible for the upregulation of IL-4 and IL-10 expression in lymphocytes. In macrophages, IL-11 was reported to inhibit IL-1 and IL-12. In addition, IL-11 was reported to activate Th2 cells but suppress Th1 axis (reviewed by Du and Williams (1997), Nandurkar et al. (1998), Schwertschlag et al. (1999), Putoczki and Ernst (2010)).

Moreover, IL-11 is known to have a considerable influence on cortical thickness and strength of long bones, increased osteoblastogenesis, regulation of stem cell development, regulation of proliferation and inhibition of apoptosis in epithelial cells, and improving tolerance to oxidative stress in endothelial cells (reviewed by Putoczki and Ernst (2010), Garbers and Scheller (2013)).

Considering its role in diseases, IL-11 was found associated with antiinflammatory and mucosal protective effects in animal models of acute and chronic inflammation, such as mucositis, inflammatory bowel disease, arthritis, and autoimmune joint disease (Trepicchio and Dorner, 1998; Walmsley et al., 1998). In addition, there is evidence that IL-11 has cardioprotective functions, as it was found involved in the reduction in the infarct size in vivo

(Kimura et al., 2007) and attenuating cardiac dysfunction through the inhibition of cardiac fibrosis (Obana et al., 2012). This cytokine is known to play a role in the regulation of autoimmune demyelination (Gurfein et al., 2009) and prevention of diabetes in vivo (Lgssiar et al., 2004). Elevated IL-11 protein level was observed in patients with psoriasis (Pietrzak et al., 2008). Finally, mRNA expression of IL-11 was significantly lower in the colon of patients with ulcerative colitis as compared to healthy controls (Verma et al., 2013).

5.2.2 The Expression of IL-11 in Cancer Cell Lines and in Human Cancers

During the last decade, quite a few studies have appeared evaluating the expression patterns of either IL-11 or IL-11Rα in patients with various malignancies. The results of these studies are interesting, considering the fact that IL-11 is rarely expressed in healthy tissues (Schwertschlag et al., 1999).

The first report investigating the abundance of IL-11 in cancer was performed by Meng et al. (2001), who demonstrated the presence of this cytokine in malignant epithelial cells from breast cancer and surrounding adipose tissue samples obtained from 25 mastectomy specimens. Interestingly, the authors observed that IL-11 inhibited differentiation of adipose fibroblasts causing accumulation around malignant breast epithelial cells. Further experiments by Ren et al. (2013) revealed that IL-11 serum levels and mRNA expression were higher in 90 patients with breast cancer metastatic to bone as compared to 90 patients with primary breast cancer. These results implicate IL-11 as a regulator of tumor progression and metastasis.

Campbell et al. (2001a) revealed the expression of IL-11Rα mRNA in cancer cells and stromal layer of 45 of 48 (93.8%) primary ovarian carcinoma samples. However, the IL-11 mRNA was expressed in only 3 of 21 malignant samples studied. In addition, the authors showed that recombinant IL-11 did not stimulate cell growth and also failed to prevent paclitaxel-induced apoptosis in human ovarian cancer cell lines SKOV-3 and OVCAR-3.

Bellone et al. (2006) examined tissue specimens from 65 patients with pancreatic cancer, comparing tumoral versus normal pancreatic tissues. The authors showed that IL-11 mRNA was markedly overexpressed in tumors versus normal tissues. In addition, the authors observed the expression of IL-11 in five pancreatic carcinoma cell lines (BxPC-3, Capan-2, PANC-1, MIAPaCa-2, and PT-45). Interestingly, high IL-11 levels correlated with longer survival among cancer patients in this study.

Ellmark et al. (2006) used antibody microarray analysis to examine the abundance of 127 proteins, among which are cytokines, chemokines, and complementary factors, among 35 malignant and normal stomach tissue samples. The authors found that tissue levels of IL-11 were significantly overexpressed in tumor tissues versus normal.

Similarly, Nakayama et al. (2007) demonstrated that among the 73 cases of gastric adenocarcinoma, 53 (72.6%) and 47 cases (64.4%) had positive staining for the IL-11 and IL-11Rα proteins in cancer cells. Furthermore, the expression of IL-11Rα did correlate with the vessel infiltration ($p < 0.01$) and grade of tumor invasion ($p < 0.05$). Additionally, the authors observed the expression of both IL-11 and IL-11Rα in four human gastric cancer cell lines, namely, MKN-1, MKN-28, NUGC-3, and SCH.

Sales et al. (2010) investigated the abundance of IL-11 and IL-11Rα in 30 endometrial adenocarcinoma tissues versus 10 normal endometrial tissues, showing elevated expression of IL-11 in tumors. Interestingly, the highest levels of IL-11 were observed in tissues with poorly differentiated adenocarcinoma, which suggests that this cytokine may be involved in tumor progression. Moreover, the authors revealed that IL-11 synthesis and release is regulated by $PGF_{2\alpha}$ via the FP receptor, and the expression of FP receptor colocalized with IL-11 and IL-11Rα protein expression in both normal and tumor tissues.

Yamazumi et al. (2006) examined the presence of IL-11 and IL-11Rα among 115 cases of surgically resected human colonic adenocarcinoma and 11 cases of colonic adenoma. It was found that 100 and 6 cases were positive for IL-11, and 87 and 4 cases were positive for IL-11Rα, respectively. Moreover, the authors identified that IL-11Rα expression correlated with the depth of tumor invasion and the histological differentiation, whereas IL-11 did not correlate with any clinicopathological characteristics.

In accordance with the previous study, Yoshizaki et al. (2006) confirmed the expression of IL-11 and IL-11Rα in the majority of 103 investigated patients with colorectal carcinoma and 24 cases of colorectal adenoma. As compared to normal colonic mucosal tissues, both IL-11 and IL-11Rα were overexpressed in malignant tissues. Furthermore, the authors revealed the expression of IL-11 by five human colorectal carcinoma cell lines, DLD-1, HT-29, Caco-2, Lovo, and Colo-320DM. Similarly to the previous report, colorectal cancer cells showed a statistically significant correlation between IL-11R·expression and the depth of invasion, and IL-11 did not correlate with any clinicopathological factors.

Lewis et al. (2009) investigated the abundance of IL-11Rα in primary osseus (*n* = 30) and pulmonary metastatic osteosarcoma (*n* = 19), showing a marked upregulation in both groups. In addition, the authors found that IL-11Rα was expressed by neither normal bone nor normal lung.

Interestingly, Wu et al. (2013) reported that intratumoral levels of IL-11 in patients with bladder cancer were lower than those in healthy subjects. However, the sample for this study was relatively low, only 27 tissue specimens from cancer patients and 32 control samples. Therefore, the results from this study should be interpreted with caution. More interestingly, the authors demonstrated that IL-11 levels in seven bladder cancer cell lines were significantly lower in comparison with primary human bladder cell culture. Finally, the expression level of IL-11 did correlate with the tumor grade and stage in patients with bladder cancer.

Finally, several groups revealed the overexpression of IL-11Rα in prostate cancer tissues and identified the involvement of this receptor in the progression of human prostate cancer (Campbell et al., 2001b; Zurita et al., 2004).

Altogether, the aforementioned studies provide strong evidence for the link between IL-11, IL-11Rα, and cancer development and progression of cancer.

5.2.3 IL-11 and Metastatic Tumor Formation

An extensive research project by Kang et al. (2003) revealed a specific set of genes mediating breast cancer metastasis to bone, among which is IL-11. The authors showed that IL-11 plays a pivotal role in invasion of tumor cells, contributing to bone metastasis. Also, the downregulation of IL-11 in a bone cancer model was associated with decreased osteoclast formation and increased metalloproteolytic activities (Luis-Ravelo et al., 2013). Further investigations conducted by multiple research groups implicated IL-11 as an important prognostic factor for bone metastasis from various primary tumor sites (Kozlow and Guise, 2005; Javelaud et al., 2007; Baselga et al., 2008; Bohn et al., 2009; Sterling et al., 2011; Xiang et al., 2011; Pollari et al., 2012).

It was also observed that recombinant IL-11 causes the overexpression of MMP-13 in SHC gastric carcinoma cells through the phosphorylation of Phosphoinositide 3-kinase (PI3K)/AKT and JAK/STAT3 (Yang et al., 2014). Similarly, Nakayama et al. (2007) showed that recombinant human IL-11 promotes the migration of SCH cells via the activation of the PI3K signal transduction pathway.

Yoshizaki et al. (2006) demonstrated that the use of recombinant human IL-11 (rhIL-11) stimulated the proliferation and migration of human colon cancer cell line HT-29 through the activation of PI3K and p44/p42 MAPK pathways.

Shen et al. (2012) identified that CD14[+] tumor associated macrophages cocultured with distant metastasis cell lines exhibited higher expression if IL-11. In addition, the authors observed significant association between the expression of IL-11 in tumor-associated macrophages and gastric cancer cell invasion speed under hypoxic conditions.

Lay et al. (2012) found that treatment of endometrial cancer cell line AN3CA with recombinant IL-11 resulted in 50% increase in cell migration. Further, the authors revealed that cell treatment with the specific IL-11 inhibitor or a STAT3 inhibitor completely abolished the observed effect.

Finally, it was found that IL-11 increases the migration and motility in human chondrosarcoma cells through the activation of PI3K, Akt, and NF-κB pathways (Li et al., 2012). Importantly, the authors found that IL-11 upregulated the expression of intercellular adhesion molecule-1, which has long been associated with metastatic formation in various cancers (Sipos et al., 2012; Liu et al., 2013; Soto et al., 2013).

5.2.4 Summary

The above-mentioned studies identify IL-11 as a major procarcinogenic agent. Considering molecular mechanisms of IL-11-mediated tumorigenesis, it is difficult to find an explanation for its behavior. First, it is known that IL-11 can activate STAT3, which has long been known to promote carcinogenesis through the stimulation of angiogenesis, promotion of migration and motility in cancer cells (Sellier et al., 2013). However, recent findings indicated that STAT3 can also possess tumor suppressor role (de la Iglesia et al., 2008; Musteanu et al., 2010; Lee et al., 2012). Second, IL-11 has also been reported to activate STAT1, which has been reported to inhibit tumor growth through the activation of proapoptotic and antiproliferative pathways in cancer cells (Kim and Lee, 2007). It is known to inhibit angiogenesis as well (Strieter et al., 1995; Li et al., 2004). The balance between STAT1 and STAT3 signaling determines antitumoral or tumorigenic response, and IL-11 is one of the most important players influencing this balance. A possible explanation of IL-11-mediated tumorigenesis is that this cytokine was reported to trigger STAT3 more intensively as compared to STAT1.

Multiple studies have indicated a marked prometastatic activity of IL-11, which is obviously due to IL-11-driven facilitation of cell motility and migration. However, as an antiinflammatory cytokine, IL-11 may restrict procarcinogenic activities of IL-1 and other proinflammatory mediators, thereby decreasing risk of cancer occurrence.

On the one hand, procarcinogenic properties of IL-11 can be partially explained by the suppression of the production of IL-12, which has been implicated as an anticancer cytokine (Yuzhalin and Kutikhin, 2012). On the other hand, however, IL-11 inhibits the expression of proinflammatory cytokine IL-1, which has been repeatedly associated with occurrence, development, and progression of various malignancies (Dinarello, 1998; Dinarello, 2010; Yuzhalin, 2011; Kasza et al., 2013).

In conclusion, there is clear evidence that IL-11 promotes carcinogenesis; however, more studies should be performed in order to identify potential antitumorigenic roles of this cytokine.

5.3 INTERLEUKIN-31

IL-31 is a four-helical 18 kDa protein composed of 141 amino acid residues, which was identified and cloned by Dillon et al. in 2004. The mature IL-31 protein is the result of 164-amino acids precursor processing. This cytokine signals through a receptor complex composed of two subunits, IL-31 receptor A (IL-31RA) and oncostatin M receptor (OSMR), which are expressed on epithelial cells and activated monocytes (Castellani et al., 2006). IL-31 is ubiquitously expressed throughout the body; small amounts of IL-31 mRNA were identified in testis, skeletal muscle, bone marrow, colon, small intestine, kidney, thymus, and trachea. The expression of IL-31 was observed in skin-homing-activated CD4+ T cells and activated CD8+ T cells but neither in resting nor in activated NK cells, monocytes and B cells (Dillon et al., 2004).

Although biological effects of IL-31 are poorly studied, multiple studies demonstrated an impact of this cytokine in skin inflammation (Dillon et al., 2004; Sonkoly et al., 2006; Bilsborough et al., 2006; Takaoka et al., 2006). IL-31 was shown to induce the expression of chemokines CXCL1, CXCL8, CCL2, and CCL1, as well as proinflammatory cytokines IL-1β and IL-6 in eosinophils (Cheung et al., 2010). Moreover, IL-31 upregulates the expression of CCL2, IL-6, IL-8, epidermal growth factor, and VEGF synergistically with either IL-4 or IL-13 in vitro (Ip et al., 2007). Signal transduction pathways of IL-31 involve ERK1/ERK2 MAP kinases, PI3K/AKT pathway, and JAK1/JAK2/STAT3/STAT5 (Fukada et al., 1996; Diveu et al., 2004; Dreuw et al., 2004).

It has been found that IL-31 can play a role in etiopathogenesis of various autoimmune diseases. Due to the fact that the expression of this cytokine is in many respects limited to skin, it has been mainly associated with autoimmune skin disorders. It was shown that either overexpression of IL-31 or subcutaneous administration of this cytokine resulted in severe pruritus, alopecia, and skin lesions in a mouse model (Dillon et al., 2004). Furthermore, IL-31Rα was found overexpressed in skin from patients with atopic dermatitis as compared to healthy skin (Bilsborough et al., 2006). In addition, serum IL-31 levels correlated with severity of disease in children with atopic dermatitis (Siniewicz-Luzeńczyk et al., 2013). Recently, It was also demonstrated that a single intradermal injection of IL-31 provokes scratching behavior in healthy NC/Nga and BALB/c mice (Arai et al., 2013). Furthermore, canine IL-31 induced pruritic behaviors in dogs when introduced through intravenous, subcutaneous, and intradermal routes (Gonzales et al., 2013).

Levels of IL-31 and IL-31RA were markedly increased in submucosal tissues across patients with allergic rhinitis and also in human airway epithelial cells (Shah et al., 2013). Elevated levels of IL-31 correlated with high disease severity in children with atopic dermatitis (Ezzat et al., 2011). In addition, IL-31 mRNA expression was elevated in the inflammatory infiltrates from skin biopsies from patients with atopic dermatitis (Nobbe et al., 2012). Furthermore, IL-31 was profoundly overexpressed in pruritic atopic in comparison with nonpruritic psoriatic skin inflammation (Sonkoly et al., 2006). Also, higher expression of IL-31R was observed in an animal model of airway hypersensitivity (Dillon et al., 2004).

Concentrations of IL-31 in various immune cells were shown to be elevated by ultraviolet B radiation and reactive oxygen species (Lüscher-Firzlaff et al., 2008; Cornelissen et al. 2011). Furthermore, staphylococcal α-toxin stimulation of peripheral blood mononuclear cells significantly enhanced the production of IL-31 in patients with atopic dermatitis (Niebuhr et al., 2011). Also, it was found that IL-31RA levels were upregulated in human dermal microvascular endothelial cells which were activated after stimulation with IFN-γ (Feld et al., 2010).

Recently, few studies have focused on the role of IL-31 in cancer, suggesting possible involvement of this cytokine in tumorigenesis.

Singer et al. (2013) examined serum of 29 patients with cutaneous T-cell lymphomas and 13 healthy and aged-matched controls for levels of IL-31 mRNA, showing a considerable difference in the expression of this cytokine. Interestingly, IL-31 concentrations were found associated with patients experiencing marked itch at the time of sample collection, which confirms the involvement of this cytokine in the development of pruritus. Moreover, serum levels of IL-31 were not detected in 92% nonpruritic patients, implicating this cytokine as a potential target for anti-itch treatment. In 2005, a National Cutaneous Lymphoma Foundation Survey revealed that 53.9% of 640 involved patients with cutaneous T-cell lymphomas are affected by pruritus, which indicates that further investigation of the relationship between IL-31 and itch in the context of cancer is absolutely reasonable.

Similar findings were reported by Ohmatsu et al. (2012), who demonstrated that serum IL-31 levels were markedly increased in 38 patients with cutaneous T-cell lymphomas than those in 23 healthy control subjects. In addition, the authors found that serum levels of IL-31 were significantly higher in patients with stage IV as compared to patients with stage I, suggesting that this cytokine may be involved in disease progression.

An interesting study was performed by Dambacher et al. (2007), who showed that IL31 at high doses and low cell density (<5000 cells/well) can induce a profound suppression of cell proliferation in the colorectal cancer cell line HCT116 through the activation of STAT1/STAT3, ERK1/ERK2, and Akt. Strikingly, IL-31 for some reason stimulated the growth of cancer cells in dense cell cultures. Moreover, the authors found that mRNA levels of IL-31, IL-31Rα, and OSMR were overexpressed in HCT116 cell line. Furthermore, the presence of LPS or proinflammatory cytokines TNF-α, IL1β, or IFN-γ in HCT116 culture significantly upregulated the synthesis of IL-31, IL-31Rα, and OSMR. IL-31, in turn, was shown to upregulate IL-8. Finally, the authors showed that IL-31 mRNA levels were increased in 22 patients with inflammatory bowel disease.

Thus far, there is a lack of studies investigating the impact of IL-31 on tumor biology; nevertheless, the existing data support the hypothesis that this cytokine may be involved in carcinogenesis. Clearly, further research is needed to verify whether IL-31 has a considerable influence on cancer development.

REFERENCES

Aka, P., Emmanuel, B., Vila, M.C., Jariwala, A., Nkrumah, F., Periago, M.V., Neequaye, J., Kiruthu, C., Levine, P.H., Biggar, R.J., Bhatia, K., Bethony, J.M., Mbulaiteye, S.M., January 6, 2014. Elevated serum levels of interleukin-6 in endemic Burkitt lymphoma in Ghana. Hematol. Oncol. http://dx.doi.org/10.1002/hon. 2121 (Epub ahead of print).

Aleksandrova, K., Boeing, H., Nöthlings, U., Jenab, M., Fedirko, V., Kaaks, R., Lukanova, A., Trichopoulou, A., Trichopoulos, D., Boffetta, P., Trepo, E., Westhpal, S., Duarte-Salles, T., Stepien, M., Overvad, K., Tjønneland, A., Halkjaer, J., Boutron-Ruault, M.C., Dossus, L., Racine, A., Lagiou, P., Bamia, C., Benetou, V., Agnoli, C., Palli, D., Panico, S., Tumino, R., Vineis, P., Bueno-de-Mesquita, B., Peeters, P.H., Gram, I.T., Lund, E., Weiderpass, E., Quirós, J.R., Agudo, A., Sánchez, M.J., Gavrila, D., Barricarte, A., Dorronsoro, M., Ohlsson, B., Lindkvist, B., Johansson, A., Sund, M., Khaw, K.T., Wareham, N., Travis, R.C., Riboli, E., Pischon, T., January 17, 2014. Inflammatory and metabolic biomarkers and risk of liver and biliary tract cancer. Hepatology. http://dx.doi.org/10.1002/hep.27016 (Epub ahead of print).

Alexandrakis, M.G., Passam, F.H., Kyriakou, D.S., Christophoridou, A.V., Perisinakis, K., Hatzivasili, A., Foudoulakis, A., Castanas, E., 2004. Serum level of interleukin-16 in multiple myeloma patients and its relationship to disease activity. Am. J. Hematol. 75 (2), 101–106.

Ando, K., Takahashi, F., Motojima, S., Nakashima, K., Kaneko, N., Hoshi, K., Takahashi, K., 2013. Possible role for tocilizumab, an anti-interleukin-6 receptor antibody, in treating cancer cachexia. J. Clin. Oncol. 31 (6), e69–e72.

Arai, I., Tsuji, M., Takeda, H., Akiyama, N., Saito, S., 2013. A single dose of interleukin-31 (IL-31) causes continuous itch-associated scratching behaviour in mice. Exp. Dermatol. 22 (10), 669–671.

Ashizawa, T., Okada, R., Suzuki, Y., Takagi, M., Yamazaki, T., Sumi, T., Aoki, T., Ohnuma, S., Aoki, T., 2005. Clinical significance of interleukin-6 (IL-6) in the spread of gastric cancer: role of IL-6 as a prognostic factor. Gastric Cancer 8 (2), 124–131.

Ataie-Kachoie, P., Badar, S., Morris, D.L., Pourgholami, M.H., 2013. Minocycline targets the NF-κB Nexus through suppression of TGF-β1-TAK1-IκB signaling in ovarian cancer. Mol. Cancer Res. 11 (10), 1279–1291.

Ataie-Kachoie, P., Pourgholami, M.H., Morris, D.L., 2013. Inhibition of the IL-6 signaling pathway: a strategy to combat chronic inflammatory diseases and cancer. Cytokine Growth Factor Rev. 24 (2), 163–173.

Bachelot, T., Ray-Coquard, I., Menetrier-Caux, C., Rastkha, M., Duc, A., Blay, J.Y., 2003. Prognostic value of serum levels of interleukin 6 and of serum and plasma levels of vascular endothelial growth factor in hormone-refractory metastatic breast cancer patients. Br. J. Cancer 88 (11), 1721–1726.

Barton, V.A., Hall, M.A., Hudson, K.R., Heath, J.K., 2000. Interleukin-11 signals through the formation of a hexameric receptor complex. J. Biol. Chem. 275 (46), 36197–36203.

Baselga, J., Rothenberg, M.L., Tabernero, J., Seoane, J., Daly, T., Cleverly, A., Berry, B., Rhoades, S.K., Ray, C.A., Fill, J., Farrington, D.L., Wallace, L.A., Yingling, J.M., Lahn, M., Arteaga, C., Carducci, M., 2008. TGF-beta signalling-related markers in cancer patients with bone metastasis. Biomarkers 13 (2), 217–236.

Bellacosa, A., Kumar, C.C., Di Cristofano, A., Testa, J.R., 2005. Activation of AKT kinases in cancer: implications for therapeutic targeting. Adv. Cancer Res. 94, 29–86.

Bellone, G., Smirne, C., Mauri, F.A., Tonel, E., Carbone, A., Buffolino, A., Dughera, L., Robecchi, A., Pirisi, M., Emanuelli, G., 2006. Cytokine expression profile in human pancreatic carcinoma cells and in surgical specimens: implications for survival. Cancer Immunol. Immunother. 55 (6), 684–698.

Bellone, S., Watts, K., Cane, S., Palmieri, M., Cannon, M.J., Burnett, A., Roman, J.J., Pecorelli, S., Santin, A.D., 2005. High serum levels of interleukin-6 in endometrial carcinoma are associated with uterine serous papillary histology, a highly aggressive and chemotherapy-resistant variant of endometrial cancer. Gynecol. Oncol. 98 (1), 92–98.

Belluco, C., Nitti, D., Frantz, M., Toppan, P., Basso, D., Plebani, M., Lise, M., Jessup, J.M., 2000. Interleukin-6 blood level is associated with circulating carcinoembryonic antigen and prognosis in patients with colorectal cancer. Ann. Surg. Oncol. 7 (2), 133–138.

Berek, J.S., Chung, C., Kaldi, K., Watson, J.M., Knox, R.M., Martínez-Maza, O., 1991. Serum interleukin-6 levels correlate with disease status in patients with epithelial ovarian cancer. Am. J. Obstet. Gynecol. 164 (4), 1038–1042. discussion 1042–3.

Bilsborough, J., Leung, D.Y., Maurer, M., Howell, M., Boguniewicz, M., Yao, L., Storey, H., LeCiel, C., Harder, B., Gross, J.A., 2006. IL-31 is associated with cutaneous lymphocyte antigen-positive skin homing T cells in patients with atopic dermatitis. J. Allergy Clin. Immunol. 117 (2), 418–425.

Bohn, O.L., Nasir, I., Brufsky, A., Tseng, G.C., Bhargava, R., MacManus, K., Chivukula, M., 2009. Biomarker profile in breast carcinomas presenting with bone metastasis. Int. J. Clin. Exp. Pathol. 3 (2), 139–146.

Borsellino, N., Belldegrun, A., Bonavida, B., 1995. Endogenous interleukin 6 is a resistance factor for cis-diamminedichloroplatinum and etoposide-mediated cytotoxicity of human prostate carcinoma cell lines. Cancer Res. 55 (20), 4633–4639.

Breen, E.C., Rezai, A.R., Nakajima, K., Beall, G.N., Mitsuyasu, R.T., Hirano, T., Kishimoto, T., Martinez-Maza, O., 1990. Infection with HIV is associated with elevated IL-6 levels and production. J. Immunol. 144 (2), 480–484.

Brighenti, E., Calabrese, C., Liguori, G., Giannone, F.A., Trerè, D., Montanaro, L., Derenzini, M., February 17, 2014. Interleukin 6 downregulates p53 expression and activity by stimulating ribosome biogenesis: a new pathway connecting inflammation to cancer. Oncogene. http://dx.doi.org/10.1038/onc.2014.1 (Epub ahead of print).

Campbell, C.L., Guardiani, R., Ollari, C., Nelson, B.E., Quesenberry, P.J., Savarese, T.M., 2001. Interleukin-11 receptor expression in primary ovarian carcinomas. Gynecol. Oncol. 80 (2), 121–127.

Campbell, C.L., Jiang, Z., Savarese, D.M., Savarese, T.M., 2001. Increased expression of the interleukin-11 receptor and evidence of STAT3 activation in prostate carcinoma. Am. J. Pathol. 158 (1), 25–32.

Castellani, M.L., Salini, V., Frydas, S., Donelan, J., Madhappan, B., Petrarca, C., Vecchiet, J., Falasca, K., Neri, G., Tete, S., 2006. Interleukin-31: a new cytokine involved in inflammation of the skin. Int. J. Immunopathol. Pharmacol. 19 (1), 1–4.

Chen, C.J., Sung, W.W., Lin, Y.M., Chen, M.K., Lee, C.H., Lee, H., Yeh, K.T., Ko, J.L., 2012. Gender difference in the prognostic role of interleukin 6 in oral squamous cell carcinoma. PLoS One 7 (11), e50104.

Chen, M.F., Chen, P.T., Lu, M.S., Lin, P.Y., Chen, W.C., Lee, K.D., 2013. IL-6 expression predicts treatment response and outcome in squamous cell carcinoma of the esophagus. Mol. Cancer 12, 26.

Chen, M.F., Lin, P.Y., Wu, C.F., Chen, W.C., Wu, C.T., 2013. IL-6 expression regulates tumorigenicity and correlates with prognosis in bladder cancer. PLoS One 8 (4), e61901.

Cheung, P.F., Wong, C.K., Ho, A.W., Hu, S., Chen, D.P., Lam, C.W., 2010. Activation of human eosinophils and epidermal keratinocytes by Th2 cytokine IL-31: implication for the immunopathogenesis of atopic dermatitis. Int. Immunol. 22 (6), 453–467.

Cho, Y.A., Sung, M.K., Yeon, J.Y., Ro, J., Kim, J., 2013. Prognostic role of interleukin-6, interleukin-8, and leptin levels according to breast cancer subtype. Cancer Res. Treat. 45 (3), 210–219.

Chuang, J.Y., Huang, Y.L., Yen, W.L., Chiang, I.P., Tsai, M.H., Tang, C.H., 2014. Syk/JNK/AP-1 signaling pathway mediates interleukin-6-promoted cell migration in oral squamous cell carcinoma. Int. J. Mol. Sci. 15 (1), 545–559.

Conze, D., Weiss, L., Regen, P.S., Bhushan, A., Weaver, D., Johnson, P., Rincón, M., 2001. Autocrine production of interleukin 6 causes multidrug resistance in breast cancer cells. Cancer Res. 61 (24), 8851–8858.

Cornelissen, C., Brans, R., Czaja, K., Skazik, C., Marquardt, Y., Zwadlo-Klarwasser, G., Kim, A., Bickers, D.R., Lüscher-Firzlaff, J., Lüscher, B., Baron, J.M., 2011. Ultraviolet B radiation and reactive oxygen species modulate interleukin-31 expression in T lymphocytes, monocytes and dendritic cells. Br. J. Dermatol. 165 (5), 966–975.

Coward, J., Kulbe, H., Chakravarty, P., Leader, D., Vassileva, V., Leinster, D.A., Thompson, R., Schioppa, T., Nemeth, J., Vermeulen, J., Singh, N., Avril, N., Cummings, J., Rexhepaj, E., Jirström, K., Gallagher, W.M., Brennan, D.J., McNeish, I.A., Balkwill, F.R., 2011. Interleukin-6 as a therapeutic target in human ovarian cancer. Clin. Cancer Res. 17 (18), 6083–6096.

Cui, X., Liu, J., Bai, L., Tian, J., Zhu, J., 2014. Interleukin-6 induces malignant transformation of rat mesenchymal stem cells in association with enhanced signaling of signal transducer and activator of transcription 3. Cancer Sci. 105 (1), 64–71.

Dambacher, J., Beigel, F., Seiderer, J., Haller, D., Göke, B., Auernhammer, C.J., Brand, S., 2007. Interleukin 31 mediates MAP kinase and STAT1/3 activation in intestinal epithelial cells and its expression is upregulated in inflammatory bowel disease. Gut 56 (9), 1257–1265.

Davidson, A.J., Freeman, S.A., Crosier, K.E., Wood, C.R., Crosier, P.S., 1997. Expression of murine interleukin 11 and its receptor alpha-chain in adult and embryonic tissues. Stem Cells 15 (2), 119–124.

de la Iglesia, N., Konopka, G., Puram, S.V., Chan, J.A., Bachoo, R.M., You, M.J., Levy, D.E., Depinho, R.A., Bonni, A., 2008. Identification of a PTEN-regulated STAT3 brain tumor suppressor pathway. Genes Dev. 22 (4), 449–462.

Dhanesuan, N., Sharp, J.A., Blick, T., Price, J.T., Thompson, E.W., 2002. Doxycycline-inducible expression of SPARC/Osteonectin/BM40 in MDA-MB-231 human breast cancer cells results in growth inhibition. Breast Cancer Res. Treat. 75 (1), 73–85.

DiCosmo, B.F., Geba, G.P., Picarella, D., Elias, J.A., Rankin, J.A., Stripp, B.R., Whitsett, J.A., Flavell, R.A., 1994. Airway epithelial cell expression of interleukin-6 in transgenic mice. Uncoupling of airway inflammation and bronchial hyperreactivity. J. Clin. Invest. 94 (5), 2028–2035.

Dillon, S.R., Sprecher, C., Hammond, A., Bilsborough, J., Rosenfeld-Franklin, M., Presnell, S.R., Haugen, H.S., Maurer, M., Harder, B., Johnston, J., Bort, S., Mudri, S., Kuijper, J.L., Bukowski, T., Shea, P., Dong, D.L., Dasovich, M., Grant, F.J., Lockwood, L., Levin, S.D., LeCiel, C., Waggie, K., Day, H., Topouzis, S., Kramer, J., Kuestner, R., Chen, Z., Foster, D., Parrish-Novak, J., Gross, J.A., 2004. Interleukin 31, a cytokine produced by activated T cells, induces dermatitis in mice. Nat. Immunol. 5 (7), 752–760.

Dinarello, C.A., 1998. Interleukin-1, interleukin-1 receptors and interleukin-1 receptor antagonist. Int. Rev. Immunol. 16 (5–6), 457–499.

Dinarello, C.A., 2010. Why not treat human cancer with interleukin-1 blockade? Cancer Metastasis Rev. 29 (2), 317–329.

Diveu, C., Lak-Hal, A.H., Froger, J., Ravon, E., Grimaud, L., Barbier, F., Hermann, J., Gascan, H., Chevalier, S., 2004. Predominant expression of the long isoform of GP130-like (GPL) receptor is required for interleukin-31 signaling. Eur. Cytokine Netw. 15 (4), 291–302.

Dorff, T.B., Goldman, B., Pinski, J.K., Mack, P.C., Lara Jr, P.N., Van Veldhuizen Jr, P.J., Quinn, D.I., Vogelzang, N.J., Thompson Jr, I.M., Hussain, M.H., 2010. Clinical and correlative results of SWOG S0354: a phase II trial of CNTO328 (siltuximab), a monoclonal antibody against interleukin-6, in chemotherapy-pretreated patients with castration-resistant prostate cancer. Clin. Cancer Res. 16 (11), 3028–3034.

Dreuw, A., Radtke, S., Pflanz, S., Lippok, B.E., Heinrich, P.C., Hermanns, H.M., 2004. Characterization of the signaling capacities of the novel gp130-like cytokine receptor. J. Biol. Chem. 279 (34), 36112–36120.

Du, X., Williams, D.A., 1997. Interleukin-11: review of molecular, cell biology, and clinical use. Blood 89 (11), 3897–3908.

Duan, Z., Feller, A.J., Penson, R.T., Chabner, B.A., Seiden, M.V., 1999. Discovery of differentially expressed genes associated with paclitaxel resistance using cDNA array technology: analysis of interleukin (IL) 6, IL-8, and monocyte chemotactic protein 1 in the paclitaxel-resistant phenotype. Clin. Cancer Res. 5 (11), 3445–3453.

Ellmark, P., Ingvarsson, J., Carlsson, A., Lundin, B.S., Wingren, C., Borrebaeck, C.A., 2006. Identification of protein expression signatures associated with *Helicobacter pylori* infection and gastric adenocarcinoma using recombinant antibody microarrays. Mol. Cell. Proteomics 5 (9), 1638–1646.

Emilie, D., Wijdenes, J., Gisselbrecht, C., Jarrousse, B., Billaud, E., Blay, J.Y., Gabarre, J., Gaillard, J.P., Brochier, J., Raphael, M., 1994. Administration of an anti-interleukin-6 monoclonal antibody to patients with acquired immunodeficiency syndrome and lymphoma: effect on lymphoma growth and on B clinical symptoms. Blood 84 (8), 2472–2479.

Ezzat, M.H., Hasan, Z.E., Shaheen, K.Y., 2011. Serum measurement of interleukin-31 (IL-31) in paediatric atopic dermatitis: elevated levels correlate with severity scoring. J. Eur. Acad. Dermatol. Venereol. 25 (3), 334–339.

Feld, M., Shpacovitch, V.M., Fastrich, M., Cevikbas, F., Steinhoff, M., 2010. Interferon-γ induces upregulation and activation of the interleukin-31 receptor in human dermal microvascular endothelial cells. Exp. Dermatol. 19 (10), 921–923.

Fizazi, K., De Bono, J.S., Flechon, A., Heidenreich, A., Voog, E., Davis, N.B., Qi, M., Bandekar, R., Vermeulen, J.T., Cornfeld, M., Hudes, G.R., 2012. Randomised phase II study of siltuximab (CNTO 328), an anti-IL-6 monoclonal antibody, in combination with mitoxantrone/prednisone versus mitoxantrone/prednisone alone in metastatic castration-resistant prostate cancer. Eur. J. Cancer 48 (1), 85–93.

Foran, E., Garrity-Park, M.M., Mureau, C., Newell, J., Smyrk, T.C., Limburg, P.J., Egan, L.J., 2010. Upregulation of DNA methyltransferase-mediated gene silencing, anchorage-independent growth, and migration of colon cancer cells by interleukin-6. Mol. Cancer Res. 8 (4), 471–481.

Fujiwara, H., Suchi, K., Okamura, S., Okamura, H., Umehara, S., Todo, M., Shiozaki, A., Kubota, T., Ichikawa, D., Okamoto, K., Ochiai, T., Kokuba, Y., Sonoyama, T., Otsuji, E., 2011. Elevated serum CRP levels after induction chemoradiotherapy reflect poor treatment response in association with IL-6 in serum and local tumor site in patients with advanced esophageal cancer. J. Surg. Oncol. 103 (1), 62–68.

Fukada, T., Hibi, M., Yamanaka, Y., Takahashi-Tezuka, M., Fujitani, Y., Yamaguchi, T., Nakajima, K., Hirano, T., 1996. Two signals are necessary for cell proliferation induced by a cytokine receptor gp130: involvement of STAT3 in anti-apoptosis. Immunity 5 (5), 449–460.

Fulciniti, M., Hideshima, T., Vermot-Desroches, C., Pozzi, S., Nanjappa, P., Shen, Z., Patel, N., Smith, E.S., Wang, W., Prabhala, R., Tai, Y.T., Tassone, P., Anderson, K.C., Munshi, N.C., 2009. A high-affinity fully human anti-IL-6 mAb, 1339, for the treatment of multiple myeloma. Clin. Cancer Res. 15 (23), 7144–7152.

Gao, S.P., Mark, K.G., Leslie, K., Pao, W., Motoi, N., Gerald, W.L., Travis, W.D., Bornmann, W., Veach, D., Clarkson, B., Bromberg, J.F., 2007. Mutations in the EGFR kinase domain mediate STAT3 activation via IL-6 production in human lung adenocarcinomas. J. Clin. Invest. 117 (12), 3846–3856.

Garbers, C., Scheller, J., 2013. Interleukin-6 and interleukin-11: same but different. Biol. Chem. 394 (9), 1145–1161.

Gonzales, A.J., Humphrey, W.R., Messamore, J.E., Fleck, T.J., Fici, G.J., Shelly, J.A., Teel, J.F., Bammert, G.F., Dunham, S.A., Fuller, T.E., McCall, R.B., 2013. Interleukin-31: its role in canine pruritus and naturally occurring canine atopic dermatitis. Vet. Dermatol. 24 (1), 48–53. e11–2.

Gurfein, B.T., Zhang, Y., López, C.B., Argaw, A.T., Zameer, A., Moran, T.M., John, G.R., 2009. IL-11 regulates autoimmune demyelination. J. Immunol. 183 (7), 4229–4240.

Hassan, H.T., Drexler, H.G., 1995. Interleukins and colony stimulating factors in human myeloid leukemia cell lines. Leuk. Lymphoma 20 (1–2), 1–15.

Hassan, W., Ding, L., Gao, R.Y., Liu, J., Shang, J., 2014. Interleukin-6 signal transduction and its role in hepatic lipid metabolic disorders. Cytokine 66 (2), 133–142.

He, G., Dhar, D., Nakagawa, H., Font-Burgada, J., Ogata, H., Jiang, Y., Shalapour, S., Seki, E., Yost, S.E., Jepsen, K., Frazer, K.A., Harismendy, O., Hatziapostolou, M., Iliopoulos, D., Suetsugu, A., Hoffman, R.M., Tateishi, R., Koike, K., Karin, M., 2013. Identification of liver cancer progenitors whose malignant progression depends on autocrine IL-6 signaling. Cell. 155 (2), 384–396.

Heike, T., Nakahata, T., 2002. Ex vivo expansion of hematopoietic stem cells by cytokines. Biochim. Biophys. Acta 1592 (3), 313–321.

Hirano, T., Yasukawa, K., Harada, H., Taga, T., Watanabe, Y., Matsuda, T., Kashiwamura, S., Nakajima, K., Koyama, K., Iwamatsu, A., et al., 1986. Complementary DNA for a novel human interleukin (BSF-2) that induces B lymphocytes to produce immunoglobulin. Nature 324 (6092), 73–76.

Hirata, H., Tetsumoto, S., Kijima, T., Kida, H., Kumagai, T., Takahashi, R., Otani, Y., Inoue, K., Kuhara, H., Shimada, K., Nagatomo, I., Takeda, Y., Goya, S., Yoshizaki, K., Kawase, I., Tachibana, I., Kishimoto, T., Kumanogoh, A., 2013. Favorable responses to tocilizumab in two patients with cancer-related cachexia. J. Pain Symptom Manage. 46 (2), e9–e13.

Hoesel, B., Schmid, J.A., 2013. The complexity of NF-κB signaling in inflammation and cancer. Mol. Cancer 12, 86.

Huang, M., Page, C., Reynolds, R.K., Lin, J., 2000. Constitutive activation of stat 3 oncogene product in human ovarian carcinoma cells. Gynecol. Oncol. 79 (1), 67–73.

Ikeguchi, M., Hatada, T., Yamamoto, M., Miyake, T., Matsunaga, T., Fukumoto, Y., Yamada, Y., Fukuda, K., Saito, H., Tatebe, S., 2009. Serum interleukin-6 and -10 levels in patients with gastric cancer. Gastric Cancer 12 (2), 95–100.

Interleukin-6 Receptor Mendelian Randomisation Analysis (IL6R MR) Consortium, Hingorani, A.D., Casas, J.P., 2012. The interleukin-6 receptor as a target for prevention of coronary heart disease: a mendelian randomization analysis. Lancet 379 (9822), 1214–1224.

Ip, W.K., Wong, C.K., Li, M.L., Li, P.W., Cheung, P.F., Lam, C.W., 2007. Interleukin-31 induces cytokine and chemokine production from human bronchial epithelial cells through activation of mitogen-activated protein kinase signalling pathways: implications for the allergic response. Immunology 122 (4), 532–541.

Ishikawa, H., Tsuyama, N., Liu, S., Abroun, S., Li, F.J., Otsuyama, K., Zheng, X., Ma, Z., Maki, Y., Iqbal, M.S., Obata, M., Kawano, M.M., 2005. Accelerated proliferation of myeloma cells by interleukin-6 cooperating with fibroblast growth factor receptor 3-mediated signals. Oncogene 24 (41), 6328–6332.

Ito, H., Takazoe, M., Fukuda, Y., Hibi, T., Kusugami, K., Andoh, A., Matsumoto, T., Yamamura, T., Azuma, J., Nishimoto, N., Yoshizaki, K., Shimoyama, T., Kishimoto, T., 2004. A pilot randomized trial of a human anti-interleukin-6 receptor monoclonal antibody in active Crohn's disease. Gastroenterology 126 (4), 989–996. discussion 947.

Jang, J.W., Oh, B.S., Kwon, J.H., You, C.R., Chung, K.W., Kay, C.S., Jung, H.S., 2012. Serum interleukin-6 and C-reactive protein as a prognostic indicator in hepatocellular carcinoma. Cytokine 60 (3), 686–693.

Javelaud, D., Mohammad, K.S., McKenna, C.R., Fournier, P., Luciani, F., Niewolna, M., André, J., Delmas, V., Larue, L., Guise, T.A., Mauviel, A., 2007. Stable overexpression of Smad7 in human melanoma cells impairs bone metastasis. Cancer Res. 67 (5), 2317–2324.

Jiang, Y., Zhu, J., Wu, L., Xu, G., Dai, J., Liu, X., 2012. Tetracycline inhibits local inflammation induced by cerebral ischemia via modulating autophagy. PLoS One 7 (11), e48672.

Kang, B.S., Chung, E.Y., Yun, Y.P., Lee, M.K., Lee, Y.R., Lee, K.S., Min, K.R., Kim, Y., 2001. Inhibitory effects of anti-inflammatory drugs on interleukin-6 bioactivity. Biol. Pharm Bull. 24 (6), 701–703.

Kang, Y., Siegel, P.M., Shu, W., Drobnjak, M., Kakonen, S.M., Cordón-Cardo, C., Guise, T.A., Massagué, J., 2003. A multigenic program mediating breast cancer metastasis to bone. Cancer Cell 3 (6), 537–549.

Karkera, J., Steiner, H., Li, W., Skradski, V., Moser, P.L., Riethdorf, S., Reddy, M., Puchalski, T., Safer, K., Prabhakar, U., Pantel, K., Qi, M., Culig, Z., 2011. The anti-interleukin-6 antibody siltuximab down-regulates genes implicated in tumorigenesis in prostate cancer patients from a phase I study. Prostate 71 (13), 1455–1465.

Kasza, A., 2013. IL-1 and EGF regulate expression of genes important in inflammation and cancer. Cytokine 62 (1), 22–33.

Kim, D.H., Sarbassov, D.D., Ali, S.M., King, J.E., Latek, R.R., Erdjument-Bromage, H., Tempst, P., Sabatini, D.M., 2002. mTOR interacts with raptor to form a nutrient-sensitive complex that signals to the cell growth machinery. Cell 110 (2), 163–175.

Kim, H.S., Lee, M.S., 2007. STAT1 as a key modulator of cell death. Cell Signal 19 (3), 454–465.

Kimura, R., Maeda, M., Arita, A., Oshima, Y., Obana, M., Ito, T., Yamamoto, Y., Mohri, T., Kishimoto, T., Kawase, I., Fujio, Y., Azuma, J., 2007. Identification of cardiac myocytes as the target of interleukin 11, a cardioprotective cytokine. Cytokine 38 (2), 107–115.

Kottke, T., Boisgerault, N., Diaz, R.M., Donnelly, O., Rommelfanger-Konkol, D., Pulido, J., Thompson, J., Mukhopadhyay, D., Kaspar, R., Coffey, M., Pandha, H., Melcher, A., Harrington, K., Selby, P., Vile, R., 2013. Detecting and targeting tumor relapse by its resistance to innate effectors at early recurrence. Nat. Med. 19 (12), 1625–1631.

Koziorowski, D., Tomasiuk, R., Szlufik, S., Friedman, A., 2012. Inflammatory cytokines and NT-proCNP in Parkinson's disease patients. Cytokine 60 (3), 762–766.

Kozlow, W., Guise, T.A., 2005. Breast cancer metastasis to bone: mechanisms of osteolysis and implications for therapy. J. Mammary Gland Biol. Neoplasia 10 (2), 169–180.

Krzystek-Korpacka, M., Matusiewicz, M., Diakowska, D., Grabowski, K., Blachut, K., Kustrzeba-Wojcicka, I., Terlecki, G., Gamian, A., 2008. Acute-phase response proteins are related to cachexia and accelerated angiogenesis in gastroesophageal cancers. Clin. Chem. Lab. Med 46 (3), 359–364.

Lay, V., Yap, J., Sonderegger, S., Dimitriadis, E., 2012 Aug. Interleukin 11 regulates endometrial cancer cell adhesion and migration via STAT3. Int. J. Oncol. 41 (2), 759–764.

Lee, J., Kim, J.C., Lee, S.E., Quinley, C., Kim, H., Herdman, S., Corr, M., Raz, E., 2012. Signal transducer and activator of transcription 3 (STAT3) protein suppresses adenoma-to-carcinoma transition in Apcmin/+ mice via regulation of Snail-1 (SNAI) protein stability. J. Biol. Chem. 287 (22), 18182–18189.

Leslie, K., Gao, S.P., Berishaj, M., Podsypanina, K., Ho, H., Ivashkiv, L., Bromberg, J., 2010. Differential interleukin-6/Stat3 signaling as a function of cellular context mediates Ras-induced transformation. Breast Cancer Res. 12 (5), R80.

Lewis, V.O., Ozawa, M.G., Deavers, M.T., Wang, G., Shintani, T., Arap, W., Pasqualini, R., 2009. The interleukin-11 receptor alpha as a candidate ligand-directed target in osteosarcoma: consistent data from cell lines, orthotopic models, and human tumor samples. Cancer Res. 69 (5), 1995–1999.

Lgssiar, A., Hassan, M., Schott-Ohly, P., Friesen, N., Nicoletti, F., Trepicchio, W.L., Gleichmann, H., 2004. Interleukin-11 inhibits NF-kappaB and AP-1 activation in islets and prevents diabetes induced with streptozotocin in mice. Exp. Biol. Med. (Maywood) 229 (5), 425–436.

Li, S., Xia, X., Mellieon, F.M., Liu, J., Steele, S., 2004. Candidate genes associated with tumor regression mediated by intratumoral IL-12 electroporation gene therapy. Mol. Ther. 9 (3), 347–354.

Li, T.M., Wu, C.M., Huang, H.C., Chou, P.C., Fong, Y.C., Tang, C.H., 2012. Interleukin-11 increases cell motility and up-regulates intercellular adhesion molecule-1 expression in human chondrosarcoma cells. J. Cell. Biochem. 113 (11), 3353–3362.

Liao, W.C., Lin, J.T., Wu, C.Y., Huang, S.P., Lin, M.T., Wu, A.S., Huang, Y.J., Wu, M.S., 2008. Serum interleukin-6 level but not genotype predicts survival after resection in stages II and III gastric carcinoma. Clin. Cancer Res. 14 (2), 428–434.

Liu, X., Chen, Q., Yan, J., Wang, Y., Zhu, C., Chen, C., Zhao, X., Xu, M., Sun, Q., Deng, R., Zhang, H., Qu, Y., Huang, J., Jiang, B., Yu, J., November 21, 2013. MiRNA-296-3p-ICAM-1 axis promotes metastasis of prostate cancer by possible enhancing survival of natural killer cell-resistant circulating tumour cells. Cell Death Dis. 4, e928.

Liu, Y., Liu, A., Li, H., Li, C., Lin, J., 2011. Celecoxib inhibits interleukin-6/interleukin-6 receptor-induced JAK2/STAT3 phosphorylation in human hepatocellular carcinoma cells. Cancer Prev. Res. (Phila) 4 (8), 1296–1305.

Ljungberg, B., Grankvist, K., Rasmuson, T., 1997. Serum interleukin-6 in relation to acute-phase reactants and survival in patients with renal cell carcinoma. Eur. J. Cancer 33 (11), 1794–1798.

Luis-Ravelo, D., Antón, I., Zandueta, C., Valencia, K., Ormazábal, C., Martínez-Canarias, S., Guruceaga, E., Perurena, N., Vicent, S., De Las Rivas, J., Lecanda, F., October 28, 2013. A gene signature of bone metastatic colonization sensitizes for tumor-induced osteolysis and predicts survival in lung cancer. Oncogene. http://dx.doi.org/10.1038/onc.2013.440 (Epub ahead of print).

Lüscher-Firzlaff, J., Gawlista, I., Vervoorts, J., Kapelle, K., Braunschweig, T., Walsemann, G., Rodgarkia-Schamberger, C., Schuchlautz, H., Dreschers, S., Kremmer, E., Lilischkis, R., Cerni, C., Wellmann, A., Lüscher, B., 2008 Feb 1. The human trithorax protein hASH2 functions as an oncoprotein. Cancer Res. 68 (3), 749–758.

Meng, L., Zhou, J., Sasano, H., Suzuki, T., Zeitoun, K.M., Bulun, S.E., 2001. Tumor necrosis factor alpha and interleukin 11 secreted by malignant breast epithelial cells inhibit adipocyte differentiation by selectively down-regulating CCAAT/enhancer binding protein alpha and peroxisome proliferator-activated receptor gamma: mechanism of desmoplastic reaction. Cancer Res. 61 (5), 2250–2255.

Middleton, K., Jones, J., Lwin, Z., Coward, J.I., 2014. Interleukin-6: an angiogenic target in solid tumours. Crit. Rev. Oncol. Hematol. 89 (1), 129–139.

Mitsunaga, S., Ikeda, M., Shimizu, S., Ohno, I., Furuse, J., Inagaki, M., Higashi, S., Kato, H., Terao, K., Ochiai, A., 2013. Serum levels of IL-6 and IL-1β can predict the efficacy of gemcitabine in patients with advanced pancreatic cancer. Br. J. Cancer 108 (10), 2063–2069.

Mitsuyama, K., Sata, M., Rose-John, S., 2006. Interleukin-6 trans-signaling in inflammatory bowel disease. Cytokine Growth Factor Rev. 17 (6), 451–461.

Mizutani, Y., Bonavida, B., Koishihara, Y., Akamatsu, K., Ohsugi, Y., Yoshida, O., 1995. Sensitization of human renal cell carcinoma cells to cis-diamminedichloroplatinum(II) by anti-interleukin 6 monoclonal antibody or anti-interleukin 6 receptor monoclonal antibody. Cancer Res. 55 (3), 590–596.

Moreau, P., Harousseau, J.L., Wijdenes, J., Morineau, N., Milpied, N., Bataille, R., 2000. A combination of anti-interleukin 6 murine monoclonal antibody with dexamethasone and high-dose melphalan induces high complete response rates in advanced multiple myeloma. Br. J. Haematol. 109 (3), 661–664.

Moreau, P., Hulin, C., Marit, G., Caillot, D., Facon, T., Lenain, P., Berthou, C., Pégourié, B., Stoppa, A.M., Casassus, P., Michallet, M., Benboubker, L., Maisonneuve, H., Doyen, C., Leyvraz, S., Mathiot, C., Avet-Loiseau, H., Attal, M., Harousseau, J.L., 2010 Jun. IFM group. Stem cell collection in patients with de novo multiple myeloma treated with the combination of bortezomib and dexamethasone before autologous stem cell transplantation according to IFM 2005-01 trial. Leukemia 24 (6), 1233–1235.

Morgan, G., 2010. Future drug developments in multiple myeloma: an overview of novel lenalidomide-based combination therapies. Blood Rev. 24 (Suppl. 1), S27–S32.

Muangchan, C., Pope, J.E., 2012. Interleukin 6 in systemic sclerosis and potential implications for targeted therapy. J. Rheumatol. 39 (6), 1120–1124.

Mudter, J., Neurath, M.F., 2007. Il-6 signaling in inflammatory bowel disease: pathophysiological role and clinical relevance. Inflamm. Bowel Dis. 13 (8), 1016–1023.

Muñoz-Cánoves, P., Scheele, C., Pedersen, B.K., Serrano, A.L., 2013. Interleukin-6 myokine signaling in skeletal muscle: a double-edged sword? FEBS J. 280 (17), 4131–4148.

Musteanu, M., Blaas, L., Mair, M., Schlederer, M., Bilban, M., Tauber, S., Esterbauer, H., Mueller, M., Casanova, E., Kenner, L., Poli, V., Eferl, R., 2010. Stat3 is a negative regulator of intestinal tumor progression in Apc(Min) mice. Gastroenterology 138 (3), 1003–1011. e1–5.

Nakayama,T.,Yoshizaki,A., Izumida, S., Suehiro,T., Miura, S., Uemura,T.,Yakata,Y., Shichijo, K.,Yamashita, S., Sekin, I., 2007. Expression of interleukin-11 (IL-11) and IL-11 receptor alpha in human gastric carcinoma and IL-11 upregulates the invasive activity of human gastric carcinoma cells. Int. J. Oncol. 30 (4), 825–833.

Nandurkar, H.H., Robb, L., Begley, C.G., 1998.The role of IL-II in hematopoiesis as revealed by a targeted mutation of its receptor. Stem Cells 16 (Suppl. 2), 53–65.

Necula, L.G., Chivu-Economescu, M., Stanciulescu, E.L., Bleotu, C., Dima, S.O., Alexiu, I., Dumitru, A., Constantinescu, G., Popescu, I., Diaconu, C.C., 2012. IL-6 and IL-11 as markers for tumor aggressiveness and prognosis in gastric adenocarcinoma patients without mutations in Gp130 subunits. J. Gastrointestin. Liver Dis. 21 (1), 23–29.

Neiva, K.G.,Warner, K.A., Campos, M.S., Zhang, Z., Moren, J., Danciu,T.E., Nör, J.E., 2014. Endothelial cell-derived interleukin-6 regulates tumor growth. BMC Cancer 14 (1), 99 (Epub ahead of print).

Neurath, M.F., Finotto, S., 2011. IL-6 signaling in autoimmunity, chronic inflammation and inflammation-associated cancer. Cytokine Growth Factor Rev. 22 (2), 83–89.

Niebuhr, M., Mamerow, D., Heratizadeh, A., Satzger, I., Werfel, T., 2011. Staphylococcal α-toxin induces a higher T cell proliferation and interleukin-31 in atopic dermatitis. Int. Arch. Allergy Immunol. 156 (4), 412–415.

Nikitakis, N.G., Hamburger, A.W., Sauk, J.J., 2002.The nonsteroidal anti-inflammatory drug sulindac causes down-regulation of signal transducer and activator of transcription 3 in human oral squamous cell carcinoma cells. Cancer Res. 62 (4), 1004–1007.

Nishimoto, N., Kanakura,Y., Aozasa, K., Johkoh,T., Nakamura, M., Nakano, S., Nakano, N., Ikeda,Y., Sasaki,T., Nishioka, K., Hara, M.,Taguchi, H., Kimura,Y., Kato,Y., Asaoku, H., Kumagai, S., Kodama, F., Nakahara, H., Hagihara, K.,Yoshizaki, K., Kishimoto,T., 2005. Humanized anti-interleukin-6 receptor antibody treatment of multicentric Castleman disease. Blood 106 (8), 2627–2632.

Nobbe, S., Dziunycz, P., Mühleisen, B., Bilsborough, J., Dillon, S.R., French, L.E., Hofbauer, G.F., 2012. IL-31 expression by inflammatory cells is preferentially elevated in atopic dermatitis. Acta Derm.Venereol. 92 (1), 24–28.

Nonomura, N., Nakayama, M., Takayama, H., Nishimura, K., Okuyama, A., 2008. Molecular-targeted therapy for prostate cancer. Hinyokika Kiyo 54 (1), 63–66 (Article in Japanese).

Obana, M., Miyamoto, K., Murasawa, S., Iwakura,T., Hayama,A.,Yamashita,T., Shiragaki, M., Kumagai, S., Miyawaki, A., Takewaki, K., Matsumiya, G., Maeda, M., Yoshiyama, M., Nakayama, H., Fujio,Y., 2012.Therapeutic administration of IL-11 exhibits the postconditioning effects against ischemia-reperfusion injury via STAT3 in the heart. Am. J. Physiol. Heart Circ. Physiol. 303 (5), H569–H577.

Oguro, T., Ishibashi, K., Sugino, T., Hashimoto, K., Tomita, S.,Takahashi, N.,Yanagida,T., Haga, N.,Aikawa, K., Suzutani,T.,Yamaguchi, O., Kojima,Y., 2013. Humanised antihuman IL-6R antibody with interferon inhibits renal cell carcinoma cell growth in vitro and in vivo through suppressed SOCS3 expression. Eur. J. Cancer 49 (7), 1715–1724.

Ohmatsu, H., Sugaya, M., Suga, H., Morimura, S., Miyagaki,T., Kai, H., Kagami, S., Fujita, H., Asano,Y., Tada,Y., Kadono, T., Sato, S., 2012. Serum IL-31 levels are increased in patients with cutaneous T-cell lymphoma. Acta Derm.Venereol. 92 (3), 282–283.

Oka, M., Yamamoto, K., Takahashi, M., Hakozaki, M., Abe, T., Iizuka, N., Hazama, S., Hirazawa, K., Hayashi, H., Tangoku, A., Hirose, K., Ishihara, T., Suzuki, T., 1996. Relationship between serum levels of interleukin 6, various disease parameters and malnutrition in patients with esophageal squamous cell carcinoma. Cancer Res. 56 (12), 2776–2780.

Okamoto, M., Kawamata, H., Kawai, K., Oyasu, R., 1995. Enhancement of transformation in vitro of a nontumorigenic rat urothelial cell line by interleukin 6. Cancer Res. 55 (20), 4581–4585.

Pang, X.H., Zhang, J.P., Zhang, Y.J., Yan, J., Pei, X.Q., Zhang, Y.Q., Li, J.Q., Zheng, L., Chen, M.S., 2011. Preoperative levels of serum interleukin-6 in patients with hepatocellular carcinoma. Hepatogastroenterology 58 (110–111), 1687–1693.

Paul, S.R., Bennett, F., Calvetti, J.A., Kelleher, K., Wood, C.R., O'Hara Jr, R.M., Leary, A.C., Sibley, B., Clark, S.C., Williams, D.A., Yang, Y.C., 1990. Molecular cloning of a cDNA encoding interleukin 11, a stromal cell-derived lymphopoietic and hematopoietic cytokine. Proc. Natl. Acad. Sci. USA 87 (19), 7512–7516.

Penson, R.T., Kronish, K., Duan, Z., Feller, A.J., Stark, P., Cook, S.E., Duska, L.R., Fuller, A.F., Goodman, A.K., Nikrui, N., MacNeill, K.M., Matulonis, U.A., Preffer, F.I., Seiden, M.V., 2000. Cytokines IL-1beta, IL-2, IL-6, IL-8, MCP-1, GM-CSF and TNFalpha in patients with epithelial ovarian cancer and their relationship to treatment with paclitaxel. Int. J. Gynecol. Cancer 10 (1), 33–41.

Pietrzak, A., Zalewska, A., Chodorowska, G., Nockowski, P., Michalak-Stoma, A., Osemlak, P., Krasowska, D., 2008. Genes and structure of selected cytokines involved in pathogenesis of psoriasis. Folia Histochem. Cytobiol. 46 (1), 11–21.

Plante, M., Rubin, S.C., Wong, G.Y., Federici, M.G., Finstad, C.L., Gastl, G.A., 1994. Interleukin-6 level in serum and ascites as a prognostic factor in patients with epithelial ovarian cancer. Cancer 73 (7), 1882–1888.

Pollari, S., Käkönen, R.S., Mohammad, K.S., Rissanen, J.P., Halleen, J.M., Wärri, A., Nissinen, L., Pihlavisto, M., Marjamäki, A., Perälä, M., Guise, T.A., Kallioniemi, O., Käkönen, S.M., 2012. Heparin-like polysaccharides reduce osteolytic bone destruction and tumor growth in a mouse model of breast cancer bone metastasis. Mol. Cancer Res. 10 (5), 597–604.

Porta, C., De Amici, M., Quaglini, S., Paglino, C., Tagliani, F., Boncimino, A., Moratti, R., Corazza, G.R., 2008. Circulating interleukin-6 as a tumor marker for hepatocellular carcinoma. Ann. Oncol. 19 (2), 353–358.

Pourgholami, M.H., Ataie-Kachoie, P., Badar, S., Morris, D.L., 2013. Minocycline inhibits malignant ascites of ovarian cancer through targeting multiple signaling pathways. Gynecol. Oncol. 129 (1), 113–119.

Pourgholami, M.H., Mekkawy, A.H., Badar, S., Morris, D.L., 2012. Minocycline inhibits growth of epithelial ovarian cancer. Gynecol. Oncol. 125 (2), 433–440.

Pu, Y.S., Hour, T.C., Chuang, S.E., Cheng, A.L., Lai, M.K., Kuo, M.L., 2004. Interleukin-6 is responsible for drug resistance and anti-apoptotic effects in prostatic cancer cells. Prostate 60 (2), 120–129.

Puchalski, T., Prabhakar, U., Jiao, Q., Berns, B., Davis, H.M., 2010. Pharmacokinetic and pharmacodynamic modeling of an anti-interleukin-6 chimeric monoclonal antibody(siltuximab) in patients with metastatic renal cell carcinoma. Clin. Cancer Res. 16 (5), 1652–1661.

Putoczki, T., Ernst, M., 2010. More than a sidekick: the IL-6 family cytokine IL-11 links inflammation to cancer. J. Leukoc. Biol. 88 (6), 1109–1117.

Qiu, Y., Ravi, L., Kung, H.J., 1998. Requirement of ErbB2 for signalling by interleukin-6 in prostate carcinoma cells. Nature 393 (6680), 83–85.

Ren, L., Wang, X., Dong, Z., Liu, J., Zhang, S., 2013. Bone metastasis from breast cancer involves elevated IL-11 expression and the gp130/STAT3 pathway. Med. Oncol. 30 (3), 634.

Robb, L., Hilton, D.J., Brook-Carter, P.T., Begley, C.G., 1997. Identification of a second murine interleukin-11 receptor alpha-chain gene (IL11Ra2) with a restricted pattern of expression. Genomics 40 (3), 387–394.

Rojas, A., Liu, G., Coleman, I., Nelson, P.S., Zhang, M., Dash, R., Fisher, P.B., Plymate, S.R., Wu, J.D., 2011. IL-6 promotes prostate tumorigenesis and progression through autocrine cross-activation of IGF-IR. Oncogene 30 (20), 2345–2355.

Romas, E., Udagawa, N., Zhou, H., Tamura, T., Saito, M., Taga, T., Hilton, D.J., Suda, T., Ng, K.W., Martin, T.J., 1996. The role of gp130-mediated signals in osteoclast development: regulation of interleukin 11 production by osteoblasts and distribution of its receptor in bone marrow cultures. J. Exp. Med. 183 (6), 2581–2591.

Rosen, D.G., Mercado-Uribe, I., Yang, G., Bast Jr, R.C., Amin, H.M., Lai, R., Liu, J., 2006. The role of constitutively active signal transducer and activator of transcription 3 in ovarian tumorigenesis and prognosis. Cancer 107 (11), 2730–2740.

Rossi, J.F., Négrier, S., James, N.D., Kocak, I., Hawkins, R., Davis, H., Prabhakar, U., Qin, X., Mulders, P., Berns, B., 2010. A phase I/II study of siltuximab (CNTO 328), an anti-interleukin-6 monoclonal antibody, in metastatic renal cell cancer. Br. J. Cancer 103 (8), 1154–1162.

Rutsch, S., Neppalli, V.T., Shin, D.M., DuBois, W., Morse 3rd, H.C., Goldschmidt, H., Janz, S., 2010. IL-6 and MYC collaborate in plasma cell tumor formation in mice. Blood 115 (9), 1746–1754.

Sales, K.J., Grant, V., Cook, I.H., Maldonado-Pérez, D., Anderson, R.A., Williams, A.R., Jabbour, H.N., 2010. Interleukin-11 in endometrial adenocarcinoma is regulated by prostaglandin F2alpha-F-prostanoid receptor interaction via the calcium-calcineurin-nuclear factor of activated T cells pathway and negatively regulated by the regulator of calcineurin-1. Am. J. Pathol. 176 (1), 435–445.

Sansone, P., Bromberg, J., 2012. Targeting the interleukin-6/Jak/stat pathway in human malignancies. J. Clin. Oncol. 30 (9), 1005–1014.

Sansone, P., Storci, G., Tavolari, S., Guarnieri, T., Giovannini, C., Taffurelli, M., Ceccarelli, C., Santini, D., Paterini, P., Marcu, K.B., Chieco, P., Bonafè, M., 2007. IL-6 triggers malignant features in mammospheres from human ductal breast carcinoma and normal mammary gland. J. Clin. Invest. 117 (12), 3988–4002.

Schwertschlag, U.S., Trepicchio, W.L., Dykstra, K.H., Keith, J.C., Turner, K.J., Dorner, A.J., 1999. Hematopoietic, immunomodulatory and epithelial effects of interleukin-11. Leukemia 13 (9), 1307–1315.

Sellier, H., Rébillard, A., Guette, C., Barré, B., Coqueret, O., 2013. How should we define STAT3 as an oncogene and as a potential target for therapy? JAKSTAT 2 (3), e24716.

Selzer, M.G., Zhu, B., Block, N.L., Lokeshwar, B.L., 1999. CMT-3, a chemically modified tetracycline, inhibits bony metastases and delays the development of paraplegia in a rat model of prostate cancer. Ann. N.Y. Acad. Sci. 878, 678–682.

Shah, S.A., Ishinaga, H., Hou, B., Okano, M., Takeuchi, K., 2013. Effects of interleukin-31 on MUC5AC gene expression in nasal allergic inflammation. Pharmacology 91 (3–4), 158–164.

Shaul, Y.D., Seger, R., 2007. The MEK/ERK cascade: from signaling specificity to diverse functions. Biochim. Biophys. Acta 1773 (8), 1213–1226.

Shen, Z., Seppänen, H., Vainionpää, S., Ye, Y., Wang, S., Mustonen, H., Puolakkainen, P., 2012. IL10, IL11, IL18 are differently expressed in CD14+ TAMs and play different role in regulating the invasion of gastric cancer cells under hypoxia. Cytokine 59 (2), 352–357.

Shimazaki, J., Goto, Y., Nishida, K., Tabuchi, T., Motohashi, G., Ubukata, H., Tabuchi, T., 2013. In patients with colorectal cancer, preoperative serum interleukin-6 level and granulocyte/lymphocyte ratio are clinically relevant biomarkers of long-term cancer progression. Oncology 84 (6), 356–361.

Shinriki, S., Jono, H., Ota, K., Ueda, M., Kudo, M., Ota, T., Oike, Y., Endo, M., Ibusuki, M., Hiraki, A., Nakayama, H., Yoshitake, Y., Shinohara, M., Ando, Y., 2009. Humanized anti-interleukin-6 receptor antibody suppresses tumor angiogenesis and in vivo growth of human oral squamous cell carcinoma. Clin. Cancer Res. 15 (17), 5426–5434.

Shinriki, S., Jono, H., Ueda, M., Ota, K., Ota, T., Sueyoshi, T., Oike, Y., Ibusuki, M., Hiraki, A., Nakayama, H., Shinohara, M., Ando, Y., 2011. Interleukin-6 signalling regulates vascular endothelial growth factor-C synthesis and lymphangiogenesis in human oral squamous cell carcinoma. J. Pathol. 225 (1), 142–150.

Singer, E.M., Shin, D.B., Nattkemper, L.A., Benoit, B.M., Klein, R.S., Didigu, C.A., Loren, A.W., Dentchev, T., Wysocka, M., Yosipovitch, G., Rook, A.H., 2013. IL-31 is produced by the malignant T-cell population in cutaneous T-Cell lymphoma and correlates with CTCL pruritus. J. Invest. Dermatol. 133 (12), 2783–2785.

Siniewicz-Luzeńczyk, K., Stańczyk-Przyłuska, A., Zeman, K., 2013. Correlation between serum interleukin-31 level and the severity of disease in children with atopic dermatitis. Postepy Dermatol. Alergol. 30 (5), 282–285.

Sipos, E., Chen, L., András, I.E., Wrobel, J., Zhang, B., Pu, H., Park, M., Eum, S.Y., Toborek, M., 2012. Proinflammatory adhesion molecules facilitate polychlorinated biphenyl-mediated enhancement of brain metastasis formation. Toxicol. Sci. 126 (2), 362–371.

Siveen, K.S., Sikka, S., Surana, R., Dai, X., Zhang, J., Kumar, A.P., Tan, B.K., Sethi, G., Bishayee, A., January 2, 2014. Targeting the STAT3 signaling pathway in cancer: role of synthetic and natural inhibitors. Biochim. Biophys. Acta 1845 (2), 136–154. http://dx.doi.org/10.1016/j.bbcan.2013.12.005 (Epub ahead of print).

Slevin, M., Krupinski, J., Slowik, A., Rubio, F., Szczudlik, A., Gaffney, J., 2000. Activation of MAP kinase (ERK-1/ERK-2), tyrosine kinase and VEGF in the human brain following acute ischaemic stroke. Neuroreport 11 (12), 2759–2764.

Songür, N., Kuru, B., Kalkan, F., Ozdilekcan, C., Cakmak, H., Hizel, N., 2004. Serum interleukin-6 levels correlate with malnutrition and survival in patients with advanced non-small cell lung cancer. Tumori 90 (2), 196–200.

Sonkoly, E., Muller, A., Lauerma, A.I., Pivarcsi, A., Soto, H., Kemeny, L., Alenius, H., Dieu-Nosjean, M.C., Meller, S., Rieker, J., Steinhoff, M., Hoffmann, T.K., Ruzicka, T., 2006. Zlotnik A, Homey B. IL-31: a new link between T cells and pruritus in atopic skin inflammation. J. Allergy Clin. Immunol. 117 (2), 411–417.

Soto, M.S., Serres, S., Anthony, D.C., Sibson, N.R., April 2013. Functional role of endothelial adhesion molecules in the early stages of brain metastasis. Neuro. Oncol. 16 (4), 540–551.

Spooren, A., Kolmus, K., Laureys, G., Clinckers, R., De Keyser, J., Haegeman, G., Gerlo, S., 2011. Interleukin-6, a mental cytokine. Brain Res. Rev. 67 (1–2), 157–183.

Sterling, J.A., Edwards, J.R., Martin, T.J., Mundy, G.R., 2011. Advances in the biology of bone metastasis: how the skeleton affects tumor behavior. Bone 48 (1), 6–15.

Strieter, R.M., Kunkel, S.L., Arenberg, D.A., Burdick, M.D., Polverini, P.J., 1995. Interferon gamma-inducible protein 10 (IP-10), a member of the C-X-C chemokine family, is an inhibitor of angiogenesis. Biochem. Biophys. Res. Commun. 210 (1), 51–57.

Swaak, A.J., van Rooyen, A., Nieuwenhuis, E., Aarden, L.A., 1988. Interleukin-6 (IL-6) in synovial fluid and serum of patients with rheumatic diseases. Scand. J. Rheumatol. 17 (6), 469–474.

Takaoka, A., Arai, I., Sugimoto, M., Honma, Y., Futaki, N., Nakamura, A., Nakaike, S., 2006. Involvement of IL-31 on scratching behavior in NC/Nga mice with atopic-like dermatitis. Exp. Dermatol. 15 (3), 161–167.

Trepicchio, W.L., Dorner, A.J., 1998. The therapeutic utility of interleukin-11 in the treatment of inflammatory disease. Expert Opin. Investig. Drugs 7 (9), 1501–1504.

Tsuboi, I., Tanaka, H., Nakao, M., Shichijo, S., Itoh, K., 1995. Nonsteroidal anti-inflammatory drugs differentially regulate cytokine production in human lymphocytes: up-regulation of TNF, IFN-gamma and IL-2, in contrast to down-regulation of IL-6 production. Cytokine 7 (4), 372–379.

Tsuchiya, K., Jo, T., Takeda, N., Al Heialy, S., Siddiqui, S., Shalaby, K.H., Risse, P.A., Maghni, K., Martin, J.G., 2010. EGF receptor activation during allergic sensitization affects IL-6-induced T-cell influx to airways in a rat model of asthma. Eur. J. Immunol. 40 (6), 1590–1602.

Ujiie, H., Tomida, M., Akiyama, H., Nakajima, Y., Okada, D., Yoshino, N., Takiguchi, Y., Tanzawa, H., 2012. Serum hepatocyte growth factor and interleukin-6 are effective prognostic markers for non-small cell lung cancer. Anticancer Res. 32 (8), 3251–3258.

Valles, S.L., Benlloch, M., Rodriguez, M.L., Mena, S., Pellicer, J.A., Asensi, M., Obrador, E., Estrela, J.M., 2013. Stress hormones promote growth of B16-F10 melanoma metastases: an interleukin 6- and glutathione-dependent mechanism. J. Transl. Med. 11, 72.

Venkiteshwaran, A., Tocilizumab, 2009. MAbs 1 (5), 432–438.

Verma, R., Verma, N., Paul, J., 2013 Jul-Sep. Expression of inflammatory genes in the colon of ulcerative colitis patients varies with activity both at the mRNA and protein level. Eur. Cytokine. Netw. 24 (3), 130–138.

Waage, A., Slupphaug, G., Shalaby, R., 1990. Glucocorticoids inhibit the production of IL6 from monocytes, endothelial cells and fibroblasts. Eur. J. Immunol. 20 (11), 2439–2443.

Walmsley, M., Butler, D.M., Marinova-Mutafchieva, L., Feldmann, M., 1998. An anti-inflammatory role for interleukin-11 in established murine collagen-induced arthritis. Immunology 95 (1), 31–37.

Wang, L.S., Chow, K.C., Wu, C.W., 1999. Expression and up-regulation of interleukin-6 in oesophageal carcinoma cells by n-sodium butyrate. Br. J. Cancer 80 (10), 1617–1622.

Wu, D., Tao, J., Ding, J., Qu, P., Lu, Q., Zhang, W., 2013. Interleukin-11, an interleukin-6-like cytokine, is a promising predictor for bladder cancer prognosis. Mol. Med. Rep. 7 (2), 684–688.

Xiang, Z.L., Zeng, Z.C., Tang, Z.Y., Fan, J., He, J., Zeng, H.Y., Zhu, X.D., 2011. Potential prognostic biomarkers for bone metastasis from hepatocellular carcinoma. Oncologist 16 (7), 1028–1039.

Yadav, A., Kumar, B., Datta, J., Teknos, T.N., Kumar, P., 2011. IL-6 promotes head and neck tumor metastasis by inducing epithelial-mesenchymal transition via the JAK-STAT3-SNAIL signaling pathway. Mol. Cancer Res. 9 (12), 1658–1667.

Yamazumi, K., Nakayama, T., Kusaba, T., Wen, C.Y., Yoshizaki, A., Yakata, Y., Nagayasu, T., Sekine, I., 2006. Expression of interleukin-11 and interleukin-11 receptor alpha in human colorectal adenocarcinoma; immunohistochemical analyses and correlation with clinicopathological factors. World J. Gastroenterol. 12 (2), 317–321.

Yang, G., Ma, F., Zhong, M., Fang, L., Peng, Y., Xin, X., Zhong, J., Zhu, W., Zhang, Y., April 2014. Interleukin-11 induces the expression of matrix metalloproteinase 13 in gastric cancer SCH cells partly via the PI3K-AKT and JAK-STAT3 pathways. Mol. Med. Rep. 9 (4), 1371–1375. http://dx.doi.org/10.3892/mmr.2014.1932 (Epub ahead of print).

Yoneda, M., Fujiwara, H., Furutani, A., Ikai, A., Tada, H., Shiozaki, A., Komatsu, S., Kubota, T., Ichikawa, D., Okamoto, K., Konishi, H., Murayama, Y., Kuriu, Y., Ikoma H., Nakanishi, M., Ochiai, T., Otsuji, E., 2013. Prognostic impact of tumor IL-6 expression after preoperative chemoradiotherapy in patients with advanced esophageal squamous cell carcinoma. Anticancer Res. 33 (6), 2699–2705.

Yoon, J.Y., Lafarge, S., Dawe, D., Lakhi, S., Kumar, R., Morales, C., Marshall, A., Gibson, S.B., Johnston, J.B., 2012. Association of interleukin-6 and interleukin-8 with poor prognosis in elderly patients with chronic lymphocytic leukemia. Leuk. Lymphoma 53 (9), 1735–1742.

Yoshizaki, A., Nakayama, T., Yamazumi, K., Yakata, Y., Taba, M., Sekine, I., 2006. Expression of interleukin (IL)-11 and IL-11 receptor in human colorectal adenocarcinoma: IL-11 up-regulation of the invasive and proliferative activity of human colorectal carcinoma cells. Int. J. Oncol. 29 (4), 869–876.

Yuzhalin, A., 2011. The role of interleukin DNA polymorphisms in gastric cancer. Hum. Immunol. 72 (11), 1128–1136.

Yuzhalin, A.E., Kutikhin, A.G., 2012. Interleukin-12: clinical usage and molecular markers of cancer susceptibility. Growth Factors 30 (3), 176–191.

Zhang, G., Tsang, C.M., Deng, W., Yip, Y.L., Lui, V.W., Wong, S.C., Cheung, A.L., Hau, P.M., Zeng, M., Lung, M.L., Chen, H., Lo, K.W., Takada, K., Tsao, S.W., 2013. Enhanced IL-6/IL-6R signaling promotes growth and malignant properties in EBV-infected premalignant and cancerous nasopharyngeal epithelial cells. PLoS One 8 (5), e62284.

Zhang, G.J., Adachi, I., 1999. Serum interleukin-6 levels correlate to tumor progression and prognosis in metastatic breast carcinoma. Anticancer Res. 19 (2B), 1427–1432.

Zhang, Y., Yan, W., Collins, M.A., Bednar, F., Rakshit, S., Zetter, B.R., Stanger, B.Z., Chung, I., Rhim, A.D., di Magliano, M.P., 2013. Interleukin-6 is required for pancreatic cancer progression by promoting MAPK signaling activation and oxidative stress resistance. Cancer Res. 73 (20), 6359–6374.

Zurita, A.J., Troncoso, P., Cardó-Vila, M., Logothetis, C.J., Pasqualini, R., Arap, W., 2004. Combinatorial screenings in patients: the interleukin-11 receptor alpha as a candidate target in the progression of human prostate cancer. Cancer Res. 64 (2), 435–439.

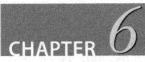

CHAPTER 6

Interleukin-10 Superfamily and Cancer

Two things fill the mind with ever-increasing wonder and awe, the more often and the more intensely the mind of thought is drawn to them: the starry heavens above me and the moral law within me.
Immanuel Kant, German philosopher (1724–1804)

6.1 INTERLEUKIN-10

6.1.1 Description of IL-10 and Overview of its Biology

In the early 1990s, the research group led by Tim R. Mossman isolated and characterized a previously unknown agent, which markedly inhibited the production of several cytokines, including interleukin (IL)-2 and interferon (IFN)-γ (Fiorentino et al., 1989; Moore et al., 1990). Due to this effect, the novel factor was initially called cytokine synthesis inhibitory factor. Today, IL-10 is the founding member of a large superfamily of cytokines, which also includes IL-19, IL-20, IL-22, IL-24, IL-26, and the unique type III IFN-γ subfamily consisting of IL-28A (IFN-γ1), IL-28B (IFN-γ2), and IL-29 (IFN-γ3). Structure analysis carried out by Zdanov et al. (1995, 1997) revealed that IL-10 represents a 37-kDa heterodimer forming a "V-shaped structure". In addition, the authors also discovered that each monomer has a molecular weight of 18.5 kDa and consists of six alpha helices. Regarding other representatives of the IL-10 superfamily, it is known that IL-19, IL-20, IL-22, and IL-24 are active as monomers and that IL-26 may act as either a dimer or a monomer (Zdanov, 2010). All the monomers of the IL-10 superfamily are topologically similar to the single chain of IL-10; however, slight differences in their molecular structure cause a wide variety of biological effects of these cytokines (Zdanov, 2010). Interestingly, numerous viral homologs of IL-10 are known, including human and simian cytomegalovirus (Kotenko et al., 2000; Lockridge et al., 2000), equine type 2 herpes virus (Rode et al., 1993), Epstein–Barr virus (Hsu et al., 1990; Vieira et al., 1991), and Orf parapoxvirus (Fleming et al., 1997, 2000). Notably, all the representatives of the IL-10 superfamily are regarded as class II cytokines, which

Interleukins in Cancer Biology
http://dx.doi.org/10.1016/B978-0-12-801121-8.00006-3

means that they have structural characteristics similar to those of type I and II IFNs (Pestka et al., 2004b; Krause and Pestka, 2005, 2007; Dunn et al., 2006; Zdanov, 2010).

All the representatives of the IL-10 superfamily operate through two closely related heterodimeric receptors IL-10R1 and IL-10R2 (Mosser and Zhang, 2008). Almost all human cells express IL-10R2, suggesting a broad spectrum of activity of the IL-10 superfamily. Binding of IL-10 to the corresponding receptor recruits JAK1 and Tyk2 to the receptor's intracellular domain. Subsequent activation of STAT3 leads to its homodimerization and translocation into the nucleus, where the regulation of numerous genes occurs (Decker and Meinke, 1997; Mosser and Zhang, 2008). However, this is the most basic and simplified mechanism of IL-10 signaling; in fact, IL-10 is able to exert its functions through different signaling pathways depending on the condition of the immune system. In addition, it should be noted that the regulation of the IL-10 synthesis is a complex process as well. A series of experiments revealed that numerous transcription factors, including Sp1 (Steinke et al., 2004), pbx1 (Chung et al., 2007), C/EBP (Liu et al., 2003; Csyka et al., 2007), nuclear factor kappa-B (NF-κB) (Wessells et al., 2004), c-Maf (Cao et al., 2005), activating transcription factor (ATF) (Rooney et al., 1994), IFN regulatory factors (IRFs) (Ziegler-Heitbrock et al., 2003), and cAMP response element-binding protein (CREB) (Hu et al., 2006) may bind to the IL-10 promoter, thereby indicating a wide range of mechanisms enhancing the production of this cytokine during the immune response (reviewed by Mosser and Zhang, 2008). Moreover, IL-10 expression is also regulated at the posttranscriptional level through class II AU-rich elements (Mosser and Zhang, 2008). It is also important to note that recently Naiyer et al. (2013) isolated and characterized a human IL-10 receptor antagonist, which currently is being actively investigated.

The major source of IL-10 are monocytes (de Waal Malefyt et al., 1991) and macrophages (Asadullah et al., 2003), but it was also found to be expressed in T regulatory cells (Vieira et al., 2004), Th1 cells (O'Gara and Vieira, 2007), Th2 cells (Fiorentino et al., 1989), B cells (Pistoia, 1997), dendritic cells (DCs) (Corinti et al., 2001), mast cells (Lin and Befus, 1997), eosinophils (Nakajima et al., 1996), and keratinocytes (Enk and Katz, 1992; Teunissen et al., 1997). The influence of IL-10 is primarily focused on DCs, Treg cells, and on macrophages. The biological effects of IL-10 are pleiotropic and include the following:

- Downregulation of all major proinflammatory cytokines, such as IL-1, IL-2, IL-6, IL-8, IL-12, IFN-γ, and tumor necrosis factor (TNF)-α in NK cells and macrophages (Cassatella et al., 1993; Jenkins et al., 1994;

Moore et al., 2001; Denys et al., 2002; Asadullah et al., 2003), thereby initiating polarization toward an antiinflammatory phenotype.

- Upregulation of antiinflammatory cytokines, including IL-1RA and soluble TNF-α receptor (Jenkins et al., 1994; Joyce et al., 1994; Hart et al., 1996).
- Inhibition of antigen-presenting cell function in DCs, macrophages, and monocytes (de Waal Malefyt et al., 1991; Romagnani, 1995).
- Suppression of proliferation and function of T cells (Matsuda et al., 1994; Tang et al., 2012; Podojil et al., 2013; Selleri et al., 2013) and differentiation and activity of DCs (Sun et al., 2012).
- Downregulation of major histocompatibility complex (MHC) class I in DCs (Corinti et al., 2001; Seliger et al., 1996), affecting their antigen presentation capability.
- Downregulation of MHC class I in B cells (Zeidler et al., 1997).
- Stimulation of proliferation and cytotoxicity of NK cells (Mocellin et al., 2003, 2004).

As seen, IL-10 possesses immunoregulatory and antiinflammatory activities and plays a great role in the modulation of the immune response (Poole et al., 1995). In particular, the release of IL-10 protects the human body during immunopathology, allergy, and autoimmune conditions. It is believed that IL-10-driven immune suppression is due to the blocking of nuclear transportation of NF-κB and its subsequent binding to the DNA strand (Wang et al., 1995; Clarke et al., 1998), but other signaling pathways are also known to be partially involved in this process (Mosser and Zhang, 2008). A more detailed description of the structure and biological effects of IL-10 are illuminated in brilliant review articles by Zdanov (2010) and Mosser and Zhang (2008).

6.1.2 Immunobiology of IL-10 in Tumor Models

In 90s and '00s, numerous basic investigations were performed in order to evaluate the impact of IL-10 on cancer in various models. Most of these were in vitro experiments, but several in vivo experiments were conducted as well. Interestingly, somewhat controversial findings were obtained during these studies, suggesting both procarcinogenic and anticarcinogenic activities of IL-10.

6.1.2.1 Models Supporting the Tumor-promoting Impact of IL-10

There is a lot of evidence supporting the procarcinogenic effects of IL-10 in tumor models. Rohrer and Coggin (1995) demonstrated that IL-10 is able to reduce tumor cytotoxic T lymphocytes (CTL) cytotoxicity and IFN-γ secretion in lymphoma cell lines. Hagenbaugh et al. (1997) injected non-small-cell lung carcinoma (NSCLC) cell culture into IL-10 trans-genic mice, and showed that these mice developed relatively large tumors. Further injection of the anti-IL-10 antibody resulted in a significant decrease in tumor size, thereby indicating the restoration of the anticancer immune response in the absence of the IL-10. In addition, Garcia-Hernandez et al. (2002) demonstrated that IL-10 markedly enhanced cell proliferation in vitro and tumor growth in vivo through direct autocrine stimulation of B16 melanoma cells. Notably, the authors also indicated that IL-10 promoted angiogenesis, decreased necrosis, and reduced the activity of macrophages. Furthermore, Kim et al. (1995) found that squamous cell carcinoma and basal cell carcinoma cell lines overexpress IL-10; moreover, the authors also indicated that tumor-infiltrating lymphocyte-driven lysis of autologous cancer cells was abrogated by IL-10. Additionally, it should be noted that multiple studies demonstrated the augmentation of anticancer immune response in vitro and enhancement of antimetastatic immunity and tumor rejection in vivo after treatment with IL-10 inhibitors such as mafosfamide (Rico et al., 2012), cyclophosphamide (Matar et al., 1998, 2000, 2001; Malvicini et al., 2009, 2011), anti-IL-10 antisense oligonucleotides (Kim et al., 2000), anti-IL-10 antibodies (Jovasevic et al., 2004; Huang et al., 2012), and anti-IL-10R antibodies (Vicari et al., 2002; Huang et al., 2012). In addition, numerous studies provided an evidence of IL-10-mediated decrease in the expression of human leukocyte antigen class I molecules in various murine tumor models (Salazar-Onfray et al., 1995, 1997; Petersson et al., 1998; Garcia-Hernandez et al., 2002) and human melanoma cell lines (Matsuda et al., 1994; Yue et al., 1997; Garcia-Hernandez et al., 2002; Kurte et al., 2004), thereby showing IL-10-mediated protection of cancer cells from attack by T cells. Similarly, Kundu and Fulton (1997) demonstrated that IL-10 inhibited tumor metastasis through the downregulation of MHC class I expression in murine mammary cell lines. Specht et al. (2001) discovered that plasmacytoma cell lines treated with anti-IL-10 antibodies showed the abrogated activation of CTLs and significantly accelerated tumor growth. Finally, a recent report by Sung et al. (2013) demonstrated that IL-10 was associated with tumor aggressiveness in lung adenocarcinoma in vivo.

6.1.2.2 Models Supporting the Anticancer Impact of IL-10

Nevertheless, there is also an enormous amount of research showing that IL-10 may also act as a tumor-suppressive agent. Gerard et al. (1996) discovered that the transfection of a B16F1 melanoma cell line with an

IL-10-containing vector resulted in a profound loss of tumorigenicity depending on the amount of IL-10 secreted. More strikingly, the authors observed the stimulation of an antitumor systemic immune response, particularly the activation of T cells and NK cells. Similarly, Giovarelli et al. (1995) observed a rejection of mammary adenocarcinoma in mice transfected with an IL-10-containing retrovirus. The authors found that the obtained effects were due to the IL-10-mediated stimulation of cytotoxic T lymphocytes, NK cells, and neutrophils. In addition, Huang et al. (1995) showed that administration of IL-10 suppressed metastasis formation as well as tumor growth in human melanoma cells. Furthermore, Kambayashi et al. (1995) revealed that high concentrations of IL-10 were associated with a profound suppression of murine peritoneal tumor-associated macrophages in vivo. All the above-mentioned results were successfully replicated by Berman et al. (1996) in murine models of melanoma, sarcoma, and colorectal carcinoma. In addition, Barth et al. (1996) demonstrated tumor rejection in mice immunized with tumor cells transfected with the *IL-10* gene. Interestingly, the authors also found that IL-10 did not induce an antitumor immune response in vitro. Consistent with previous findings, several groups indicated that IL-10 inhibited metastasis by enhancing the activity of NK cells in melanoma models in vivo and in murine mammary tumor cell lines (Kundu et al., 1996; Zheng et al., 1996; Huang et al., 1999). In their further investigations, Kundu et al. (1998) demonstrated a marked decrease in cancer growth and metastasis, which were due to the IL-10-mediated upregulation of the synthesis of an inducible isoform of nitric oxide synthase (iNOS). We discuss the relationship among IL-10, iNOS, and cancer in another paragraph. Adris et al. (1999) showed that IL-10 enhanced an antitumor immunity in murine CT26 colon carcinoma cells infected with an IL-10-containing retrovirus. It was indicated that the expression of IL-10 stimulated CD4$^+$ and CD8$^+$ T cells, inhibited the growth capability of tumor cells, and reduced their metastatic potential as well. Finally, several findings suggested that IL-10 may promote tumor neovascularization. In particular, it was reported that recombinant human and viral IL-10 are both able to inhibit vascular endothelial growth factor (VEGF)-mediated angiogenesis in the model of Burkitt lymphoma in vitro (Cervenak et al., 2000). Moreover, Zeng et al. (2010) demonstrated that lung tumor cell lines expressing IL-10 showed a fourfold increase in tumor microvessel density and also exhibited a significant resistance to apoptosis. Further experiments devoted to this issue obtained similar results in melanoma (Huang et al., 1999), glioma (Segal et al., 2002), and in other models (Groux et al., 1999; Emmerich et al., 2012).

6.1.3 Expression of IL-10 in Patients with Cancer

In the last 15 years, a massive amount of research was performed in order to evaluate the levels of IL-10 in patients with different malignancies. Elevated concentrations of IL-10 were detected in subjects with colorectal carcinoma (Szkaradkiewicz et al., 2009; Stanilov et al., 2010; Toiyama et al., 2010; Svobodova et al., 2011; Kemik et al., 2012), esophageal cancer (Kemik et al., 2012), malignant melanoma (Kruger-Krasagakes et al., 1994; Fortis et al., 1996), pancreatic and gastric adenocarcinomas (Kemik et al., 2012; Dummer et al., 1996; Fortis et al., 1996), renal cell carcinoma (Menetrier-Caux et al., 1999; Wittke et al., 1999), prostate cancer (Dwivedi et al., 2011), ovarian cancer (Mustea et al., 2009; Zhu et al., 2010; Rabinovich et al., 2010), non-small-cell lung cancer (Zhao et al., 2013a), superficial transitional cell carcinoma of the bladder (Agarwal et al., 2010; Lang et al., 2012), premalignant cervical lesions (Mindiola et al., 2008; Torres-Poveda et al., 2012), various lymphomas (Cortes et al., 1995; Asadullah et al., 1997, 2000; Cortes and Kurzrock, 1997; Sarris et al., 1999; Vassilakopoulos et al., 2001; Fayad et al., 2001; Nacinović-Duletić et al., 2008; Guney et al., 2009; Labidi et al., 2010; Gaiolla et al., 2011; Purdue et al., 2011; Charbonneau et al., 2012; Gupta et al., 2012; Mellgren et al., 2012), malignant pleural effusions (Klimatsidas et al., 2012), and rare peritoneal malignancies (Vlaeminck-Guillem et al., 2013).

Moreover, increased levels of IL-10 were associated with disease progression, recurrence, poor prognosis, and poor outcome in patients with oral squamous cell carcinoma (Chen et al., 2013a), colorectal carcinoma (Bobe et al., 2010; Toiyama et al., 2010), gastric cancer (Ikeguchi et al., 2009; Szaflarska et al., 2009), prostate cancer (Dwivedi et al., 2011), ovarian cancer (Zhu et al., 2010), chronic lymphocytic leukemia (Lech-Maranda et al., 2012), laryngeal and pharyngeal carcinomas (Alhamarneh et al., 2011), various lymphomas (Blay et al., 1993; Stasi, 1994a,b; Cortes et al., 1995), and pediatric soft tissue sarcomas (Bien et al., 2013). In addition, high concentrations of IL-10 in tumor associated macrophages (TAMs) correlated with a stage, tumor size, lymph node metastasis, lymphovascular invasion, or poor histologic differentiation in subjects with lung cancer (Wang et al., 2011a). It should also be mentioned that serum IL-10 levels were not associated with clinical pathological factors, treatment response, and overall survival in subjects with nasopharyngeal carcinoma (Lu et al., 2012) and breast cancer (Pockaj et al., 2004; Pooja et al., 2012). Interestingly, low IL-10 levels were also reported to be associated with a poor outcome in patients with stage I non-small-cell lung cancer (Soria et al., 2003). Additionally, it was also observed that in patients with hepatocellular carcinoma (HCC), IL-10 contributed to the Treg-mediated suppression of the cytotoxic activities and IFN-γ production by γδT cells (Yi et al., 2013). Finally, conflicting results were obtained regarding the association between serum concentrations of IL-10 and head and neck squamous cell carcinoma (Melinceanu et al., 2011; Mojtahedi et al., 2012; Hamzavi et al., 2013) and HCC (Jang et al., 2012; Welling et al., 2012).

An interesting study was conducted by Svenson et al. (2013) who found that elevated peripheral levels of IL-10 were associated with an increased telomere length in the blood cells of patients with renal cell tumors. The authors speculated that this observation may indicate the reduced cell division rate in leukocytes, thereby reflecting the IL-10-mediated suppression of immunity. However, the statistical power of this study was relatively low, so the results obtained should be interpreted with caution.

As seen, the results from multiple observations suggest that an overexpression of IL-10 may be associated with the development and progression of cancer. Possibly, serum levels of IL-10 may serve as indicators for the detection of certain malignancies, and this cytokine therefore could become a significant cancer-predicting biomarker.

6.1.4 IL-10-Signaling Pathways in Cancer

6.1.4.1 IL-10 is Implicated in Tumorigenesis through Multiple Signaling Pathways

The investigation of the basic properties and effects of the IL-10 in malignant disease has begun more than 10 years ago; nevertheless, the understanding of molecular mechanisms involved in these processes started shaping up only recently. The activation of IL-10 expression is known to be mediated by toll-like receptor (TLR)2, TLR3, and TLR4 in the presence of an infectious agent or pathogen-associated molecular patterns (PAMPs) (Bogunovic et al., 2011; Chang et al., 2012; Ying et al., 2013). It was found that IL-10 promotes tumor aggressiveness through the upregulation of CIP2A, an oncoprotein correlated with an accelerated cell growth and cancer progression (Sung et al., 2013). Moreover, Gupta et al. (2012) revealed that IL-10 constitutively induces the activation of the JAK2/STAT3 pathway in diffuse large B cell lymphoma cells but not in normal cells. Other groups observed the presence of aberrant JAK2 mutants among patients with B cell lymphoma (Steensma et al., 2006), primary mediastinal lymphoma (Melzner et al., 2006), and Hodgkin lymphoma (Melzner et al., 2006). Importantly, it should be noted that the JAK2/STAT3 pathway is known to play a major role in hematological malignancies (reviewed by Ferrajoli et al., 2006;Valentino and Pierre, 2006). In addition, Chang et al. (2012) revealed that the production of IL-10 in human monocyte-derived DCs from patients with gastric cancer is dependent on p38 mitogen-activated protein kinase (MAPK) signaling and on NF-κB activation. Consistent with previous reports, Ying et al. (2013) demonstrated that the activation of MAPK, c-Jun, N-terminal kinase (JNK - Janus kinase), and signal transducer and activator of transcription 3 (STAT3) was associated with an increased IL-10 production in bladder epithelial cells. Finally, a recent study by Sanda et al. (2013) revealed that T cell acute lymphoblastic leukemia cell lines and tissue samples showed the activation of a pathway involving TYK2, STAT1, and bcl-2, an antiapoptotic protein associated with numerous cancers (Barille-Nion et al., 2012). As seen, IL-10 has complex interactions with various transcription factors within cancer cells. Here, we discuss the relationship between IL-10 and the molecules involved in cancer development and progression.

6.1.4.2 IL-10 and Transforming Growth Factor Beta

Transforming growth factor beta (TGF-β) is a ubiquitous protein involved in cell differentiation and proliferation. In addition, it is believed to play a major role in apoptosis and cell adhesion (reviewed by Wu and Hill, 2009). The connection between TGF-β and numerous human diseases, including cancer, has been established long ago (Blobe et al., 2000). On the one hand, TGF-β inhibits the development of tumors at early stages due to the suppression of apoptosis and reduction of cell proliferation rate (reviewed by Levy and Hill, 2006). On the other hand, however, a lot of malignant tumors have been found to overexpress this cytokine, thereby promoting cell invasiveness and metastasis formation (reviewed by Pardali and Moustakas, 2007). An important role in the regulation of TGF-β is played by IL-10. It was demonstrated that IL-10 is able to upregulate the expression of TGF-β in both normal cells (Wei et al., 2013) and in cancer cells (Jin et al., 2013). In addition, TGF-β was shown to increase the synthesis of IL-10 in a positive-feedback loop in various models, including cutaneous leishmaniasis, influenza A virus infection, allergic asthma, and cervical carcinoma (Hejazi et al., 2012; Chen et al., 2012; Srivastava et al., 2012; Yalcin et al., 2012). Furthermore, IL-10 was found to enhance the expression of the TGF-β receptor, thereby increasing the responsiveness to this cytokine (Cottrez and

Groux, 2001). Possibly, all these findings may indicate a possible involvement of the IL-10/TGF-β axis in the development of cancer; however, there is currently a lack of in-depth studies devoted to this problem.

6.1.4.3 IL-10 and Cyclooxygenase 2/Prostaglandin 2

There is accumulating evidence of the relationship between IL-10 and cyclooxygenase 2 (COX-2), and prostaglandin 2 (PGE2). PGE2 is an important regulator of numerous vital processes in the human body, and it is produced from arachidonic acid due to the activity of an enzyme COX-2. It is to be noted that COX-2 and PGE2 were numerously reported to promote carcinogenesis through stimulation of cell invasion, angiogenesis, cell growth, and survival (Hida et al., 2000; Dohadwala et al., 2002; Castelao et al., 2003; Pold et al., 2004; Wang and Dubois, 2006). The major signaling pathways of COX-2/PGE$_2$-driven carcinogenesis include EGFR–PI3K–Akt, Ras–MAPK, and Wnt (Wang and Dubois, 2006). Numerous reports demonstrated that the concentrations of COX-2 and PGE2 were markedly elevated in malignant disease (Pugh and Thomas, 1994; Sano et al., 1995; Thill et al., 2010; Cordes et al., 2012; Hogendorf et al., 2012; Rasmuson et al., 2012). Poole et al. (1995) discovered that human peripheral blood mononuclear cells treated with an IL-10 demonstrated a decrease in PGE2 production in a dose-dependent manner. Likewise, Niiro et al. (1997) revealed that IL-10 is able to inhibit the production of COX-2 and PGE2 in human neutrophils. In accordance with previous reports, Berg et al. (2001) found that the lipopolysaccharide (LPS)-induced production of COX-2 mRNA and intracellular PGE2 from IL-10-deficient spleen cell line was more than five times greater in comparison with that from wild-type spleen cells. Furthermore, a series of subsequent studies indicated that treatment with IL-10 showed an inhibitory effect on COX-2 mRNA concentrations and PGE2 release in rat microglial cultures (Minghetti et al., 1998), human osteoarthritis synovial fibroblasts (Alaaeddine et al., 1999), intact fetal membranes (Brown et al., 2000), mouse and human keratinocytes (Ramaswamy et al., 2000), human peripheral blood mononuclear cells (Endo et al., 1998; Maloney et al., 1998; Pyeon et al., 2000; Inoue et al., 2004), astroglial murine cultures (Molina-Holgado et al., 2002), and in human placental explants (Hanna et al., 2006; Bayraktar et al., 2009).

All these findings suggest a possible protective role of IL-10 in cancer through inhibition of the COX-2/PGE2 axis; however, there is a lack of studies investigating the link between IL-10 and COX-2/PGE2 in malignant disease. In addition, it should also be mentioned that COX-2/PGE2 may have an impact on the endogenous production of IL-10 as well. It was reported that recombinant or LPS-induced COX-2/PGE2 enhanced the transcriptional rate of IL-10 mRNA in human non-small-lung cancer cells (Huang et al., 1996), human microglia (Levi et al., 1998), LLC cell cultures (Stolina et al., 2000), bone marrow-derived dendritic cells (DC) (Harizi et al., 2002), and chitosan- and LPS-treated mouse leukemic "macrophage" cell lines (Chou et al., 2003). In addition, Michelin et al. (2002) found that PGE2 released by COX-2 stimulated the IL-10-driven immunosuppression in splenocytes from mice infected by *Paracoccidioides brasiliensis*. Additionally, transgenic mice expressing COX-2 in the liver exhibited a 4.4-fold increase in serum IL-10 levels, according to a recent study by Yu et al. (2007). However, in contrast to the above-mentioned observations, it was also reported that PGE_2 did not regulate the production of IL-10 by human dendritic cells (Teloni et al., 2007). Finally, it was found that IL-10 may activate COX-2/PGE2 by the suppression of IL-1 (Al-Ashy et al., 2006).

The exact signaling mechanisms of the crosstalk between IL-10 and COX-2/PGE2 are not well investigated until now. Inoue et al. (2004) revealed that IL-10 suppressed the activation of p38 MAPK, extracellular signal-related kinase (ERK), and MKK3/6 in CD40-stimulated human peripheral blood monocytes, thereby inhibiting the production of COX-2/PGE2. Furthermore, Yu et al. (2007) observed the NF-κb-dependent upregulation of IL-10 in COX-2 transgenic mice. In addition, it was recently shown that IL-10 synthesis was regulated by COX-2 through ERK and p38 in patients with NSCLC (Patel et al., 2012). Nevertheless, all these data should be replicated for better reliability. Undoubtedly, further research is required to shed light on the signaling mechanisms and the relationship between IL-10 and COX-2/PGE2 in the context of cancer.

6.1.4.4 IL-10 and iNOS

It was already mentioned that IL-10 was demonstrated to inhibit tumor growth through the upregulation of iNOS (Kundu et al., 1998). In addition, it was also found that IL-10 upregulated NO production in activated macrophages in a dose-dependent manner (Jacobs et al., 1998); possibly, this effect was due to the IL-10-mediated upregulation of iNOS. Multiple research groups reported that the iNOS-dependent generation of nitric oxide suppressed tumorigenicity, abrogated metastasis, and promoted the apoptotic destruction of cancer cells (Thomsen et al., 1995; Xie et al., 1995; Juang et al., 1998; Garban and Bonavida, 1999). On the other hand, there is evidence that intracellular NO may contribute to impaired DNA repair by upregulating p53, poly(ADP-ribose) polymerase (PARP), and the DNA-dependent protein kinase, and moreover promote angiogenesis by upregulating VEGF (reviewed by Xu et al., 2002).

However, in contrast to the findings of Kundu et al. (1998) and Jacobs et al. (1998), it was also shown that IL-10 downregulated the mRNA expression of iNOS in vitro (Goff et al., 1998). So, the interactions between IL-10 and iNOS and their roles in cancer development are still the subject of debates.

6.1.4.5 IL-10 and E-selectin

An investigation of the impact of IL-10 on endothelial cells revealed a significant upregulation of the expression of a cell adhesion protein E-selectin (Vora et al., 1996). Likewise, mice injected with an IL-10-containing vector were reported to produce an increased amount of E-selectin mRNA (Myers et al., 2003). Multiple research studies demonstrated that E-selectin is able to increase the adhesion of cancer cells to epithelial cells, thereby promoting metastasis formation. Functional selectin ligands were found in various malignancies, including in colon cancer, gastric carcinoma, bladder cancer, pancreatic cancer, breast carcinoma, and prostate cancer (reviewed by St Hill, 2011). Moreover, the expression patterns of selectin ligands in tumor cells correlated with a poor prognosis and metastasis formation in subjects with different cancers (reviewed by Laubli and Borsig, 2010). However, according to the results obtained by several research groups, it seems that there are no straightforward connections between IL-10 and E-selectin. By contrast to previous findings, Noble et al. (2000) found that IL-10 reduced the amounts of monocyte-derived endothelial E-selectin in vitro. In addition, it was revealed that mice transferred with IL-10-bearing lentivirus demonstrated decreased patterns of E-selectin expression in models of venous thrombosis (Henke et al., 2000) and liver ischemia-reperfusion injury (Ke et al., 2007). Moreover, IL-10 inhibited the production of E-selectin in a cerebral ischemia-reperfusion rat model (Du et al., 2009). Finally, IL-10 did not change the expression of E-selectin, neither in LPS-treated mice (Morise et al., 1999) nor in human endothelial cell cultures exposed to LPS or *Borrelia burgdorferi* (Lisinski and Furie, 2002). As seen, the above-mentioned contradictory findings question the definite role of IL-10 in the regulation of E-selectin, and further in-depth research is needed to illuminate this issue.

6.1.4.6 IL-10 and Programed Cell Death Ligands

Programed cell death ligands (PD-L, B7-H) represent a class of costimulatory molecules involved in the regulation of the immune response through the upregulation and downregulation of certain cytokines (Loke and Allison, 2003). Importantly, almost all members of the B7-H family primarily exert an inhibitory effect on the immune system (reviewed by Francisco et al., 2010). For instance, B7-H1 may lead to T cell exhaustion (Day et al., 2006; Francisco et al., 2010), inhibition of macrophage and DC response to TLR agonists and microorganisms (Huang et al., 2009a; Yao et al., 2009), and blocking of PI3K and Akt signaling pathways (Parsa et al., 2007; Francisco et al., 2010). In addition, multiple research groups demonstrated that high expression of B7-H ligands were correlated with an increased tumor aggressiveness; elevated risk of death; and poor prognosis among patients with renal cell carcinoma (Thompson et al., 2004), ovarian cancer (Hamanishi et al., 2007), and pancreatic carcinoma (Huang et al., 2009b). Moreover, levels of B7-H1, B7-H3, and B7-H4 were found to be significantly increased in patients with various cancers, including non-small-cell lung cancer (Sun et al., 2006), glioma (Bloch et al., 2013), ductal and lobular breast cancer (Tringler et al., 2005), renal cell carcinoma (Krambeck et al., 2006; Crispen et al., 2008), and prostate cancer (Zang et al., 2007). However, there are also several reports indicating that certain representatives of the B7-H family, in particular, B7-H3, may elicit a protective antitumor effect and be a beneficial factor for anticancer immunity (reviewed by Yi and Chen, 2009). Thus, it seems that the role of B7-H ligands in cancer is at least ambiguous.

Several recent discoveries have established a link between IL-10 and B7-H ligands in the context of cancer. There are numerous reports indicating that IL-10 is able to upregulate the expression of B7-H1 and B7-H4 in macrophages, monocytes, DCs, and in the tumor microenvironment (Zou, 2005; Kryczek et al., 2007; Yi and Chen, 2009). In particular, Chen et al. (2013b) demonstrated that IL-10 produced by TAMs directly stimulates the expression of B7-H3 in lung cancer cell lines. In addition, Bloch et al. (2013) demonstrated that human gliomas can upregulate B7-H1 expression in circulating monocytes and in tumor-infiltrative macrophages through IL-10 signaling, thereby promoting immunosuppression. Furthermore, the simultaneous increase in the levels of IL-10 and B7-H1 was observed in 60 HCC tissues and in 40 pancreatic carcinoma samples, according to the results of Geng et al. (2008, 2011). Additionally, similar findings were obtained by Huang et al. (2009a,b) in 35 pancreatic cancer tissues. Interestingly, it was also observed that tumor Treg cells and antigen-presenting cells but not primary tumor cells trigger the spontaneous production of IL-10 with the subsequent upregulation of B7-H ligands (Kryczek et al., 2007). Finally, consistent with these results, Fujimura et al. (2012) observed that the depletion of human

Treg cells resulted in the decreased production of IL-10 as well as of B7-H1, B7-H3, and B7-H4 in myeloid-derived suppressor cells in ret melanomas. All these observations indicate the presence of complicated interactions among Treg cells, IL-10, and B7-H representatives; however, the signaling pathways of IL-10-mediated upregulation of B7-H ligands are still unknown. We suggest that further investigations in the field should (1) determine the most precise role of each B7-H representative (at least B7-H1, B7-H3, and B7-H4) in cancer, (2) clarify the exact mechanism of IL-10-driven expression of B7-H ligands, and (3) evaluate the impact of simultaneous IL-10 and B7-H blockade on cancer development and progression in preclinical studies.

6.1.4.7 IL-10 and VEGF

As known, VEGF is a key regulator of tumor angiogenesis (Kieran et al., 2012). Huang et al. (1996) provided the first evidence of the IL-10-mediated inhibition of VEGF in tumor models. The authors demonstrated that the human melanoma cell line A375P transfected with a vector containing full-length murine IL-10 DNA showed significantly lower amounts of VEGF, thereby promoting the suppression of tumor growth and metastasis formation. Similarly, Matsumoto (1997) observed the IL-10-mediated inhibition of the production of VEGF in peripheral blood mononuclear cells among Japanese patients with lipoid nephrosis. Interestingly, in their next paper, the authors indicated a synergistic effect of IL-10 and IL-13 on VEGF suppression (Matsumoto et al., 1997). Further investigations by Matsumoto et al. (1999) showed that recombinant IL-10 was found to reduce VEGF release in a dose-dependent manner, and moreover, it was observed that IL-10 synergized with IL-4 to promote VEGF inhibition. Di Carlo et al. (1998) subcutaneously injected a mouse mammary adenocarcinoma cell line containing IL-10 DNA into syngeneic BALB/c mice, and showed a profound downregulation of the VEGF expression in the tumor area. Several subsequent studies devoted to this issue only confirmed the findings obtained in previous experiments. Silvestre et al. (2000) showed that IL-10-deficient mice developed more evident ischemia-induced angiogenesis in comparison with that in control IL-10$^{+/+}$ mice. In addition, the authors observed that IL-10-deficient mice exhibited 80% increased levels of VEGF, as compared to those exhibited by control animals. Similarly, Kawakami et al. (2001) showed that IL-10 expression significantly correlated with a decreased neovascularization in 53 Japanese patients with colon cancer and Cervenak et al. (2000) indicated that IL-10 suppressed the VEGF-mediated proliferation of microvascular endothelial cells in vitro. Finally, IL-10-driven inhibition of angiogenesis was demonstrated in mice bearing VEGF-producing ovarian cancer cells (Kohno et al., 2003).

Some investigators, however, reported an opposite impact of IL-10 on VEGF production and tissue neovascularization. For instance, Trompezinski et al. (2002) found that IL-10 was unable to reduce the expression of VEGF in human activated keratinocytes. Similarly, Choi et al. (2002) demonstrated that VEGF production and release by the human first trimester trophoblast cell line were not affected by IL-10. In addition, Nagata et al. (2002) revealed that the expression of IL-10 correlated with *VEGF* gene expression in 45 Japanese patients with esophageal cancer. It was also found that the treatment of healthy monocytes with exogenous VEGF resulted in increased intracellular IL-10 levels, according to the results of Sugai et al. (2004). Furthermore, Sakamoto et al. (2006) reported that IL-10 was associated with a high microvessel density among 109 Japanese patients with gastric cancer. Hatanaka et al. (2001) found that non-small-cell lung cancer cells producing IL-10 showed marked stromal vascularization through the expression of proteins playing a dramatic role in vascular development, including angiopoietin (Ang)-1, Ang-2, and TIE2. Finally, Dace et al. (2008) demonstrated that IL-10 promoted retinal angiogenesis by the upregulating VEGF expression in a mouse model of oxygen-induced retinopathy.

These controversial findings indicate a highly complex relationship between IL-10 and VEGF-mediated neovascularization.

6.1.5 Clinical Trials

Administration of human recombinant IL-10 to healthy volunteers showed transient dose-dependent alterations in neutrophil and platelet counts as well as in various subpopulations of lymphocytes. Importantly, these experiments demonstrated that IL-10 was well tolerated and that there were no adverse symptoms even at high doses of this cytokine (Chernoff et al., 1995; Huhn et al., 1996, 1997). Regarding the usage of recombinant IL-10 in disease treatment, numerous phase I and II clinical trials were performed in order to test this cytokine in patients with inflammatory and autoimmune diseases, including rheumatoid arthritis (Keystone et al., 1998), psoriasis (reviewed by Asadullah et al., 2004), and Crohn's disease (reviewed by Lindsay and Hodgson, 2001; Herfarth and Scholmerich, 2002). Although IL-10 demonstrated a tendency toward clinical improvement in all these trials, promising results were shown only for the treatment of psoriasis. Currently, there are no clinical trials of IL-10 in cancer treatment; possibly, it makes sense to conduct this research in the future.

6.1.6 Brief Summary and Future Directions

It is currently unclear whether IL-10 may be an effective agent against cancer. Different studies show controversial results regarding the impact of this cytokine on cancer development and progression. Moreover, IL-10 has a complex relationship with numerous mediators involved in tumorigenesis, and many of them are not yet well studied. Undoubtedly, more basic and clinical investigations are required to clarify this issue; therefore, we suggest that the most attractive and promising targets for further research on the IL-10 signaling in cancer are the following: TGF-β, iNOS, E-selectin, COX-2/PGE2, and programed cell death ligands.

IL-10 can initiate an effective anticancer immune response through the activation of NK cells, and suppression of COX-2/PGE2; at the same time, IL-10-driven immunosuppression may weaken the immunity, thereby contributing to successful tumor development. The interactions between IL-10 and many factors playing a dramatic role in oncogenesis, such as VEGF, iNOS, and E-selectin, are still obscured, and these relationships should be elucidated in the nearest future. Finally, we suggest that there is a need to conduct clinical trials in order to test IL-10 in patients with malignant tumors.

6.2 INTERLEUKIN-19

6.2.1 Overview of IL-19

Having considered the role of IL-10 in cancer biology, we shall now turn our attention to its recently discovered cousin named IL-19. This IL is characterized as a 21-kDa α-helical monomeric cytokine containing a hydrophobic core formed by two disulfide bonds. Although IL-19 has a 30% homology with IL-10, it is significantly more similar in structure and sequence to IL-20 and IL-24 (>40% of homology). For this reason, IL-19, IL-20, and IL-24 are commonly characterized as members of the IL-19 subfamily of the IL-10 superfamily (Fickenscher et al., 2002; Pestka et al., 2004a; Sabat et al., 2007).

IL-19 is known to be derived from various cells, including B cells, monocytes, macrophages, epithelial cells, and endothelial cells (Gallagher et al., 2000; Gallagher, 2010; Wolk et al., 2002). Additionally, IL-19 was also found to be expressed in keratinocytes (Kunz et al., 2006) smooth muscle cells (Tian et al., 2008), fetal membranes (Menon et al., 2006), and synovial tissue (Alanärä et al., 2010). IL-19 exerts its biological effects through the IL-20R1/IL-20R2 heterodimeric receptor. It is important to note that alongside IL-19, the IL-20R1/IL-20R2 receptor is also shared by IL-20 and IL-24 with a different binding affinity (Parrish-Novak et al., 2002). The binding of IL-19 to the corresponding receptor leads to the activation and nuclear translocation of STAT1 and STAT3 (Parrish-Novak et al., 2002). In addition, recent in vitro assays showed that IL-19 activates JNK, ERK, AKT, and NFκB as well (Hsing et al., 2012).

Most biological effects of IL-19 are still being actively investigated. To date, numerous reports provided evidence that IL-19 exerts a proinflammatory activity (Fickenscher et al., 2002; Gallagher, 2010; Hsing et al., 2008a). In particular, IL-19 was reported to upregulate the expression of proinflammatory cytokines L-6 and TNF-α (Liao et al., 2002; Hsing et al., 2006), induce apoptosis in macrophages (Liao et al., 2002) and lung epithelium cells (Hsing et al., 2008b), and to promote reactive oxygen species (ROS) production (Liao et al., 2002). An association between IL-9 and autoimmune diseases has been established not long ago. In particular, IL-19 was suspected to play an important role in psoriasis through the upregulation of the keratinocyte growth factor (Li et al., 2005; Wang et al., 2012a). Moreover, a link between IL-19 and rheumatoid arthritis was also identified recently (Sakurai et al., 2008). In addition, it was recently found that IL-19 blockade attenuated collagen-induced arthritis in rats (Hsu et al., 2012a,b).

However, several reports demonstrated that IL-19 elicited a profound antiinflammatory response in vascular smooth muscle cell pathophysiological processes (Cuneo et al., 2010), vascular inflammation (England and Autieri, 2012), and experimental model of colitis (Azuma et al., 2010). In addition, it was also found that macrophages from IL-19-deficient mice demonstrated significantly enhanced production of proinflammatory cytokines upon TLR activation. Possibly, these antiinflammatory effects may be due to the IL-19-dependent upregulation of antiinflammatory cytokines IL-4, IL-10, and IL-13 in human monocytes (Liao et al., 2002; Oral et al., 2006).

As seen, biological effects of IL-19 are pleiotropic and have a profound impact on the immune system. Multiple reports indicate that IL-19 may play a role in the pathogenesis of various human diseases, including that of asthma (Liao et al., 2004), uremia (Hsing et al., 2007), endotoxic shock (Hsing et al., 2008c), psoriasis (Li et al., 2005; Wang et al., 2012a), and rheumatoid arthritis (Sakurai et al., 2008). More interestingly, recent discoveries revealed that this cytokine may be of great importance in the context of cancer development.

6.2.2 Possible Role of IL-19 in Cancer Development

Nowadays, the data on the impact of IL-19 on cancer are limited. However, recent findings devoted to this issue have shown very important clues that may clarify the overall picture. First, various tumor tumors have been reported to express IL-19. Hsing et al. (2008a,b) used anti-IL-19 monoclonal antibody to reveal the expression patterns of this cytokine in malignant tumors, and showed that IL-19 was strongly stained in ovarian cancer and squamous cell carcinoma of the tongue, esophagus, and buccal mucosa. Moderate concentrations of IL-19 were found in HCC, renal cell carcinoma, breast cancer, lung cancer, and squamous cell carcinoma of the skin. Thyroid papillary carcinoma, thymic carcinoma, and B cell lymphoma were weakly stained for IL-19. Importantly, the authors found no evidence of IL-19 in healthy tissues and moreover indicated that IL-19 contributed to cell proliferation in squamous cell carcinoma of the oral cavity. Second, in their subsequent investigations, Hsing et al. (2012) demonstrated that IL-19 derived from breast cancer cells contributed to the proliferation and migration of tumor cells through metastasis formation and provided a microenvironment for tumor growth. In particular, the authors indicated that IL-19 upregulated the expression of prometastatic agents matrix metalloproteinases (MMP)-2 and MMP-9, proliferative mediator TGF-β, and pro-inflammatory cytokine IL-1β. Interestingly, it was also found that IL-19 contributed to a production and assembly of fibronectin. Fibronectin is a glycoprotein of the extracellular matrix, and it is known to be involved in metastasis formation, tumor angiogenesis, and cancer progression (reviewed by Van Obberghen-Schilling et al., 2011). In addition, the researchers also indicated the IL-19-driven upregulation of a chemokine receptor CXCR4, which is constantly expressed in tumors. In particular, CXCR4 is involved in metastasis formation in breast cancer, angiogenesis in glioblastoma, and in the development and progression of gastric cancer (reviewed by Domanska et al., 2013). Finally, the authors also indicated that IL-19 promoted the expression of IL-6 in breast cancer cells (Hsing et al., 2012). Regarding molecular mechanisms of the IL-19-mediated cancer development, it was revealed that all the same factors, namely, STAT3, JNK, ERK, AKT, and NF-κb, were involved in signaling (Hsing et al., 2013).

As seen, the only study devoted to the investigation of the role of IL-19 in cancer provided a substantial evidence to believe that this cytokine exerts a marked effect on tumor development. To conclude based on a single example, we assume that IL-19 may modulate cancer progression in many ways, including (1) MMP- and fibronectin-driven formation of metastasis, (2) TGF-β-mediated increase in cell proliferation, and

(3) CXCR4-dependent promotion of angiogenesis. No doubt, further research should be focused on IL-19 in order to clarify these issues.

6.3 INTERLEUKIN-20

We are now moving toward IL-20, a novel cytokine, which is also being actively investigated nowadays and which was found to be associated with various abnormal conditions within the body. IL-20 represents an α-helical cytokine with a molecular weight of 17.7 kDa. It is expressed on the surface of epithelial and endothelial cells, and on monocytes as well. IL-20 elicits its biological effects through two distinct receptor complexes. The first receptor complex comprises of 33.5-kDa IL-20R1 and 26.4-kDa IL-20R2 subunits, thereby constituting a 77.7-kDa receptor complex. The second complex consists of IL-22R1 and IL-20R2 subunits. Binding of IL-20 to its corresponding complexes causes elevated proinflammatory activity in mesangial cells, keratinocytes, endothelial cells, synovial fibroblasts, and renal epithelial cells (Blumberg et al., 2001; Otkjaer et al., 2007). An inflammatory-promoting activity of IL-20 was found to be markedly associated with features of development and pathogenesis of various diseases and conditions (Hofmann et al., 2012), including those of rheumatoid arthritis (Hsu et al., 2006; Kragstrup et al., 2008; Hsu and Chang, 2010), atherosclerosis (Caligiuri et al., 2006; Chen et al., 2006; Kleemann et al., 2008), psoriasis (Wei et al., 2005; Sa et al., 2007; Wang et al., 2012b), brain injury (Chen and Chang, 2009), ulcerative colitis (Fonseca-Camarillo et al., 2013), and renal failure (Li et al., 2008a). In addition, IL-20 overexpression in transgenic mice resulted in neonatal lethality with skin abnormalities including aberrant epidermal differentiation (Blumberg et al., 2001). So far, the regulation of the expression of IL-20 is poorly studied; however, some knowledge of this process is available. It was reported that the administration of LPS triggered the expression of the IL-20 mRNA through MAPK and MyD88 signaling pathways (Hosoi et al., 2004). In addition, it was also found that proinflammatory IL-1β is able to upregulate IL-20 through stress-activated kinase 1 (MSK1) NF-κB- and MAPK-dependent mechanisms (Otkjaer et al., 2007). Interestingly, other investigators demonstrated that IL-20 downregulated IL-1β and IL-17A, thereby promoting infection in mice (Myles et al., 2013). Finally, IL-20 was associated with Jak/STAT3 expression and signaling in nonlesional psoriatic skin (Andrés et al., 2013).

To date, there are several reports indicating a possible link between IL-20 and cancer development. First, it was demonstrated that IL-20 is able to promote tumor angiogenesis through the upregulation of basic fibroblast growth factor (bFGF) and VEGF (Hsieh et al., 2006). Second, a marked increase in the expression patterns of IL-20 and IL-20R1 was found in 233 tissue samples collected from patients with bladder cancer, according to the study of Lee et al. (2012). Moreover, the authors indicated that this cytokine significantly promoted the migration and invasion of cancer cells, and it was revealed that these activities were associated with an IL-20-dependent upregulation of MMP-9 through NF-κB and AP-1. Interestingly, these data are consistent with the findings of Hsieh et al. (2006), who reported that IL-20 increased the migration of endothelial cells through the upregulation of MMP-2 and MMP-9. In addition, Lee et al. (2012) indicated that IL-20 stimulated the activation of MAPK, JAK1, JAK2, STAT1, STAT2, and STAT5 in bladder cancer cells. It is also important to note that the authors successfully replicated their previous results in subsequent investigations and demonstrated that the procarcinogenic effects of IL-20 were due to the cell cycle inhibitor p21 (WAF1). In particular, it was found that IL-20 directly activated p21 without altering cell cycle progression (Lee et al., 2013). Moreover, the inhibition of p21 resulted in a significant suppression of MMP-9 expression and total blockade of ERK and NF-κB signaling, thereby removing procarcinogenic effects (Lee et al., 2013). Third, Jung et al. (2009) revealed that the expression profile of IL-20 was increased in a murine bladder cancer model. Similarly, Hsu et al. (2012a) observed a significant elevation in IL-10 levels in human primary and bone-metastatic breast cancer. Similarly to previous findings, the authors reported that cell proliferation and migration, as well as advanced tumor stage and metastasis, were associated with higher amounts of IL-20. Additionally, the authors demonstrated that these procarcinogenic effects were due to the upregulation of MMP-9, MMP-12, cathepsin G, and cathepsin K. By investigating the molecular mechanisms, the authors showed that IL-20 stimulated the activation of STAT3, ERK, JNK, and Bcl-XL. It is interesting to note that the authors did not indicate the IL-20-mediated activation of NF-κB, which is contrary to the data of Lee et al. (2012). In addition, Hsu et al. (2012a) found that treatment with anti-IL-20 monoclonal antibodies resulted in a marked suppression of tumor growth and in the prevention of metastasis in vivo. Finally, in their further investigations, Hsu et al. (2012b) revealed that treatment with IL-20 increased the migration and proliferation of oral cancer cell lines through activated STAT3, AKT, JNK, and ERK. In addition, IL-20 was found to upregulate TNF-α, IL-1β, monocyte chemotactic protein-1, CCR4, CXCR4 and to promote ROS production. As predicted, the administration of anti-IL-20 antibodies resulted in the significant suppression of tumor growth and inflammation, thereby confirming previous results.

However, other reports indicate that IL-20 may exert antitumor activities as well. First, Heuze-Vourc'h et al. (2005) showed that IL-20 is able to suppress angiogenesis and downregulate COX-2 and PGE2 in human bronchial epithelial and endothelial cells, which may be evidence of the anticancer potential of this cytokine. Second, Baird et al. (2011) demonstrated that treatment of non-small lung cancer cells with recombinant IL-20 caused a marked decrease in the expression of the VEGF mRNA, and thereby suggested another mechanism of IL-20-mediated inhibition of angiogenesis.

To conclude, there are many reasons to believe that IL-20 may play a great role in cancer progression; however, some contradictory results make it necessary to perform further an in-depth analysis of (1) the effect of IL-20 on COX-2/PGE2 in cancer cells and (2) the role of IL-20 in angiogenesis.

6.4 INTERLEUKIN-22

6.4.1 Overview

The cloning and purification of IL-22 are associated with a series of experiments conducted by Dumoutier et al. (2000a,b). Initially, this molecule was characterized as a hepatocyte-stimulating factor and originally designated a human IL-10-related T cell-derived inducible factor. Despite the fact that this cytokine was discovered 14 years ago, its investigation in the context of cancer and other diseases has started very recently.

IL-22 is a 20-kDa α-helical cytokine and consists of 179 amino acid residues. It has a quite limited homology as compared to other family members, as the sequence identity between human IL-22 and IL-10 is only 22%. IL-22 is expressed by various immune cells, including mast cells, splenocytes, γδ T cells, NK cells, DCs, lymphoid tissue inducer (LTi) cells, and LTi-like cells. The biological effects of IL-22 are exerted through a heterodimeric receptor composed of IL-22R1 and IL-10Rβ subunits. The latter subunit is shared by IL-10R2 with other representatives of the superfamily family, IL-10, IL-26, IL-28, and IL-29. It is important to note that IL-22R is predominantly expressed by the epithelium, including epithelial cells of the skin, colon, and lung; therefore, the activity of this cytokine is aimed predominantly on epithelial tissues. In addition, among cells that respond to IL-22 are hepatocytes and pancreocytes (Kotenko et al., 2001). Upon binding to a corresponding receptor, IL-22 triggers JAK1, Tyk2, and MAPKs, followed by the activation of transcription factors, such as STAT1, STAT3, and STAT5 (Dumoutier et al., 2000a). Furthermore, IL-22 has also been reported to activate Akt, and MAPK signaling pathways, involving ERK1/2, MEK1/2, JNK, and p38 kinase (Lejeune et al., 2002; Sonnenberg et al., 2010). The production of IL-22 is known to be enhanced by RAR-related orphan receptor gamma (RORγt), ligand-dependent transcription factor (aryl hydrocarbon receptor (AHR)), and B cell-activating transcription factor Batf (Ivanov et al., 2006; Schraml et al., 2009; Veldhoen et al., 2009). In addition, certain cytokines, such as IL-6, IL-21, and IL-23, have been shown to trigger the synthesis of IL-22 in T helper cells (Rutz and Ouyang, 2011). Furthermore, the expression of IL-22 has shown in vivo to be activated by PAMPs, such as LPS (Dumoutier et al., 2000b), and by anti-CD3 stimulation in T cells (Xie et al., 2000). The suppression of IL-22 is due to c-Maf and IRF4 (Rutz et al., 2011; Valdez et al., 2012). The detailed overview of IL-22 signaling pathways in mice and humans can be found in a brilliant review article by Rutz et al. (2013).

IL-22 can be characterized as a pleiotropic cytokine with a versatile spectrum of biological effects. One of the most important functions of this cytokine is to maintain tissue homeostasis as well as to support tissue repair and wound healing. This is provided by the IL-22-driven increase in the MAPK-dependent proliferation of epithelial cells (reviewed by Rutz et al., 2013). It has also been shown that IL-22 regulates the expression of genes involved in cell differentiation and mobility (Wolk et al., 2006). Additionally, it is well known that by eliciting its effects on epithelial cells, IL-22 creates a defense barrier against various pathogens. Multiple studies have shown that this cytokine is able to contribute to the production and release of antimicrobial peptides such as defensins and S-100 proteins, thereby having a considerable influence on the antimicrobial defense of the body (Liang et al., 2006; Wolk et al., 2006; Van Belle et al., 2012). IL-22 is also known to upregulate the expression of acute phase proteins in the liver, such as serum α1-antichymotrypsin, amyloid A, and haptoglobin. This cytokine was also found to promote osteoclastogenesis through triggering the receptor activator of NF-κB ligand in human synovial fibroblasts (Kim et al., 2012). Interestingly, the administration of mouse IL-22 resulted in decreased body weight, serum albumin, and red blood cells levels (Pittmann et al., 2011).

Multiple studies indicate that IL-22 plays a pivotal role in innate and adaptive immunity. Interestingly, it can act as either a proinflammatory agent through the upregulation of IL-6, G-CSF, and TNF or it can have a protective impact on inflammation. Furthermore, IL-22 has been reported to play a role in various autoinflammatory diseases. Increased levels of IL-22 were found to be associated with lupus erythematosus (Zhao et al., 2013b), Sjogren's syndrome (Ciccia et al., 2012), Behcet's disease (Cai et al., 2013), asthma (Pennino et al., 2013; Manni et al., 2014), atopic dermatitis (Nograles et al., 2009), multiple sclerosis (Beyeen et al., 2010), psoriasis (Ouyang, 2010; Hao, 2013), inflammatory bowel disease (ibd) (Seiderer and Brand, 2009; Ouyang, 2010), and rheumatoid arthritis (da Rocha, 2012; Xie et al., 2012). It is interesting, however, that multiple experiments on animal models showed that IL-22 may exert either a pathogenic impact or a protective impact on the above-mentioned diseases (Yang and Zheng, 2014). In particular, two different groups independently observed that IL-22 is a survival factor for hepatocytes during acute liver inflammation (Radaeva et al., 2004; Zenewicz et al., 2007). On the contrary, the administration of an endogenous IL-22 promoted inflammation in mice with collagen-induced arthritis, thereby exacerbating the disease (Geboes et al., 2009). Also, the use of anti–IL-22 antibodies profoundly decreased bone erosion and inflammation in IL-1Ra-defecient mice with arthritis (Marijnissen et al., 2011).

Recent studies identified a specific CD4$^+$ T cell subset that produces IL-22, called Th22 (Duhen et al., 2009; Eyerich et al., 2009). These cells are different from Th1 or Th17 subsets as they do not express IL-17 or IFN-γ and Th17 and the Th1-affiliated transcription factors T-bet and RORγt. The priming of Th22 cell differentiation can be triggered by either IL-6 or TNF-α with or without the help of DCs (Eyerich et al., 2009; Trifari et al., 2009). Some researchers argue that Th22 is the main source of secreted IL-22, although this cytokine is known to be expressed by other immune cells. Importantly, Th22 cells have been found to be involved in the pathogenesis of autoimmune diseases (Kagami et al., 2010; Qin et al., 2011; Zhang et al., 2011) and cancers (Ye et al., 2012; Liu et al., 2012). Nonetheless, the origin and functions of these cells have been poorly investigated so far and require further research.

Despite the fact that IL-22 is a double-edged sword in immunity, some researchers argue that this cytokine can be considered as a potential therapeutic for autoimmune diseases. So far, several groups have managed to suppress autoimmune diseases by using the anticytokine vaccination. Indeed, this approach seems quite promising, although the following in-depth studies are still needed.

6.4.2 IL-22 and Cancer

Quite a few studies on the association between IL-22 and cancer have appeared in recent years, suggesting the possible involvement of this cytokine in tumorigenesis.

Zhang et al. (2008) investigated the possible involvement of IL-22 in lung cancer. The authors found that high levels of this cytokine were observed in primary tumor tissue, malignant pleural effusions, and in the serum of 19 patients with NSCLC. Moreover, posttranscriptional silencing of the IL-22 gene caused by RNA interference profoundly suppressed xenograft tumor growth in BALB/c nude mice, thereby suggesting a pivotal role of IL-22 in lung cancer. By investigating the molecular mechanisms of IL-22-mediated oncogenesis, Zhang et al. showed that this cytokine significantly inhibits apoptosis in lung cancer cells by the activation of STAT3 and ERK1/2 signaling pathways. Another study exploring the role of IL-22 in lung cancer was recently conducted by Kobold et al. (2013). The authors found that IL-22 was expressed in 58% of small-cell lung cancer cases and in 46% of large-cell lung cancer cases (a total of 103 patients) and promoted growth in chemotherapy-resistant cancer cells. Also, the expression of IL-22R1 was observed in six of seven different lung cancer cell lines, although the activation of STAT3 was observed only in one cell line.

Several recently published articles suggest that IL-22 can potentially be involved in colorectal carcinogenesis. The assumption is that IL-22-mediated production of antimicrobial peptides can possibly lead to changes in gut microbiota, and thereby promote intestinal inflammation and cancer development. In addition, an interesting study conducted by Ziesché et al. (2007) identified that IL-22 triggers the expression of inducible nitric oxide synthase in human colon carcinoma cells, suggesting the involvement of NO-mediated mechanism in colon tumorigenesis. Further, Petanidis et al. (2013) analyzed the abundance of IL-22 in 92 patients with colorectal cancer and 54 age- and sex-matched healthy volunteers. The authors observed raised protein and mRNA levels in colorectal cancer patients as compared to that in controls. Interestingly, the levels of IL-22 were significantly higher in the tissues of patients without K-ras mutation in comparison with that of patients bearing the K-ras mutation. Furthermore, as compared to the K-ras negative group, mRNA levels of IL-22 were lower in the K-ras positive group. Consistently with previous reports, Jiang et al. (2013) showed that the concentration of IL-22 was significantly elevated in tissues from 82 patients with colon cancer and in 40 patients with ulcerative colitis. In addition, IL-22 stimulated tumor growth in vivo through the promotion of proliferation and inhibition of apoptosis. Furthermore, Kirchberger et al. (2013) demonstrated that the expression of IL-22 mRNA was more than twofold higher in colon cancer tissue versus that in normal tissue in 58% of pairs. Also, the authors found that IL-22 was associated with the development and maintenance of invasive colorectal cancer. It was revealed that colonic innate lymphoid cells are the major source of IL-22 in their samples and that these cells are responsible for bacteria-driven colon carcinogenesis. The depletion of these cells in mice with invasive colon cancer resulted in a marked reduction of inflammation with a further amelioration of the disease. Moreover, the authors showed that IL-22 blockade significantly suppressed tumor maintenance, and thereby suggested a critical role of this cytokine in colorectal tumorigenesis. Finally, Wu et al. (2013a) recently found that increased serum levels of IL-22 are associated with a chemoresistant condition of colorectal cancer in 87 patients.

There is also evidence suggesting a considerable impact of IL-22 on HCC. Brand et al. (2007) discovered that the expression of IL-22 is associated with an accelerated proliferation of hepatic cells. In order to clarify the role of IL-22 in hepatic tumorigenesis, Park et al. (2011a) generated a strain of transgenic mice overexpressing IL-22 in the liver. The authors demonstrated that IL-22 transgenic mice were prone to diethylnitrosamine-induced liver tumorigenesis. The animals exhibited a bigger tumor size and a higher liver weight ratio in comparison with those exhibited by healthy wild-type mice 9 months post diethylnitrosamine injection. Further, Jiang et al. (2011) identified significantly higher serum concentrations of IL-22 in 109 patients with HCC as compared to that in 48 controls with benign disease. In addition, the authors demonstrated in vitro that tumorigenic effects of IL-22 are due to the STAT3-driven promotion of antiapoptotic activities and proliferation of cancer cells. Feng et al. (2012) examined liver samples from 64 patients with chronic hepatitis B virus (HBV), and showed that IL-22 promotes the proliferation of liver stem/progenitor cells, which are believed to be a major source of liver cancer stem cells (Barker et al., 2009). Finally, Kim et al. (2013) found that IL-22 levels were decreased in 83 patients with HCC as compared to those in 33 healthy controls; however, the concentration of this cytokine increased early after transarterial chemoembolization in 63 cancer patients.

An interesting study was recently conducted by Wang et al. (2011b), who examined the impact of IL-22 on adipose tissue. The authors generated a transgenic mouse model with adipose-specific expression of IL-22, and these mice had no phenotype or metabolic alterations when fed with a high fat diet. Unexpectedly, 100% of transgenic mice developed spontaneous liposarcomas within 4 months of a high fat diet. Further analysis showed that IL-22 promoted the production of proinflammatory cytokines, such as IL-1β,

TNF-α, IL-6, IL-10, and IFN-γ through the activation of ERK pathway in adipose tissue and adipocytes. The results of this study suggest that obesity and IL-22-mediated inflammatory response may jointly contribute to cancer occurrence and development.

Several studies examined the role of IL-22-expressing Th22 cells in tumor specimens. Ye et al. (2012) found increased proportions of Th22 cells in malignant pleural effusions from 32 patients with newly diagnosed lung cancer. The levels of IL-22 were also significantly higher in pleural fluid as compared to that in serum. Furthermore, the authors showed that the recruitment of Th22 cells into pleural fluid was induced by chemokines CCL20, CCL22, and CCL27. Similarly to previous findings, the authors showed that IL-22 exhibited antiapoptotic activities in adenocarcinomic human alveolar basal epithelial cell line A549. Additionally, IL-22 stimulated the migration of A549 cells induced by primary mesenchyme cells and enhanced the intercellular adherent activity of cancer cells. Another study conducted by Liu et al. (2012) showed that increased circulating Th22 cells correlated with tumor progression and poor survival in 32 patients with human gastric cancer as compared to that in 19 healthy controls. Moreover, the frequencies of Th22 were markedly increased in stage III–IV gastric cancer patients versus that in stage I–II cancer and correlated with the overall survival rate. Similarly, Zhuang et al. (2012) found that Th22 cells were associated with tumor progression and predicted a poorer patient survival among 76 patients with gastric cancer.

There are several studies investigating the impact of IL-22 on hematological malignancies. Cao et al. (2010) determined high levels of IL-22 in plasma and culture supernatants of 10 multiple myeloma cell lines but not in the peripheral blood samples of 30 patients with multiple myeloma. Gangemi et al. (2013) found IL-22 overexpressed in 51 patients with B-chronic lymphocytic leukemia in comparison with 24 age- and sex-matched healthy controls. Similarly, Miyagaki et al. (2011) showed that the levels of IL-22 were markedly increased in skin biopsies and in the sera from 21 patients with cutaneous T cell lymphoma as compared to that of 24 healthy control subjects. Finally, Gelebart et al. (2011) revealed that IL-22RA1 is aberrantly expressed in mantle cell lymphoma cell lines and tumors.

Long-standing data implicate inherited variations in IL genes as important modificators of tumorigenesis (Yuzhalin, 2011; Kutikhin et al., 2014). Recent reports indicate that IL-22 gene polymorphisms can also play a role in cancer risk. Thompson et al. (2010) performed a case–control study in order to explore the role of seven single nucleotide polymorphisms (SNPs) within the IL-22 gene in 561 colon cancer cases and 722 population controls. The authors showed that the presence of heterozygous genotype and homozygous for the G allele for the rs1179251 polymorphism is associated with a 46% increased risk of developing colon cancer (odds ratio (OR) = 1.46; 95% confidence interval (CI) = 1.04–2.05 and OR = 2.10; 95% CI = 0.66–6.66, respectively) after adjustment for sex, age, and race. More associations were revealed by Eun et al. (2013), who indicated that the rs2227485 SNP correlates with the risk and the multifocality of papillary thyroid cancer in a sample of 94 cancer patients and in 213 healthy controls (codominant model, OR = 2.39, 95% CI = 1.21–4.71, p = 0.012; dominant model, OR = 1.89, 95% CI 1.08–3.31, p = 0.022).

6.4.3 Summary

Despite the fact that the biology of Th22 cells and IL-22 has not yet been fully understood, considerable attention has been paid to the investigation of the impact of this cytokine in cancer biology. The findings shown above identify a link between IL-22 and various malignancies, including lung cancer, colorectal carcinoma, gastric cancer, HCC, and hematological malignancies. Among the molecular mechanisms of IL-22-driven tumorigenesis is the inhibition of apoptosis and increased mitogenic activity. In addition, the proinflammatory activity of IL-22 and IL-22-mediated stimulation of NO synthesis may also contribute to carcinogenesis; however, more studies are needed to validate these hypotheses. Finally, the IL-22-mediated production of antimicrobial peptides can potentially stimulate bacteria-related colon tumorigenesis. Further research is necessarily to provide a better understanding of the role of this pleiotropic and extremely diverse cytokine is cancer biology.

6.5 INTERLEUKIN-24

6.5.1 Overview

In the early 1990s, Jiang and Fisher used a relatively new differentiation induction subtraction hybridization approach to identify a novel gene whose expression was highly different in normal and malignant melanocytes (Jiang and Fisher, 1993; Jiang et al., 1993, 1994). The authors indicated that the amount of the mRNA of this gene was high in normal cells, but was very low in cancer cells. In their subsequent research, Jiang et al. (1996) demonstrated that it acts as a negative growth regulator for tumor cells, thereby showing an attractive perspective for its therapeutic usage. This novel gene was initially called melanoma differentiation-associated 7 (*mda-7*), and later, several research groups were able to expand the knowledge of this agent and reveal its close relationship with the IL-10 cytokine superfamily and show profound anticancer activities in melanoma cells (Huang et al., 2001; Ekmekcioglu et al., 2001; Ellerhorst et al., 2002; Sarkar et al., 2002; Pestka et al., 2004a). Thus, because of functions, sequence homology, and chromosomal localization of the *mda-7* gene, it was decided to give this cytokine a new name, IL-24 (Sauane et al., 2003).

This cytokine represents a 24-kDa protein expressed on the surface of most immune cells as well on melanocytes and keratinocytes (Jiang et al., 1995; Huang et al., 2001; Wolk et al., 2002). Similarly to IL-20, IL-24 interacts with both IL-20R1/IL-20R2 and IL-22R1/IL-20R2 receptor complexes (Parrish-Novak et al., 2002) to elicit its biological effects, which are (1) cell growth inhibition; induction of (2) apoptosis; and (3) autophagy; and (4) proanginogenic activity. Historically, most investigations on IL-24 were focused primarily on cancer, as strong tumor suppressor activities of this cytokine have been revealed.

A series of early experiments showed that the level of IL-24 was significantly decreased in metastatic tumors, suggesting its potential impact on carcinogenesis (Jiang et al., 1995; Huang et al., 2001; Wolk et al., 2002). Further studies have demonstrated that IL-24 leads to the stimulation of cell growth arrest with subsequent cell death (Saito et al., 2005; Xue et al., 2006; Pataer et al., 2007), triggered by the activation of apoptosis (Su et al., 1998; Sarkar et al., 2002), inhibition of angiogenesis (Xie et al., 2008), and induction of autophagy (Yacoub et al., 2008a; Bhutia et al., 2010). Obviously, all these effects are inextricably linked with malignant disease, which caught the attention of many cancer biologists; therefore, a huge amount of research was performed on this issue during the last decade. Here we discuss the main achievements of these studies in detail, focusing on (1) cell growth inhibition, (2) apoptosis, (3) angiogenesis, and (4) autophagy.

6.5.2 IL-24 and Cell Growth Inhibition

It was mentioned before that the active research in the field of IL-24 was started after the discovery of the fact that IL-24 exerts a growth suppressive effect on melanoma cells (Jiang et al., 1995, 1996). Further investigations successfully replicated these findings and demonstrated a marked suppression of cancer cell growth in different transgenic cell and murine models, including those of breast carcinoma, various gliomas, prostate carcinoma, pancreatic cancer, renal cell carcinoma, lung cancer, gastric carcinoma, leukemia, osteosarcoma, ovarian cancer, and colorectal carcinoma (Table 6.1). In addition, these studies demonstrated a plethora of interesting observations. In particular, it was indicated that IL-24 promotes the suppression of cell growth only in tumor tissues but not in normal (healthy) tissues.

Table 6.1 Much Research has Demonstrated IL-24-mediated Suppression of Tumor Growth in Various Cancers

Malignancy	Reference
Gliomas	Su et al. (2003); Yacoub et al. (2003a,b); Yacoub et al. (2004); Park et al. (2008); Yacoub et al. (2008a,b,c); Hamed et al. (2010a,b); Yacoub et al. (2010); Wang et al. (2013)
Pancreatic cancer	Lebedeva et al. (2008); Pan et al. (2008a,b); Wang et al. (2008); Xue et al. (2010); Cai et al. (2012); He et al. (2013)
Breast carcinoma	Su et al. (1998); Sarkar et al. (2005); Bocangel et al. (2006); Chada et al. (2006); Zheng et al. (2007); Ni et al. (2008); Patani et al. (2010); Zhu et al. (2012); Zhao et al. (2012); Bhutia et al. (2013); Li et al. (2013a,b)
Ovarian cancer	Leath et al. (2004); Gopalan et al. (2005); Gopalan et al. (2007); Shanker et al. (2007); Emdad et al. (2006); Mahasreshti et al. (2006); Xiong et al. (2007)
Prostate cancer	Lebedeva et al. (2003); Sauane et al. (2004, 2006, 2008, 2010); Saito et al. (2005); Su et al. (2006); Sarkar et al. (2007); Bhutia et al. (2010); Dash et al. (2010)
HCC	Xie et al. (2011); Wang et al. (2012a,b)
Renal cell carcinoma	Yacoub et al. (2003c); Park et al. (2009, 2011a,b); Eulitt et al. (2010)
Lung cancer	Saeki et al. (2000); Saeki et al. (2002); Nishikawa et al. (2004); Ramesh et al. (2004a,b); Sieger et al. (2004); Oida et al. (2005); Emdad et al. (2007a,b); Inoue et al. (2007); Gupta et al. (2008); Xie et al. (2008); Zhong et al. (2010); Huang et al. (2011); Zhu et al. (2011)
Gastric cancer	Bao et al. (2009); Wei et al. (2010); Yan et al. (2010)
Osteosarcoma	Han et al. (2009)
Cervical cancer	Huang et al. (2001); Shi et al. (2007); Li et al. (2011)
Colon and rectal cancers	Emdad et al. (2007a,b); Chang et al. (2009, 2011); Azab et al. (2012); Xu et al. (2013)
Leukemia	Dong et al. (2008); Sainz-Perez et al. (2008); Rahmani et al. (2010)

Further research revealed that IL-24 does not evoke apoptosis in noncancer cells, but selectively provided the initiation of apoptotic cell destruction in tumor cells. This interesting phenomenon was called the "bystander antitumor effect".

Treatment of human non-small-cell lung cancer with IL-24 was found to be very effective in combination with a drug gefitinib, a selective reversible EGFR inhibitor (Emdad et al., 2007a). In addition, good results were obtained when using IL-24 in combination with angiogenesis inhibitor bevacizumab, nonsteroidal antiinflammatory medication sulindac, inhibitor of certain tyrosine and Raf kinases sorafenib, and apoptosis activator cisplatin for the treatment of lung cancer, renal cell carcinoma, and cervical cancer (Oida et al., 2005; Inoue et al., 2007; Eulitt et al., 2010; Li et al., 2011). More recently, several studies reported a successful experience of treating various cancers with oncolytic adenoviruses ZD55, MUD55, and SG600 harboring the IL-24 gene (Wei et al., 2010; Xue et al., 2010; Cai et al., 2013; He et al., 2013). Profound antitumor activity against colon cancer cells was demonstrated using an adenovirus containing the IL-24 gene and the anti-VEGF ribozyme gene (Chang et al., 2009). Finally, it was also recently revealed that IL-24 containing retrovirus has more evident anticancer effects in combination with a dietary agent perillyl alcohol (Lebedeva et al., 2008).

6.5.3 IL-24 and Apoptosis

Multiple studies implicate IL-24 as a major enhancer of apoptosis, although the mechanisms of this phenomenon have not been fully understood so far. In particular, numerous studies performed on various models, including those of breast cancer, melanoma, prostate cancer, malignant glioma, ovarian cancer, and cervical cancer, have shown that IL-24 is able to shift a balance in proapoptotic (BAX and BAK) and antiapoptotic (BCL-2 and BCL-X_L) representatives of the BCL family, and thereby promote programed cell death (reviewed by Fisher, 2005; Gupta et al., 2006; Fisher et al., 2007). Interestingly, it was found that IL-24 induces apoptosis exclusively in cancer cells without affecting normal cells (Sarkar et al., 2002). The activation of IL-24-induced apoptosis has not been associated with p53, pRB, and p21 (Lebedeva et al., 2003, 2005), although p38 MAPK has been found to be highly phosphorylated in chronic lymphocytic leukemia B cells with IL-24-driven apoptosis (Sainz-Perez et al., 2006). In addition, some groups showed that IL-24-induced apoptosis has been associated with the activation of double stranded RNA-activated kinase and protein kinase R, which in turn contributed to an increase in the phosphorylation of eIF2 alpha

(Pataer et al., 2002, 2005). Furthermore, proteins involved in the regulation of mitochondrial integrity and endoplasmic reticulum stress have also been related to IL-24-dependent apoptosis in numerous studies (Gupta et al., 2006; Park et al., 2009; Hamed et al., 2010a;Yacoub et al., 2010). However, further studies are necessary to explore the role of IL-24 in apoptosis.

6.5.4 IL-24 and Angiogenesis

An increasing amount of evidence indicates that apart from apoptosis IL-24 may inhibit tumor growth through the regulation of angiogenesis as well. Saeki et al. (2002) investigated an adenovirus-mediated overexpression of IL-24 in p53-wild-typ lung cell lines inoculated in nude mice. The authors observed a profound tumor growth inhibition through the induction of apoptosis and inhibition of epithelial cell proliferation. The researchers indicated a reduced tumor microvessel density and decreased amounts of VEGF and TGF-β, major mediators of neovascularization. In addition, CD31, a commonly used marker of angiogenesis, was significantly downregulated in tumor cells. Similarly, Nishikawa et al. (2004) showed that treatment with IL-24 decreased microvessel density in an NSCLC xenograft tumor model. Interestingly, the effect was more evident when combining the therapy with radiation (4.4-fold reduction in density). Additionally, the basal expression of VEGF and bFGF was also suppressed by IL-24.

Ramesh et al. (2004a) evaluated the antiangiogenic activity of IL-24 in vitro and in vivo, and showed that this cytokine inhibits the differentiation and migration of endothelial cells but not cell proliferation. It is interesting that the treatment of cells with various concentrations of IL-24 (1, 5, 10, and 50 ng/mL) showed the same result. Further, the authors indicated that treatment with IL-24 inhibits angiogenesis and tumor growth both in vivo and in vitro and that IP-10 and IFN-γ did not have an impact on IL-24-driven antiangiogenic activity. Finally, the researchers showed that IL-24 activated the STAT3 signaling pathway.

Tong et al. (2005) studied advanced cancer patients who received an intratumoral injection of INGN 241, a nonreplicating adenovirus vector carrying the *IL-24* transgene. An average of 28% reduction in CD31 staining was observed among tissue specimen on day 30 in comparison with that for pretreatment, thereby indicating the antiangiogenic activity of IL-24. Sarkar et al. (2007) investigated whether the injection of a virus containing the *IL-24* gene into nude mice inoculated with prostate cancer cells would affect tumor growth. The subsequent staining for CD31 revealed that IL-24 significantly inhibited angiogenesis in all the samples. Recently, Xie et al. (2011)

found that the adenovirus-mediated ING4 and IL-24 expression caused a significant downregulation of CD31, VEGF microvessel density in two models of HCC. Finally, Frewer et al. (2013) analyzed the abundance of IL-24 and other factors in 127 human breast cancer tissue samples, and demonstrated that a higher expression of vascular endothelial growth factor receptor-3 and VEGF-C correlated with a lower expression of intratumoral IL-24.

The importance of the impact of neovascularization on tumor growth is obvious. Together, the above-mentioned findings provide strong support for the antiangiogenic factor in IL-24-mediated antitumor effects. Based on the findings, it can be concluded that the research devoted to the impact of IL-24 on angiogenesis has been very successful.

6.5.5 IL-24 and Autophagy

Having discussed the role of IL-24 in apoptosis and angiogenesis, we suppose it is also important to mention the impact of this cytokine on yet another important mechanism, that is, autophagy. Autophagy is a basic catabolic process involving the bulk degradation of cellular components of all eukaryotes through the lysosomal machinery, particularly in response to various stress stimuli, such as starvation, chemotherapy, infection, and hormone treatments. However, autophagy happens under normal conditions as well. One major point that distinguishes this process from apoptosis is that autophagy plays a normal part in cell growth, development, and homeostasis. For example, autophagy is well known to be an essential part of tissue remodeling during the normal development of an organism. At the cellular level, the stages of autophagy include (1) formation of double-membraned vesicles containing cytoplasmic material, (2) fusion of these vesicles with lysosomes, and (3) lysosome-induced degradation of the material. At the molecular level, autophagy is mediated by >15 genes called autophagy-related genes. In brief, the formation of a phagophore (double membrane that encloses and isolates the cytoplasmic components) starts with the inhibition of mammalian target of rapamycin complex 1 kinase, which activates the ULK1 kinase complex consisting of ULK1, Atg13, and Atg17. This process is also modulated by Vps34, Beclin-1, ATG5, Ambra, Bif1, and Bcl-2. Upon formation, the phagophore is further maturated and elongated by LC-3-II. Once an autophagosome has finally formed, it fuses its external membrane with lysosomes to degrade the cargo.

Autophagy may exert both positive and negative effects on cancer cells (Jin and White, 2007). On the one hand, autophagy can promote tumor survival through the degradation of damaged mitochondria and buffering of oxidative stress. Further, autophagy may help to overcome hypoxia and nutrient deprivation in tumor cells, thereby contributing to their survival as well (Degenhardt et al., 2006). During 2004–2014, autophagy has been shown to protect tumors from radiation therapy (Ogier-Denis and Codogno, 2003) and chemotherapy (Kanzawa et al., 2004). Finally, DNA damage and genomic instability in response to stress in the absence of autophagy can result in an increased mutation rate and in cancer occurrence. To illustrate the effect of autophagy on tumors, it is worthwhile to mention an experiment performed by Mathew et al. (2009), who clearly demonstrated that autophagy-proficient cells (i.e., normally expressing autophagy-related genes) have been demonstrated to potentiate tumor survival as compared to autophagy-deficient ones, which have been deficient in *beclin-1* and *ATG5* genes. A deficiency of autophagy genes has been found associated with an enhanced tumorigenesis in vivo (Qu et al., 2003). It has also been recently found that the inhibition of autophagy significantly decreased tumorigenic growth of pancreatic cancer in vivo (Yang et al., 2011). On the other hand, multiple studies showed that autophagy can be induced by molecules with tumor-suppressive functions, such as beclin-1, ATG4C, ambra1, and UVRAG. In addition, autophagy has been found to inhibit necrosis and chronic inflammation through the activation of proinflammatory high-mobility group protein B1 (HMGB1), and thereby protect against tumorigenesis in certain conditions (Tang et al., 2010).

IL-24 has been demonstrated to have a considerable influence on autophagy. A series of pioneer experiments performed by Yacoub et al. (2008a,b, 2010) revealed that IL-24 profoundly inhibited the cell survival of primary human glioma cells in vitro through the promotion of autophagy via a protein kinase R–like endoplasmic reticulum kinase (PERK)- and cathepsin B-dependent mechanism. Activation of PERK promoted the vesicularization of an LC-3 that in turn activated LC-3 (ATG8) and increased the expression of other autophagy regulatory proteins Beclin-1 and ATG5 (Yacoub, 2008a,b). Similar effects of IL-24 were shown in malignant renal carcinoma cells through the same signaling pathway, involving ceramide, C95 and PERK (Park et al., 2009). In addition, the authors demonstrated that IL-24-driven autophagy was modulated by the p38 MAPK and JNK1/2 signaling pathways, and correlated with the inactivation of ERK1/2. Further investigations performed by Bhutia et al. (2011) on prostate cancer cells confirmed that IL-24-induced autophagy involves PERK but acts neither through serine/threonine–protein kinase/endoribonuclease (IRE1) nor through ATF6. Interestingly, the authors also revealed that

IL-24-driven autophagy ultimately culminated in apoptosis, and when apoptosis was blocked by the overexpression of Bcl-2 or Bcl-xL, autophagy increased. Further, Dash et al. (2011) found that the combination of IL-24 with Mcl-1 inhibitor Sabutoclax induced beclin-1- and ATG5-mediated autophagy followed by apoptosis. These results emphasize the importance of autophagy in the promotion of apoptosis during anticancer response. The switch between autophagy and apoptosis is currently being actively investigated, and certain autophagy-related genes such as beclin-1 have been so far found to be involved in apoptosis initiation (Maiuri et al., 2007; Djavaheri-Mergny et al., 2010).

Another study conducted by Yang et al. (2010) transfected chronic lymphocytic leukemia B cells with constantly replicating adenovirus containing the *IL-24* gene, showing that the inhibition of autophagy through the overexpression of IL-24 strongly augmented the antileukemia activity both in vitro and in vivo. In addition, it was found that the combination of IL-24 with a covalent inhibitor of phosphoinositide 3-kinases wortmanin showed profound anticancer effects in established leukemia xenografts. Recently, Hamed et al. (2010b) showed that the autophagy-inducing drug OSU-03012 increased the toxicity of IL-24 against glioblastoma multiforme cells. Consistent with previous findings, the authors observed that the toxic effects of IL-24 were due to the initiation of PERK-dependent autophagy. Further experiments performed by Hamed et al. (2013a,b) demonstrated that combining histone deacetylase inhibitors with IL-24 resulted in growth inhibition in multiple cancer cell lines through autophagic flux. Moreover, the authors also demonstrated that the knockdown of key genes involved in autophagy (ATG5, CD95, beclin-1) caused the reduction of IL-24-mediated toxicity, confirming the results obtained previously.

Collectively, these findings indicate that although little is known about the role of IL-24 in cancer-related autophagy, it is certainly true that this cytokine may affect autophagy in tumor cells through defined pathways. While the initial findings are intriguing and promising, further research devoted to this problem is necessary.

6.5.6 Summary

Concluding this section, we can say that IL-24 is currently one of the most promising candidates to treat cancer in the future. Multiple studies have been done to validate IL-24 as a major antitumor agent, acting through (1) inhibition of proliferation; (2) promotion of apoptosis; (3) suppression of angiogenesis; and (4) stimulation of autophagy. Importantly, IL-24 has a unique ability to affect tumor cells while having almost no effect on normal cells, which can be extremely useful in the clinical application of this cytokine. More research should be performed to elucidate the exact mechanism of such an unusual effect.

In 2005, a Phase I dose-escalation clinical trial was performed to investigate the impact of IL-24 on human cancer (Tong et al., 2005). The authors demonstrated the direct tumor growth inhibition and bystander antitumor effects when administered a nonreplicating adenoviral construct expressing the IL-24 transgene to 22 patients with advanced cancer. Currently, Phase II clinical trials are being conducted by different groups. Hopefully, these studies will help to establish IL-24 as a valid anticancer therapeutic agent.

6.6 INTERLEUKIN-26

IL-26 is a newly discovered member of the IL-10 superfamily, which shares a 24.7% amino acid identity and 47% similarity with IL-10. However, IL-26 shares an 85–95% amino acid sequence homology with its own mammalian paralogs. This cytokine was initially discovered in human T cells after growth transformation by the rhadinovirus herpes virus *Saimiri* or simian γ_2-herpes virus. IL-26 may act as either a monomer or homodimer, which is able to adhere to glycosaminoglycans on cell surfaces, because of its positive charge (Braum et al., 2012). So far, IL-26 has been found to be expressed by NK cells, activated T cells, macrophage-like synoviocytes from rheumatoid arthritis joints and in peripheral mononuclear blood cells. In addition, IL-26 was found to be coexpressed with IL-22 (Donnelly et al., 2010).

The biological effects of IL-26 are exerted through the heterodimeric receptor complex that comprises IL-20R1 and IL-10R2 subunits. Both subunits are widely expressed by various tissues and cell types, especially by hematopoietic cells. IL-20R1 is responsible for the specific binding with IL-26, whereas IL-10R2 is necessary for the signal transduction. Upon binding, IL-26 induces the phosphorylation of Tyk1 and Jak1, followed by the activation of STAT1 and STAT3 (Sheikh et al., 2004; Hör et al., 2004; Yoon et al., 2006, 2010). In addition, the triggering of IL-26 was associated with the activation of ERK-1/2 and stress-activated protein kinase (SAPK)/ JNK, and MAPKs (Dambacher et al., 2009).

Due to the lack of research devoted to this problem, little is known about the primary functions of IL-26. Recently, it was demonstrated that IL-26 is overexpressed in rheumatoid arthritis and promotes the synthesis of proinflammatory cytokines and Th17 cell generation (Corvaisier et al., 2012). Further, IL-26 levels were increased in serum and lesional skin of patients with psoriasis (Michalak-Stoma et al., 2011). Interestingly, certain SNPs within the IL-26 gene were found to be associated with multiple sclerosis and rheumatoid arthritis (Goris et al., 2001; Vandenbroeck et al., 2003). Intestinal epithelial cell lines were shown to express both IL-26 receptor subunits IL-20R1 and IL-10R2. Finally, inflamed colonic lesions from patients with Crohn's disease exhibited an elevated IL-26 mRNA level of IL-26, and it was significantly associated with the expression of IL-8 and IL-22 (Dambacher et al., 2009).

There is little evidence to suggest that IL-26 can be implemented in cancer development. Recently, You et al. (2013) investigated the prosurvival and proliferative effects of IL-24 in vitro. The researchers found that IL-24 enhanced cell proliferation and provided an antiapoptotic effect on MKN45 and SGC-7901 cell lines through the activation of STAT1 and STAT3. Further, real-time polymerase chain reaction analysis revealed that IL-26 serum levels and mRNA in 60 fresh human gastric cancer tissues were significantly overexpressed in comparison with that in normal gastric tissues. Finally, IL-20R1 was shown to be overexpressed in gastric cancer tissues as compared to that in normal ones.

This study has gone some way toward understanding the impact of IL-26 on cancer. Undoubtedly, further research will be required to extend the existing knowledge on this problem.

6.7 TYPE III IFNS: IL-28A, IL-28B, AND IL-29

6.7.1 Overview

IL-28A (IFN-γ1), IL-28B (IFN-γ2), and IL-29 (IFN-γ3) belong to the type III IFN subfamily and exhibit a very high level of homology in the amino acid sequence. While the amino acid identity between IL-28A and IL-28B is around 96%, this indicator, however, is very low between type I and type III IFNs, and ranges from 15% to 20%. This group of proteins was discovered in 2003 by two independent groups and initially described as a new IFN subtype, since they shared common expression patterns and signaling pathways with those of type I and II IFNs (Kotenko et al., 2003; Sheppard et al., 2003).

Multiple cell types are known to produce type I and type III IFNs in response to viral infection, including Th1, NK, and NKT-cell subsets. However, the biological effects of IL-28A, IL-28B, and IL-29 are mainly directed on epithelial cells, which unlike other cell types exhibit the highest abundance of IFN-λ receptor on their surface. Thus, the majority of authors consider all cells of epithelial origin as primary targets for IFN-λs. However, some researchers claim that cellular targets for type III IFNs may also include hepatocytes (Doyle et al., 2006), colon cells (Lasfar et al., 2006), adipocytes (Witte et al., 2009), and neurons (Zitzmann et al., 2006). In addition, some studies indicate that IFN-γ can also induce a weak response in certain immune cells, such as macrophages, plasmacytoid cells, monocyte-derived dendritic cells, peripheral blood mononuclear cells, and bone marrow cells (Coccia et al., 2004; Lasfar et al., 2006; Donelly and Kotenko, 2010). Of these, DCs have shown an especially high level of response to IL-28A, IL-28B, and IL-29.

The receptor for type III IFNs is a heterodimeric complex that comprises the unique IFN-λR1 subunit (IL-28RA) and the IL-10R2 subunit, which is shared with other family representatives IL-10, IL-22, and IL-26. Binding of IFN-λs to the corresponding receptor results in the phosphorylation of Jak1 and Tyk1, which in turn leads to the activation of STAT1, STAT2, STAT3, STAT4, or STAT5 depending on cell type. In addition, IFN-γs were reported to trigger the signaling of Akt/PI3K, MAPK, ERK1, ERK2, SAPK, JNK, and p38 kinase (Brand et al., 2005; Zhou et al., 2007). According to the results of recent studies, the transcriptional regulation of IL-28A, IL-28B, and IL-29 syntheses is regulated through IRFs, NF-κB and AP-1 signaling pathways (Onoguchi et al., 2007; Thomson et al., 2009). These regulation patterns are very similar to those in type I and IFNs, although some studies reported that type I and type II IFN antiviral systems act independently of each other (Zhou et al., 2007; Ank et al., 2008; Wang et al., 2009).

Much research has been done in recent years to investigate the biological effects of IFN-γs within the body. As mentioned above, type III IFNs elicit antimicrobial functions that are typical for all IFNs. The expression of type III IFNs in response to various TLR agonists and viruses was shown in multiple in vivo and in vitro studies (Coocia et al., 2004; Ank et al., 2006; Onoguchi et al., 2007; Donnelly and Kotenko, 2010). Further, IL-28A, IL-28B, and IL-29 demonstrated considerable antiviral activity against hepatitis C virus, hepatitis B virus, and vesicular stomatitis virus, Newcastle disease virus, measles virus, Sendai virus, mumps virus, parainfluenzae virus III, influenza A virus, Sindbis virus, encephalomyocarditis virus, and coxsackievirus B1 (Robek et al., 2005; Yang et al., 2005; Marcello et al., 2006). In addition, it was recently found that IFN-γs can activate the antiviral pathway in either human NT2-N neurons infected with herpes simplex virus type 1 or human IFN-$\gamma^{+/+}$ blood monocyte-derived macrophages infected with human immunodeficiency virus type 1 (Hou et al., 2009; Zhou et al., 2011). However, researchers failed to demonstrate antiviral activities of type III IFNs in mice infected with either hepatotropic Thogotovirus (Mordstein et al., 2008) or lymphocytic choriomeningitis virus (Ank et al., 2006). Additionally, no response to IFN-γs was observed in DCs and in macrophages infected with the Lassa virus (Baize et al., 2006). It is important to mention that clinical data from a phase 1 trial study showed profound antiviral effects of recombinant IL-29 administered for the treatment of patients with hepatitis C virus (Miller et al., 2009), suggesting the therapeutic application of this cytokine.

Considering the particular impact of IFN-γs on the immune system, we should bear in mind the fact that these factors predominantly act as immunomodulatory agents. Although there is still no clear picture of how type III IFNs influence immune cells, numerous studies reported that these cytokines have a considerable role in immunity. A series of experiments revealed that IFN-γs can profoundly suppress Th2 and Th17 responses in various immune cells (Jordan et al., 2007; Dai et al., 2009; Koltsida et al., 2011). Moreover, IL-28A was reported to promote Th1 immune skewing and to alleviate allergic airway disease in lung DCs (Koltsida et al., 2011). Quite recently, it was discovered that IL-28A, IL-28B, and IL-29 have the potential to induce apoptosis (Li et al., 2008b). The signaling induced by these cytokines in colorectal adenocarcinoma cell lines resulted in immediate senescence followed by DNA fragmentation and release of caspase-3, caspase-8, and caspase-9. This important finding highlighted the major role of these cytokines in pathological processes, such as cancer, and since then active investigations in this field have begun. Another research study suggested that these cytokines may enhance antigen presentation. In particular, IL-28A, IL-28B, and IL-29 were found to upregulate the expression of MHC I molecules in several cell lines, thereby indicating a great role of these cytokines in presentation of viral components (Kotenko et al., 2003; Sato et al., 2006). Further investigations showed that the maturation and migration capacity of human DCs were found to be increased after treatment with IFN-γ; furthermore, DCs treated with IFN-λs exhibited a marked increase in the IL-2-dependent proliferation of CD4$^+$CD25$^+$ regulatory T cells (Mennechet and Uzé, 2006). Several studies demonstrated that type III IFNs can affect the expression of chemokines and of other cytokines. In particular, IL-29 was recently shown to induce the production of

TNF and IL-12p40 in macrophages; however, treatment with IL-29 did not affect monocytes or monocyte-derived dendritic cells (Liu et al., 2011). Of note, both TNF and IL-12 possess marked antitumor activities (Yuzhalin and Kutikhin, 2012); thus, this finding may have a sense in the context of cancer research. Expression of IL-28 was upregulated by IFN-λs in intestinal epithelial cells (Brand et al., 2005). Moreover, IL-28A elevated the mRNA of MIG/CXCL9, IP-10/CXCL10, and TAC/CXCL11, which are chemoattractants involved in multiple immune reactions and angiogenesis (Pekarek et al., 2007). It was also revealed that IL-29 upregulated the expression of TLR3 and enhanced the response to TLR3 stimulation through a positive-feedback loop, thereby amplifying antiviral defense in keratinocytes (Wolk et al., 2008). Additionally, IFN-λs downregulated IL-4, IL-5, IL-6, IL-10, and IL-13 in human peripheral blood mononuclear cells in a series of experiments (Jordan et al., 2007; Srinivas et al., 2008; Dai et al., 2009). Finally, there is little evidence that suggests the engagement of type III IFNs in autoimmune diseases. It was recently shown that patients with systemic lupus erythematosus and rheumatoid arthritis had significantly higher amounts of IL-28 protein in sera and mRNA in peripheral blood mononucleated cells as compared to those of normal controls (Lin et al., 2012; Wu et al., 2013b).

6.7.2 IL-28A, IL-28B, IL-29, and Cancer

A plethora of studies have been performed to investigate the impact of type III IFNs on tumor development, showing that these cytokines have a considerable role in tumor growth inhibition. For the first time the importance of IFN-λs in anticancer defense was demonstrated by Dumoutier et al. (2004), who found that IFN-λ1 inhibited the proliferation of IL-28R/LICR2-expressing human lymphoma cells through the activation of STAT2, STAT3, and STAT4. Further, Meager et al. (2005) reported that the proliferation of human astrocytoma/glioblastoma-derived cell lines was markedly inhibited by IL-28A and IL-29. According to the authors, these cytokines may be considered as "weak" type IFNs since relatively high concentrations of these cytokines were required to induce a response as compared to that of type I IFNs. Moreover, it is important to mention an interesting study performed by Sato et al. (2006), who investigated the impact of type III IFNs on murine melanoma and colon cancer cell lines, showing that the overproduction of IFN-λ inhibited cell growth in vitro in vivo. More importantly, the researchers showed that the formation of pulmonary metastasis was totally prevented in IFN-λ-treated mice as compared to that in controls. Further, targeting therapy of liver metastasis by injection of IFN-λ cDNA resulted in partial tumor regression and in significantly better mice survival. Lasfar et al. (2006) transfected human melanoma cell line B16 with adenovirus containing the *IL-28A* gene, demonstrating a marked suppression of tumor growth after subcutaneous injection into mice. In another report, Numasaki et al. (2007) demonstrated that retroviral IL-28-expressing mice exhibited a significant decrease in fibrosarcoma tumor growth and in lung metastasis formation. In addition, the researchers indicated that IL-28 prolonged the survival of tumor-bearing mice and observed that IL-12 enhanced the IFN-λ-modulated antitumor response in the presence or absence of IFN-γ.

Currently, the exact mechanisms of anticancer activities of IL-28A, IL-28B, and of IL-29 are not clearly understood. Nevertheless, one of these mechanisms is apparently associated with the proapoptotic activities of these cytokines. The first study in this field was performed by Zitzmann et al. (2006), and contained a number of new and important insights. First, the authors showed that the treatment of human neuroendocrine tumor cell lines with IL-28A and IL-29 significantly reduced the cell number, by 20% and 30%, respectively. Phosphorylation of STAT1, STAT2, and STAT3 was observed immediately after treatment. More interestingly, the authors revealed that both IL-28A and IL-29 activated apoptotic pathways in cancer cells. After 44 h of incubation, treated cells exhibited a high level of DNA fragmentation as well as considerable amounts of cleaved caspase-3 and PARP products, which are the commonly used markers of apoptosis. Also, Zinzmann et al. found that suppressor of cytokine signaling 1 and 3 (SOCS1 and SOCS3) could act as negative regulators of IFN-λ signaling, completely abolishing the antitumor activities of these cytokines. Of note, numerous studies demonstrated the critical roles of SOCS1 and SOCS3 in various tumors (reviewed by Inagaki-Ohara et al., 2013).

Maher et al. (2008) determined the impact of the anticancer response caused by IFN-λ in the immortal human keratinocyte line, mouse melanoma cells, and human fibrosarcoma cell line. Incubation of treated cells for 72 h led to a 50% decrease in the cell proliferation; furthermore, IFN-λ-treated cells underwent programed cell death as shown by annexin-V and propidium iodide staining. In addition, the authors revealed that antiproliferative and antiapoptotic effects were due to JAK/STAT pathway activation. Although IFN-λ was more effective than IFN-α was in inducing an antiproliferative effect that overlapped with the activation of apoptosis, the combination of these two agents resulted in a profound antiproliferative activity, suggesting the joint use of these cytokines for cancer treatment.

It was mentioned above that previous investigations by Li et al. (2008a) also clearly demonstrated the proapoptotic activities of type III IFNs in the human colorectal adenocarcinoma cell line. Further, Li et al. (2010) examined whether IFN-λ1 could inhibit the growth of esophageal carcinoma cells. Moreover, the researchers demonstrated that IFN-λ1 promoted the Rb- and p21-mediated cell cycle arrest at G1 phase followed by apoptosis. Interestingly, the authors observed a profound suppression of esophageal carcinoma development after treatment with IFN-λ1 together with commonly used chemotherapy drugs cisplatin and fluorouracil. This finding may suggest the further usage of this cytokine for cancer therapy. Further studies by Li et al. (2012) revealed that various bladder cancer tissues and cell lines express IL-28A; moreover, this cytokine was reported to induce wound healing migration of bladder cancer cells through NF-κB-modulated MMP-9 expression triggering the MAPK signaling pathway. Treatment of cells and tissues with anti-IL-28 antibodies or IFN-λ receptor knockdown resulted in the abrogation of IL-28A-mediated triggering of MMP-9 production as well as in the activation of MAPK and NF-κB. Interestingly, the results obtained by Li et al. may suggest that IL-28A can promote tumor metastasis, which is in disagreement with previous reports indicating IFN-λ-dependent suppression of metastatic activity (Sato et al., 2006; Numasaki et al., 2007).

Recent studies provided more support for the link between type III IFNs and apoptosis. Tezuka et al. (2012) reported that murine IL-28A suppressed the tumor growth of B16 melanoma cells in vitro through the activation of apoptosis. The authors detected a significant increase in caspase-3 and caspase-7 activities 48 h after IFN-λ2 treatment, and the apoptotic activity was completely blocked in the presence of anti-IFN-λ I monoclonal antibodies. In accordance with previous findings, Yan et al. (2013) reported that IL-28A-expressing mice with lung adenosarcoma exhibited a profound decrease in the tumor growth, promotion of tumor apoptosis, subcutaneous tumor necrosis, and cystic degeneration. Further, the authors found that IL-28A treatment was associated with an increased number of CD3+CD4+, CD3+CD8+, and NK CD3−CD49+ cells.

It was mentioned previously that IL-28A was found to upregulate MIG/CXCL9, IP-10/CXCL10, and TAC/CXCL11 (Pekarek et al., 2007). As known, these chemokines play a crucial role in the prevention of tumor neovascularization, and also contribute to a number of other tumor-related processes (Zhu et al., 2012). The results obtained by Pekarek et al. highlight the need for the further continuation of the investigation of the impact of type III cytokines and angiogenesis, and this connection should be elaborated in the follow-up studies.

Finally, it can be suggested that the determination of serum levels of IFN-λs may be of clinical significance. Support for this comes from the recent study of Naumnik et al. (2012), who examined the clinical usefulness of the assessment of IL-29 in 45 Polish patients with advanced stages of lung cancer. The authors found that the abundance of IL-29 in serum was significantly higher than in bronchoalveolar lavage fluid. In addition, IL-29 levels were higher at stage III as compared to that at stage IV.

6.7.3 Summary

In the last 10 years, a growing interest has been devoted to the expanding knowledge about IL-28A, IL-28B, and IL-29. The comparison between type I and type III IFNs is outside the scope of this book. Although these two IFN classes share common patterns of regulation and signaling pathways, their biological effects seem to be different (Li et al., 2013a). Multiple studies demonstrated that IFN-λs possess profound antiviral and immunomodulatory functions and that they can also play a role in the development of autoimmune diseases. More importantly, IL-28A, IL-28B, and IL-29 also provide significant proapoptotic and antiproliferative effects, which is extremely relevant in the context of cancer. A series of in vitro and in vivo experiments showed that type III IFNs can markedly suppress the development of cultured cancer cell lines and established tumors. To conclude, further experiments on IL-28A, IL-28B, and IL-29 could involve clinical trials evaluating the usefulness of these cytokines in patients with cancers.

REFERENCES

Adris, S., Klein, S., Jasnis, M., Chuluyan, E., Ledda, M., Bravo, A., Carbone, C., Chernajovsky, Y., Podhajcer, O., 1999. IL-10 expression by CT26 colon carcinoma cells inhibits their malignant phenotype and induces a T cell-mediated tumor rejection in the context of a systemic Th2 response. Gene Ther. 6 (10), 1705–1712.

Agarwal, A., Agrawal, U., Verma, S., Mohanty, N.K., Saxena, S., 2010. Serum Th1 and Th2 cytokine balance in patients of superficial transitional cell carcinoma of bladder pre- and post-intravesical combination immunotherapy. Immunopharmacol. Immunotoxicol. 32 (2), 348–356.

Al-Ashy, R., Chakroun, I., El-Sabban, M.E., Homaidan, F.R., 2006. The role of NF-kappaB in mediating the anti-inflammatory effects of IL-10 in intestinal epithelial cells. Cytokine 36 (1–2), 1–8.

Alaaeddine, N., Di Battista, J.A., Pelletier, J.P., Kiansa, K., Cloutier, J.M., Martel-Pelletier, J., 1999. Inhibition of tumor necrosis factor alpha-induced prostaglandin E2 production by the antiinflammatory cytokines interleukin-4, interleukin-10, and interleukin-13 in osteoarthritic synovial fibroblasts: distinct targeting in the signaling pathways. Arthritis Rheum. 42 (4), 710–718.

Alanärä, T., Karstila, K., Moilanen, T., Silvennoinen, O., Isomäki, P., 2010. Expression of IL-10 family cytokines in rheumatoid arthritis: elevated levels of IL-19 in the joints. Scand. J. Rheumatol. 39 (2), 118–126.

Alhamarneh, O., Agada, F., Madden, L., Stafford, N., Greenman, J., 2011. Serum IL10 and circulating CD4(+) CD25(high) regulatory T cell numbers as predictors of clinical outcome and survival in patients with head and neck squamous cell carcinoma. Head Neck 33 (3), 415–423.

Andrés, R.M., Hald, A., Johansen, C., Kragballe, K., Iversen, L., 2013. Studies of Jak/STAT3 expression and signalling in psoriasis identifies STAT3-Ser727 phosphorylation as a modulator of transcriptional activity. Exp. Dermatol. 22 (5), 323–328.

Ank, N., West, H., Bartholdy, C., Eriksson, K., Thomsen, A.R., Paludan, S.R., 2006. Lambda interferon (IFN-lambda), a type III IFN, is induced by viruses and IFNs and displays potent antiviral activity against select virus infections in vivo. J. Virol. 80 (9), 4501–4509.

Ank, N., Iversen, M.B., Bartholdy, C., Staeheli, P., Hartmann, R., Jensen, U.B., Dagnaes-Hansen, F., Thomsen, A.R., Chen, Z., Haugen, H., Klucher, K., Paludan, S.R., Feb 15, 2008. An important role for type III interferon (IFN-lambda/IL-28) in TLR-induced antiviral activity. J. Immunol. 180 (4), 2474–2485.

Asadullah, K., Gellrich, S., Haeussler-Quade, A., Friedrich, M., Docke, W.D., Jahn, S., Volk, H.D., Sterry, W., 2000. Cytokine expression in primary cutaneous germinal center cell lymphomas. Exp. Dermatol. 9 (1), 71–76.

Asadullah, K., Sterry, W., Volk, H.D., 2003. Interleukin-10 therapy—review of a new approach. Pharmacol. Rev. 55 (2), 241–269.

Asadullah, K., Friedrich, M., Docke, W.D., Jahn, S., Volk, H.D., Sterry, W., 1997. Enhanced expression of T-cell activation and natural killer cell antigens indicates systemic antitumor response in early primary cutaneous T-cell lymphoma. J. Invest. Dermatol. 108 (5), 743–747.

Asadullah, K., Sabat, R., Friedrich, M., Volk, H.D., Sterry, W., 2004. Interleukin-10: an important immunoregulatory cytokine with major impact on psoriasis. Curr. Drug Targets Inflamm. Allergy 3 (2), 185–192.

Azab, B., Dash, R., Das, S.K., Bhutia, S.K., Shen, X.N., Quinn, B.A., Sarkar, S., Wang, X.Y., Hedvat, M., Dmitriev, I.P., Curiel, D.T., Grant, S., Dent, P., Reed, J.C., Pellecchia, M., Sarkar, D., Fisher, P.B., 2012. Enhanced delivery of mda-7/IL-24 using a serotype chimeric adenovirus (Ad.5/3) in combination with the apogossypol derivative BI-97C1 (Sabutoclax) improves therapeutic efficacy in low CAR colorectal cancer cells. J. Cell. Physiol. 227 (5), 2145–2153.

Azuma, Y.T., Matsuo, Y., Kuwamura, M., Yancopoulos, G.D., Valenzuela, D.M., Murphy, A.J., Nakajima, H., Karow, M., Takeuchi, T., 2010. Interleukin-19 protects mice from innate-mediated colonic inflammation. Inflamm. Bowel. Dis. 16 (6), 1017–1028.

Baird, A.M., Gray, S.G., O'Byrne, K.J., 2011. IL-20 is epigenetically regulated in NSCLC and down regulates the expression of VEGF. Eur. J. Cancer 47 (12), 1908–1918.

Baize, S., Pannetier, D., Faure, C., Marianneau, P., Marendat, I., Georges-Courbot, M.C., Deubel, V., 2006. Role of interferons in the control of Lassa virus replication in human dendritic cells and macrophages. Microbes Infect. 8 (5), 1194–1202.

Bao, W., Miao, J., Sheng, W., Shan, Y., Li, Z., Wang, X., Jing, Y., Han, Y., Yang, J., 2009. Adenovirus mediated IL-24 gene expression suppresses gastric cancer cell growth in vitro. Shengwu Gongcheng Xuebao 25 (10), 1586–1592. [Article in Chinese].

Barille-Nion, S., Bah, N., Vequaud, E., Juin, P., 2012. Regulation of cancer cell survival by BCL2 family members upon prolonged mitotic arrest: opportunities for anticancer therapy. Anticancer Res. 32 (10), 4225–4233.

Barker, N., Ridgway, R.A., van Es, J.H., van de Wetering, M., Begthel, H., van den Born, M., Danenberg, E., Clarke, A.R., Sansom, O.J., Clevers, H., 2009. Crypt stem cells as the cells-of-origin of intestinal cancer. Nature 457 (7229), 608–611.

Barth Jr, R.J., Coppola, M.A., Green, W.R., 1996. In vivo effects of locally secreted IL-10 on the murine antitumor immune response. Ann. Surg. Oncol. 3 (4), 381–386.

Bayraktar, M., Peltier, M., Vetrano, A., Arita, Y., Gurzenda, E., Joseph, A., Kazzaz, J., Sharma, S., Hanna, N., 2009. IL-10 modulates placental responses to TLR ligands. Am. J. Reprod. Immunol. 62 (6), 390–399.

Berg, D.J., Zhang, J., Lauricella, D.M., Moore, S.A., 2001. Il-10 is a central regulator of cyclooxygenase-2 expression and prostaglandin production. J. Immunol. 166 (4), 2674–2680.

Berman, R.M., Suzuki, T., Tahara, H., Robbins, P.D., Narula, S.K., Lotze, M.T., 1996. Systemic administration of cellular IL-10 induces an effective, specific, and long-lived immune response against established tumors in mice. J. Immunol. 157 (1), 231–238.

Beyeen, A.D., Adzemovic, M.Z., Ockinger, J., Stridh, P., Becanovic, K., Laaksonen, H., Lassmann, H., Harris, R.A., Hillert, J., Alfredsson, L., Celius, E.G., Harbo, H.F., Kockum, I., Jagodic, M., Olsson, T., 2010. IL-22RA2 associates with multiple sclerosis and macrophage effector mechanisms in experimental neuroinflammation. J. Immunol. 185 (11), 6883–6890.

Bhutia, S.K., Dash, R., Das, S.K., Azab, B., Su, Z.Z., Lee, S.G., Grant, S., Yacoub, A., Dent, P., Curiel, D.T., Sarkar, D., Fisher, P.B., 2010. Mechanism of autophagy to apoptosis switch triggered in prostate cancer cells by antitumor cytokine melanoma differentiation-associated gene 7/interleukin-24. Cancer Res. 70 (9), 3667–3676.

Bhutia, S.K., Das, S.K., Azab, B., Menezes, M.E., Dent, P., Wang, X.Y., Sarkar, D., Fisher, P.B., May 30, 2013. Targeting breast cancer initiating/stem cells with melanoma differentiation associated gene-7/interleukin-24 (mda-7/IL-24). Int. J. Cancer http://dx.doi.org/10.1002/ijc.28289. [Epub ahead of print].

Bhutia, S.K., Das, S.K., Azab, B., Dash, R., Su, Z.Z., Lee, S.G., Dent, P., Curiel, D.T., Sarkar, D., Fisher, P.B., 2011. Autophagy switches to apoptosis in prostate cancer cells infected with melanoma differentiation associated gene-7/interleukin-24 (mda-7/IL-24). Autophagy 7 (9), 1076–1077.

Bien, E., Krawczyk, M., Izycka–Swieszewska, E., Trzonkowski, P., Kazanowska, B., Adamkiewicz–Drozynska, E., Balcerska, A., 2013. Deregulated systemic IL-10/IL-12 balance in advanced and poor prognosis paediatric soft tissue sarcomas. Biomarkers 18 (3), 204–215.

Blay, J.Y., Burdin, N., Rousset, F., Lenoir, G., Biron, P., Philip, T., Banchereau, J., Favrot, M.C., 1993. Serum interleukin-10 in non-Hodgkin's lymphoma: a prognostic factor. Blood 82 (7), 2169–2174.

Blobe, G.C., Schiemann, W.P., Lodish, H.F., 2000. Role of transforming growth factor beta in human disease. N. Engl. J. Med. 342 (18), 1350–1358.

Bloch, O., Crane, C.A., Kaur, R., Safaee, M., Rutkowski, M.J., Parsa, A.T., May 29, 2013. Gliomas promote immunosuppression through induction of B7-H1 expression in tumor-associated macrophages. Clin. Cancer Res. [Epub ahead of print].

Blumberg, H., Conklin, D., Xu, W.F., Grossmann, A., Brender, T., Carollo, S., Eagan, M., Foster, D., Haldeman, B.A., Hammond, A., Haugen, H., Jelinek, L., Kelly, J.D., Madden, K., Maurer, M.F., Parrish-Novak, J., Prunkard, D., Sexson, S., Sprecher, C., Waggie, K., West, J., Whitmore, T.E., Yao, L., Kuechle, M.K., Dale, B.A., Chandrasekher, Y.A., 2001. Interleukin 20: discovery, receptor identification, and role in epidermal function. Cell 104 (1), 9–19.

Bobe, G., Murphy, G., Albert, P.S., Sansbury, L.B., Lanza, E., Schatzkin, A., Colburn, N.H., Cross, A.J., 2010. Serum cytokine concentrations, flavonol intake and colorectal adenoma recurrence in the polyp prevention trial. Br. J. Cancer 103 (9), 1453–1461.

Bocangel, D., Zheng, M., Mhashilkar, A., Liu, Y., Ramesh, R., Hunt, K.K., Chada, S., 2006. Combinatorial synergy induced by adenoviral-mediated mda-7 and herceptin in Her-2+ breast cancer cells. Cancer Gene Ther. 13 (10), 958–968.

Bogunovic, D., Manches, O., Godefroy, E., Yewdall, A., Gallois, A., Salazar, A.M., Marie, I., Levy, D.E., Bhardwaj, N., 2011. TLR4 engagement during TLR3-induced proinflammatory signaling in dendritic cells promotes IL-10-mediated suppression of antitumor immunity. Cancer Res. 71 (16), 5467–5476.

Brand, S., Dambacher, J., Beigel, F., Zitzmann, K., Heeg, M.H., Weiss, T.S., Prüfer, T., Olszak, T., Steib, C.J., Storr, M., Göke, B., Diepolder, H., Bilzer, M., Thasler, W.E., Auernhammer, C.J., 2007. IL-22-mediated liver cell regeneration is abrogated by SOCS-1/3 overexpression in vitro. Am. J. Physiol. Gastrointest. Liver Physiol. 292 (4), G1019–G1028.

Brand, S., Beigel, F., Olszak, T., Zitzmann, K., Eichhorst, S.T., Otte, J.M., Diebold, J., Diepolder, H., Adler, B., Auernhammer, C.J., Göke, B., Dambacher, J., 2005. IL-28A and IL-29 mediate antiproliferative and antiviral signals in intestinal epithelial cells and murine CMV infection increases colonic IL-28A expression. Am. J. Physiol. Gastrointest. Liver Physiol. 289 (5), G960–G968.

Braum, O., Pirzer, H., Fickenscher, H., 2012. Interleukin-26, a highly cationic T-cell cytokine targeting epithelial cells. Antiinflamm. Antiallergy Agents Med. Chem. 11 (3), 221–229.

Brown, N.L., Alvi, S.A., Elder, M.G., Bennett, P.R., Sullivan, M.H., 2000. The regulation of prostaglandin output from term intact fetal membranes by anti-inflammatory cytokines. Immunology 99 (1), 124–133.

Cai, T., Wang, Q., Zhou, Q., Wang, C., Hou, S., Qi, J., Kijlstra, A., Yang, P., 2013. Increased expression of IL-22 is associated with disease activity in Behcet's disease. PLoS One 8 (3), e59009.

Cai, Y., Liu, X., Huang, W., Zhang, K., Liu, X.Y., 2012. Synergistic antitumor effect of TRAIL and IL-24 with complete eradication of hepatoma in the CTGVT-DG strategy. Acta Biochim. Biophys. Sin. (Shanghai) 44 (6), 535–543.

Caligiuri, G., Kaveri, S.V., Nicoletti, A., 2006. IL-20 and atherosclerosis: another brick in the wall. Arterioscler. Thromb. Vasc. Biol. 26 (9), 1929–1930.

Cao, S., Liu, J., Song, L., Ma, X., 2005. The protooncogene c–Maf is an essential transcription factor for IL-10 gene expression in macrophages. J. Immunol. 174 (6), 3484–3492.

Cao, Y., Luetkens, T., Kobold, S., Hildebrandt, Y., Gordic, M., Lajmi, N., Meyer, S., Bartels, K., Zander, A.R., Bokemeyer, C., Kröger, N., Atanackovic, D., 2010. The cytokine/chemokine pattern in the bone marrow environment of multiple myeloma patients. Exp. Hematol. 38 (10), 860–867.

Cassatella, M.A., Meda, L., Bonora, S., Ceska, M., Constantin, G., 1993. Interleukin 10 (IL-10) inhibits the release of proinflammatory cytokines from human polymorphonuclear leukocytes. Evidence for an autocrine role of tumor necrosis factor and IL-1 beta in mediating the production of IL-8 triggered by lipopolysaccharide. J. Exp. Med. 178 (6), 2207–2211.

Castelao, J.E., Bart 3rd, R.D., DiPerna, C.A., Sievers, E.M., Bremner, R.M., 2003. Lung cancer and cyclooxygenase-2. Ann. Thorac. Surg. 76 (4), 1327–1335.

Cervenak, L., Morbidelli, L., Donati, D., Donnini, S., Kambayashi, T., Wilson, J.L., Axelson, H., Castacos-Velez, E., Ljunggren, H.G., Malefyt, R.D., Granger, H.J., Ziche, M., Bejarano, M.T., 2000. Abolished angiogenicity and tumorigenicity of Burkitt lymphoma by interleukin-10. Blood 96 (7), 2568–2573.

Chada, S., Mhashilkar, A.M., Liu, Y., Nishikawa, T., Bocangel, D., Zheng, M., et al., 2006. mda-7 gene transfer sensitizes breast carcinoma cells to chemotherapy, biologic therapies and radiotherapy: correlation with expression of bcl-2 family members. Cancer Gene Ther. 13, 490–502.

Chang, S., Chen, W., Yang, J., Xie, Y., Sheng, W., 2009. Antitumor activity of an adenovirus harboring two therapeutic genes, anti-VEGF ribozyme and human IL-24, in colon cancer. Mol. Med. Rep. 2 (5), 693–700.

Chang, L.L., Wang, S.W., Wu, I.C., Yu, F.J., Su, Y.C., Chen, Y.P., Wu, D.C., Kuo, C.H., Hung, C.H., 2012. Impaired dendritic cell maturation and IL-10 production following H. pylori stimulation in gastric cancer patients. Appl. Microbiol. Biotechnol. 96 (1), 211–220.

Charbonneau, B., Maurer, M.J., Ansell, S.M., Slager, S.L., Fredericksen, Z.S., Ziesmer, S.C., Macon, W.R., Habermann, T.M., Witzig, T.E., Link, B.K., Cerhan, J.R., Novak, A.J., 2012. Pretreatment circulating serum cytokines associated with follicular and diffuse large B-cell lymphoma: a clinic-based case–control study. Cytokine 60 (3), 882–889.

Chen, C., Shen, Y., Qu, Q.X., Chen, X.Q., Zhang, X.G., Huang, J.A., 2013. Induced expression of B7-H3 on the lung cancer cells and macrophages suppresses T-cell mediating anti-tumor immune response. Exp. Cell Res. 319 (1), 96–102.

Chen, C.J., Sung, W.W., Su, T.C., Chen, M.K., Wu, P.R., Yeh, K.T., Ko, J.L., Lee, H., 2013. High expression of interleukin 10 might predict poor prognosis in early stage oral squamous cell carcinoma patients. Clin. Chim. Acta 415, 25–30.

Chen, W.Y., Cheng, B.C., Jiang, M.J., Hsieh, M.Y., Chang, M.S., 2006. IL-20 is expressed in atherosclerosis plaques and promotes atherosclerosis in apolipoprotein E-deficient mice. Arterioscler. Thromb. Vasc. Biol. 26 (9), 2090–2095.

Chen, W.Y., Chang, M.S., 2009. IL-20 is regulated by hypoxia-inducible factor and up-regulated after experimental ischemic stroke. J. Immunol. 182 (8), 5003–5012.

Chen, Z.F., Xu, Q., Ding, J.B., Zhang, Y., Du, R., Ding, Y., 2012. CD4+CD25+Foxp3+ Treg and TGF-beta play important roles in pathogenesis of Uygur cervical carcinoma. Eur. J. Gynaecol. Oncol. 33 (5), 502–507.

Chernoff, A.E., Granowitz, E.V., Shapiro, L., Vannier, E., Lonnemann, G., Angel, J.B., Kennedy, J.S., Rabson, A.R., Wolff, S.M., Dinarello, C.A., 1995. A randomized, controlled trial of IL-10 in humans. Inhibition of inflammatory cytokine production and immune responses. J. Immunol. 154 (10), 5492–5499.

Choi, S.J., Park, J.Y., Lee, Y.K., Choi, H.I., Lee, Y.S., Koh, C.M., Chung, I.B., 2002. Effects of cytokines on VEGF expression and secretion by human first trimester trophoblast cell line. Am. J. Reprod. Immunol. 48 (2), 70–76.

Chou, T.C., Fu, E., Shen, E.C., 2003. Chitosan inhibits prostaglandin E2 formation and cyclooxygenase-2 induction in lipopolysaccharide-treated RAW 264.7 macrophages. Biochem. Biophys. Res. Commun. 308 (2), 403–407.

Chung, E.Y., Liu, J., Homma, Y., Zhang, Y., Brendolan, A., Saggese, M., Han, J., Silverstein, R., Selleri, L., Ma, X., 2007. Interleukin-10 expression in macrophages during phagocytosis of apoptotic cells is mediated by homeodomain proteins Pbx1 and Prep-1. Immunity 27 (6), 952–964.

Ciccia, F., Guggino, G., Rizzo, A., Ferrante, A., Raimondo, S., Giardina, A., Dieli, F., Campisi, G., Alessandro, R., Triolo, G., 2012. Potential involvement of IL-22 and IL-22-producing cells in the inflamed salivary glands of patients with Sjogren's syndrome. Ann. Rheum. Dis. 71 (2), 295–301.

Clarke, C.J., Hales, A., Hunt, A., Foxwell, B.M., 1998. IL-10-mediated suppression of TNF-alpha production is independent of its ability to inhibit NF kappa B activity. Eur. J. Immunol. 28 (5), 1719–1726.

Coccia, E.M., Severa, M., Giacomini, E., Monneron, D., Remoli, M.E., Julkunen, I., Cella, M., Lande, R., Uzé, G., 2004. Viral infection and toll-like receptor agonists induce a differential expression of type I and lambda interferons in human plasmacytoid and monocyte-derived dendritic cells. Eur. J. Immunol. 34 (3), 796–805.

Cordes, T., Hoellen, F., Dittmer, C., Salehin, D., Kümmel, S., Friedrich, M., Köster, F., Becker, S., Diedrich, K., Thill, M., 2012. Correlation of prostaglandin metabolizing enzymes and serum PGE2 levels with vitamin D receptor and serum 25(OH)2D3 levels in breast and ovarian cancer. Anticancer Res. 32 (1), 351–357.

Corinti, S., Albanesi, C., la Sala, A., Pastore, S., Girolomoni, G., 2001. Regulatory activity of autocrine IL-10 on dendritic cell functions. J. Immunol. 166 (7), 4312–4318.

Cortes, J., Kurzrock, R., 1997. Interleukin-10 in non-Hodgkin's lymphoma. Leuk. Lymphoma 26 (3–4), 21–29.

Cortes, J.E., Talpaz, M., Cabanillas, F., Seymour, J.F., Kurzrock, R., 1995. Serum levels of interleukin-10 in patients with diffuse large cell lymphoma: lack of correlation with prognosis. Blood 85 (9), 2516–2520.

Corvaisier, M., Delneste, Y., Jeanvoine, H., Preisser, L., Blanchard, S., Garo, E., Hoppe, E., Barré, B., Audran, M., Bouvard, B., Saint-André, J.P., Jeannin, P., 2012. IL-26 is overexpressed in rheumatoid arthritis and induces proinflammatory cytokine production and Th17 cell generation. PLoS Biol. 10 (9), e1001395.

Cottrez, F., Groux, H., 2001. Regulation of TGF-beta response during T cell activation is modulated by IL-10. J. Immunol. 167 (2), 773–778.

Crispen, P.L., Sheinin, Y., Roth, T.J., Lohse, C.M., Kuntz, S.M., Frigola, X., Thompson, R.H., Boorjian, S.A., Dong, H., Leibovich, B.C., Blute, M.L., Kwon, E.D., 2008. Tumor cell and tumor vasculature expression of B7-H3 predict survival in clear cell renal cell carcinoma. Clin. Cancer Res. 14 (16), 5150–5157.

Csyka, B., Nemeth, Z.H., Virag, L., Gergely, P., Leibovich, S.J., Pacher, P., Sun, C.X., Blackburn, M.R., Vizi, E.S., Deitch, E.A., Hasky, G., 2007. A2A adenosine receptors and C/EBPbeta are crucially required for IL-10 production by macrophages exposed to Escherichia coli. Blood 110 (7), 2685–2695.

Cuneo, A.A., Herrick, D., Autieri, M.V., 2010. Il-19 reduces VSMC activation by regulation of mRNA regulatory factor HuR and reduction of mRNA stability. J. Mol. Cell. Cardiol. 49 (4), 647–654.

da Rocha Jr, L.F., Duarte, Â.L., Dantas, A.T., Mariz, H.A., Pitta Ida, R., Galdino, S.L., Pitta, M.G., 2012. Increased serum interleukin 22 in patients with rheumatoid arthritis and correlation with disease activity. J. Rheumatol. 39 (7), 1320–1325.

Dace, D.S., Khan, A.A., Kelly, J., Apte, R.S., 2008. Interleukin-10 promotes pathological angiogenesis by regulating macrophage response to hypoxia during development. PLoS One 3 (10), e3381.

Dai, J., Megjugorac, N.J., Gallagher, G.E., Yu, R.Y., Gallagher, G., 2009. IFN-lambda1 (IL-29) inhibits GATA3 expression and suppresses Th2 responses in human naive and memory T cells. Blood 113 (23), 5829–5838.

Dambacher, J., Beigel, F., Zitzmann, K., De Toni, E.N., Göke, B., Diepolder, H.M., Auernhammer, C.J., Brand, S., 2009. The role of the novel Th17 cytokine IL-26 in intestinal inflammation. Gut 58 (9), 1207–1217.

Dash, R., Azab, B., Quinn, B.A., Shen, X., Wang, X.Y., Das, S.K., Rahmani, M., Wei, J., Hedvat, M., Dent, P., Dmitriev, I.P., Curiel, D.T., Grant, S., Wu, B., Stebbins, J.L., Pellecchia, M., Reed, J.C., Sarkar, D., Fisher, P.B., 2011. Apogossypol derivative BI-97C1 (Sabutoclax) targeting Mcl-1 sensitizes prostate cancer cells to mda-7/IL-24-mediated toxicity. Proc. Natl. Acad. Sci. U S A 108 (21), 8785–8790.

Dash, R., Richards, J.E., Su, Z.Z., Bhutia, S.K., Azab, B., Rahmani, M., Dasmahapatra, G., Yacoub, A., Dent, P., Dmitriev, I.P., Curiel, D.T., Grant, S., Pellecchia, M., Reed, J.C., Sarkar, D., Fisher, P.B., 2010. Mechanism by which Mcl-1 regulates cancer-specific apoptosis triggered by mda-7/IL-24, an IL-10-related cytokine. Cancer Res. 70 (12), 5034–5045.

Day, C.L., Kaufmann, D.E., Kiepiela, P., Brown, J.A., Moodley, E.S., Reddy, S., Mackey, E.W., Miller, J.D., Leslie, A.J., DePierres, C., Mncube, Z., Duraiswamy, J., Zhu, B., Eichbaum, Q., Altfeld, M., Wherry, E.J., Coovadia, H.M., Goulder, P.J., Klenerman, P., Ahmed, R., Freeman, G.J., Walker, B.D., 2006. PD-1 expression on HIV-specific T cells is associated with T-cell exhaustion and disease progression. Nature 443 (7109), 350–354.

de Waal Malefyt, R., Abrams, J., Bennett, B., Figdor, C.G., de Vries, J.E., 1991. Interleukin 10(IL-10) inhibits cytokine synthesis by human monocytes: an autoregulatory role of IL-10 produced by monocytes. J. Exp. Med. 174 (5), 1209–1220.

Decker, T., Meinke, A., 1997. Jaks, stats and the immune system. Immunobiology 198 (1–3), 99–111.

Degenhardt, K., Mathew, R., Beaudoin, B., Bray, K., Anderson, D., Chen, G., Mukherjee, C., Shi, Y., Gélinas, C., Fan, Y., Nelson, D.A., Jin, S., White, E., 2006. Autophagy promotes tumor cell survival and restricts necrosis, inflammation, and tumorigenesis. Cancer Cell 10 (1), 51–64.

Denys, A., Udalova, I.A., Smith, C., Williams, L.M., Ciesielski, C.J., Campbell, J., Andrews, C., Kwaitkowski, D., Foxwell, B.M., 2002. Evidence for a dual mechanism for IL-10 suppression of TNF-alpha production that does not involve inhibition of p38 mitogen-activated protein kinase or NF-kappa B in primary human macrophages. J. Immunol. 168 (10), 4837–4845.

Di Carlo, E., Coletti, A., Modesti, A., Giovarelli, M., Forni, G., Musiani, P., 1998. Local release of interleukin-10 by transfected mouse adenocarcinoma cells exhibits pro- and anti-inflammatory activity and results in a delayed tumor rejection. Eur. Cytokine Netw. 9 (1), 61–68.

Djavaheri-Mergny, M., Maiuri, M.C., Kroemer, G., 2010. Cross talk between apoptosis and autophagy by caspase-mediated cleavage of Beclin 1. Oncogene 29 (12), 1717–1719.

Dohadwala, M., Batra, R.K., Luo, J., Lin, Y., Krysan, K., Pold, M., Sharma, S., Dubinett, S.M., 2002. Autocrine/paracrine prostaglandin E2 production by non-small cell lung cancer cells regulates matrix metalloproteinase-2 and CD44 in cyclooxygenase-2-dependent invasion. J. Biol. Chem. 277 (52), 50828–50833.

Domanska, U.M., Kruizinga, R.C., Nagengast, W.B., Timmer-Bosscha, H., Huls, G., de Vries, E.G., Walenkamp, A.M., 2013. A review on CXCR4/CXCL12 axis in oncology: no place to hide. Eur. J. Cancer 49 (1), 219–230.

Dong, C.Y., Zhang, F., Duan, Y.J., Yang, B.X., Lin, Y.M., Ma, X.T., 2008. mda-7/IL-24 inhibits the proliferation of hematopoietic malignancies in vitro and in vivo. Exp. Hematol. 36 (8), 938–946.

Donnelly, R.P., Kotenko, S.V., 2010. Interferon-lambda: a new addition to an old family. J. Interferon. Cytokine Res. 30 (8), 555–564.

Donnelly, R.P., Sheikh, F., Dickensheets, H., Savan, R., Young, H.A., Walter, M.R., 2010. Interleukin-26: an IL-10-related cytokine produced by Th17 cells. Cytokine Growth Factor Rev. 21 (5), 393–401.

Doyle, S.E., Schreckhise, H., Khuu-Duong, K., Henderson, K., Rosler, R., Storey, H., Yao, L., Liu, H., Barahmand-pour, F., Sivakumar, P., Chan, C., Birks, C., Foster, D., Clegg, C.H., Wietzke-Braun, P., Mihm, S., Klucher, K.M., 2006. Interleukin-29 uses a type 1 interferon-like program to promote antiviral responses in human hepatocytes. Hepatology 44 (4), 896–906.

Du, H.W., Liu, N., Wu, Z.H., Chen, R.H., Weng, J.S., Huang, H.P., 2009. Inhibiting effects of interleukin-10 on expression of E-selectin and L-selectin in cerebral ischemia–reperfusion: experiment with rats. Zhonghua Yixue Zazhi 89 (1), 59–62. [Article in Chinese].

Duhen, T., Geiger, R., Jarrossay, D., Lanzavecchia, A., Sallusto, F., 2009. Production of interleukin 22 but not interleukin 17 by a subset of human skin-homing memory T cells. Nat. Immunol. 10 (8), 857–863.

Dummer, W., Bastian, B.C., Ernst, N., Schanzle, C., Schwaaf, A., Brocker, E.B., 1996. Interleukin-10 production in malignant melanoma: preferential detection of IL-10-secreting tumor cells in metastatic lesions. Int. J. Cancer 66 (5), 607–610.

Dumoutier, L., Van Roost, E., Colau, D., Renauld, J.C., 2000. Human interleukin-10-related T cell-derived inducible factor: molecular cloning and functional characterization as an hepatocyte-stimulating factor. Proc. Natl. Acad. Sci. USA 97 (18), 10144–10149.

Dumoutier, L., Louahed, J., Renauld, J.C., 2000. Cloning and characterization of IL-10-related T cell-derived inducible factor (IL-TIF), a novel cytokine structurally related to IL-10 and inducible by IL-9. J. Immunol. 164 (4), 1814–1819.

Dumoutier, L., Tounsi, A., Michiels, T., Sommereyns, C., Kotenko, S.V., Renauld, J.C., 2004. Role of the interleukin (IL)-28 receptor tyrosine residues for antiviral and antiproliferative activity of IL-29/interferon-lambda 1: similarities with type I interferon signaling. J. Biol. Chem. 279 (31), 32269–32274.

Dunn, G.P., Koebel, C.M., Schreiber, R.D., 2006. Interferons, immunity, and cancer immunoediting. Nat. Rev. Immunol. 6 (11), 836–848.

Dwivedi, S., Goel, A., Natu, S.M., Mandhani, A., Khattri, S., Pant, K.K., 2011. Diagnostic and prognostic significance of prostate specific antigen and serum interleukin 18 and 10 in patients with locally advanced prostate cancer: a prospective study. Asian Pac. J. Cancer Prev. 12 (7), 1843–1848.

Ekmekcioglu, S., Ellerhorst, J., Mhashilkar, A.M., Sahin, A.A., Read, C.M., Prieto, V.G., Chada, S., Grimm, E.A., 2001. Down-regulated melanoma differentiation associated gene (mda-7) expression in human melanomas. Int. J. Cancer 94 (1), 54–59.

Ellerhorst, J.A., Prieto, V.G., Ekmekcioglu, S., Broemeling, L., Yekell, S., Chada, S., et al., 2002. Loss of MDA-7 expression with progression of melanoma. J. Clin. Oncol. 20, 1069–1074.

Emdad, L., Lebedeva, I.V., Su, Z.Z., Sarkar, D., Dent, P., Curiel, D.T., Fisher, P.B., 2007. Melanoma differentiation associated gene-7/interleukin-24 reverses multidrug resistance in human colorectal cancer cells. Mol. Cancer Ther. 6 (11), 2985–2994.

Emdad, L., Sarkar, D., Lebedeva, I.V., Su, Z.Z., Gupta, P., Mahasreshti, P.J., Dent, P., Curiel, D.T., Fisher, P.B., 2006. Ionizing radiation enhances adenoviral vector expressing mda-7/IL-24-mediated apoptosis in human ovarian cancer. J. Cell. Physiol. 208 (2), 298–306.

Emdad, L., Lebedeva, I.V., Su, Z.Z., Gupta, P., Sarkar, D., Settleman, J., Fisher, P.B., 2007. Combinatorial treatment of non-small-cell lung cancers with gefitinib and Ad.mda-7 enhances apoptosis-induction and reverses resistance to a single therapy. J. Cell. Physiol. 210 (2), 549–559.

Emmerich, J., Mumm, J.B., Chan, I.H., LaFace, D., Truong, H., McClanahan, T., Gorman, D.M., Oft, M., 2012. IL-10 directly activates and expands tumor-resident CD8(+) T cells without de novo infiltration from secondary lymphoid organs. Cancer Res. 72 (14), 3570–3581.

Endo, T., Ogushi, F., Kawano, T., Sone, S., 1998. Comparison of the regulations by Th2-type cytokines of the arachidonic-acid metabolic pathway in human alveolar macrophages and monocytes. Am. J. Respir. Cell Mol. Biol. 19 (2), 300–307.

England, R.N., Autieri, M.V., 2012. Anti-inflammatory effects of interleukin-19 in vascular disease. Int. J. Inflam. 2012, 253583.

Enk, A.H., Katz, S.I., 1992. Identification and induction of keratinocyte-derived IL-10. J. Immunol. 149 (1), 92–95.

Eulitt, P.J., Park, M.A., Hossein, H., Cruikshanks, N., Yang, C., Dmitriev, I.P., Yacoub, A., Curiel, D.T., Fisher, P.B., Dent, P., 2010. Enhancing mda-7/IL-24 therapy in renal carcinoma cells by inhibiting multiple protective signaling pathways using sorafenib and by Ad.5/3 gene delivery. Cancer Biol. Ther. 10 (12), 1290–1305.

Eun, Y.G., Shin, I.H., Lee, Y.C., Shin, S.Y., Kim, S.K., Chung, J.H., Kwon, K.H., 2013. Interleukin 22 polymorphisms and papillary thyroid cancer. J. Endocrinol. Invest. 36 (8), 584–587.

Eyerich, S., Eyerich, K., Pennino, D., Carbone, T., Nasorri, F., Pallotta, S., Cianfarani, F., Odorisio, T., Traidl-Hoffmann, C., Behrendt, H., Durham, S.R., Schmidt-Weber, C.B., Cavani, A., 2009. Th22 cells represent a distinct human T cell subset involved in epidermal immunity and remodeling. J. Clin. Invest. 119 (12), 3573–3585.

Fayad, L., Keating, M.J., Reuben, J.M., O'Brien, S., Lee, B.N., Lerner, S., Kurzrock, R., 2001. Interleukin-6 and interleukin-10 levels in chronic lymphocytic leukemia: correlation with phenotypic characteristics and outcome. Blood 97 (1), 256–263.

Feng, D., Kong, X., Weng, H., Park, O., Wang, H., Dooley, S., Gershwin, M.E., Gao, B., 2012. Interleukin-22 promotes proliferation of liver stem/progenitor cells in mice and patients with chronic hepatitis B virus infection. Gastroenterology 143 (1), 188–198. e7.

Ferrajoli, A., Faderl, S., Ravandi, F., Estrov, Z., 2006. The JAK–STAT pathway: a therapeutic target in hematological malignancies. Curr. Cancer Drug. Targets 6 (8), 671–679.

Fickenscher, H., Hor, S., Kupers, H., Knappe, A., Wittmann, S., Sticht, H., 2002. The interleukin-10 family of cytokines. Trends Immunol. 23 (2), 89–96.

Fiorentino, D.F., Bond, M.W., Mosmann, T.R., 1989. Two types of mouse T helper cell. IV. Th2 clones secrete a factor that inhibits cytokine production by Th1 clones. J. Exp. Med. 170, 2081–2095.

Fisher, P.B., Sarkar, D., Lebedeva, I.V., Emdad, L., Gupta, P., Sauane, M., Su, Z.Z., Grant, S., Dent, P., Curiel, D.T., Senzer, N., Nemunaitis, J., 2007. Melanoma differentiation associated gene-7/interleukin-24 (mda-7/IL-24): novel gene therapeutic for metastatic melanoma. Toxicol. Appl. Pharmacol. 224 (3), 300–307.

Fisher, P.B., 2005. Is mda-7/IL-24 a "magic bullet" for cancer? Cancer Res. 65 (22), 10128–10138.

Fleming, S.B., Haig, D.M., Nettleton, P., Reid, H.W., McCaughan, C.A., Wise, L.M., Mercer, A., 2000. Sequence and functional analysis of a homolog of interleukin-10 encoded by the parapox virus orf virus. Virus Genes 21 (1–2), 85–95.

Fleming, S.B., McCaughan, C.A., Andrews, A.E., Nash, A.D., Mercer, A.A., 1997. A homolog of interleukin-10 is encoded by the poxvirus orf virus. J. Virol. 71 (6), 4857–4861.

Fonseca-Camarillo, G., Furuzawa-Carballeda, J., Llorente, L., Yamamoto-Furusho, J.K., 2013. IL-10– and IL-20–expressing epithelial and inflammatory cells are increased in patients with ulcerative colitis. J. Clin. Immunol. 33 (3), 640–648.

Fortis, C., Foppoli, M., Gianotti, L., Galli, L., Citterio, G., Consogno, G., Gentilini, O., Braga, M., 1996. Increased interleukin-10 serum levels in patients with solid tumours. Cancer Lett. 104 (1), 1–5.

Francisco, L.M., Sage, P.T., Sharpe, A.H., 2010. The PD-1 pathway in tolerance and autoimmunity. Immunol. Rev. 236, 219–242.

Frewer, N.C., Ye, L., Sun, P.H., Owen, S., Ji, K., Frewer, K.A., Hargest, R., Jiang, W.G., 2013. Potential implication of IL-24 in lymphangiogenesis of human breast cancer. Int. J. Mol. Med. 31 (5), 1097–1104.

Fujimura, T., Ring, S., Umansky, V., Mahnke, K., Enk, A.H., 2012. Regulatory T cells stimulate B7-H1 expression in myeloid-derived suppressor cells in ret melanomas. J. Invest. Dermatol. 132 (4), 1239–1246.

Gaiolla, R.D., Domingues, M.A., Niero–Melo, L., de Oliveira, D.E., 2011. Serum levels of interleukins 6, 10, and 13 before and after treatment of classic Hodgkin lymphoma. Arch. Pathol. Lab. Med. 135 (4), 483–489.

Gallagher, G., 2010. Interleukin-19: multiple roles in immune regulation and disease. Cytokine Growth Factor Rev. 21 (5), 345–352.

Gallagher, G., Dickensheets, H., Eskdale, J., Izotova, L.S., Mirochnitchenko, O.V., Peat, J.D., Vazquez, N., Pestka, S., Donnelly, R.P., Kotenko, S.V., 2000. Cloning, expression and initial characterization of interleukin-19 (IL-19), a novel homologue of human interleukin-10 (IL-10). Genes Immun. 1 (7), 442–450.

Gangemi, S., Allegra, A., Alonci, A., Pace, E., Ferraro, M., Cannavò, A., Penna, G., Saitta, S., Gerace, D., Musolino, C., 2013. Interleukin 22 is increased and correlated with CD38 expression in patients with B-chronic lymphocytic leukemia. Blood Cells Mol. Dis. 50 (1), 39–40.

Garban, H.J., Bonavida, B., May 1999. Nitric oxide sensitizes ovarian tumor cells to Fas-induced apoptosis. Gynecol. Oncol. 73 (2), 257–264.

Garcia-Hernandez, M.L., Hernandez-Pando, R., Gariglio, P., Berumen, J., 2002. Interleukin-10 promotes B16-melanoma growth by inhibition of macrophage functions and induction of tumour and vascular cell proliferation. Immunology 105 (2), 231–243.

Geboes, L., Dumoutier, L., Kelchtermans, H., Schurgers, E., Mitera, T., Renauld, J.C., Matthys, P., 2009. Proinflammatory role of the Th17 cytokine interleukin-22 in collagen-induced arthritis in C57BL/6 mice. Arthritis Rheum. 60 (2), 390–395.

Gelebart, P., Zak, Z., Dien-Bard, J., Anand, M., Lai, R., 2011. Interleukin 22 signaling promotes cell growth in mantle cell lymphoma. Transl. Oncol. 4 (1), 9–19.

Geng, L., Deng, J., Jiang, G., Song, P., Wang, Z., Jiang, Z., Zhang, M., Zheng, S., 2011. B7-H1 up-regulated expression in human hepatocellular carcinoma tissue: correlation with tumor interleukin-10 levels. Hepatogastroenterology 58 (107–108), 960–964.

Geng, L., Huang, D., Liu, J., Qian, Y., Deng, J., Li, D., Hu, Z., Zhang, J., Jiang, G., Zheng, S., 2008. B7-H1 up-regulated expression in human pancreatic carcinoma tissue associates with tumor progression. J. Cancer Res. Clin. Oncol. 134 (9), 1021–1027.

Gerard, C.M., Bruyns, C., Delvaux, A., Baudson, N., Dargent, J.L., Goldman, M., Velu, T., 1996. Loss of tumorigenicity and increased immunogenicity induced by interleukin-10 gene transfer in B16 melanoma cells. Hum. Gene Ther. 7 (1), 23–31.

Giovarelli, M., Musiani, P., Modesti, A., Dellabona, P., Casorati, G., Allione, A., Consalvo, M., Cavallo, F., di Pierro, F., De Giovanni, C., et al., 1995. Local release of IL-10 by transfected mouse mammary adenocarcinoma cells does not suppress but enhances antitumor reaction and elicits a strong cytotoxic lymphocyte and antibody-dependent immune memory. J. Immunol. 155 (6), 3112–3123.

Goff, W.L., Johnson, W.C., Cluff, C.W., 1998. *Babesia bovis* immunity. In vitro and in vivo evidence for IL-10 regulation of IFN-gamma and iNOS. Ann. N Y Acad. Sci. 849, 161–180.

Gopalan, B., Litvak, A., Sharma, S., Mhashilkar, A.M., Chada, S., Ramesh, R., 2005. Activation of the Fas-FasL signaling pathway by MDA-7/IL-24 kills human ovarian cancer cells. Cancer Res. 65, 3017–3024.

Gopalan, B., Shanker, M., Chada, S., Ramesh, R., 2007. MDA-7/IL-24 suppresses human ovarian carcinoma growth in vitro and in vivo. Mol. Cancer 6, 11.

Goris, A., Marrosu, M.G., Vandenbroeck, K., 2001. Novel polymorphisms in the IL-10 related AK155 gene (chromosome 12q15). Genes Immun. 2 (5), 284–286.

Groux, H., Cottrez, F., Rouleau, M., Mauze, S., Antonenko, S., Hurst, S., McNeil, T., Bigler, M., Roncarolo, M.G., Coffman, R.L., 1999. A transgenic model to analyze the immunoregulatory role of IL-10 secreted by antigen-presenting cells. J. Immunol. 162 (3), 1723–1729.

Guney, N., Soydinc, H.O., Basaran, M., Bavbek, S., Derin, D., Camlica, H., Yasasever, V., Topuz, E., 2009. Serum levels of interleukin-6 and interleukin-10 in Turkish patients with aggressive non–Hodgkin's lymphoma. Asian Pac. J. Cancer Prev. 10 (4), 669–674.

Gupta, P., Su, Z.Z., Lebedeva, I.V., Sarkar, D., Sauane, M., Emdad, L., Bachelor, M.A., Grant, S., Curiel, D.T., Dent, P., Fisher, P.B., 2006. mda-7/IL-24: Multifunctional cancer-specific apoptosis-inducing cytokine. Pharmacol. Ther. 111, 596–628.

Gupta, P., Emdad, L., Lebedeva, I.V., Sarkar, D., Dent, P., Curiel, D.T., Settleman, J., Fisher, P.B., 2008. Targeted combinatorial therapy of non-small cell lung carcinoma using a GST-fusion protein of full-length or truncated MDA-7/IL-24 with Tarceva. J. Cell. Physiol. 215 (3), 827–836.

Gupta, M., Han, J.J., Stenson, M., Maurer, M., Wellik, L., Hu, G., Ziesmer, S., Dogan, A., Witzig, T.E., 2012. Elevated serum IL-10 levels in diffuse large B-cell lymphoma: a mechanism of aberrant JAK2 activation. Blood 119 (12), 2844–2853.

Hör, S., Pirzer, H., Dumoutier, L., Bauer, F., Wittmann, S., Sticht, H., Renauld, J.C., de Waal Malefyt, R., Fickenscher, H., 2004. The T-cell lymphokine, interleukin-26, targets epithelial cells through the interleukin-20 receptor 1 and interleukin-10 receptor 2 chains. J. Biol. Chem. 279, 33343–33351.

Hagenbaugh, A., Sharma, S., Dubinett, S.M., Wei, S.H., Aranda, R., Cheroutre, H., Fowell, D.J., Binder, S., Tsao, B., Locksley, R.M., Moore, K.W., Kronenberg, M., 1997. Altered immune responses in interleukin 10 transgenic mice. J. Exp. Med. 185 (12), 2101–2110.

Hamanishi, J., Mandai, M., Iwasaki, M., Okazaki, T., Tanaka, Y., Yamaguchi, K., Higuchi, T., Yagi, H., Takakura, K., Minato, N., Honjo, T., Fujii, S., 2007. Programmed cell death 1 ligand 1 and tumor-infiltrating CD8+ T lymphocytes are prognostic factors of human ovarian cancer. Proc. Natl. Acad. Sci. U S A 104 (9), 3360–3365.

Hamed, H.A.,Yacoub, A., Park, M.A., Eulitt, P., Sarkar, D., Dimitrie, I.P., Chen, C.S., Grant, S., Curiel, D.T., Fisher, P.B., Dent, P., 2010. OSU-03012 enhances Ad.7-induced GBM cell killing via ER stress and autophagy and by decreasing expression of mitochondrial protective proteins. Cancer Biol.Ther. 9 (7), 526–536.

Hamed, H.A.,Yacoub, A., Park, M.A., Eulitt, P.J., Dash, R., Sarkar, D., Dmitriev, I.P., Lesniak, M.S., Shah, K., Grant, S., Curiel, D.T., Fisher, P.B., Dent, P., 2010. Inhibition of multiple protective signaling pathways and Ad.5/3 delivery enhances mda-7/IL-24 therapy of malignant glioma. Mol.Ther. 18 (6), 1130–1142.

Hamed, H.A., Das, S.K., Sokhi, U.K., Park, M.A., Cruickshanks, N., Archer, K., Ogretmen, B., Grant, S., Sarkar, D., Fisher, P.B., Dent, P., 2013 Aug 28. Combining histone deacety-lase inhibitors with MDA-7/IL-24 enhances killing of renal carcinoma cells. Cancer Biol.Ther. 14 (11). [Epub ahead of print].

Hamed, H.A.,Yacoub, A., Park, M.A., Archer, K., Das, S.K., Sarkar, D., Grant, S., Fisher, P.B., Dent, P., 2013. Histone deacetylase inhibitors interact with melanoma differentiation associated-7/interleukin-24 to kill primary human glioblastoma cells. Mol. Pharmacol. 84 (2), 171–181.

Hamzavi, M.,Tadbir, A.A., Rezvani, G., Ashraf, M.J., Fattahi, M.J., Khademi, B., Sardari, Y., Jeirudi, N., 2013.Tissue expression, serum and salivary levels of IL-10 in patients with head and neck squamous cell carcinoma. Asian Pac. J. Cancer Prev. 14 (3), 1681–1685.

Han,Y., Miao, J., Sheng, W.,Wang, X., Jing,Y., Shan,Y., Liu,T., Bao,W.,Yang, J., 2009. Inter-leukin 24 inhibits growth and induces apoptosis of osteosarcoma cells MG-63 in vitro and in vivo. Shengwu Gongcheng Xuebao 25 (10), 1538–1545. [Article in Chinese].

Hanna, N., Bonifacio, L., Weinberger, B., Reddy, P., Murphy, S., Romero, R., Sharma, S., 2006. Evidence for interleukin-10-mediated inhibition of cyclo-oxygenase-2 expression and prostaglandin production in preterm human placenta. Am. J. Reprod. Immunol. 55 (1), 19–27.

Hao, J.Q.,Aug 25, 2013.Targeting interleukin-22 in psoriasis. Inflammation. 37 (1), 94–99.

Harizi, H., Juzan, M., Pitard, V., Moreau, J.F., Gualde, N., 2002. Cyclooxygenase-2-issued prostaglandin e(2) enhances the production of endogenous IL-10, which down-regu-lates dendritic cell functions. J. Immunol. 168 (5), 2255–2263.

Hart, P.H., Hunt, E.K., Bonder, C.S., Watson, C.J., Finlay-Jones, J.J., 1996. Regulation of surface and soluble TNF receptor expression on human monocytes and synovial fluid macrophages by IL-4 and IL-10. J. Immunol. 157 (8), 3672–3680.

Hatanaka, H.,Abe,Y., Naruke, M.,Tokunaga,T., Oshika,Y., Kawakami,T., Osada, H., Nagata, J., Kamochi, J.,Tsuchida,T., Kijima, H.,Yamazaki, H., Inoue, H., Ueyama,Y., Nakamura, M., 2001. Significant correlation between interleukin 10 expression and vascularization through angiopoietin/TIE2 networks in non-small cell lung cancer. Clin. Cancer Res. 7 (5), 1287–1292.

He, B., Huang, X., Liu, X., Xu, B., Sep 2013. Cancer targeting gene-viro-therapy for pancre-atic cancer using oncolytic adenovirus ZD55-IL-24 in immune-competent mice. Mol. Biol. Rep. 40 (9), 5397–5405.

Hejazi, Sh, Hoseini, S., Javanmard, Sh, Zarkesh, Sh, Khamesipour, A., 2012. Interleukin-10 and transforming growth factor-β in early and late lesions of patients with leishmania major induced cutaneous leishmaniasis. Iran. J. Parasitol. 7 (3), 16–23.

Henke, P.K., DeBrunye, L.A., Strieter, R.M., Bromberg, J.S., Prince, M., Kadell,A.M., Sarkar, M., Londy, F., Wakefield, T.W., 2000.Viral IL-10 gene transfer decreases inflammation and cell adhesion molecule expression in a rat model of venous thrombosis. J. Immunol. 164 (4), 2131–2141.

Herfarth, H., Scholmerich, J., 2002. IL-10 therapy in Crohn's disease: at the crossroads.Treat-ment of Crohn's disease with the anti-inflammatory cytokine interleukin 10. Gut 50 (2), 14–67.

Heuze-Vourc'h, N., Liu, M., Dalwadi, H., Baratelli, F.E., Zhu, L., Goodglick, L., Pold, M., Sharma, S., Ramirez, R.D., Shay, J.W., Minna, J.D., Strieter, R.M., Dubinett, S.M., 2005. IL-20, an anti-angiogenic cytokine that inhibits COX-2 expression. Biochem. Biophys. Res. Commun. 333 (2), 470–475.

Hida, T., Kozaki, K., Muramatsu, H., Masuda, A., Shimizu, S., Mitsudomi, T., Sugiura, T., Ogawa, M., Takahashi, T., 2000. Cyclooxygenase-2 inhibitor induces apoptosis and enhances cytotoxicity of various anticancer agents in non–small cell lung cancer cell lines. Clin. Cancer Res. 6 (5), 2006–2011.

Hofmann, S.R., Rösen-Wolff, A., Tsokos, G.C., Hedrich, C.M., 2012. Biological properties and regulation of IL-10 related cytokines and their contribution to autoimmune disease and tissue injury. Clin. Immunol. 143 (2), 116–127.

Hogendorf, P., Durczyński, A., Kumor, A., Strzelczyk, J., 2012. Prostaglandin E2 (PGE2) in portal blood in patients with pancreatic tumor—a single institution series. J. Invest. Surg. 25 (1), 8–13.

Hosoi, T., Wada, S., Suzuki, S., Okuma, Y., Akira, S., Matsuda, T., Nomura, Y., 2004. Bacterial endotoxin induces IL-20 expression in the glial cells. Brain Res. Mol. Brain Res. 130 (1–2), 23–29.

Hou, W., Wang, X., Ye, L., Zhou, L., Yang, Z.Q., Riedel, E., Ho, W.Z., 2009. Lambda interferon inhibits human immunodeficiency virus type 1 infection of macrophages. J. Virol. 83 (8), 3834–3842.

Hsieh, M.Y., Chen, W.Y., Jiang, M.J., Cheng, B.C., Huang, T.Y., Chang, M.S., 2006. Interleukin-20 promotes angiogenesis in a direct and indirect manner. Genes Immun. 7 (3), 234–242.

Hsing, C.H., Chiu, C.J., Chang, L.Y., Hsu, C.C., Chang, M.S., 2008. IL-19 is involved in the pathogenesis of endotoxic shock. Shock 29 (1), 7–15.

Hsing, C.H., Li, H.H., Hsu, Y.H., Ho, C.L., Chuang, S.S., Lan, K.M., Chang, M.S., 2008. The distribution of interleukin-19 in healthy and neoplastic tissue. Cytokine 44 (2), 221–228.

Hsing, C.H., Cheng, H.C., Hsu, Y.H., Chan, C.H., Yeh, C.H., Li, C.F., Chang, M.S., Feb 1, 2012. Upregulated IL-19 in breast cancer promotes tumor progression and affects clinical outcome. Clin. Cancer Res. 18 (3), 713–725.

Hsing, C.H., Kwok, F.A., Cheng, H.C., Li, C.F., Chang, M.S., Oct 9, 2013. Inhibiting interleukin-19 activity ameliorates esophageal squamous cell carcinoma progression. PLoS One 8 (10), e75254.

Hsing, C.H., Hsu, C.C., Chen, W.Y., Chang, L.Y., Hwang, J.C., Chang, M.S., 2007. Expression of IL-19 correlates with Th2 cytokines in uraemic patients. Nephrol. Dial. Transplant. 22 (8), 2230–2238.

Hsing, C.H., Hsieh, M.Y., Chen, W.Y., Cheung So, E., Cheng, B.C., Chang, M.S., 2006. Induction of interleukin-19 and interleukin-22 after cardiac surgery with cardiopulmonary bypass. Ann. Thorac. Surg. 81 (6), 2196–2201.

Hsu, D.H., de Waal Malefyt, R., Fiorentino, D.F., Dang, M.N., Vieira, P., de Vries, J., Spits, H., Mosmann, T.R., Moore, K.W., 1990. Expression of interleukin-10 activity by Epstein–Barr virus protein BCRF1. Science 250 (4982), 830–832.

Hsu, Y.H., Chang, M.S., 2010. Interleukin-20 antibody is a potential therapeutic agent for experimental arthritis. Arthritis Rheum. 62 (11), 3311–3321.

Hsu, Y.H., Hsieh, P.P., Chang, M.S., 2012a. Interleukin-19 blockade attenuates collagen-induced arthritis in rats. Rheumatology (Oxford) 51 (3), 434–442.

Hsu, Y.H., Hsing, C.H., Li, C.F., Chan, C.H., Chang, M.C., Yan, J.J., Chang, M.S., 2012b. Anti-IL-20 monoclonal antibody suppresses breast cancer progression and bone osteolysis in murine models. J. Immunol. 188 (4), 1981–1991.

Hsu, Y.H., Li, H.H., Hsieh, M.Y., Liu, M.F., Huang, K.Y., Chin, L.S., Chen, P.C., Cheng, H.H., Chang, M.S., 2006. Function of interleukin-20 as a proinflammatory molecule in rheumatoid and experimental arthritis. Arthritis Rheum. 54 (9), 2722–2733.

Hu, X., Paik, P.K., Chen, J., Yarilina, A., Kockeritz, L., Lu, T.T., Woodgett, J.R., Ivashkiv, L.B., 2006. IFN-gamma suppresses IL-10 production and synergizes with TLR2 by regulating GSK3 and CREB/AP-1 proteins. Immunity 24 (5), 563–574.

Huang, D.S., Liu, J.W., Geng, L., Jiang, G.P., Shen, G.L., Yao, W.F., 2009. Role of B7–H1 in pancreatic carcinoma immune evasion. Zhonghua Waike Zazhi 47 (4), 282–285. Article in Chinese.

Huang, S., Xie, K., Bucana, C.D., Ullrich, S.E., Bar-Eli, M., 1996. Interleukin 10 suppresses tumor growth and metastasis of human melanoma cells: potential inhibition of angiogenesis. Clin. Cancer Res. 2 (12), 1969–1979.

Huang, J.H., Ling, C.H., Yang, J.C., Zhao, D.G., Xie, Y.F., Sheng, W.H., 2011. The in vitro and in vivo effects of adenovirus-mediated inhibitor of growth 4 and interleukin-24 co-expression on the radiosensitivity of human lung adenocarcinoma. Zhonghua Jiehe He Huzi Zazhi 34 (6), 413–418. [Article in Chinese].

Huang, Z., Zhang, Z., Jiang, Y., Zhang, D., Chen, J., Dong, L., Zhang, J., 2012. Targeted delivery of oligonucleotides into tumor-associated macrophages for cancer immunotherapy. J. Control. Release 158 (2), 286–292.

Huang, E.Y., Madireddi, M.T., Gopalkrishnan, R.V., Leszczyniecka, M., Su, Z., Lebedeva, I.V., Kang, D., Jiang, H., Lin, J.J., Alexandre, D., Chen, Y., Vozhilla, N., Mei, M.X., Christiansen, K.A., Sivo, F., Goldstein, N.I., Mhashilkar, A.B., Chada, S., Huberman, E., Pestka, S., Fisher, P.B., 2001. Genomic structure, chromosomal localization and expression profile of a novel melanoma differentiation associated (mda-7) gene with cancer specific growth suppressing and apoptosis inducing properties. Oncogene 20 (48), 7051–7063.

Huang, S., Ullrich, S.E., Bar-Eli, M., 1999. Regulation of tumor growth and metastasis by interleukin-10: the melanoma experience. J. Interferon. Cytokine Res. 19 (7), 697–703.

Huang, M., Wang, J., Lee, P., Sharma, S., Mao, J.T., Meissner, H., Uyemura, K., Modlin, R., Wollman, J., Dubinett, S.M., 1995. Human non–small cell lung cancer cells express a type 2 cytokine pattern. Cancer Res. 55 (17), 3847–3853.

Huang, X., Venet, F., Wang, Y.L., Lepape, A., Yuan, Z., Chen, Y., Swan, R., Kherouf, H., Monneret, G., Chung, C.S., Ayala, A., 2009. PD-1 expression by macrophages plays a pathologic role in altering microbial clearance and the innate inflammatory response to sepsis. Proc. Natl. Acad. Sci. U S A 106 (15), 6303–6308.

Huhn, R.D., Radwanski, E., O'Connell, S.M., Sturgill, M.G., Clarke, L., Cody, R.P., Affrime, M.B., Cutler, D.L., 1996. Pharmacokinetics and immunomodulatory properties of intravenously administered recombinant humaninterleukin-10 in healthy volunteers. Blood 87 (2), 699–705.

Huhn, R.D., Radwanski, E., Gallo, J., Affrime, M.B., Sabo, R., Gonyo, G., Monge, A., Cutler, D.L., 1997. Pharmacodynamics of subcutaneous recombinant human interleukin-10 in healthy volunteers. Clin. Pharmacol. Ther. 62 (2), 171–180.

Ikeguchi, M., Hatada, T., Yamamoto, M., Miyake, T., Matsunaga, T., Fukumoto, Y., Yamada, Y., Fukuda, K., Saito, H., Tatebe, S., 2009. Serum interleukin-6 and -10 levels in patients with gastric cancer. Gastric Cancer 12 (2), 95–100.

Inagaki-Ohara, K., Kondo, T., Ito, M., Yoshimura, A., 2013. SOCS, inflammation, and cancer. JAKSTAT 2 (3), e24053.

Inoue, S., Hartman, A., Branch, C.D., Bucana, C.D., Bekele, B.N., Stephens, L.C., Chada, S., Ramesh, R., 2007. mda-7 In combination with bevacizumab treatment produces a synergistic and complete inhibitory effect on lung tumor xenograft. Mol. Ther. 15 (2), 287–294.

Inoue,Y., Otsuka,T., Niiro, H., Nagano, S.,Arinobu,Y., Ogami, E.,Akahoshi, M., Miyake, K., Ninomiya, I., Shimizu, S., Nakashima, H., Harada, M., 2004. Novel regulatory mechanisms of CD40-induced prostanoid synthesis by IL-4 and IL-10 in human monocytes. J. Immunol. 172 (4), 2147–2154.

Ivanov, I.I., McKenzie, B.S., Zhou, L.,Tadokoro, C.E., Lepelley,A., Lafaille,J.J., Cua, D.J., Littman, D.R., 2006.The orphan nuclear receptor RORgammat directs the differentiation program of proinflammatory IL-17+ T helper cells. Cell 126 (6), 1121–1133.

Jacobs, F., Chaussabel, D.,Truyens, C., Leclerq,V., Carlier,Y., Goldman, M.,Vray, B., 1998. IL-10 up-regulates nitric oxide (NO) synthesis by lipopolysaccharide (LPS)-activated macrophages: improved control of *Trypanosoma cruzi* infection. Clin. Exp. Immunol. 113 (1), 59–64.

Jang,J.W., Oh, B.S., Kwon,J.H.,You, C.R., Chung, K.W., Kay, C.S.,Jung, H.S., 2012. Serum interleukin-6 and C-reactive protein as a prognostic indicator in hepatocellular carcinoma. Cytokine 60 (3), 686–693.

Jenkins, J.K., Malyak, M., Arend, W.P., 1994. The effects of interleukin-10 on interleukin-1 receptor antagonist and interleukin-1 beta production in human monocytes and neutrophils. Lymphokine Cytokine Res. 13 (1), 47–54.

Jiang, H., Fisher, P.B., 1993. Use of a sensitive and efficient subtraction hybridization protocol for the identification of genes differentially regulated during the induction of differentiation in human melanoma cells. Mol. Cell. Differ. 1, 285–299.

Jiang, H., Su, Z.Z., Lin, J.J., Goldstein, N.I.,Young, C.S., Fisher, P.B., Aug 20, 1996. The melanoma differentiation associated gene mda-7 suppresses cancer cell growth. Proc. Natl.Acad. Sci. U S A 93 (17), 9160–9165.

Jiang, R.,Wang, H., Deng, L., Hou,J., Shi, R.,Yao, M.,Wang, X.,Yu, L., Sun, B., 2013. IL-22 is related to development of human colon cancer by activation of STAT3. BMC Cancer 13, 59.

Jiang, H., Lin, J., Fisher, P.B., 1994.A molecular definition of terminal cell differentiation in human melanoma cells. Mol. Cell. Differ. 2, 221–239.

Jiang, R.,Tan, Z., Deng, L., Chen,Y., Xia,Y., Gao,Y.,Wang, X., Sun, B., 2011. Interleukin-22 promotes human hepatocellular carcinoma by activation of STAT3. Hepatology 54 (3), 900–909.

Jiang, H., Su, Z.Z., Boyd, J., Fisher, P.B., 1993. Gene expression changes associated with reversible growth suppression and the induction of terminal differentiation in human melanoma cells. Mol. Cell. Differ. 1, 41–66.

Jiang, H., Lin, J.J., Su, Z.Z., Goldstein, N.I., Fisher, P.B., 1995. Subtraction hybridization identifies a novel melanoma differentiation associated gene, *mda*-7, modulated during human melanoma differentiation, growth and progression. Oncogene 11, 2477–2486.

Jin, S., White, E., 2007. Role of autophagy in cancer: management of metabolic stress. Autophagy 3 (1), 28–31.

Jin,Y., Liu, R., Xie, J., Xiong, H., He, J.C., Chen, N., Jul 2013. Interleukin-10 deficiency aggravates kidney inflammation and fibrosis in the unilateral ureteral obstruction mouse model. Lab. Invest. 93 (7), 801–811. http://dx.doi.org/10.1038/labinvest.2013.64.

Jordan, W.J., Eskdale, J., Srinivas, S., Pekarek,V., Kelner, D., Rodia, M., Gallagher, G., 2007. Human interferon lambda-1 (IFN-lambda1/IL-29) modulates the Th1/Th2 response. Genes Immun. 8 (3), 254–261.

Jovasevic,V.M., Gorelik, L., Bluestone, J.A., Mokyr, M.B., 2004. Importance of IL-10 for CTLA-4-mediated inhibition of tumor-eradicating immunity. J. Immunol. 172 (3), 1449–1454.

Joyce, D.A., Gibbons, D.P., Green, P., Steer, J.H., Feldmann, M., Brennan, F.M., 1994. Two inhibitors of pro-inflammatory cytokine release, interleukin-10 and interleukin-4, have contrasting effects on release of soluble p75 tumor necrosis factor receptor by cultured monocytes. Eur. J. Immunol. 24 (11), 2699–2705.

Juang, S.H., Xie, K., Xu, L., Shi, Q., Wang, Y., Yoneda, J., Fidler, I.J., 1998. Suppression of tumorigenicity and metastasis of human renal carcinoma cells by infection with retroviral vectors harboring the murine inducible nitric oxide synthase gene. Hum. Gene Ther. 9 (6), 845–854.

Jung, M.Y., Kim, S.H., Cho, D., Kim, T.S., 2009. Analysis of the expression profiles of cytokines and cytokine-related genes during the progression of breast cancer growth in mice. Oncol. Rep. 22 (5), 1141–1147.

Kagami, S., Rizzo, H.L., Lee, J.J., Koguchi, Y., Blauvelt, A., 2010. Circulating Th17, Th22, and Th1 cells are increased in psoriasis. J. Invest. Dermatol. 130 (5), 1373–1383.

Kambayashi, T., Alexander, H.R., Fong, M., Strassmann, G., 1995. Potential involvement of IL-10 in suppressing tumor-associated macrophages. Colon-26-derived prostaglandin E2 inhibits TNF-alpha release via a mechanism involving IL-10. J. Immunol. 154 (7), 3383–3390.

Kanzawa, T., Germano, I.M., Komata, T., Ito, H., Kondo, Y., Kondo, S., 2004. Role of autophagy in temozolomide-induced cytotoxicity for malignant glioma cells. Cell Death Differ. 11 (4), 448–457.

Kawakami, T., Tokunaga, T., Hatanaka, H., Tsuchida, T., Tomii, Y., Osada, H., Onoda, N., Morino, F., Nagata, J., Kijima, H., Yamazaki, H., Abe, Y., Osamura, Y., Ueyama, Y., Nakamura, M., 2001. Interleukin 10 expression is correlated with thrombospondin expression and decreased vascular involvement in colon cancer. Int. J. Oncol. 18 (3), 487–491.

Ke, B., Shen, X.D., Tsuchihashi, S., Gao, F., Araujo, J.A., Busuttil, R.W., Ritter, T., Kupiec–Weglinski, J.W., 2007. Viral interleukin-10 gene transfer prevents liver ischemia–reperfusion injury: Toll-like receptor-4 and heme oxygenase-1 signaling in innate and adaptive immunity. Hum. Gene Ther. 18 (4), 355–366.

Kemik, O., Kemik, A.S., Begenik, H., Erdur, F.M., Emre, H., Sumer, A., Purisa, S., Tuzun, S., Kotan, C., 2012. The relationship among acute-phase response proteins, cytokines, and hormones in various gastrointestinal cancer types patients with cachectic. Hum. Exp. Toxicol. 31 (2), 117–125.

Keystone, E., Wherry, J., Grint, P., 1998. IL-10 as a therapeutic strategy in the treatment of rheumatoid arthritis. Rheum. Dis. Clin. North Am. 24 (3), 629–639.

Kieran, M.W., Kalluri, R., Cho, Y.J., 2012. The VEGF pathway in cancer and disease: responses, resistance, and the path forward. Cold Spring Harb. Perspect. Med. 2 (12), a006593.

Kim, K.W., Kim, H.R., Park, J.Y., Park, J.S., Oh, H.J., Woo, Y.J., Park, M.K., Cho, M.L., Lee, S.H., 2012. Interleukin-22 promotes osteoclastogenesis in rheumatoid arthritis through induction of RANKL in human synovial fibroblasts. Arthritis Rheum. 64 (4), 1015–1023.

Kim, J., Modlin, R.L., Moy, R.L., Dubinett, S.M., McHugh, T., Nickoloff, B.J., Uyemura, K., 1995. IL-10 production in cutaneous basal and squamous cell carcinomas. A mechanism for evading the local T cell immune response. J. Immunol. 155 (4), 2240–2247.

Kim, M.J., Jang, J.W., Oh, B.S., Kwon, J.H., Chung, K.W., Jung, H.S., Jekarl, D.W., Lee, S., 2013. Change in inflammatory cytokine profiles after transarterial chemotherapy in patients with hepatocellular carcinoma. Cytokine 64 (2), 516–522.

Kim, B.G., Joo, H.G., Chung, I.S., Chung, H.Y., Woo, H.J., Yun, Y.S., 2000. Inhibition of interleukin-10 (IL-10) production from MOPC 315 tumor cells by IL-10 antisense oligodeoxynucleotides enhances cell-mediated immune responses. Cancer Immunol. Immunother. 49 (8), 433–440.

Kirchberger, S., Royston, D.J., Boulard, O., Thornton, E., Franchini, F., Szabady, R.L., Harrison, O., Powrie, F., 2013. Innate lymphoid cells sustain colon cancer through production of interleukin-22 in a mouse model. J. Exp. Med. 210 (5), 917–931.

Kleemann, R., Zadelaar, S., Kooistra, T., 2008. Cytokines and atherosclerosis: a comprehensive review of studies in mice. Cardiovasc. Res. 79 (3), 360–376.

Klimatsidas, M., Anastasiadis, K., Foroulis, C., Tossios, P., Bisiklis, A., Papakonstantinou, C., Rammos, K., 2012. Elevated levels of anti inflammatory IL-10 and pro inflammatory IL-17 in malignant pleural effusions. J. Cardiothorac. Surg. 7, 104.

Kobold, S.,Völk, S., Clauditz,T., Küpper, N.J., Minner, S.,Tufman,A., Düwell, P., Lindner, M., Koch, I., Heidegger, S., Rothenfuer, S., Schnurr, M., Huber, R.M.,Wilczak,W., Endres, S., 2013. Interleukin-22 is frequently expressed in small- and large-cell lung cancer and promotes growth in chemotherapy-resistant cancer cells. J.Thorac. Oncol. 8 (8), 1032–1042.

Kohno,T., Mizukami, H., Suzuki, M., Saga,Y.,Takei,Y., Shimpo, M., Matsushita,T., Okada,T., Hanazono,Y., Kume,A., Sato, I., Ozawa, K., 2003. Interleukin-10-mediated inhibition of angiogenesis and tumor growth in mice bearingVEGF-producing ovarian cancer. Cancer Res. 63 (16), 5091–5094.

Koltsida, O., Hausding, M., Stavropoulos,A., Koch, S.,Tzelepis, G., Ubel, C., Kotenko, S.V., Sideras, P., Lehr, H.A.,Tepe, M., Klucher, K.M., Doyle, S.E., Neurath, M.F., Finotto, S., Andreakos, E., 2011. IL-28A (IFN-λ2) modulates lung DC function to promote Th1 immune skewing and suppress allergic airway disease. EMBO Mol. Med. 3 (6), 348–361.

Kotenko, S.V., Saccani, S., Izotova, L.S., Mirochnitchenko, O.V., Pestka, S., 2000. Human cytomegalovirus harbors its own unique IL-10 homolog (cmvIL-10). Proc. Natl. Acad. Sci. U S A 97 (4), 1695–1700.

Kotenko, S.V., Gallagher, G., Baurin,V.V., Lewis-Antes,A., Shen, M., Shah, N.K., Langer, J.A., Sheikh, F., Dickensheets, H., Donnelly, R.P., 2003. IFN-lambdas mediate antiviral protection through a distinct class II cytokine receptor complex. Nat. Immunol. 4 (1), 69–77.

Kotenko, S.V., Izotova, L.S., Mirochnitchenko, O.V., Esterova, E., Dickensheets, H., Donnelly, R.P., Pestka, S., 2001. Identification of the functional interleukin-22 (IL-22) receptor complex: the IL-10R2 chain (IL-10Rbeta) is a common chain of both the IL-10 and IL-22 (IL-10-relatedT cell-derived inducible factor, IL-TIF) receptor complexes. J. Biol. Chem. 276 (4), 2725–2732.

Kragstrup,T.W., Otkjaer, K., Holm, C., Jørgensen,A., Hokland, M., Iversen, L., Deleuran, B., 2008. The expression of IL-20 and IL-24 and their shared receptors are increased in rheumatoid arthritis and spondyloarthropathy. Cytokine 41 (1), 16–23.

Krambeck,A.E.,Thompson, R.H., Dong, H., Lohse, C.M., Park, E.S., Kuntz, S.M., Leibovich, B.C., Blute, M.L., Cheville, J.C., Kwon, E.D., 2006. B7–H4 expression in renal cell carcinoma and tumor vasculature: associations with cancer progression and survival. Proc. Natl.Acad. Sci. U S A 103 (27), 10391–10396.

Krause, C.D., Pestka, S., 2007. Historical developments in the research of interferon receptors. Cytokine Growth Factor Rev. 18 (5–6), 473–482.

Krause, C.D., Pestka, S., 2005. Evolution of the class 2 cytokines and receptors, and discovery of new friends and relatives. Pharmacol.Ther. 106 (3), 299–346.

Kruger-Krasagakes, S., Krasagakis, K., Garbe, C., Schmitt, E., Huls, C., Blankenstein,T., Diamantstein,T., 1994. Expression of interleukin 10 in human melanoma. Br. J. Cancer 70 (6), 1182–1185.

Kryczek, I.,Wei, S., Zhu, G., Myers, L., Mottram, P., Cheng, P., Chen, L., Coukos, G., Zou, W., 2007. Relationship between B7-H4, regulatory T cells, and patient outcome in human ovarian carcinoma. Cancer Res. 67 (18), 8900–8905.

Kundu, N., Fulton, A.M., 1997. Interleukin-10 inhibits tumor metastasis, downregulates MHC class I, and enhances NK lysis. Cell. Immunol. 180 (1), 55–61.

Kundu, N., Dorsey, R., Jackson, M.J., Guiterrez, P., Wilson, K., Fu, S., Ramanujam, K., Thomas, E., Fulton,A.M., 1998. Interleukin-10 gene transfer inhibits murine mammary tumors and elevates nitric oxide. Int. J. Cancer 76 (5), 713–719.

Kundu, N., Beaty,T.L., Jackson, M.J., Fulton,A.M., 1996.Antimetastatic and antitumor activities of interleukin 10 in a murine model of breast cancer. J. Natl. Cancer Inst. 88 (8), 536–541.

Kunz, S., Wolk, K., Witte, E., Witte, K., Doecke, W.D., Volk, H.D., Sterry, W., Asadullah, K., Sabat, R., 2006. Interleukin (IL)-19, IL-20 and IL-24 are produced by and act on keratinocytes and are distinct from classical ILs. Exp. Dermatol. 15 (12), 991–1004.

Kurte, M., Lypez, M., Aguirre, A., Escobar, A., Aguillyn, J.C., Charo, J., Larsen, C.G., Kiessling, R., Salazar-Onfray, F., 2004. A synthetic peptide homologous to functional domain of human IL-10 down-regulates expression of MHC class I and transporter associated with antigen processing 1/2 in human melanoma cells. J. Immunol. 173 (3), 1731–1737.

Kutikhin, A.G., Yuzhalin, A.E., Volkov, A.N., Zhivotovskiy, A.S., Brusina, E.B., January 21, 2014. Correlation between genetic polymorphisms within IL-1B and TLR4 genes and cancer risk in a Russian population: a case-control study. Tumour Biol. 35 (5), 4821–4830.

Labidi, S.I., Ménétrier–Caux, C., Chabaud, S., Chassagne, C., Sebban, C., Gargi, T., Biron, P., Blay, J.Y., Ghesquières, H., 2010. Serum cytokines in follicular lymphoma. Correlation of TGF-β and VEGF with survival. Ann. Hematol. 89 (1), 25–33.

Lang, F., Linlin, M., Ye, T., Yuhai, Z., 2012. Alterations of dendritic cell subsets and TH1/TH2 cytokines in the peripheral circulation of patients with superficial transitional cell carcinoma of the bladder. J. Clin. Lab. Anal. 26 (5), 365–371.

Lasfar, A., Lewis-Antes, A., Smirnov, S.V., Anantha, S., Abushahba, W., Tian, B., Reuhl, K., Dickensheets, H., Sheikh, F., Donnelly, R.P., Raveche, E., Kotenko, S.V., 2006. Characterization of the mouse IFN-lambda ligand-receptor system: IFN-lambdas exhibit antitumor activity against B16 melanoma. Cancer Res. 66 (8), 4468–4477.

Laubli, H., Borsig, L., 2010. Selectins promote tumor metastasis. Semin. Cancer Biol. 20 (3), 169–177.

Leath 3rd, C.A., Kataram, M., Bhagavatula, P., Gopalkrishnan, R.V., Dent, P., Fisher, P.B., Pereboev, A., Carey, D., Lebedeva, I.V., Haisma, H.J., Alvarez, R.D., Curiel, D.T., Mahasreshti, P.J., 2004. Infectivity enhanced adenoviral-mediated mda-7/IL-24 gene therapy for ovarian carcinoma. Gynecol. Oncol. 94 (2), 352–362.

Lebedeva, I.V., Su, Z.Z., Sarkar, D., Gopalkrishnan, R.V., Waxman, S., Yacoub, A., Dent, P., Fisher, P.B., 2005. Induction of reactive oxygen species renders mutant and wild-type K-ras pancreatic carcinoma cells susceptible to Ad.mda-7-induced apoptosis. Oncogene 24 (4), 585–596.

Lebedeva, I.V., Su, Z.Z., Vozhilla, N., Chatman, L., Sarkar, D., Dent, P., Athar, M., Fisher, P.B., 2008. Mechanism of in vitro pancreatic cancer cell growth inhibition by melanoma differentiation-associated gene-7/interleukin-24 and perillyl alcohol. Cancer Res. 68 (18), 7439–7447.

Lebedeva, I.V., Sarkar, D., Su, Z.Z., Kitada, S., Dent, P., Stein, C.A., Reed, J.C., Fisher, P.B., 2003. Bcl-2 and Bcl-x(L) differentially protect human prostate cancer cells from induction of apoptosis by melanoma differentiation associated gene-7, mda-7/IL-24. Oncogene 22 (54), 8758–8773.

Lech-Maranda, E., Grzybowska–Izydorczyk, O., Wyka, K., Mlynarski, W., Borowiec, M., Antosik, K., Cebula–Obrzut, B., Makuch–Lasica, H., Nowak, G., Klimkiewicz–Wojciechowska, G., Wawrzyniak, E., Bilinski, P., Robak, T., Warzocha, K., 2012. Serum tumor necrosis factor-α and interleukin-10 levels as markers to predict outcome of patients with chronic lymphocytic leukemia in different risk groups defined by the IGHV mutation status. Arch. Immunol. Ther. Exp. (Warsz) 60 (6), 477–486.

Lee, S.J., Cho, S.C., Lee, E.J., Kim, S., Lee, S.B., Lim, J.H., Choi, Y.H., Kim, W.J., Moon, S.K., 2013. Interleukin-20 promotes migration of bladder cancer cells through extracellular signal-regulated kinase (ERK)-mediated MMP-9 protein expression leading to nuclear factor (NF-κB) activation by inducing the up-regulation of p21(WAF1) protein expression. J. Biol. Chem. 288 (8), 5539–5552.

Lee, S.J., Lee, E.J., Kim, S.K., Jeong, P., Cho, Y.H., Yun, S.J., Kim, S., Kim, G.Y., Choi, Y.H., Cha, E.J., Kim, W.J., Moon, S.K., 2012. Identification of pro-inflammatory cytokines associated with muscle invasive bladder cancer; the roles of IL-5, IL-20, and IL-28A. PLoS One 7 (9), e40267.

Lejeune, D., Dumoutier, L., Constantinescu, S., Kruijer, W., Schuringa, J.J., Renauld, J.C., 2002. Interleukin-22 (IL-22) activates the JAK/STAT, ERK, JNK, and p38 MAP kinase pathways in a rat hepatoma cell line. Pathways that are shared with and distinct from IL-10. J. Biol. Chem. 277 (37), 33676–33682.

Levi, G., Minghetti, L., Aloisi, F., 1998. Regulation of prostanoid synthesis in microglial cells and effects of prostaglandin E2 on microglial functions. Biochimie 80 (11), 899–904.

Levy, L., Hill, C.S., 2006. Alterations in components of the TGF-beta superfamily signaling pathways in human cancer. Cytokine Growth Factor Rev. 17 (1–2), 41–58.

Li, Y.J., Liu, G., Li, Y., Vecchiarelli-Federico, L.M., Liu, J.C., Zacksenhaus, E., Shan, S.W., Yang, B.B., Li, Q., Dash, R., Fisher, P.B., Archer, M.C., Ben-David, Y., 2013. mda-7/IL-24 expression inhibits breast cancer through upregulation of growth arrest-specific gene 3 (gas3) and disruption of β1 integrin function. Mol. Cancer Res. 11 (6), 593–603.

Li, L., Wang, Z.X., Wang, Z.H., 2011. Combination of IL-24 and cisplatin inhibits cervical cancer growth in a xenograft nude mice model. Asian Pac. J. Cancer Prev. 12 (12), 3293–3298.

Li, W., Lewis-Antes, A., Huang, J., Balan, M., Kotenko, S.V., 2008. Regulation of apoptosis by type III interferons. Cell. Prolif. 41 (6), 960–979.

Li, H.H., Lin, Y.C., Chen, P.J., Hsiao, C.H., Lee, J.Y., Chen, W.C., Chang, M.S., 2005. Interleukin-19 upregulates keratinocyte growth factor and is associated with psoriasis. Br. J. Dermatol. 153 (3), 591–595.

Li, Q., Kawamura, K., Tada, Y., Shimada, H., Hiroshima, K., Tagawa, M., 2013. Novel type III interferons produce anti-tumor effects through multiple functions. Front. Biosci. (Landmark Ed) 18, 909–918.

Li, Q., Kawamura, K., Ma, G., Iwata, F., Numasaki, M., Suzuki, N., Shimada, H., Tagawa, M., 2010. Interferon-lambda induces G1 phase arrest or apoptosis in oesophageal carcinoma cells and produces anti-tumour effects in combination with anti-cancer agents. Eur. J. Cancer 46 (1), 180–190.

Li, H.H., Hsu, Y.H., Wei, C.C., Lee, P.T., Chen, W.C., Chang, M.S., 2008. Interleukin-20 induced cell death in renal epithelial cells and was associated with acute renal failure. Genes Immun. 9 (5), 395–404.

Liang, S.C., Tan, X.Y., Luxenberg, D.P., Karim, R., Dunussi-Joannopoulos, K., Collins, M., Fouser, L.A., 2006. Interleukin (IL)-22 and IL-17 are coexpressed by Th17 cells and cooperatively enhance expression of antimicrobial peptides. J. Exp. Med. 203 (10), 2271–2279.

Liao, S.C., Cheng, Y.C., Wang, Y.C., Wang, C.W., Yang, S.M., Yu, C.K., Shieh, C.C., Cheng, K.C., Lee, M.F., Chiang, S.R., Shieh, J.M., Chang, M.S., 2004. IL-19 induced Th2 cytokines and was up-regulated in asthma patients. J. Immunol. 173 (11), 6712–6718.

Liao, Y.C., Liang, W.G., Chen, F.W., Hsu, J.H., Yang, J.J., Chang, M.S., 2002. IL-19 induces production of IL-6 and TNF-alpha and results in cell apoptosis through TNF-alpha. J. Immunol. 169 (8), 4288–4297.

Lin, S.C., Kuo, C.C., Tsao, J.T., Lin, L.J., 2012. Profiling the expression of interleukin (IL)-28 and IL-28 receptor α in systemic lupus erythematosus patients. Eur. J. Clin. Invest. 42 (1), 61–69.

Lin, T.J., Befus, A.D., 1997. Differential regulation of mast cell function by IL-10 and stem cell factor. J. Immunol. 159 (8), 4015–4023.

Lindsay, J.O., Hodgson, H.J., 2001. Review article: the immunoregulatory cytokine interleukin-10—a therapy for Crohn's disease? Aliment. Pharmacol. Ther. 15 (11), 1709–1716.

Lisinski, T.J., Furie, M.B., 2002. Interleukin-10 inhibits proinflammatory activation of endothelium in response to Borrelia burgdorferi or lipopolysaccharide but not interleukin-1beta or tumor necrosis factor alpha. J. Leukoc. Biol. 72 (3), 503–511.

Liu, T., Peng, L., Yu, P., Zhao, Y., Shi, Y., Mao, X., Chen, W., Cheng, P., Wang, T., Chen, N., Zhang, J., Liu, X., Li, N., Guo, G., Tong, W., Zhuang, Y., Zou, Q., Dec 2012. Increased circulating Th22 and Th17 cells are associated with tumor progression and patient survival in human gastric cancer. J. Clin. Immunol. 32 (6), 1332–1339.

Liu, B.S., Janssen, H.L., Boonstra, A., 2011. IL-29 and IFNα differ in their ability to modulate IL-12 production by TLR-activated human macrophages and exhibit differential regulation of the IFNγ receptor expression. Blood 117 (8), 2385–2395.

Liu, Y.W., Tseng, H.P., Chen, L.C., Chen, B.K., Chang, W.C., 2003. Functional cooperation of simian virus 40 promoter factor 1 and CCAAT/enhancer–binding protein beta and delta in lipopolysaccharide-induced gene activation of IL-10 in mouse macrophages. J. Immunol. 171 (2), 821–828.

Lockridge, K.M., Zhou, S.S., Kravitz, R.H., Johnson, J.L., Sawai, E.T., Blewett, E.L., Barry, P.A., 2000. Primate cytomegaloviruses encode and express an IL-10–like protein. Virology 268 (2), 272–280.

Loke, P., Allison, J.P., 2003. PD-L1 and PD-L2 are differentially regulated by Th1 and Th2 cells. Proc. Natl. Acad. Sci. USA 100 (9), 5336–5341.

Lu, K., Feng, X., Deng, Q., Sheng, L., Liu, P., Xu, S., Su, D., 2012. Prognostic role of serum cytokines in patients with nasopharyngeal carcinoma. Onkologie 35 (9), 494–498.

Mahasreshti, P.J., Kataram, M., Wu, H., Yalavarthy, L.P., Carey, D., Fisher, P.B., Chada, S., Alvarez, R.D., Haisma, H.J., Dent, P., Curiel, D.T., 2006. Ovarian cancer targeted adenoviral-mediated mda-7/IL-24 gene therapy. Gynecol. Oncol. 100 (3), 521–532.

Maher, S.G., Sheikh, F., Scarzello, A.J., Romero-Weaver, A.L., Baker, D.P., Donnelly, R.P., Gamero, A.M., 2008. IFNalpha and IFNlambda differ in their antiproliferative effects and duration of JAK/STAT signaling activity. Cancer Biol. Ther. 7 (7), 1109–1115.

Maiuri, M.C., Zalckvar, E., Kimchi, A., Kroemer, G., 2007. Self-eating and self-killing: crosstalk between autophagy and apoptosis. Nat. Rev. Mol. Cell. Biol. 8 (9), 741–752.

Maloney, C.G., Kutchera, W.A., Albertine, K.H., McIntyre, T.M., Prescott, S.M., Zimmerman, G.A., 1998. Inflammatory agonists induce cyclooxygenase type 2 expression by human neutrophils. J. Immunol. 160 (3), 1402–1410.

Malvicini, M., Rizzo, M., Alaniz, L., Picero, F., Garcia, M., Atorrasagasti, C., Aquino, J.B., Rozados, V., Scharovsky, O.G., Matar, P., Mazzolini, G., 2009. A novel synergistic combination of cyclophosphamide and gene transfer of interleukin-12 eradicates colorectal carcinoma in mice. Clin. Cancer Res. 15 (23), 7256–7265.

Malvicini, M., Ingolotti, M., Piccioni, F., Garcia, M., Bayo, J., Atorrasagasti, C., Alaniz, L., Aquino, J.B., Espinoza, J.A., Gidekel, M., Scharovsky, O.G., Matar, P., Mazzolini, G., 2011. Reversal of gastrointestinal carcinoma-induced immunosuppression and induction of antitumoural immunity by a combination of cyclophosphamide and gene transfer of IL-12. Mol. Oncol. 5 (3), 242–255.

Manni, M.L., Robinson, K.R., Alcorn, J.F., 2014. A tale of two cytokines: IL-17 and IL-22 in asthma and infection. Expert Rev. Respir. Med. 8 (1), 25–42.

Marcello, T., Grakoui, A., Barba-Spaeth, G., Machlin, E.S., Kotenko, S.V., MacDonald, M.R., Rice, C.M., 2006. Interferons alpha and lambda inhibit hepatitis C virus replication with distinct signal transduction and gene regulation kinetics. Gastroenterology 131 (6), 1887–1898.

Marijnissen, R.J., Koenders, M.I., Smeets, R.L., Stappers, M.H., Nickerson-Nutter, C., Joosten, L.A., Boots, A.M., van den Berg, W.B., 2011. Increased expression of interleukin-22 by synovial Th17 cells during late stages of murine experimental arthritis is controlled by interleukin-1 and enhances bone degradation. Arthritis Rheum. 63 (10), 2939–2948.

Matar, P., Rozados, V.R., Gonzalez, A.D., Dlugovitzky, D.G., Bonfil, R.D., Scharovsky, O.G., 2000. Mechanism of antimetastatic immunopotentiation by low-dose cyclophosphamide. Eur. J. Cancer 36 (8), 1060–1066.

Matar, P., Rozados,V.R., Roggero, E.A., Bonfil, R.D., Scharovsky, O.G., 1998. Modulation of the antimetastatic effect of a single low dose of cyclophosphamide on rat lymphoma. Tumour Biol. 19 (2), 69–76.

Matar, P., Rozados,V.R., Gervasoni, S.I., Scharovsky, O.G., 2001. Down regulation of T-cell-derived IL-10 production by low-dose cyclophosphamide treatment in tumor-bearing rats restores in vitro normal lymphoproliferative response. Int. Immunopharmacol. 1 (2), 307–319.

Mathew, R., Karp, C.M., Beaudoin, B.,Vuong, N., Chen, G., Chen, H.Y., Bray, K., Reddy,A., Bhanot, G., Gelinas, C., Dipaola, R.S., Karantza-Wadsworth,V.,White, E., 2009. Autophagy suppresses tumorigenesis through elimination of p62. Cell 137 (6), 1062–1075.

Matsuda, M., Salazar, F., Petersson, M., Masucci, G., Hansson, J., Pisa, P., Zhang, Q.J., Masucci, M.G., Kiessling, R., 1994. Interleukin 10 pretreatment protects target cells from tumor- and allo-specific cytotoxic T cells and downregulates HLA class I expression. J. Exp. Med. 180 (6), 2371–2376.

Matsumoto, K., Ohi, H., Kanmatsuse, K., 1997. Interleukin 10 and interleukin 13 synergize to inhibit vascular permeability factor release by peripheral blood mononuclear cells from patients with lipoid nephrosis. Nephron 77 (2), 212–218.

Matsumoto, K., Ohi, H., Kanmatsuse, K., 1999. Interleukin-4 cooperates with interleukin-10 to inhibit vascular permeability factor release by peripheral blood mononuclear cells from patients with minimal-change nephrotic syndrome. Am. J. Nephrol. 19 (1), 21–27.

Matsumoto, K., 1997. Interleukin 10 inhibits vascular permeability factor release by peripheral blood mononuclear cells in patients with lipoid nephrosis. Nephron 75 (2), 154–159.

Meager, A.,Visvalingam, K., Dilger, P., Bryan, D., Wadhwa, M., 2005. Biological activity of interleukins-28 and -29: comparison with type I interferons. Cytokine 31 (2), 109–118.

Melinceanu, L., Lerescu, L.,Tucureanu, C., Caras, I., Pitica, R., Sarafoleanu, C., Salageanu,A., 2011. Serum perioperative profile of cytokines in patients with squamous cell carcinoma of the larynx. J. Otolaryngol. Head Neck Surg. 40 (2), 143–150.

Mellgren, K., Hedegaard, C.J., Schmiegelow, K., Muller, K., 2012. Plasma cytokine profiles at diagnosis in pediatric patients with non–Hodgkin lymphoma. J. Pediatr. Hematol. Oncol. 34 (4), 271–275.

Melzner, I.,Weniger, M.A., Menz, C.K., Moller, P., 2006. Absence of the JAK2V617F activating mutation in classical Hodgkin lymphoma and primary mediastinal B-cell lymphoma. Leukemia 20 (1), 157–158.

Menetrier-Caux, C., Bain, C., Favrot, M.C., Duc, A., Blay, J.Y., 1999. Renal cell carcinoma induces interleukin 10 and prostaglandin E2 production by monocytes. Br. J. Cancer 79 (1), 119–130.

Mennechet, F.J., Uzé, G., 2006. Interferon-lambda-treated dendritic cells specifically induce proliferation of FOXP3-expressing suppressor T cells. Blood 107 (11), 4417–4423.

Menon, R., Ismail, L., Ismail, D., Merialdi, M., Lombardi, S.J., Fortunato, S.J., 2006. Human fetal membrane expression of IL-19 and IL-20 and its differential effect on inflammatory cytokine production. J. Matern. Fetal Neonatal Med. 19 (4), 209–214.

Michalak-Stoma, A., Pietrzak,A., Szepietowski, J.C., Zalewska-Janowska, A., Paszkowski,T., Chodorowska, G., 2011. Cytokine network in psoriasis revisited. Eur. Cytokine Netw. 22 (4), 160–168.

Michelin, M.A., Figueiredo, F., Cunha, F.Q., 2002. Involvement of prostaglandins in the immunosuppression occurring during experimental infection by Paracoccidioides brasiliensis. Exp. Parasitol. 102 (3–4), 170–177.

Miller, D.M., Klucher, K.M., Freeman, J.A., Hausman, D.F., Fontana, D.,Williams, D.E., 2009. Interferon lambda as a potential new therapeutic for hepatitis C. Ann. N Y Acad. Sci. 1182, 80–87.

Mindiola, R., Caulejas, D., Núcez–Troconis, J., Araujo, M., Delgado, M., Mosquera, J., 2008. Increased number of IL-2, IL-2 receptor and IL-10 positive cells in premalignant lesions of the cervix. Invest. Clin. 49 (4), 533–545.

Minghetti, L., Polazzi, E., Nicolini, A., Levi, G., 1998. Opposite regulation of prostaglandin E2 synthesis by transforming growth factor-beta1 and interleukin 10 in activated microglial cultures. J. Neuroimmunol. 82 (1), 31–39.

Miyagaki, T., Sugaya, M., Suga, H., Kamata, M., Ohmatsu, H., Fujita, H., Asano, Y., Tada, Y., Kadono, T., Sato, S., 2011. IL-22, but not IL-17, dominant environment in cutaneous T-cell lymphoma. Clin. Cancer Res. 17 (24), 7529–7538.

Mocellin, S., Panelli, M.C., Wang, E., Nagorsen, D., Marincola, F.M., 2003. The dual role of IL-10. Trends Immunol. 24 (1), 36–43.

Mocellin, S., Panelli, M., Wang, E., Rossi, C.R., Pilati, P., Nitti, D., Lise, M., Marincola, F.M., 2004. IL-10 stimulatory effects on human NK cells explored by gene profile analysis. Genes Immun. 5 (8), 621–630.

Mojtahedi, Z., Khademi, B., Yehya, A., Talebi, A., Fattahi, M.J., Ghaderi, A., 2012. Serum levels of interleukins 4 and 10 in head and neck squamous cell carcinoma. J. Laryngol. Otol. 126 (2), 175–179.

Molina-Holgado, E., Arevalo-Martin, A., Ortiz, S., Vela, J.M., Guaza, C., 2002. Theiler's virus infection induces the expression of cyclooxygenase-2 in murine astrocytes: inhibition by the anti-inflammatory cytokines interleukin-4 and interleukin-10. Neurosci. Lett. 324 (3), 237–241.

Moore, K.W., Vieira, P., Fiorentino, D.F., Trounstine, M.L., Khan, T.A., Mosmann, T.R., 1990. Homology of cytokine synthesis inhibitory factor (IL-10) to the Epstein–Barr virus gene BCRFI. Science 248, 1230–1234.

Moore, K.W., de Waal Malefyt, R., Coffman, R.L., O'Garra, A., 2001. Interleukin-10 and the interleukin-10 receptor. Annu. Rev. Immunol. 19, 683–765.

Mordstein, M., Kochs, G., Dumoutier, L., Renauld, J.C., Paludan, S.R., Klucher, K., Staeheli, P., 2008. Interferon-lambda contributes to innate immunity of mice against influenza A virus but not against hepatotropic viruses. PLoS Pathog. 4 (9), e1000151.

Morise, Z., Eppihimer, M., Granger, D.N., Anderson, D.C., Grisham, M.B., 1999. Effects of lipopolysaccharide on endothelial cell adhesion molecule expression in interleukin-10 deficient mice. Inflammation 23 (2), 99–110.

Mosser, D.M., Zhang, X., 2008. Interleukin-10: new perspectives on an old cytokine. Immunol. Rev. 226, 205–218.

Mustea, A., Braicu, E.I., Koensgen, D., Yuan, S., Sun, P.M., Stamatian, F., Lichtenegger, W., Chen, F.C., Chekerov, R., Sehouli, J., 2009. Monitoring of IL-10 in the serum of patients with advanced ovarian cancer: results from a prospective pilot-study. Cytokine 45 (1), 8–11.

Myers Jr, D.D., Hawley, A.E., Farris, D.M., Chapman, A.M., Wrobleski, S.K., Henke, P.K., Wakefield, T.W., 2003. Cellular IL-10 is more effective than viral IL-10 in decreasing venous thrombosis. J. Surg. Res. 112 (2), 168–174.

Myles, I.A., Fontecilla, N.M., Valdez, P.A., Vithayathil, P.J., Naik, S., Belkaid, Y., Ouyang, W., Datta, S.K., Aug 2013. Signaling via the IL-20 receptor inhibits cutaneous production of IL-1β and IL-17A to promote infection with methicillin-resistant Staphylococcus aureus. Nat. Immunol. 14 (8), 804–811. http://dx.doi.org/10.1038/ni.2637.

Nacinović–Duletić, A., Stifter, S., Dvornik, S., Skunca, Z., Jonjić, N., 2008. Correlation of serum IL-6, IL-8 and IL-10 levels with clinicopathological features and prognosis in patients with diffuse large B–cell lymphoma. Int. J. Lab. Hematol. 30 (3), 230–239.

Nagata, J., Kijima, H., Hatanaka, H., Tokunaga, T., Takagi, A., Mine, T., et al., 2002. Correlation between interleukin 10 and vascular endothelial growth factor expression in human esophageal cancer. Int. J. Mol. Med. 10 (2), 169–172.

Naiyer, M.M., Saha, S., Hemke,V., Roy, S., Singh, S., Musti, K.V., Saha, B., 2013. Identification and characterization of a human IL-10 receptor antagonist. Hum. Immunol. 74 (1), 28–31.

Nakajima, H., Gleich, G.J., Kita, H., 1996. Constitutive production of IL-4 and IL-10 and stimulated production of IL-8 by normal peripheral blood eosinophils. J. Immunol. 156 (12), 4859–4866.

Naumnik, W., Naumnik, B., Niewiarowska, K., Ossolinska, M., Chyczewska, E., 2012. Novel cytokines: IL-27, IL-29, IL-31 and IL-33. Can they be useful in clinical practice at the time diagnosis of lung cancer? Exp. Oncol. 34 (4), 348–353.

Ni, Q.C., Yang, L., Zhang, C.H., Zhou, F., Zhu, H.J., Huang, J.F., 2008. Effects of adenoviral-mediated melanoma differentiation associated gene-7/IL-24 on growth and apoptosis of breast cancer cells. Zhonghua Yixue Zazhi 88 (42), 3008–3011.

Niiro, H., Otsuka, T., Izuhara, K., Yamaoka, K., Ohshima, K., Tanabe, T., Hara, S., Nemoto, Y., Tanaka, Y., Nakashima, H., Niho, Y., Mar 1, 1997. Regulation by interleukin-10 and interleukin-4 of cyclooxygenase-2 expression in human neutrophils. Blood 89 (5), 1621–1628.

Nishikawa, T., Ramesh, R., Munshi, A., Chada, S., Meyn, R.E., 2004. Adenovirus-mediated mda-7 (IL24) gene therapy suppresses angiogenesis and sensitizes NSCLC xenograft tumors to radiation. Mol. Ther. 9 (6), 818–828.

Noble, K.E., Harkness, D., Yong, K.L., 2000. Interleukin 10 regulates cellular responses in monocyte/endothelial cell co-cultures. Br. J. Haematol. 108 (3), 497–504.

Nograles, K.E., Zaba, L.C., Shemer, A., Fuentes-Duculan, J., Cardinale, I., Kikuchi, T., Ramon, M., Bergman, R., Krueger, J.G., Guttman-Yassky, E., 2009. IL-22-producing "T22" T cells account for upregulated IL-22 in atopic dermatitis despite reduced IL-17-producing TH17 T cells. J. Allergy Clin. Immunol. 123 (6), 1244–1252. e2.

Numasaki, M., Tagawa, M., Iwata, F., Suzuki, T., Nakamura, A., Okada, M., Iwakura, Y., Aiba, S., Yamaya, M., 2007. IL-28 elicits antitumor responses against murine fibrosarcoma. J. Immunol. 178 (8), 5086–5098.

O'Garra, A., Vieira, P., 2007. T(H)1 cells control themselves by producing interleukin-10. Nat. Rev. Immunol. 7 (6), 425–428.

Ogier-Denis, E., Codogno, P., 2003. Autophagy: a barrier or an adaptive response to cancer. Biochim. Biophys. Acta 1603 (2), 113–128.

Oida, Y., Gopalan, B., Miyahara, R., Inoue, S., Branch, C.D., Mhashilkar, A.M., Lin, E., Bekele, B.N., Roth, J.A., Chada, S., Ramesh, R., 2005. Sulindac enhances adenoviral vector expressing mda-7/IL-24-mediated apoptosis in human lung cancer. Mol. Cancer Ther. 4 (2), 291–304.

Onoguchi, K., Yoneyama, M., Takemura, A., Akira, S., Taniguchi, T., Namiki, H., Fujita, T., 2007. Viral infections activate types I and III interferon genes through a common mechanism. J. Biol. Chem. 282 (10), 7576–7581.

Oral, H.B., Kotenko, S.V., Yilmaz, M., Mani, O., Zumkehr, J., Blaser, K., Akdis, C.A., Akdis, M., 2006. Regulation of T cells and cytokines by the interleukin-10 (IL-10)-family cytokines IL-19, IL-20, IL-22, IL-24, and IL-26. Eur. J. Immunol. 36 (2), 380–388.

Otkjaer, K., Kragballe, K., Johansen, C., Funding, A.T., Just, H., Jensen, U.B., Sørensen, L.G., Nørby, P.L., Clausen, J.T., Iversen, L., 2007. IL-20 gene expression is induced by IL-1beta through mitogen-activated protein kinase and NF-kappaB-dependent mechanisms. J. Invest. Dermatol. 127 (6), 1326–1336.

Ouyang, W., 2010. Distinct roles of IL-22 in human psoriasis and inflammatory bowel disease. Cytokine Growth Factor Rev. 21 (6), 435–441.

Pan, X.T., Zhu, Q.Y., Li, D.C., Yang, J.C., Zhang, Z.X., Zhu, X.G., Zhao, H., 2008. Effect of recombinant adenovirus vector mediated human interleukin-24 gene transfection on pancreatic carcinoma growth. Chin. Med. J. (Engl) 121 (20), 2031–2036.

Pan, X., Sheng, W., Zhu, Q., Xie, Y., Ye, Z., Xiang, J., Li, D., Yang, J., 2008. Inhibition of pancreatic carcinoma growth by adenovirus-mediated human interleukin-24 expression in animal model. Cancer Biother. Radiopharm. 23 (4), 425–434.

Pardali, K., Moustakas, A., 2007. Actions of TGF-beta as tumor suppressor and pro-metastatic factor in human cancer. Biochim. Biophys. Acta 1775 (1), 21–62.

Park, M.A., Yacoub, A., Sarkar, D., Emdad, L., Rahmani, M., Spiegel, S., Koumenis, C., Graf, M., Curiel, D.T., Grant, S., Fisher, P.B., Dent, P., 2008. PERK-dependent regulation of MDA-7/IL-24-induced autophagy in primary human glioma cells. Autophagy 4 (4), 513–515.

Park, M.A., Hamed, H.A., Mitchell, C., Cruickshanks, N., Dash, R., Allegood, J., Dmitriev, I.P., Tye, G., Ogretmen, B., Spiegel, S., Yacoub, A., Grant, S., Curiel, D.T., Fisher, P.B., Dent, P., 2011. A serotype 5/3 adenovirus expressing MDA-7/IL-24 infects renal carcinoma cells and promotes toxicity of agents that increase ROS and ceramide levels. Mol. Pharmacol. 79 (3), 368–380.

Park, M.A., Walker, T., Martin, A.P., Allegood, J., Vozhilla, N., Emdad, L., Sarkar, D., Rahmani, M., Graf, M., Yacoub, A., Koumenis, C., Spiegel, S., Curiel, D.T., Voelkel-Johnson, C., Grant, S., Fisher, P.B., Dent, P., 2009. MDA-7/IL-24-induced cell killing in malignant renal carcinoma cells occurs by a ceramide/CD95/PERK-dependent mechanism. Mol. Cancer Ther. 8 (5), 1280–1291.

Park, O., Wang, H., Weng, H., Feigenbaum, L., Li, H., Yin, S., Ki, S.H., Yoo, S.H., Dooley, S., Wang, F.S., Young, H.A., Gao, B., 2011. In vivo consequences of liver-specific interleukin-22 expression in mice: implications for human liver disease progression. Hepatology 54 (1), 252–261.

Parrish-Novak, J., Xu, W., Brender, T., Yao, L., Jones, C., West, J., Brandt, C., Jelinek, L., Madden, K., McKernan, P.A., Foster, D.C., Jaspers, S., Chandrasekher, Y.A., 2002. Interleukins 19, 20, and 24 signal through two distinct receptor complexes. Differences in receptor-ligand interactions mediate unique biological functions. J. Biol. Chem. 277 (49), 47517–47523.

Parsa, A.T., Waldron, J.S., Panner, A., Crane, C.A., Parney, I.F., Barry, J.J., Cachola, K.E., Murray, J.C., Tihan, T., Jensen, M.C., Mischel, P.S., Stokoe, D., Pieper, R.O., 2007. Loss of tumor suppressor PTEN function increases B7-H1 expression and immunoresistance in glioma. Nat. Med. 13 (1), 84–88.

Pataer, A., Vorburger, S.A., Barber, G.N., Chada, S., Mhashilkar, A.M., Zou-Yang, H., Stewart, A.L., Balachandran, S., Roth, J.A., Hunt, K.K., Swisher, S.G., 2002. Adenoviral transfer of the melanoma differentiation-associated gene 7 (mda7) induces apoptosis of lung cancer cells via up-regulation of the double-stranded RNA-dependent protein kinase (PKR). Cancer Res. 62 (8), 2239–2243.

Pataer, A., Vorburger, S.A., Chada, S., Balachandran, S., Barber, G.N., Roth, J.A., Hunt, K.K., Swisher, S.G., 2005. Melanoma differentiation-associated gene-7 protein physically associates with the double-stranded RNA-activated protein kinase PKR. Mol. Ther. 11 (5), 717–723.

Pataer, A., Bocangel, D., Chada, S., Roth, J.A., Hunt, K.K., Swisher, S.G., 2007. Enhancement of adenoviral MDA-7-mediated cell killing in human lung cancer cells by geldanamycin and its 17-allylamino-17-demethoxy analogue. Cancer Gene Ther. 14, 12–18.

Patani, N., Douglas-Jones, A., Mansel, R., Jiang, W., Mokbel, K., 2010. Tumour suppressor function of MDA-7/IL-24 in human breast cancer. Cancer Cell. Int. 10, 29.

Patel, S., Vetale, S., Teli, P., Mistry, R., Chiplunkar, S., 2012. IL-10 production in non-small cell lung carcinoma patients is regulated by ERK, P38, and COX-2. J. Cell. Mol. Med. 16 (3), 531–544.

Pekarek, V., Srinivas, S., Eskdale, J., Gallagher, G., 2007. Interferon lambda-1 (IFN-lambda1/IL-29) induces ELR(-) CXC chemokine mRNA in human peripheral blood mononuclear cells, in an IFN-gamma-independent manner. Genes Immun. 8 (2), 177–180.

Pennino, D., Bhavsar, P.K., Effner, R., Avitabile, S., Venn, P., Quaranta, M., Marzaioli, V., Cifuentes, L., Durham, S.R., Cavani, A., Eyerich, K., Chung, K.F., Schmidt-Weber, C.B., Eyerich, S., 2013. IL-22 suppresses IFN-γ-mediated lung inflammation in asthmatic patients. J. Allergy Clin. Immunol. 131 (2), 562–570.

Pestka, S., Krause, C.D., Sarkar, D., Walter, M.R., Shi, Y., Fisher, P.B., 2004. Interleukin-10 and related cytokines and receptors. Annu. Rev. Immunol. 22, 929–979.

Pestka, S., Krause, C.D., Walter, M.R., 2004. Interferons, interferon-like cytokines, and their receptors. Immunol. Rev. 202, 8–32.

Petanidis, S., Anestakis, D., Argyraki, M., Hadzopoulou-Cladaras, M., Salifoglou, A., 2013. Differential expression of IL-17, 22, and 23 in the progression of colorectal cancer in patients with K-ras mutation: ras signal inhibition and crosstalk with GM-CSF and IFN-γ. PLoS One 8 (9), e73616.

Petersson, M., Charo, J., Salazar-Onfray, F., Noffz, G., Mohaupt, M., Qin, Z., Klein, G., Blankenstein, T., Kiessling, R., 1998. Constitutive IL-10 production accounts for the high NK sensitivity, low MHC class I expression, and poor transporter associated with antigen processing (TAP)-1/2 function in the prototype NK target YAC-1. J. Immunol. 161 (5), 2099–2105.

Pistoia, V., Jul 1997. Production of cytokines by human B cells in health and disease. Immunol. Today 18 (7), 343–350.

Pittmann, D.D., Goad, B., Lambert, A.J., Clark, E., Tan, X.Y., Spaulding, V., et al., 2011. IL-22 is a tightly-regulated IL-10- like molecule that induces as acute-phase response and renal tubular basophilia. Genes Immun. 2, 172 (Abstr.).

Pockaj, B.A., Basu, G.D., Pathangey, L.B., Gray, R.J., Hernandez, J.L., Gendler, S.J., Mukherjee, P., 2004. Reduced T-cell and dendritic cell function is related to cyclooxygenase–2 overexpression and prostaglandin E2 secretion in patients with breast cancer. Ann. Surg. Oncol. 11 (3), 328–339.

Podojil, J.R., Liu, L.N., Marshall, S.A., Chiang, M.Y., Goings, G.E., Chen, L., Langermann, S., Miller, S.D., Aug 2013. B7–H4Ig inhibits mouse and human T-cell function and treats EAE via IL-10/Treg-dependent mechanisms. J. Autoimmun. 44, 71–81.

Põld, M., Krysan, K., Põld, A., Dohadwala, M., Heuze-Vourc'h, N., Mao, J.T., Riedl, K.L., Sharma, S., Dubinett, S.M., Sep 15, 2004. Cyclooxygenase-2 modulates the insulin-like growth factor axis in non-small-cell lung cancer. Cancer Res. 64 (18), 6549–6555.

Pold, M., Zhu, L.X., Sharma, S., Burdick, M.D., Lin, Y., Lee, P.P., Pxld, A., Luo, J., Krysan, K., Dohadwala, M., Mao, J.T., Batra, R.K., Strieter, R.M., Dubinett, S.M., 2004. Cyclooxygenase-2–dependent expression of angiogenic CXC chemokines ENA–78/CXC Ligand (CXCL) 5 and interleukin-8/CXCL8 in human non–small cell lung cancer. Cancer Res. 64 (5), 1853–1860.

Pooja, S., Chaudhary, P., Nayak, L.V., Rajender, S., Saini, K.S., Deol, D., Kumar, S., Bid, H.K., Konwar, R., 2012. Polymorphic variations in IL-1β, IL-6, and IL-10 genes, their circulating serum levels and breast cancer risk in Indian women. Cytokine 60 (1), 122–128.

Poole, S., Cunha, F.Q., Selkirk, S., Lorenzetti, B.B., Ferreira, S.H., 1995. Cytokine-mediated inflammatory hyperalgesia limited by interleukin-10. Br. J. Pharmacol. 115 (4), 684–688.

Pugh, S., Thomas, G.A., 1994. Patients with adenomatous polyps and carcinomas have increased colonic mucosal prostaglandin E2. Gut 35 (5), 675–678.

Purdue, M.P., Lan, Q., Bagni, R., Hocking, W.G., Baris, D., Reding, D.J., Rothman, N., 2011. Prediagnostic serum levels of cytokines and other immune markers and risk of non–Hodgkin lymphoma. Cancer Res. 71 (14), 4898–4907.

Pyeon, D., Diaz, F.J., Splitter, G.A., 2000. Prostaglandin E(2) increases bovine leukemia virus tax and pol mRNA levels via cyclooxygenase 2: regulation by interleukin-2, interleukin-10, and bovine leukemia virus. J. Virol. 74 (12), 5740–5745.

Qin, W.Z., Chen, L.L., Pan, H.F., Leng, R.X., Zhai, Z.M., Wang, C., Li, R.J., Wang, S., Wang, H.P., Ye, D.Q., 2011. Expressions of IL-22 in circulating CD4+/CD8+ T cells and their correlation with disease activity in SLE patients. Clin. Exp. Med. 11 (4), 245–250.

Qu, X., Yu, J., Bhagat, G., Furuya, N., Hibshoosh, H., Troxel, A., Rosen, J., Eskelinen, E.L., Mizushima, N., Ohsumi,Y., Cattoretti, G., Levine, B., 2003. Promotion of tumorigenesis by heterozygous disruption of the beclin 1 autophagy gene. J. Clin. Invest. 112 (12), 1809–1820.

Rabinovich, A., Medina, L., Piura, B., Huleihel, M., 2010. Expression of IL-10 in human normal and cancerous ovarian tissues and cells. Eur. Cytokine Netw. 21 (2), 122–128.

Radaeva, S., Sun, R., Pan, H.N., Hong, F., Gao, B., 2004. Interleukin 22 (IL-22) plays a protective role in T cell-mediated murine hepatitis: IL-22 is a survival factor for hepatocytes via STAT3 activation. Hepatology 39 (5), 1332–1342.

Rahmani, M., Mayo, M., Dash, R., Sokhi, U.K., Dmitriev, I.P., Sarkar, D., Dent, P., Curiel, D.T., Fisher, P.B., Grant, S., 2010. Melanoma differentiation associated gene-7/interleukin-24 potently induces apoptosis in human myeloid leukemia cells through a process regulated by endoplasmic reticulum stress. Mol. Pharmacol. 78 (6), 1096–1104.

Ramaswamy, K., Kumar, P., He,Y.X., 2000. A role for parasite-induced PGE2 in IL-10-mediated host immunoregulation by skin stage schistosomula of Schistosoma mansoni. J. Immunol. 165 (8), 4567–4574.

Ramesh, R., Ito, I., Gopalan, B., Saito,Y., Mhashilkar,A.M., Chada, S., 2004. Ectopic production of MDA-7/IL-24 inhibits invasion and migration of human lung cancer cells. Mol. Ther. 9 (4), 510–518.

Ramesh, R., Ito, I., Saito,Y.,Wu, Z., Mhashikar,A.M.,Wilson, D.R., Branch, C.D., Roth,J.A., Chada, S., 2004. Local and systemic inhibition of lung tumor growth after nanoparticle-mediated mda-7/IL-24 gene delivery. DNA Cell. Biol. 23 (12), 850–857.

Rasmuson, A., Kock, A., Fuskeveg, O.M., Kruspig, B., Simyn–Santamaria, J., Gogvadze,V., Johnsen,J.I., Kogner, P., Sveinbjornsson, B., 2012. Autocrine prostaglandin E2 signaling promotes tumor cell survival and proliferation in childhood neuroblastoma. PLoS One 7 (1), e29331.

Rico, M.J., Matar, P., Scharovsky, O.G., 2012. Modulation of IL-10/IL-10R expression by mafosfamide, a derivative of 4-hydroxycyclophosphamide, in a rat B-cell lymphoma. Biocell 36 (2), 91–95.

Robek, M.D., Boyd, B.S., Chisari, F.V., 2005. Lambda interferon inhibits hepatitis B and C virus replication. J.Virol. 79 (6), 3851–3854.

Rode, H.J., Janssen, W., Rosen–Wolff, A., Bugert, J.J., Thein, P., Becker,Y., Darai, G., 1993. The genome of equine herpesvirus type 2 harbors an interleukin 10 (IL10)–like gene. Virus Genes 7 (1), 111–116.

Rohrer, J.W., Coggin Jr, J.H., 1995. CD8 T cell clones inhibit antitumor T cell function by secreting IL-10. J. Immunol. 155 (12), 5719–5727.

Romagnani, S., 1995. Biology of human TH1 and TH2 cells. J. Clin. Immunol. 15 (3), 121–129.

Rooney, J.W., Hodge, M.R., McCaffrey, P.G., Rao, A., Glimcher, L.H., 1994. A common factor regulates both Th1- and Th2-specific cytokine gene expression. EMBO J. 13 (3), 625–633.

Rutz, S., Ouyang, W., 2011. Regulation of interleukin-10 and interleukin-22 expression in T helper cells. Curr. Opin. Immunol. 23 (5), 605–612.

Rutz, S., Noubade, R., Eidenschenk, C., Ota, N., Zeng,W., Zheng,Y., Hackney, J., Ding, J., Singh, H., Ouyang,W., 2011.Transcription factor c-Maf mediates the TGF-β-dependent suppression of IL-22 production in T(H)17 cells. Nat. Immunol. 12 (12), 1238–1245.

Rutz, S., Eidenschenk, C., Ouyang,W., 2013. IL-22, not simply a Th17 cytokine. Immunol. Rev. 252 (1), 116–132.

Sa, S.M.,Valdez, P.A.,Wu, J.,Jung, K., Zhong, F., Hall, L., Kasman, I.,Winer, J., Modrusan, Z., Danilenko, D.M., Ouyang,W., 2007.The effects of IL-20 subfamily cytokines on reconstituted human epidermis suggest potential roles in cutaneous innate defense and pathogenic adaptive immunity in psoriasis. J. Immunol. 178 (4), 2229–2240.

Sabat, R., Wallace, E., Endesfelder, S., Wolk, K., 2007. IL-19 and IL-20: two novel cytokines with importance in inflammatory diseases. Expert Opin. Ther. Targets 11 (5), 601–612.

Saeki, T., Mhashilkar, A., Swanson, X., Zou-Yang, X.H., Sieger, K., Kawabe, S., Branch, C.D., Zumstein, L., Meyn, R.E., Roth, J.A., Chada, S., Ramesh, R., 2002. Inhibition of human lung cancer growth following adenovirus-mediated mda-7 gene expression in vivo. Oncogene 21 (29), 4558–4566.

Saeki, T., Mhashilkar, A., Chada, S., Branch, C., Roth, J.A., Ramesh, R., 2000. Tumor-suppressive effects by adenovirus-mediated mda-7 gene transfer in non-small cell lung cancer cell in vitro. Gene Ther. 7 (23), 2051–2057.

Sainz-Perez, A., Gary-Gouy, H., Portier, A., Davi, F., Merle-Beral, H., Galanaud, P., Dalloul, A., 2006. High Mda-7 expression promotes malignant cell survival and p38 MAP kinase activation in chronic lymphocytic leukemia. Leukemia 20 (3), 498–504.

Sainz-Perez, A., Gary-Gouy, H., Gaudin, F., Maarof, G., Marfaing-Koka, A., de Revel, T., Dalloul, A., 2008. IL-24 induces apoptosis of chronic lymphocytic leukemia B cells engaged into the cell cycle through dephosphorylation of STAT3 and stabilization of p53 expression. J. Immunol. 181 (9), 6051–6060.

Saito, Y., Miyahara, R., Gopalan, B., Litvak, A., Inoue, S., Shanker, M., Branch, C.D., Mhashilkar, A.M., Roth, J.A., Chada, S., Ramesh, R., 2005. Selective induction of cell cycle arrest and apoptosis in human prostate cancer cells through adenoviral transfer of the melanoma differentiation-associated-7 (mda-7)/interleukin-24 (IL-24) gene. Cancer Gene Ther. 12 (3), 238–247.

Sakamoto, T., Saito, H., Tatebe, S., Tsujitani, S., Ozaki, M., Ito, H., Ikeguchi, M., 2006. Interleukin-10 expression significantly correlates with minor CD8+ T-cell infiltration and high microvessel density in patients with gastric cancer. Int. J. Cancer 118 (8), 1909–1914.

Sakurai, N., Kuroiwa, T., Ikeuchi, H., Hiramatsu, N., Maeshima, A., Kaneko, Y., Hiromura, K., Nojima, Y., 2008. Expression of IL-19 and its receptors in RA: potential role for synovial hyperplasia formation. Rheumatology (Oxford) 47 (6), 815–820.

Salazar-Onfray, F., Petersson, M., Franksson, L., Matsuda, M., Blankenstein, T., Karre, K., Kiessling, R., 1995. IL-10 converts mouse lymphoma cells to a CTL-resistant, NK-sensitive phenotype with low but peptide-inducible MHC class I expression. J. Immunol. 154 (12), 6291–6298.

Salazar-Onfray, F., Charo, J., Petersson, M., Freland, S., Noffz, G., Qin, Z., Blankenstein, T., Ljunggren, H.G., Kiessling, R., 1997. Down-regulation of the expression and function of the transporter associated with antigen processing in murine tumor cell lines expressing IL-10. J. Immunol. 159 (7), 3195–3202.

Sanda, T., Tyner, J.W., Gutierrez, A., Ngo, V.N., Glover, J., Chang, B.H., Yost, A., Ma, W., Fleischman, A.G., Zhou, W., Yang, Y., Kleppe, M., Ahn, Y., Tatarek, J., Kelliher, M.A., Neuberg, D.S., Levine, R.L., Moriggl, R., Muller, M., Gray, N.S., Jamieson, C.H., Weng, A.P., Staudt, L.M., Druker, B.J., Look, A.T., 2013. TYK2-STAT1-BCL2 pathway dependence in T-cell acute lymphoblastic leukemia. Cancer Discov. 3 (5), 564–577.

Sano, H., Kawahito, Y., Wilder, R.L., Hashiramoto, A., Mukai, S., Asai, K., Kimura, S., Kato, H., Kondo, M., Hla, T., 1995. Expression of cyclooxygenase-1 and -2 in human colorectal cancer. Cancer Res. 55 (17), 3785–3789.

Sarkar, D., Su, Z.Z., Lebedeva, I.V., Sauane, M., Gopalkrishnan, R.V., Valerie, K., Dent, P., Fisher, P.B., 2002. mda-7 (IL-24) Mediates selective apoptosis in human melanoma cells by inducing the coordinated overexpression of the GADD family of genes by means of p38 MAPK. Proc. Natl. Acad. Sci. USA 99 (15), 10054–10059.

Sarkar, D., Su, Z.Z., Vozhilla, N., Park, E.S., Gupta, P., Fisher, P.B., 2005. Dual cancer-specific targeting strategy cures primary and distant breast carcinomas in nude mice. Proc. Natl. Acad. Sci. U S A 102, 14034–14039.

Sarkar, D., Lebedeva, I.V., Su, Z.Z., Park, E.S., Chatman, L.,Vozhilla, N., Dent, P., Curiel, D.T., Fisher, P.B., 2007. Eradication of therapy-resistant human prostate tumors using a cancer terminator virus. Cancer Res. 67 (11), 5434–5442.

Sarris, A.H., Kliche, K.O., Pethambaram, P., Preti, A.,Tucker, S.,Jackow, C., Messina, O., Pugh, W., Hagemeister, F.B., McLaughlin, P., Rodriguez, M.A., Romaguera, J., Fritsche, H., Witzig, T., Duvic, M., Andreeff, M., Cabanillas, F., 1999. Interleukin-10 levels are often elevated in serum of adults with Hodgkin's disease and are associated with inferior failure-free survival. Ann. Oncol. 10 (4), 433–440.

Sato, A., Ohtsuki, M., Hata, M., Kobayashi, E., Murakami, T., 2006. Antitumor activity of IFN-lambda in murine tumor models. J. Immunol. 176 (12), 7686–7694.

Sauane, M., Gopalkrishnan, R.V., Choo, H.T., Gupta, P., Lebedeva, I.V.,Yacoub, A., Dent, P., Fisher, P.B., 2004. Mechanistic aspects of mda-7/IL-24 cancer cell selectivity analysed via a bacterial fusion protein. Oncogene 23 (46), 7679–7690.

Sauane, M., Su, Z.Z., Gupta, P., Lebedeva, I.V., Dent, P., Sarkar, D., Fisher, P.B., 2008. Autocrine regulation of mda-7/IL-24 mediates cancer-specific apoptosis. Proc. Natl. Acad. Sci. USA 105 (28), 9763–9768.

Sauane, M., Su, Z.Z., Dash, R., Liu, X., Norris, J.S., Sarkar, D., Lee, S.G.,Allegood, J.C., Dent, P., Spiegel, S., Fisher, P.B., 2010. Ceramide plays a prominent role in MDA-7/IL-24-induced cancer-specific apoptosis. J. Cell. Physiol. 222 (3), 546–555.

Sauane, M., Gupta, P., Lebedeva, I.V., Su, Z.Z., Sarkar, D., Randolph, A.,Valerie, K., Gopalkrishnan, R.V., Fisher, P.B., 2006. N-glycosylation of MDA-7/IL-24 is dispensable for tumor cell-specific apoptosis and "bystander" antitumor activity. Cancer Res. 66 (24), 11869–11877.

Sauane, M., Gopalkrishnan, R.V., Sarkar, D., Su, Z.Z., Lebedeva, I.V., Dent, P., Pestka, S., Fisher, P.B., 2003. MDA-7/IL-24: novel cancer growth suppressing and apoptosis inducing cytokine. Cytokine Growth Factor Rev. 14 (1), 35–51.

Schraml, B.U., Hildner, K., Ise, W., Lee, W.L., Smith, W.A., Solomon, B., Sahota, G., Sim, J., Mukasa, R., Cemerski, S., Hatton, R.D., Stormo, G.D.,Weaver, C.T., Russell, J.H., Murphy, T.L., Murphy, K.M., 2009. The AP-1 transcription factor Batf controls T(H)17 differentiation. Nature 460 (7253), 405–409.

Segal, B.M., Glass, D.D., Shevach, E.M., 2002. Cutting Edge: IL-10-producing CD4+ T cells mediate tumor rejection. J. Immunol. 168 (1), 1–4.

Seiderer, J., Brand, S., 2009. IL-22: a two-headed cytokine in IBD? Inflamm. Bowel. Dis. 15 (3), 473–474.

Seliger, B., Hohne, A., Knuth, A., Bernhard, H., Meyer, T., Tampe, R., Momburg, F., Huber, C., 1996. Analysis of the major histocompatibility complex class I antigen presentation machinery in normal and malignant renal cells: evidence for deficiencies associated with transformation and progression. Cancer Res. 56 (8), 1756–1760.

Selleri, S., Dieng, M.M., Nicoletti, S., Louis, I., Beausejour, C., Le Deist, F., Haddad, E., 2013. Cord-blood-derived mesenchymal stromal cells downmodulate CD4+ T-cell activation by inducing IL-10-producing Th1 cells. Stem Cells Dev. 22 (7), 1063–1075.

Shanker, M., Gopalan, B., Patel, S., Bocangel, D., Chada, S., Ramesh, R., 2007.Vitamin E succinate in combination with mda-7 results in enhanced human ovarian tumor cell killing through modulation of extrinsic and intrinsic apoptotic pathways. Cancer Lett. 254, 217–226.

Sheikh, F., Baurin,V.V., Lewis-Antes, A., Shah, N.K., Smirnov, S.V.,Anantha, S., Dickensheets, H., Dumoutier, L., Renauld, J.C., Zdanov, A., Donnelly, R.P., Kotenko, S.V., 2004. Cutting edge: IL-26 signals through a novel receptor complex composed of IL-20 receptor-1 and IL-10 receptor-2. J. Immunol. 172, 2006–2010.

Sheppard, P., Kindsvogel, W., Xu, W., Henderson, K., Schlutsmeyer, S.,Whitmore, T.E., Kuestner, R., Garrigues, U., Birks, C., Roraback, J., Ostrander, C., Dong, D., Shin, J., Presnell, S., Fox, B., Haldeman, B., Cooper, E., Taft, D., Gilbert, T., Grant, F.J.,Tackett, M., Krivan, W., McKnight, G., Clegg, C., Foster, D., Klucher, K.M., 2003. IL-28, IL-29 and their class II cytokine receptor IL-28R. Nat. Immunol. 4 (1), 63–68.

Shi, H., Wei, L.L., Yuan, C.F., Yang, J.X., Yi, F.P., Ma, Y.P., Song, F.Z., 2007. Melanoma differentiation-associated gene-7/interleukin 24 inhibits invasion and migration of human cervical cancer cells in vitro. Saudi Med. J. 28 (11), 1671–1675.

Sieger, K.A., Mhashilkar, A.M., Stewart, A., Sutton, R.B., Strube, R.W., Chen, S.Y., Pataer, A., Swisher, S.G., Grimm, E.A., Ramesh, R., Chada, S., 2004. The tumor suppressor activity of MDA-7/IL-24 is mediated by intracellular protein expression in NSCLC cells. Mol. Ther. 9 (3), 355–367.

Silvestre, J.S., Mallat, Z., Duriez, M., Tamarat, R., Bureau, M.F., Scherman, D., Duverger, N., Branellec, D., Tedgui, A., Levy, B.I., 2000. Antiangiogenic effect of interleukin-10 in ischemia-induced angiogenesis in mice hindlimb. Circ. Res. 87 (6), 448–452.

Sonnenberg, G.F., Fouser, L.A., Artis, D., 2010. Functional biology of the IL-22-IL-22R pathway in regulating immunity and inflammation at barrier surfaces. Adv. Immunol. 107, 1–29.

Soria, J.C., Moon, C., Kemp, B.L., Liu, D.D., Feng, L., Tang, X., Chang, Y.S., Mao, L., Khuri, F.R., 2003. Lack of interleukin-10 expression could predict poor outcome in patients with stage I non–small cell lung cancer. Clin. Cancer Res. 9 (5), 1785–1791.

Specht, C., Bexten, S., Kolsch, E., Pauels, H.G., 2001. Prostaglandins, but not tumor–derived IL-10, shut down concomitant tumor-specific CTL responses during murine plasmacytoma progression. Int. J. Cancer 91 (5), 705–712.

Srinivas, S., Dai, J., Eskdale, J., Gallagher, G.E., Megjugorac, N.J., Gallagher, G., 2008. Interferon-lambda1 (interleukin-29) preferentially down-regulates interleukin-13 over other T helper type 2 cytokine responses in vitro. Immunology 125 (4), 492–502.

Srivastava, V., Khanna, M., Sharma, S., Kumar, B., 2012. Resolution of immune response by recombinant transforming growth factor-beta (rTGF-β) during influenza A virus infection. Indian J. Med. Res. 136 (4), 641–648.

St Hill, C.A., 2011. Interactions between endothelial selectins and cancer cells regulate metastasis. Front. Biosci. 16, 323351.

Stanilov, N., Miteva, L., Stankova, N., Jovchev, J., Deliyski, T., Stanilova, S., 2010. Role of IL-12P40 and IL-10 in progression of colorectal cancer. Khirurgiia (Sofiia) (4–5), 26–29. [Article in Bulgarian].

Stasi, R., Zinzani, P.L., Galieni, P., Lauta, V.M., Damasio, E., Dispensa, E., Dammacco, F., Papa, G., Tura, S., 1994. Prognostic value of serum IL-10 and soluble IL-2 receptor levels in aggressive non-Hodgkin's lymphoma. Br. J. Haematol. 88 (4), 770–777.

Stasi, R., Zinzani, L., Galieni, P., Lauta, V.M., Damasio, E., Dispensa, E., Dammacco, F., Tura, S., Papa, G., 1994. Detection of soluble interleukin-2 receptor and interleukin-10 in the serum of patients with aggressive non-Hodgkin's lymphoma. Identification of a subset at high risk of treatment failure. Cancer 74 (6), 1792–1800.

Steensma, D.P., McClure, R.F., Karp, J.E., Tefferi, A., Lasho, T.L., Powell, H.L., DeWald, G.W., Kaufmann, S.H., 2006. JAK2V617F is a rare finding in de novo acute myeloid leukemia, but STAT3 activation is common and remains unexplained. Leukemia 20 (6), 971–978.

Steinke, J.W., Barekzi, E., Hagman, J., Borish, L., Sep 1, 2004. Functional analysis of -571 IL-10 promoter polymorphism reveals a repressor element controlled by sp1. J Immunol 173 (5), 3215–3222.

Stolina, M., Sharma, S., Lin, Y., Dohadwala, M., Gardner, B., Luo, J., Zhu, L., Kronenberg, M., Miller, P.W., Portanova, J., Lee, J.C., Dubinett, S.M., 2000. Specific inhibition of cyclooxygenase 2 restores antitumor reactivity by altering the balance of IL-10 and IL-12 synthesis. J. Immunol. 164 (1), 361–370.

Su, Z.Z., Madireddi, M.T., Lin, J.J., Young, C.S., Kitada, S., Reed, J.C., Goldstein, N.I., Fisher, P.B., 1998. The cancer growth suppressor gene mda-7 selectively induces apoptosis in human breast cancer cells and inhibits tumor growth in nude mice. Proc. Natl. Acad. Sci. USA 95 (24), 14400–14405.

Su, Z.Z., Lebedeva, I.V., Sarkar, D., Emdad, L., Gupta, P., Kitada, S., Dent, P., Reed, J.C., Fisher, P.B., 2006. Ionizing radiation enhances therapeutic activity of mda-7/IL-24: overcoming radiation- and mda-7/IL-24-resistance in prostate cancer cells overexpressing the antiapoptotic proteins bcl-xL or bcl-2. Oncogene 25 (16), 2339–2348.

Su, Z.Z., Lebedeva, I.V., Sarkar, D., Gopalkrishnan, R.V., Sauane, M., Sigmon, C.,Yacoub, A.,Valerie, K., Dent, P., Fisher, P.B., 2003. Melanoma differentiation associated gene-7, mda-7/IL-24, selectively induces growth suppression, apoptosis and radiosensitization in malignant gliomas in a p53-independent manner. Oncogene 22 (8), 1164–1180.

Sugai, H., Kono, K., Takahashi, A., Ichihara, F., Kawaida, H., Fujii, H., Matsumoto, Y., 2004. Characteristic alteration of monocytes with increased intracellular IL-10 and IL-12 in patients with advanced-stage gastric cancer. J. Surg. Res. 116 (2), 277–287.

Sun, Z., Zhang, R.,Wang, H., Jiang, P., Zhang, J., Zhang, M., Gu, L.,Yang, X., Zhang, M., Ji, X., 2012. Serum IL-10 from systemic lupus erythematosus patients suppresses the differentiation and function of monocyte-derived dendritic cells. J. Biomed. Res. 26 (6), 456–466.

Sun,Y.,Wang,Y., Zhao, J., Gu, M., Giscombe, R., Lefvert, A.K.,Wang, X., 2006. B7-H3 and B7-H4 expression in non-small-cell lung cancer. Lung Cancer 53 (2), 143–151.

Sung,W.W.,Wang,Y.C., Lin, P.L., Cheng,Y.W., Chen, C.Y.,Wu,T.C., Lee, H.,Aug 2013. IL-10 promotes tumor aggressiveness via upregulation of CIP2A transcription in lung adenocarcinoma. Clin. Cancer Res. 19 (15), 4092–4103.

Svenson, U., Gronlund, E., Soderstrom, I., Sitaram, R.T., Ljungberg, B., Roos, G., 2013. Telomere length in relation to immunological parameters in patients with renal cell carcinoma. PLoS One 8 (2), e55543.

Svobodova, S.,Topolcan, O., Holubec Jr, L., Levy, M., Pecen, L., Svacina, S., 2011. Parameters of biological activity in colorectal cancer. Anticancer Res. 31 (1), 373–378.

Szaflarska, A., Szczepanik, A., Siedlar, M., Czupryna, A., Sierzega, M., Popiela, T., Zembala, M., 2009. Preoperative plasma level of IL-10 but not of proinflammatory cytokines is an independent prognostic factor in patients with gastric cancer. Anticancer Res. 29 (12), 5005–5012.

Szkaradkiewicz, A., Marciniak, R., Chudzicka–Strugała, I., Wasilewska, A., Drews, M., Majewski, P., Karpiński, T., Zwoździak, B., 2009. Proinflammatory cytokines and IL-10 in inflammatory bowel disease and colorectal cancer patients. Arch. Immunol.Ther. Exp. (Warsz) 57 (4), 291–294.

Tang, J.F., Guan, S.H.,Wang, Z.G., 2012. Roles of interleukin-10 differentiated dendritic cell of allergic asthma patients in T-lymphocyte proliferation in vitro. Zhonghua Yixue Zazhi 92 (40), 2851–2854. [Article in Chinese].

Tang, D., Kang, R., Livesey, K.M., Cheh, C.W., Farkas,A., Loughran, P., Hoppe, G., Bianchi, M.E., Tracey, K.J., Zeh 3rd, H.J., Lotze, M.T., 2010. Endogenous HMGB1 regulates autophagy. J. Cell. Biol. 190 (5), 881–892.

Teloni, R., Giannoni, F., Rossi, P., Nisini, R., Gagliardi, M.C., 2007. Interleukin-4 inhibits cyclo-oxygenase-2 expression and prostaglandin E production by human mature dendritic cells. Immunology 120 (1), 83–89.

Teunissen, M.B., Koomen, C.W., Jansen, J., de Waal Malefyt, R., Schmitt, E.,Van den Wijngaard, R.M., Das, P.K., Bos, J.D., 1997. In contrast to their murine counterparts, normal human keratinocytes and human epidermoid cell lines A431 and HaCaT fail to express IL-10 mRNA and protein. Clin. Exp. Immunol. 107 (1), 213–223.

Tezuka,Y., Endo, S., Matsui, A., Sato, A., Saito, K., Semba, K., Takahashi, M., Murakami, T., 2012. Potential anti-tumor effect of IFN-λ2 (IL-28A) against human lung cancer cells. Lung Cancer 78 (3), 185–192.

Thill, M., Fischer, D., Kelling, K., Hoellen, F., Dittmer, C., Hornemann, A., Salehin, D., Diedrich, K., Friedrich, M., Becker, S., 2010. Expression of vitamin D receptor (VDR), cyclooxygenase–2 (COX-2) and 15-hydroxyprostaglandin dehydrogenase (15-PGDH) in benign and malignant ovarian tissue and 25-hydroxycholecalciferol (25(OH2)D3) and prostaglandin E2 (PGE2) serum level in ovarian cancer patients. J. Steroid Biochem. Mol. Biol. 121 (1–2), 387–390.

Thompson, R.H., Gillett, M.D., Cheville, J.C., Lohse, C.M., Dong, H., Webster, W.S., Krejci, K.G., Lobo, J.R., Sengupta, S., Chen, L., Zincke, H., Blute, M.L., Strome, S.E., Leibovich, B.C., Kwon, E.D., 2004. Costimulatory B7-H1 in renal cell carcinoma patients: Indicator of tumor aggressiveness and potential therapeutic target. Proc. Natl. Acad. Sci. USA 101 (49), 17174–17179.

Thompson, C.L., Plummer, S.J., Tucker, T.C., Casey, G., Li, L., 2010. Interleukin-22 genetic polymorphisms and risk of colon cancer. Cancer Causes Control 21 (8), 1165–1170.

Thomsen, L.L., Miles, D.W., Happerfield, L., Bobrow, L.G., Knowles, R.G., Moncada, S., 1995. Nitric oxide synthase activity in human breast cancer. Br. J. Cancer 72 (1), 41–44.

Thomson, S.J., Goh, F.G., Banks, H., Krausgruber, T., Kotenko, S.V., Foxwell, B.M., Udalova, I.A., 2009. The role of transposable elements in the regulation of IFN-lambda1 gene expression. Proc. Natl. Acad. Sci. USA 106 (28), 11564–11569.

Tian, Y., Sommerville, L.J., Cuneo, A., Kelemen, S.E., Autieri, M.V., 2008. Expression and suppressive effects of interleukin-19 on vascular smooth muscle cell pathophysiology and development of intimal hyperplasia. Am. J. Pathol. 173 (3), 901–909.

Toiyama, Y., Miki, C., Inoue, Y., Minobe, S., Urano, H., Kusunoki, M., 2010. Loss of tissue expression of interleukin-10 promotes the disease progression of colorectal carcinoma. Surg. Today 40 (1), 46–53.

Tong, A.W., Nemunaitis, J., Su, D., Zhang, Y., Cunningham, C., Senzer, N., Netto, G., Rich, D., Mhashilkar, A., Parker, K., Coffee, K., Ramesh, R., Ekmekcioglu, S., Grimm, E.A., van Wart Hood, J., Merritt, J., Chada, S., 2005. Intratumoral injection of INGN 241, a non-replicating adenovector expressing the melanoma-differentiation associated gene-7 (mda-7/IL24): biologic outcome in advanced cancer patients. Mol. Ther. 11 (1), 160–172.

Torres-Poveda, K., Burguete–Garcia, A.I., Cruz, M., Martinez–Nava, G.A., Bahena–Roman, M., Ortiz–Flores, E., Ramirez–Gonzalez, A., Lypez–Estrada, G., Delgado–Romero, K., Madrid–Marina, V., 2012. The SNP at −592 of human IL-10 gene is associated with serum IL-10 levels and increased risk for human papillomavirus cervical lesion development. Infect. Agent. Cancer 7 (1), 32.

Trifari, S., Kaplan, C.D., Tran, E.H., Crellin, N.K., Spits, H., 2009. Identification of a human helper T cell population that has abundant production of interleukin 22 and is distinct from T(H)-17, T(H)1 and T(H)2 cells. Nat. Immunol. 10 (8), 864–871.

Tringler, B., Zhuo, S., Pilkington, G., Torkko, K.C., Singh, M., Lucia, M.S., Heinz, D.E., Papkoff, J., Shroyer, K.R., 2005. B7-h4 is highly expressed in ductal and lobular breast cancer. Clin. Cancer Res. 11 (5), 1842–1848.

Trompezinski, S., Denis, A., Schmitt, D., Viac, J., 2002. IL-10 is unable to downregulate VEGF expression in human activated keratinocytes. Arch. Dermatol. Res. 294 (8), 377–379.

Valdez, P.A., Vithayathil, P.J., Janelsins, B.M., Shaffer, A.L., Williamson, P.R., Datta, S.K., 2012. Prostaglandin E2 suppresses antifungal immunity by inhibiting interferon regulatory factor 4 function andinterleukin-17 expression in T cells. Immunity 36 (4), 668–679.

Valentino, L., Pierre, J., 2006. JAK/STAT signal transduction: regulators and implication in hematological malignancies. Biochem. Pharmacol. 71 (6), 713–721.

Van Belle, A.B., de Heusch, M., Lemaire, M.M., Hendrickx, E., Warnier, G., Dunussi-Joannopoulos, K., Fouser, L.A., Renauld, J.C., Dumoutier, L., 2012. IL-22 is required for imiquimod-induced psoriasiform skin inflammation in mice. J. Immunol. 188 (1), 462–469.

Van Obberghen-Schilling, E., Tucker, R.P., Saupe, F., Gasser, I., Cseh, B., Orend, G., 2011. Fibronectin and tenascin-C: accomplices in vascular morphogenesis during development and tumor growth. Int. J. Dev. Biol. 55 (4–5), 511–525.

Vandenbroeck, K., Cunningham, S., Goris, A., Alloza, I., Heggarty, S., Graham, C., Bell, A., Rooney, M., 2003. Polymorphisms in the interferon-gamma/interleukin-26 gene region contribute to sex bias in susceptibility to rheumatoid arthritis. Arthritis Rheum. 48 (10), 2773–2778.

Vassilakopoulos,T.P., Nadali, G.,Angelopoulou, M.K., Siakantaris, M.P., Dimopoulou, M.N., Kontopidou, F.N., Rassidakis, G.Z., Doussis–Anagnostopoulou, I.A., Hatzioannou, M., Vaiopoulos, G., Kittas, C., Sarris,A.H., Pizzolo, G., Pangalis, G.A., 2001. Serum interleukin-10 levels are an independent prognostic factor for patients with Hodgkin's lymphoma. Haematologica 86 (3), 274–281.

Veldhoen, M., Hirota, K., Christensen,J., O'Garra,A., Stockinger, B., 2009. Natural agonists for aryl hydrocarbon receptor in culture medium are essential for optimal differentiation ofTh17 T cells. J. Exp. Med. 206 (1), 43–49.

Vicari, A.P., Chiodoni, C.,Vaure, C., Ait-Yahia, S., Dercamp, C., Matsos, F., Reynard, O., Taverne, C., Merle, P., Colombo, M.P., O'Garra, A., Trinchieri, G., Caux, C., 2002. Reversal of tumor-induced dendritic cell paralysis by CpG immunostimulatory oligonucleotide and anti-interleukin 10 receptor antibody. J. Exp. Med. 196 (4), 541–549.

Vieira, P., de Waal–Malefyt, R., Dang, M.N., Johnson, K.E., Kastelein, R., Fiorentino, D.F., deVries, J.E., Roncarolo, M.G., Mosmann, T.R., Moore, K.W., 1991. Isolation and expression of human cytokine synthesis inhibitory factor cDNA clones: homology to Epstein–Barr virus open reading frame BCRFI. Proc. Natl. Acad. Sci. USA 88 (4), 1172–1176.

Vieira, P.L., Christensen, J.R., Minaee, S., O'Neill, E.J., Barrat, F.J., Boonstra,A., Barthlott,T., Stockinger, B.,Wraith, D.C., O'Garra, A., 2004. IL-10–secreting regulatory T cells do not express Foxp3 but have comparable regulatory function to naturally occurring CD4+CD25+ regulatory T cells. J. Immunol. 172 (10), 5986–5993.

Vlaeminck-Guillem,V., Bienvenu, J., Isaac, S., Grangier, B., Golfier, F., Passot, G., Bakrin, N., Rodriguez–Lafrasse, C., Gilly, F.N., Glehen, O.,Aug 2013. Intraperitoneal cytokine level in patients with peritoneal surface malignancies.A study of the RENAPE (French Network for Rare Peritoneal Malignancies). Ann. Surg. Oncol. 20 (8), 2655–2662.

Vora, M., Romero, L.I., Karasek, M.A., 1996. Interleukin-10 induces E-selectin on small and large blood vessel endothelial cells. J. Exp. Med. 184 (3), 821–829.

Wang, C., Xue, X.,Yi, J.,Wu, Z., Chen, K., Zheng, J., Ji, W.,Yu,Y., Feb 2008. Replication-incompetent adenovirus vector-mediated MDA-7/IL-24 selectively induces growth suppression and apoptosis of hepatoma cell Line SMMC-7721. J. Huazhong Univ. Sci. Technolog. Med. Sci. 28 (1), 80–83.

Wang, C.J., Xiao, C.W.,You,T.G., Zheng,Y.X., Gao,W., Zhou, Z.Q., Chen,J., Xue, X.B., Fan, J., Zhang, H., 2012. Interferon-alpha enhances antitumor activities of oncolytic adenovirus-mediated IL-24 expression in hepatocellular carcinoma. Mol. Cancer 11 (1), 31.

Wang, D., Dubois, R.N., 2006. Prostaglandins and cancer. Gut 55 (1), 115–122.

Wang, F., Smith, N., Maier, L., Xia,W., Hammerberg, C., Chubb, H., Chen, C., Riblett, M., Johnston, A., Gudjonsson, J.E., Helfrich,Y., Kang, S., Fisher, G.J.,Voorhees, J.J., 2012. Etanercept suppresses regenerative hyperplasia in psoriasis by acutely downregulating epidermal expression of interleukin (IL)-19, IL-20 and IL-24. Br. J. Dermatol. 167 (1), 92–102.

Wang, J., Oberley-Deegan, R.,Wang, S., Nikrad, M., Funk, C.J., Hartshorn, K.L., Mason, R.J., 2009. Differentiated human alveolar type II cells secrete antiviral IL-29 (IFN-lambda 1) in response to influenza A infection. J. Immunol. 182 (3), 1296–1304.

Wang, P.,Wu, P., Siegel, M.I., Egan, R.W., Billah, M.M., 1995. Interleukin (IL)-10 inhibits nuclear factor kappa B (NF kappa B) activation in human monocytes. IL-10 and IL-4 suppress cytokine synthesis by different mechanisms. J. Biol. Chem. 270 (16), 9558–9563.

Wang, Q., Zhu,Y.,Yang, P.,Aug 2013. Is Mda-7/IL-24 a potential target and biomarker for enhancing drug sensitivity in human glioma U87 cell line? Anat. Rec. (Hoboken). 296 (8), 1154–1560. http://dx.doi.org/10.1002/ar.22723.

Wang, R., Lu, M., Zhang, J., Chen, S., Luo, X., Qin,Y., Chen, H., 2011. Increased IL-10 mRNA expression in tumor–associated macrophage correlated with late stage of lung cancer. J. Exp. Clin. Cancer Res. 30, 62.

Wang, Z., Yang, L., Jiang, Y., Ling, Z.Q., Li, Z., Cheng, Y., Huang, H., Wang, L., Pan, Y., Wang, Z., Yan, X., Chen, Y., 2011. High fat diet induces formation of spontaneous liposarcoma in mouse adipose tissue with overexpression of interleukin 22. PLoS One 6 (8), e23737.

Wei, C.C., Chen, W.Y., Wang, Y.C., Chen, P.J., Lee, J.Y., Wong, T.W., Chen, W.C., Wu, J.C., Chen, G.Y., Chang, M.S., Lin, Y.C., 2005. Detection of IL-20 and its receptors on psoriatic skin. Clin. Immunol. 117 (1), 65–72.

Wei, N., Fan, J.K., Gu, J.F., Liu, X.Y., 2010. Double-regulated oncolytic adenovirus-mediated interleukin-24 overexpression exhibits potent antitumor activity on gastric adenocarcinoma. Hum. Gene Ther. 21 (7), 855–864.

Wei, H., Yang, M., Zhao, T., Wang, X., Zhou, H., 2013. Functional expression and characterization of grass carp IL-10: an essential mediator of TGF-β1 immune regulation in peripheral blood lymphocytes. Mol. Immunol. 53 (4), 313–320.

Welling, T.H., Fu, S., Wan, S., Zou, M., Marrero, J.A., 2012. Elevated serum IL-8 is associated with the presence of hepatocellular carcinoma and independently predicts survival. Cancer Invest. 30 (10), 689–697.

Wessells, J., Baer, M., Young, H.A., Claudio, E., Brown, K., Siebenlist, U., Johnson, P.F., 2004. BCL-3 and NF-kappaB p50 attenuate lipopolysaccharide-induced inflammatory responses in macrophages. J. Biol. Chem. 279 (48), 49995–50003.

Witte, K., Gruetz, G., Volk, H.D., Looman, A.C., Asadullah, K., Sterry, W., Sabat, R., Wolk, K., 2009. Despite IFN-lambda receptor expression, blood immune cells, but not keratinocytes or melanocytes, have an impaired response to type III interferons: implications for therapeutic applications of these cytokines. Genes Immun. 10 (8), 702–714.

Wittke, F., Hoffmann, R., Buer, J., Dallmann, I., Oevermann, K., Sel, S., Wandert, T., Ganser, A., Atzpodien, J., 1999. Interleukin 10 (IL-10): an immunosuppressive factor and independent predictor in patients with metastatic renal cell carcinoma. Br. J. Cancer 79 (7–8), 1182–1184.

Wolk, K., Witte, E., Wallace, E., Döcke, W.D., Kunz, S., Asadullah, K., Volk, H.D., Sterry, W., Sabat, R., 2006. IL-22 regulates the expression of genes responsible for antimicrobial defense, cellular differentiation, and mobility in keratinocytes: a potential role in psoriasis. Eur. J. Immunol. 36 (5), 1309–1323.

Wolk, K., Witte, K., Witte, E., Proesch, S., Schulze-Tanzil, G., Nasilowska, K., Thilo, J., Asadullah, K., Sterry, W., Volk, H.D., Sabat, R., 2008. Maturing dendritic cells are an important source of IL-29 and IL-20 that may cooperatively increase the innate immunity of keratinocytes. J. Leukoc. Biol. 83 (5), 1181–1193.

Wolk, K., Kunz, S., Asadullah, K., Sabat, R., 2002. Cutting edge: immune cells as sources and targets of the IL-10 family members? J. Immunol. 168 (11), 5397–5402.

Wu, T., Cui, L., Liang, Z., Liu, C., Liu, Y., Li, J., 2013. Elevated serum IL-22 levels correlate with chemoresistant condition of colorectal cancer. Clin. Immunol. 147 (1), 38–39.

Wu, Q., Yang, Q., Sun, H., Li, M., Zhang, Y., La Cava, A., 2013. Serum IFN-λ1 is abnormally elevated in rheumatoid arthritis patients. Autoimmunity 46 (1), 40–43.

Wu, M.Y., Hill, C.S., 2009. Tgf-beta superfamily signaling in embryonic development and homeostasis. Dev. Cell. 16 (3), 329–343.

Xie, K., Huang, S., Dong, Z., Juang, S.H., Gutman, M., Xie, Q.W., Nathan, C., Fidler, I.J., 1995. Transfection with the inducible nitric oxide synthase gene suppresses tumorigenicity and abrogates metastasis by K-1735 murine melanoma cells. J. Exp. Med. 181 (4), 1333–1343.

Xie, M.H., Aggarwal, S., Ho, W.H., Foster, J., Zhang, Z., Stinson, J., Wood, W.I., Goddard, A.D., Gurney, A.L., Oct 6, 2000. Interleukin (IL)-22, a novel human cytokine that signals through the interferon receptor-related proteins CRF2-4 and IL-22R. J. Biol. Chem. 275 (40), 31335–31339.

Xie, Q., Wang, S.C., Li, J., 2012. Interleukin 22, a potential therapeutic target for rheumatoid arthritis. J. Rheumatol. 39 (11), 2220. author reply 2221.

Xie, Y., Lv, H., Sheng, W., Miao, J., Xiang, J., Yang, J., 2011. Synergistic tumor suppression by adenovirus-mediated inhibitor of growth 4 and interleukin-24 gene cotransfer in hepatocarcinoma cells. Cancer Biother. Radiopharm. 26 (6), 681–695.

Xie, Y., Sheng, W., Xiang, J., Ye, Z., Zhu, Y., Chen, X., Yang, J., 2008. Recombinant human IL-24 suppresses lung carcinoma cell growth via induction of cell apoptosis and inhibition of tumor angiogenesis. Cancer Biother. Radiopharm. 23 (3), 310–320.

Xiong, J., Peng, Z.L., Tan, X., Liu, S.L., 2007. Ad. mda-7/IL-24 construction and expression in infected drug resistant cell line of human ovarian cancer. Sichuan Da Xue Xue Bao Yi Xue Ban 38 (1), 14–17. [Article in Chinese].

Xu, S., Oshima, T., Imada, T., Masuda, M., Debnath, B., Grande, F., Garofalo, A., Neamati, N., 2013. Stabilization of MDA-7/IL-24 for colon cancer therapy. Cancer Lett. 335 (2), 421–430.

Xu, W., Liu, L.Z., Loizidou, M., Ahmed, M., Charles, I.G., 2002. The role of nitric oxide in cancer. Cell. Res. 12 (5–6), 311–320.

Xue, X.B., Zheng, J.W., Wang, C.J., Chen, K., Hu, H.Y., Hu, H., Yu, Y., Wu, Z.D., 2006. Adenovirus vector expressing MDA-7/IL-24 selectively induces growth arrests and apoptosis in human hepatocellular carcinoma cell lines independent of the state of p53 gene. Zhonghua Gan Zang Bing Za Zhi 14 (9), 670–675. [Article in Chinese].

Xue, X.B., Xiao, C.W., Zhang, H., Lu, A.G., Gao, W., Zhou, Z.Q., Guo, X.L., Zhong, M.A., Yang, Y., Wang, C.J., 2010. Oncolytic adenovirus SG600-IL24 selectively kills hepatocellular carcinoma cell lines. World J. Gastroenterol. 16 (37), 4677–4684.

Yacoub, A., Mitchell, C., Brannon, J., Rosenberg, E., Qiao, L., McKinstry, R., Linehan, W.M., Su, Z.S., Sarkar, D., Lebedeva, I.V., Valerie, K., Gopalkrishnan, R.V., Grant, S., Fisher, P.B., Dent, P., 2003. MDA-7 (interleukin-24) inhibits the proliferation of renal carcinoma cells and interacts with free radicals to promote cell death and loss of reproductive capacity. Mol. Cancer Ther. 2 (7), 623–632.

Yacoub, A., Gupta, P., Park, M.A., Rhamani, M., Hamed, H., Hanna, D., Zhang, G., Sarkar, D., Lebedeva, I.V., Emdad, L., Koumenis, C., Curiel, D.T., Grant, S., Fisher, P.B., Dent, P., 2008. Regulation of GST-MDA-7 toxicity in human glioblastoma cells by ERBB1, ERK1/2, PI3K, and JNK1-3 pathway signaling. Mol. Cancer Ther. 7 (2), 314–329.

Yacoub, A., Mitchell, C., Lebedeva, I.V., Sarkar, D., Su, Z.Z., McKinstry, R., Gopalkrishnan, R.V., Grant, S., Fisher, P.B., Dent, P., 2003. mda-7 (IL-24) Inhibits growth and enhances radiosensitivity of glioma cells in vitro via JNK signaling. Cancer Biol. Ther. 2 (4), 347–353.

Yacoub, A., Mitchell, C., Hong, Y., Gopalkrishnan, R.V., Su, Z.Z., Gupta, P., Sauane, M., Lebedeva, I.V., Curiel, D.T., Mahasreshti, P.J., Rosenfeld, M.R., Broaddus, W.C., James, C.D., Grant, S., Fisher, P.B., Dent, P., 2004. MDA-7 regulates cell growth and radiosensitivity in vitro of primary (non-established) human glioma cells. Cancer Biol. Ther. 3 (8), 739–751.

Yacoub, A., Hamed, H.A., Allegood, J., Mitchell, C., Spiegel, S., Lesniak, M.S., Ogretmen, B., Dash, R., Sarkar, D., Broaddus, W.C., Grant, S., Curiel, D.T., Fisher, P.B., Dent, P., 2010. PERK-dependent regulation of ceramide synthase 6 and thioredoxin play a key role in mda-7/IL-24-induced killing of primary human glioblastoma multiforme cells. Cancer Res. 70 (3), 1120–1129.

Yacoub, A., Hamed, H., Emdad, L., Dos Santos, W., Gupta, P., Broaddus, W.C., Ramakrishnan, V., Sarkar, D., Shah, K., Curiel, D.T., Grant, S., Fisher, P.B., Dent, P., 2008. MDA-7/IL-24 plus radiation enhance survival in animals with intracranial primary human GBM tumors. Cancer Biol. Ther. 7 (6), 917–933.

Yacoub, A., Mitchell, C., Lister, A., Lebedeva, I.V., Sarkar, D., Su, Z.Z., Sigmon, C., McKinstry, R., Ramakrishnan, V., Qiao, L., Broaddus, W.C., Gopalkrishnan, R.V., Grant, S., Fisher, P.B., Dent, P., 2003. Melanoma differentiation-associated 7 (interleukin 24) inhibits growth and enhances radiosensitivity of glioma cells in vitro and in vivo. Clin. Cancer Res. 9 (9), 3272–3281.

Yacoub, A., Park, M.A., Gupta, P., Rahmani, M., Zhang, G., Hamed, H., Hanna, D., Sarkar, D., Lebedeva, I.V., Emdad, L., Sauane, M., Vozhilla, N., Spiegel, S., Koumenis, C., Graf, M., Curiel, D.T., Grant, S., Fisher, P.B., Dent, P., 2008. Caspase-, cathepsin-, and PERK-dependent regulation of MDA-7/IL-24-induced cell killing in primary human glioma cells. Mol. Cancer Ther. 7 (2), 297–313.

Yalcin, A.D., Bisgin, A., Gorczynski, R.M., 2012. IL-8, IL-10, TGF-β, and GCSF levels were increased in severe persistent allergic asthma patients with the anti-IgE treatment. Mediators Inflamm. 2012, 720976.

Yan, S., Zhang, H., Xie, Y., Sheng, W., Xiang, J., Ye, Z., Chen, W., Yang, J., 2010. Recombinant human interleukin-24 suppresses gastric carcinoma cell growth in vitro and in vivo. Cancer Invest. 28 (1), 85–93.

Yan, Y., Zhang, J., Liu, Y., Zhu, T., Yuan, L., Ge, Y., Ding, H., Bu, X., 2013. Inhibition of lung adenocarcinoma transfected with interleukin 28A recombinant adenovirus (Ad-mIFN-λ2) in vivo. Cancer Biother. Radiopharm. 28 (2), 124–130.

Yang, S., Wang, X., Contino, G., Liesa, M., Sahin, E., Ying, H., Bause, A., Li, Y., Stommel, J.M., Dell'antonio, G., Mautner, J., Tonon, G., Haigis, M., Shirihai, O.S., Doglioni, C., Bardeesy, N., Kimmelman, A.C., 2011. Pancreatic cancers require autophagy for tumor growth. Genes Dev. 25 (7), 717–729.

Yang, X., Zheng, S.G., Jan 10, 2014. Interleukin-22: A likely target for treatment of autoimmune diseases. Autoimmun. Rev.. 13 (6), 615–620.

Yang, C., Tong, Y., Ni, W., Liu, J., Xu, W., Li, L., Liu, X., Meng, H., Qian, W., 2010. Inhibition of autophagy induced by overexpression of mda-7/interleukin-24 strongly augments the antileukemia activity in vitro and in vivo. Cancer Gene Ther. 17 (2), 109–119.

Yang, K., Puel, A., Zhang, S., Eidenschenk, C., Ku, C.L., Casrouge, A., Picard, C., von Bernuth, H., Senechal, B., Plancoulaine, S., Al-Hajjar, S., Al-Ghonaium, A., Maródi, L., Davidson, D., Speert, D., Roifman, C., Garty, B.Z., Ozinsky, A., Barrat, F.J., Coffman, R.L., Miller, R.L., Li, X., Lebon, P., Rodriguez-Gallego, C., Chapel, H., Geissmann, F., Jouanguy, E., Casanova, J.L., 2005. Human TLR-7-, -8-, and -9-mediated induction of IFN-alpha/beta and -lambda Is IRAK-4 dependent and redundant for protective immunity to viruses. Immunity 23 (5), 465–478.

Yao, S., Wang, S., Zhu, Y., Luo, L., Zhu, G., Flies, S., Xu, H., Ruff, W., Broadwater, M., Choi, I.H., Tamada, K., Chen, L., 2009. PD-1 on dendritic cells impedes innate immunity against bacterial infection. Blood 113 (23), 5811–5818.

Ye, Z.J., Zhou, Q., Yin, W., Yuan, M.L., Yang, W.B., Xiang, F., Zhang, J.C., Xin, J.B., Xiong, X.Z., Shi, H.Z., 2012. Interleukin 22-producing CD4+ T cells in malignant pleural effusion. Cancer Lett. 326 (1), 23–32.

Yi, K.H., Chen, L., 2009. Fine tuning the immune response through B7-H3 and B7-H4. Immunol. Rev. 229 (1), 145–151.

Yi, Y., He, H.W., Wang, J.X., Cai, X.Y., Li, Y.W., Zhou, J., Cheng, Y.F., Jin, J.J., Fan, J., Qiu, S.J., 2013. The functional impairment of HCC-infiltrating γδ T cells, partially mediated by regulatory T cells in a TGFβ- and IL-10–dependent manner. J. Hepatol. 58 (5), 977–983.

Ying, H., Da, L., Yu-Xiu, S., Yu, X., Li-Xia, L., Li-Mei, X., Wei-Dong, R., Oct 2013. TLR4 mediates MAPK-STAT3 axis activation in bladder epithelial cells. Inflammation. 36 (5), 1064–1074.

Yoon, S.I., Logsdon, N.J., Sheikh, F., Donnelly, R.P., Walter, M.R., 2006. Conformational changes mediate interleukin-10 receptor 2 (IL-10R2) binding to IL-10 and assembly of the signaling complex. J. Biol. Chem. 281, 35088–35096.

Yoon, S.I., Jones, B.C., Logsdon, N.J., Harris, B.D., Deshpande, A., Radaeva, S., Halloran, B.A., Gao, B., Walter, M.R., 2010. Structure and mechanism of receptor sharing by the IL-10R2 common chain. Structure 18 (5), 638–648.

You, W., Tang, Q., Zhang, C., Wu, J., Gu, C., Wu, Z., Li, X., May 21, 2013. IL-26 promotes the proliferation and survival of human gastric cancer cells by regulating the balance of STAT1 and STAT3 activation. PLoS One 8 (5), e63588.

Yu, J., Hui, A.Y., Chu, E.S., Cheng, A.S., Go, M.Y., Chan, H.L., Leung, W.K., Cheung, K.F., Ching, A.K., Chui, Y.L., Chan, K.K., Sung, J.J., 2007. Expression of a cyclo–oxygenase–2 transgene in murine liver causes hepatitis. Gut 56 (7), 991–999.

Yue, F.Y., Dummer, R., Geertsen, R., Hofbauer, G., Laine, E., Manolio, S., Burg, G., 1997. Interleukin-10 is a growth factor for human melanoma cells and down-regulates HLA class–I, HLA class–II and ICAM-1 molecules. Int. J. Cancer 71 (4), 630–637.

Yuzhalin, A., 2011. The role of interleukin DNA polymorphisms in gastric cancer. Hum. Immunol. 72 (11), 1128–1136.

Yuzhalin, A.E., Kutikhin, A.G., 2012. Interleukin-12: clinical usage and molecular markers of cancer susceptibility. Growth Factors 30 (3), 176–191.

Zang, X., Thompson, R.H., Al-Ahmadie, H.A., Serio, A.M., Reuter, V.E., Eastham, J.A., Scardino, P.T., Sharma, P., Allison, J.P., 2007. B7–H3 and B7x are highly expressed in human prostate cancer and associated with disease spread and poor outcome. Proc. Natl. Acad. Sci. U S A 104 (49), 19458–19463.

Zdanov, A., 2010. Structural analysis of cytokines comprising the IL-10 family. Cytokine Growth Factor Rev. 21 (5), 325–330.

Zdanov, A., Schalk–Hihi, C., Gustchina, A., Tsang, M., Weatherbee, J., Wlodawer, A., 1995. Crystal structure of interleukin-10 reveals the functional dimer with an unexpected topological similarity to interferon gamma. Structure (Lond) 3, 591–601.

Zdanov, A., Schalk–Hihi, C., Menon, S., Moore, K.W., Wlodawer, A., 1997. Crystal structure of Epstein–Barr virus protein BCRF1, a homolog of cellular interleukin–10. J. Mol. Biol. 268, 460–467.

Zeidler, R., Eissner, G., Meissner, P., Uebel, S., Tampe, R., Lazis, S., Hammerschmidt, W., 1997. Downregulation of TAP1 in B lymphocytes by cellular and Epstein–Barr virus-encoded interleukin–10. Blood 90 (6), 2390–2397.

Zenewicz, L.A., Yancopoulos, G.D., Valenzuela, D.M., Murphy, A.J., Karow, M., Flavell, R.A., 2007. Interleukin-22 but not interleukin-17 provides protection to hepatocytes during acute liver inflammation. Immunity 27 (4), 647–659.

Zeng, L., O'Connor, C., Zhang, J., Kaplan, A.M., Cohen, D.A., 2010. IL-10 promotes resistance to apoptosis and metastatic potential in lung tumor cell lines. Cytokine 49 (3), 294–302.

Zhang, L., Li, J.M., Liu, X.G., Ma, D.X., Hu, N.W., Li, Y.G., Li, W., Hu, Y., Yu, S., Qu, X., Yang, M.X., Feng, A.L., Wang, G.H., 2011. Elevated Th22 cells correlated with Th17 cells in patients with rheumatoid arthritis. J Clin. Immunol. 31 (4), 606–614.

Zhang, W., Chen, Y., Wei, H., Zheng, C., Sun, R., Zhang, J., Tian, Z., 2008. Antiapoptotic activity of autocrine interleukin-22 and therapeutic effects of interleukin-22-small interfering RNA on human lung cancer xenografts. Clin. Cancer Res. 14 (20), 6432–6439.

Zhao, Y., Li, Z., Sheng, W., Miao, J., Yang, J., 2012. Adenovirus-mediated ING4/IL-24 double tumor suppressor gene co-transfer enhances antitumor activity in human breast cancer cells. Oncol. Rep. 28 (4), 1315–1324.

Zhao, L., Jiang, Z., Jiang, Y., Ma, N., Wang, K., Zhang, Y., Feng, L., 2013. IL-22+CD4+ T-cells in patients with active systemic lupus erythematosus. Exp. Biol. Med. (Maywood) 238 (2), 193–199.

Zhao, L., Yang, J., Wang, H.P., Liu, R.Y., 2013. Imbalance in the Th17/Treg and cytokine environment in peripheral blood of patients with adenocarcinoma and squamous cell carcinoma. Med. Oncol. 30 (1), 461.

Zheng, L.M., Ojcius, D.M., Garaud, F., Roth, C., Maxwell, E., Li, Z., Rong, H., Chen, J., Wang, X.Y., Catino, J.J., King, I., 1996. Interleukin-10 inhibits tumor metastasis through an NK cell–dependent mechanism. J. Exp. Med. 184 (2), 579–584.

Zheng, M., Bocangel, D., Doneske, B., Mhashilkar, A., Ramesh, R., Hunt, K.K., Ekmekcio-glu, S., Sutton, R.B., Poindexter, N., Grimm, E.A., Chada, S., 2007. Human interleukin 24 (MDA-7/IL-24) protein kills breast cancer cells via the IL-20 receptor and is antago-nized by IL-10. Cancer Immunol. Immunother. 56, 205–215.

Zhong, S., Yu, D., Wang, Y., Qiu, S., Wu, S., Liu, X.Y., 2010. An armed oncolytic adenovirus ZD55-IL-24 combined with ADM or DDP demonstrated enhanced antitumor effect in lung cancer. Acta Oncol. 49 (1), 91–99.

Zhou, Z., Hamming, O.J., Ank, N., Paludan, S.R., Nielsen, A.L., Hartmann, R., 2007. Type III interferon (IFN) induces a type I IFN-like response in a restricted subset of cells through signaling pathways involving both the Jak-STAT pathway and the mitogen-activated protein kinases. J. Virol. 81 (14), 7749–7758.

Zhou, L., Li, J., Wang, X., Ye, L., Hou, W., Ho, J., Li, H., Ho, W., 2011. IL-29/IL-28A suppress HSV-1 infection of human NT2-N neurons. J. Neurovirol. 17 (3), 212–219.

Zhu, X., Ying, L.S., Xu, S.H., Zhu, C.H., Xie, J.B., 2010. Clinicopathologic and prognostic significance of serum levels of cytokines in patients with advanced serous ovarian cancer prior to surgery. Zhonghua Bing Li Xue Za Zhi 39 (10), 666–670. [Article in Chinese].

Zhu, Y., Lv, H., Xie, Y., Sheng, W., Xiang, J., Yang, J., 2011. Enhanced tumor suppression by an ING4/IL-24 bicistronic adenovirus-mediated gene cotransfer in human non-small cell lung cancer cells. Cancer Gene Ther. 18 (9), 627–636.

Zhu, W., Wei, L., Zhang, H., Chen, J., Qin, X., 2012. Oncolytic adenovirus armed with IL-24 inhibits the growth of breast cancer in vitro and in vivo. J. Exp. Clin. Cancer Res. 31, 51.

Zhuang, Y., Peng, L.S., Zhao, Y.L., Shi, Y., Mao, X.H., Guo, G., Chen, W., Liu, X.F., Zhang, J.Y., Liu, T., Luo, P., Yu, P.W., Zou, Q.M., 2012. Increased intratumoral IL-22-producing CD4(+) T cells and Th22 cells correlate with gastric cancer progression and predict poor patient survival. Cancer Immunol. Immunother. 61 (11), 1965–1975.

Ziegler-Heitbrock, L., Lotzerich, M., Schaefer, A., Werner, T., Frankenberger, M., Benkhart, E., 2003. IFN-alpha induces the human IL-10 gene by recruiting both IFN regulatory factor 1 and Stat3. J. Immunol. 171 (1), 285–290.

Ziesché, E., Bachmann, M., Kleinert, H., Pfeilschifter, J., Mühl, H., 2007. The interleukin-22/STAT3 pathway potentiates expression of inducible nitric-oxide synthase in human colon carcinoma cells. J. Biol. Chem. 282 (22), 16006–16015.

Zitzmann, K., Brand, S., Baehs, S., Göke, B., Meinecke, J., Spöttl, G., Meyer, H., Auernham-mer, C.J., 2006. Novel interferon-lambdas induce antiproliferative effects in neuroendo-crine tumor cells. Biochem. Biophys. Res. Commun. 344 (4), 1334–1341.

Zou, W., 2005. Immunosuppressive networks in the tumour environment and their thera-peutic relevance. Nat. Rev. Cancer 5 (4), 263–274.

CHAPTER 7

Interleukin-12 Superfamily and Cancer

The scientist does not study nature because it is useful; he studies it because he delights in it, and he delights in it because it is beautiful. If nature were not beautiful, it would not be worth knowing, and if nature were not worth knowing, life would not be worth living.

Henri Poincaré, French mathematician (1854–1912)

7.1 MIGHTY INTERLEUKIN-12. ATTRACTIVE CANDIDATE FOR CANCER TREATMENT?

7.1.1 Brief Description of IL-12 and Its Anticancer Properties

In 1989, a research group headed by Giorgio Trinchieri identified and purified a previously unknown molecule from the conditioned medium of B-lymphoblastoid cell line (Kobayashi et al., 1989). This 70-kDa molecule was named natural killer cell stimulatory factor (NKSF) because of its ability to enhance NK-cell-mediated cytotoxicity. When it became clear that NKSF belongs to the family of interleukins (ILs), it was renamed IL-12. This novel IL was described as a disulfide-bonded heterodimer, comprising two subunits, namely, the light 35-kDa chain (IL-12A) and the heavy 40 kDa chain (IL-12B). Additionally, the IL-12 family includes other heterodimeric cytokines, such as IL-23, IL-27, and IL-35, whose subunits consist of either or both the light and heavy chains as well (Abbas et al., 2011). The biological response of IL-12 is mediated by the IL-12 receptor (IL-12R), which is also a heterodimer, formed by IL-12R-b1 and IL-12R-b2 subunits (Wang et al., 2000). Upon binding, IL-12R-b2 is tyrosine phosphorylated and provides binding sites for the Tyk2 and Jak2 kinases, which subsequently trigger the transcription factors signal transducer and activator of transcription (STAT)3 and STAT4. Activated STATs dissociate from the receptor and form dimers before translocating to the nucleus, where they regulate the transcription of selected genes (Wang et al., 2000). IL-12 is produced in response to antigenic stimulation mainly by macrophages, human B-lymphoblastoid, and dendritic cells, and possesses an enormous variety of functions that are obligatory for the implementation of an effective immune response. First, IL-12 upregulates interferon gamma (IFN-γ) synthesis by

223

NK cells and T cells; simultaneously, it downregulates the IL-4-mediated suppression of IFN-γ production by other immune cells (Gately et al., 1998; Kobayashi et al., 1989). This property of IL-12 is of paramount importance, as IFN-γ induces a strong protection against cancer development (Ikeda et al., 2002). Particularly, IFN-γ stimulates endothelial cells, monocytes, and fibroblasts to produce chemokines with antiangiogenic activity, such as CXCL9 (Mig) and CXCL10 (IP-10) (Sgadari et al., 1996). It was found that in vivo treatment with IL-12 results in the expression of CXCL10 and CXCL9 genes in cancer cells, thereby preventing the formation of new vessels surrounding the tumor (Kanegane et al., 1998). In addition, the IL-12-induced synthesis of IFN-γ results in an increase in the activity of p53, which subsequently leads to tumor suppression due to the induction of apoptosis in cancer cells (Takaoka et al., 2003). IFN therapy has long been used as a treatment for many cancers, including leukemia and various lymphomas, such as hairy cell leukemia, chronic myeloid leukemia, nodular lymphoma, and cutaneous T-cell lymphoma (Goldstein and Laszlo, 1988). Therefore, the IL-12-driven increase in IFN-γ synthesis may provide a timely and efficient anticancer immune response.

Aside from the upregulation of IFN-γ expression, IL-12 has been reported to stimulate the secretion of the IFN regulatory factors 1 (IRF1) and 4 (IRF4), which are compulsory for the differentiation of Th1 cells (Lehtonen et al., 2003). Contemporary research on IRF1 has shown its tumor suppressor activities in the breast cancer cell line in vitro (Bouker et al., 2005). Moreover, it has been demonstrated that IRF1 is able to decrease the tumorigenicity of cells inoculated into athymic nude mice (Bowie et al., 2008). Likewise, IRF4 has recently been found to inhibit BCR/ABL-induced B-cell acute lymphoblastic leukemia and c-Myc-induced leukemia in animal models (Acquaviva et al., 2008; Pathak et al., 2011).

Furthermore, IL-12 is known to upregulate the expression of the IL-2 receptor (IL-2R), whose production at a sufficient amount is mandatory for the development of an effective anticancer immune response, especially during IL-2 immunotherapy (Yanagida et al., 1994). Another significant feature of IL-12 is that it starts the development of a protective Th1-cell-mediated immune response due to the triggering of the transcription of IL-12RB2 and IL-18 receptor 1 (IL-18RB1) (Yoshimoto et al., 1998; Nakahira et al., 2001; Becskei and Grusby, 2007). Thus, an IL-12-mediated Th1 immune response results in the triggering of antigen-specific cytotoxic T lymphocytes (CTLs) that induce apoptosis in cancer cells by displaying specific antigens on their surface (Yoshimoto et al., 1998; Nakahira et al., 2001; Becskei and Grusby, 2007). In addition, it has been recently reported that IL-12 triggers the expression of the Fas ligand within immune cells, thereby stimulating their antitumor activity (Kerkar et al., 2013). Lastly, IL-12 is known to stimulate the proliferation of T cells by recruiting STAT4 and the transcription factor c-Jun to the promoter of the IL-2R (Yanagida et al., 1994; Foukas et al., 2004) and to enhance lymphocytes to downregulate the secretion of vascular endothelial growth factor (VEGF) in tumor cells, which can be considered as another major mechanism of the IL-12-driven inhibition of angiogenesis (Cavallo et al., 2001).

Certainly, the signaling pathways of IL-12 utterly highlight the potential of this cytokine as a rational candidate for antitumor therapies (Figure 7.1).

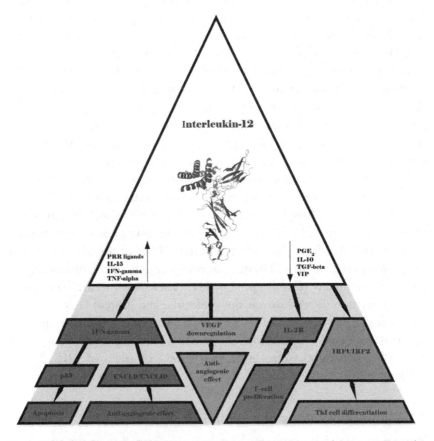

Figure 7.1 IL-12 signaling pathways involved in antitumor immune response. (For color version of this figure, the reader is referred to the online version of this book.)

7.1.2 Regulation of IL-12 Production

It is important to understand that healthy cells and tissues should either contain small amounts of IL-12 or not contain it at all. The synthesis of IL-12 is generally triggered by pattern recognition receptors (toll-like receptors, RIG-I-like receptors, C-type lectin receptors, and NOD-like receptors) that recognize structurally conserved molecules derived from microorganisms, named pathogen-associated molecular patterns (PAMPs) (Abbas et al., 2011). The most common PAMPs include lipopolysaccharide (LPS), flagellin, lipoteichoic acid, and peptidoglycan. Furthermore, the secretion of IL-12 can be triggered by IL-15 and IFN-γ produced by NK cells and/or T cells in a positive-feedback-loop manner (Kuwajima et al., 2006; Abbas et al., 2011). Furthermore, it has been recently discovered that the signal peptide peptidase homologs, SPPL2a and SPPL2b, stimulate the release of the tumor necrosis factor alpha (TNF-α) intracellular domain, which in turn promotes the production of IL-12 by activated dendritic cells (Friedmann et al., 2006). Additionally, it is necessary to mention some agents that have been reported to downregulate IL-12 synthesis. Mitsuhashi et al. (2004) demonstrated that prostaglandin E2 (PGE$_2$) secreted by cancer cells or tumor-associated host cells (macrophages, stromal cells, and endothelial cells) suppress the transcription of IL-12. Recently, several research groups have discovered that the vasoactive intestinal peptide, a neuropeptide presented in the nervous system and a ligand for G-protein-coupled receptors, suppresses the synthesis of IL-12 in macrophages triggered with bacterial antigens in a cyclic adenosine 3',5'-monophosphate-dependent manner (Xin and Sriram, 1998; Delgado and Ganea, 1999). Lastly, some immunosuppressive factors such as IL-10 and transforming growth factor-β (TGF-β) are able to inhibit the production of the IL-12 light or heavy chains, thereby contributing to tumor development (Cavallo et al., 2001). Therefore, the mechanisms of IL-12 regulation depend on various molecular and protein factors, which may alter the effectiveness of IL-12 during antitumor immune responses, and it is reasonable to consider them when forming study designs for further experiments on evaluating the impact of IL-12 on carcinogenesis.

7.1.3 Immunobiology of IL-12 in Tumor Models

Numerous animal experiments have been performed to analyze the role of IL-12 in carcinogenesis (Ma and Trinchieri, 2001). Boggio et al. (2000)

demonstrated that the administration of IL-12 to young BALB–NeuT mice carrying the activated Her-2/neu oncogene delayed the appearance of tumors and reduced the number of mammary glands involved. Moreover, the authors indicated a 50% decrease in tumor incidence across IL-12-treated FVB–NeuN mice carrying the HER-2/neu protooncogene. Next, Noguchi et al. (1996) revealed that IL-12 inhibited the carcinogenesis of 3-methylcholanthrene in mice via the release of cytokines, mediators, and nonspecific immune mechanisms. Nanni et al. (2001) demonstrated that IL-12 alone produced a significant delay in tumor latency and a dramatic reduction in tumor multiplicity across tumor-prone BALB–NeuT mice, but it did not affect tumor incidence. In addition, the combination of an allogeneic cell vaccine (Neu/H-2q cells expressing high surface levels of both p185neu and H-2q class I molecules) with systemic IL-12 prevented the onset of mammary carcinoma: mouse lifespan was more than doubled, whereas the quality of life was not impaired. In addition, this combined treatment elicited a marked specific humoral immune response. Anti-p185neu antibodies in the sera of treated mice may impair carcinogenesis by inducing a functional block of p185neu receptor function, downregulating its expression on the cell membrane, and impeding its ability to form the homodimer or heterodimer that spontaneously transduce proliferative signals to the cells (Nanni et al., 2001). A series of experiments, conducted by different groups (Brunda et al., 1993; Nastala et al., 1994; Hill et al., 2002; Hess et al., 2003; Nair et al., 2006), indicated that the injection of IL-12 directly into subcutaneous tumors resulted in a vigorous NK and cytotoxic T-cell response against the tumor and metastases in mice. Next, the antiangiogenic properties of IL-12 were observed by Voest et al. (1995), who demonstrated that IL-12 treatment almost completely inhibited corneal neovascularization in immunocompetent C57BL/6 mice, severe combined immune-deficient mice, NK-cell-deficient beige mice, and T-cell-deficient nude mice. Later, Sgadari et al. (1996) replicated this finding. Recently, Watkins et al. (2007, 2009) discovered that IL-12 dramatically decreased tumor-supportive activities of tumor-associated macrophages (TAMs), which are involved in tumor angiogenesis as well as in the initiation and progression of metastasis (van-Netten et al., 1993; Sunderkotter et al., 1994). Apparently, IL-12 is able to somehow reprogram TAMs from a tumor-supportive and immunosuppressive functional phenotype to an inflammatory tumor-suppressive phenotype (Watkins et al., 2007, 2009). However, it should be noted that the fundamental

IL-12 mechanisms that influence TAMs remain obscure and require further investigations.

7.1.4 Clinical Trials, Gene Therapy, and Further Prospects

Thus, the majority of experimental data suggest that IL-12 plays a crucial role in the anticancer immune response. However, clinical experience with IL-12 in humans is limited. First, several experiments in nonhuman primate tumor models revealed adverse side effects with IL-12 administration, including prominent hyperplasia of hematopoietic and lymphohistiocytic tissues, reversible thrombocytopenia, and anemia (Bree et al., 1994; Sarmiento et al., 1994). IL-12 has shown some clinical activity in phase I clinical trials conducted by Portielje et al. (1999). Administration of IL-12 resulted in the stabilization of disease in several renal cancer patients and partial regression of a metastatic lesion, but it has not proceeded further in clinical development due to toxicities, including fever, vomiting, mental depression, leukopenia, oral mucositis, and elevation of hepatic enzymes (Portielje et al., 1999). Motzer et al. (2001) reported that the clinical trials of IL-12 administration were closed to accrual based on the low-response proportion (only two patients out of 30 had a positive response). Likewise, the clinical trials of IL-12 administration in combination with rituximab in patients with B-cell non-Hodgkin lymphoma (NHL) have not progressed beyond phase I (Ansell et al., 2002). According to a phase I clinical study conducted by Parihar et al. (2004), the addition of IL-12 to trastuzumab therapy did not appear to enhance the efficacy of this antibody treatment. However, the authors indicated that there was one complete response in a patient with HER3[+] breast cancer metastatic to the axillary, mediastinal, and supraclavicular nodes, and two patients with stabilization of bone disease lasting 10–12 months (Parihar et al., 2004). Atkins et al. (1997) performed a phase I trial of IL-12 administration in patients with advanced colorectal cancer (CRC), melanoma, and renal cell carcinoma. Of the 37 enrolled cases, the authors indicated only one partial response (renal cell cancer) and one transient complete response (melanoma), both in previously untreated patients. However, toxicities such as fever/chills, fatigue, nausea, vomiting, and headache were common in this study. Nevertheless, several clinical studies revealed bright results with IL-12 administration. Younes et al. (2004) showed that during IL-12 treatment in patients with NHL, 21% of the patients had a partial or complete response with no evident side effects, except flu-like symptoms. Similarly, Rook et al. (1999) demonstrated that a subcutaneous dosing resulted in complete responses in

56% of the treated patients with cutaneous T-cell lymphoma with minor adverse effects observed (fever, headache). Furthermore, clinical trials on metastatic melanoma revealed that IL-12 administration induces tumor shrinkage, boosts the frequency of circulating antitumor cytotoxic lymphocytes, and enhances the expression of ligand receptor pairs contributing to the lymphocyte function-associated antigen-1/intercellular cell adhesion molecule (ICAM-1), very late antigen-4/vascular cell adhesion molecule 1, and cutaneous lymphocyte antigen/E-selectin adhesion pathways (Bajetta et al., 1998; Mortarini et al., 2000). Accordingly, the current clinical application of IL-12 is limited due to the toxicity or low efficacy of this cytokine against certain tumors. It is necessary to mention the investigations of Lenzi et al. (2002) and Weiss et al. (2003), who conducted locoregional tumor treatment with IL-12 in an effort to prevent toxicities emerging after the systematic administration of this cytokine; however, they both failed to demonstrate any positive effect.

To conclude, the low efficacy of IL-12 in the above-mentioned clinical investigations may be due to an immune suppression-dominated microenvironment in advanced tumors (Beyer and Schultze, 2006); the immunosuppressive effects of other cytokines involved in the immune response, especially those induced by IL-12 such as IL-10 (Meyaard et al., 1996); environmental and dietary factors that may alter the effectiveness of anticancer immunity across enrolled participants; differences in the sample size/age/gender/ethnic/racial differences; and chance. Currently, the development of new experimental drugs based on IL-12 is ongoing with the key focus of reducing observed toxicities and side effects. In July 2011, the National Institutes of Health approved the phase I clinical trials of the new experimental drug NHS-IL-12 for the treatment of solid tumors. The investigational hypothesis is to reduce the toxicity associated with the systemic administration of recombinant human IL-12 by selectively targeting the IL-12 delivery to tumors (http://clinicaltrials.gov/ct2/show/NCT01417546). The new NHS-IL-12 immunomodulator is composed of two IL-12 heterodimers, each fused to one of the H-chains of the NHS76 antibody, which has an affinity for both single-stranded and double-stranded DNA. Thus, NHS-IL-12 targets delivery to regions of tumor necrosis where DNA has become exposed. Potentially, the administration of NHS-IL-12 would help to avoid unwanted side effects and increase IL-12 activities. In addition, IL-12 was effective as an adjuvant for vaccination in several clinical studies. Alatrash et al. (2004) reported that the simultaneous administration of IL-12 and IFN-α2b resulted in a partial positive response in patients affected by metastatic melanoma and metastatic renal cell carcinoma. Gollob et al. (2003) indicated that the administration of recombinant human IL-12 plus low-dose IL-2 in patients with melanoma or renal cell carcinoma resulted in a partial objective response due to the increase in the production of IFN-γ and NK cells. Peterson et al. (2003) observed that the immunization with Melan-A peptide-pulsed peripheral blood mononuclear cells plus recombinant human IL-12 induced clinical activity and T-cell responses in patients with advanced melanoma. An interesting study was recently conducted by Jahn et al. (2012), who created a tumor-targeted IL-12–IL-2 fusion protein and tested it in mice with Hodgkin lymphoma. The authors demonstrated that the use of IL-12–IL-2 dual cytokine targeting to lymphoma cells provided a highly effective anticancer immune response due to the activation and recruitment of NK cells and T cells. The abovementioned findings also testify in favor of potential future therapeutical applications of IL-12. Lastly, IL-12-based immunotherapy should be tested with other anticancer drugs, including the small-molecule-targeted inhibitors sunitinib, temsirolimus, sorafenib, and the monoclonal antibody bevacizumab (Motzer and Bukowski 2006).

It is also important to discuss the possible use of IL-12 for gene therapy. The first thoughts on this issue were put forward by Wagner et al. (2004), who demonstrated that the transport of IL-12 by Epstein–Barr virus-specific CTLs resulted in a significant antitumor response against Hodgkin tumor cells in vitro. Further investigations conducted by Chinnasamy et al. (2012), Kerkar et al. (2010, 2011) and Kerkar and Restifo (2012) elaborated this problem and confirmed that CTLs engineered to release induced or single-chain IL-12 are able to effectively reduce cancer development in mice and can therefore be used as therapeutic agents for the treatment of tumors. Especially significant tumor regression was observed when using T cells simultaneously expressing IL-12 and anti-VEGF2-R chimeric antigen receptor (Chinnasamy et al., 2012). In 2011, Zhang et al. revealed that human T lymphocytes engineered to synthesize IL-12 and T-cell receptor (TCR) greatly enhance the recognition of tumor cells by TCR due to secretion of higher amounts of IFN-γ in vitro. It is important to note that several clinical trials were conducted to test the effectiveness of IL-12-based gene therapy (Table 7.1). Kang et al. (2001) performed a phase I dose-escalation clinical trial of peritumoral injections of IL-12-transduced autologous fibroblasts in nine Korean cancer patients for 7 days. Four out of 9 cases have demonstrated a transient decrease in tumor size; however, in total, no dramatic changes have been observed. Heinzerling et al. (2005)

Table 7.1 Clinical Trials for IL-12 Gene Therapy

Author, Year	Cancer Type	Patients	Dose	Response	Side Effects, Toxicity
Kang et al. (2001)	Various late stage cancers	9 Korean (Asian)	300, 1000, 3000, and 5000 ng/24 h	All patients had a transient response	Mild to moderate pain at the injection site
Heinzerling et al. (2005)	Stage IV melanoma	9 German (Caucasian)	Low (2 mg), medium (4 mg), and high (10–20 mg)	One patient had a complete response; 2 patients had stable disease; 5 patients had a transient response	Well tolerated
Mahvi et al. (2007)	Stage IV melanoma and renal cell carcinoma	12 US (Mixed)	50 mcg plasmid was injected 3 times a week for 3 weeks plus the second course with the same regimen	Three patients had stable disease; 5 patients had a partial response	Two patients had grade I local toxicity
Daud et al. (2008)	Stage IV melanoma	24 US (Mixed)	0.1, 0.25, 0.5, 1.0, and 1.6 mg/mL	Three patients had a complete response; 6 patients had stable disease	Minimal systemic toxicity: Temporal pain during the electroporation procedure or bleeding in the site of treatment

injected IL-12-containing DNA plasmid into nine German patients with stage IV melanoma. Two subjects had a stable disease, and one had a complete response, while all the others except one had a transient response at the site of the injection. Mahvi et al. (2007) administered an intratumoral injection of IL-12 plasmid DNA into 12 US patients with either metastatic melanoma or renal cell carcinoma. The authors observed a partial response (>30% tumor reduction) in five patients accompanied by a local but not a systemic antitumor response. Finally, Daud et al. (2008) performed an intratumoral delivery of a DNA plasmid designed to express IL-12 by in vivo electroporation in 24 US patients with metastatic melanoma. Three individuals experienced a complete response with hypopigmentation and gradual appearance of sites of regressed lesions. Six patients had a stable disease with no lesions developing.

According to Table 7.1, IL-12 shows some beneficial effect in all the experiments. Importantly, IL-12 gene therapy causes minimal toxicities and adverse side effects or even does not cause it at all, unlike treatment with recombinant IL-12. Undoubtedly, further clinical and biological studies in the field of IL-12 gene therapy are necessary. As in the case of clinical trials based on recombinant IL-12, further investigations should include the administration of modern anticancer drugs and adjuvant vaccines. To summarize, IL-12 is one of the most encouraging candidates for tumor immunotherapy, and it could soon become a promising agent for therapeutic application. Although we know much about major anticancer properties of IL-12, we still have no unified strategy for the application of this cytokine, which includes the preferred dosage, regimen, way of delivery (vector or plasmid), etc. The reason for this is a lack of studies, primarily large-scale studies. Hopefully, further in-depth and large-scaled research on the mighty IL-12 will bring us closer to the victory over cancer.

For further reading, the authors recommend the high-quality review articles by Airoldi and Ribatti (2011), Klinke (2010), and Waldner and Neurath (2009). The authors also note that some data in this chapter were borrowed from their recent article on this issue (Yuzhalin and Kutikhin, 2012).

7.2 INTERLEUKIN-23

7.2.1 Brief Overview of IL-23 and Its Role in Immunity

We now turn our gaze to a close relative of IL-12, a cytokine called IL-23. This IL represents a heterodimeric molecule discovered in 2000 by Oppmann et al. It is produced mainly by macrophages, monocytes, and

DCs, and composed of the p40 chain, which is shared with IL-12, and the unique p19 chain (Croxford et al., 2012). Almost all cell types express IL-23; however, the major source of this cytokine is macrophages and DCs of the skin, intestinal mucosa, and lung. The expression of IL-23 is regulated through JAK2, TYK2, extracellular signal-regulated kinase, nuclear factor kappaB (NF-κB), and probably STAT3 and STAT4 (Engel and Neurath, 2010; Xia et al., 2012). The biological effects of IL-23 are exerted via IL-23 receptor (IL-23R), which is known to be expressed on the surface of monocytes, DCs, T cells, NK cells, and microglia cells (Oppmann et al., 2000). Recent data demonstrate that IL-23 is essential for the proper functioning of the immune system. First, IL-23 was numerously reported to be a key factor for human Th17 differentiation (Hoeve et al., 2006; Stritesky et al., 2008; Volpe et al., 2008; Gerosa et al., 2008). It was demonstrated that the IL-23-mediated shift of the adaptive Immune response toward the Th17 axis may lead to the development of autoimmune and inflammatory conditions. In particular, IL-23 was implicated in the development of arthritis (Guo et al., 2013), colitis (Tang and Iwakura, 2012), diabetes (Abbasi et al., 2012), psoriasis (Lowes et al., 2013), and gastritis (Koussoulas et al., 2009). Additionally, it was also found that the lack of IL-23 correlated with the lack of Th17 cell percentage (Maloy, 2008). Second, IL-23 is known to markedly enhance the expression patterns of IL-17 in various cell types (Murphy et al., 2003). The IL-23-mediated upregulation of IL-17 activates the protective immune response against bacterial infections. Furthermore, an important crosstalk between IL-23 and transcriptional factor T-bet has been discovered recently. Reppert et al. (2011) demonstrated that the levels of IL-23 are markedly increased in lungs from tumor-bearing mice deficient in the *T-bet* gene in comparison with that of control animals. Moreover, IL-23 was also reported to directly activate an innate immune response in the presence of bacterial flagellin and other PAMPs (Kinnebrew et al., 2012). In addition, it was found that both IL-23A and IL-23B are able to regulate tumor-associated antigen presentation of DC in vivo (Ichikawa et al., 2012). Finally, multiple in vivo experiments demonstrated that the IL-23-dependent stimulation of the Th17 axis and upregulation of IL-17 resulted in a protection from numerous bacteria and fungi.

7.2.2 Expression of IL-23 in Patients with Cancer

As in the case of many other ILs, IL-23 was found to be overexpressed in patients with cancer. In 2010, Ljujic et al. reported that the serum levels of IL-23 were dramatically increased in 40 Serbian subjects with colorectal carcinoma as compared to that in 37 cancer-free controls. Wang et al. (2010) indicated that the serum concentrations of IL-23A were markedly elevated in 61 Chinese patients with hepatocellular carcinoma (HCC) as compared to that in 38 healthy volunteers. Furthermore, Adamo et al. (2011) recruited 25 Italian patients with resected CRC, who demonstrated increased circulating levels of IL-23 after but not before chemotherapy in comparison with those of 20 sex- and age-matched healthy blood donors. Similarly, Iida et al. (2011) reported that the intratumoral concentrations of IL-23 were greatly increased in 82 Japanese individuals with gastric cancer as compared to those of adjacent healthy tissues. Consistent with previous reports, Lan et al. (2011) found that the expression patterns of IL-23A and IL-23R were significantly increased in 13 Chinese patients with colorectal carcinoma and 26 subjects with intestinal polyps as compared to those of disease-free volunteers. Stanilov et al. (2012) demonstrated that the expression profile for IL-23A was altered in the monocytes of 30 subjects with CRC. Furthermore, Paladugu et al. (2013) indicated that glioma-associated monocytes produced significant amounts of IL-23 in patients with malignant gliomas as well as in cell lines. Shen et al. (2012) observed a significant increase in the serum levels of Th17-related cytokines, including IL-23, in 30 Chinese patients with multiple myeloma as compared to that in 14 healthy blood donors. In addition, Baird et al. (2013) reported that IL-23A levels were markedly increased in macrophages and in cancer cells of patients with non-small-cell lung carcinoma. Moreover, the authors indicated that post-translational genome modifications, in particular DNA CpG methylation, were associated with an altered IL-23A expression. Li et al. (2012a) observed that IL-23B was overexpressed in metastatic HCC cell line. He et al. (2011) demonstrated that IL-23 concentrations were increased in the serum of 20 Chinese patients with pancreatic cancer as compared to that of healthy volunteers. Furthermore, the authors indicated that the levels of this cytokine were higher in patients at stages III–IV as compared to those at stages I–II. Finally, Gangemi et al. (2012) reported that the serum levels of IL-23 were significantly elevated in 50 Italian women with breast cancer in comparison with those in 38 healthy controls.

7.2.3 Studies Demonstrating Tumor-Promoting Effects of IL-23

Multiple research groups reported that IL-23 plays a critical role in cancer development. On the one hand, there is accumulating evidence of procarcinogenic activities of this cytokine. For instance, it was recently discovered that IL-23 has prometastatic activities. First, Teng et al. (2011) indicated that monoclonal antibodies to IL-23 markedly inhibited B16F10 melanoma lung metastases. In addition, in vivo experiments conducted by Li et al. (2012a) demonstrated that this cytokine directly promoted the migration and invasion of HCC cells through the NF-κB-mediated upregulation of matrix metallopeptidase 9 (MMP9), a key modulator of extracellular matrix destruction. In their further investigations, Li et al. (2013) found that the concentrations of IL-23 were inversely proportional to the proliferation of cancer cells in vitro. The authors revealed that low amounts of IL-23 stimulated the proliferation of lung cancer cell lines A549 and SPCA-1, whereas high doses of this cytokine markedly suppressed the proliferative activity of these cells. Moreover, the authors demonstrated that the IL-23-dependent regulation of cancer cell proliferation was associated with a transcription factor STAT3 and Ki-67, a protein involved in cell proliferation (Bullwinkel et al., 2006; Mrklić et al., 2013). In addition, mice deficient in the *IL-23* gene showed a profound decrease in metastatic activity in the study conducted by Teng et al. (2010). The authors also observed that IL-23 significantly suppressed the activity of NK cells. Consistent with the above-mentioned studies, Langowski et al. (2006) indicated that IL-23 upregulated the expression of the MMP9, and also promoted angiogenesis in human tumors. Moreover, these findings were successfully replicated by Zhang et al. (2012), who found that the IL-23-mediated production of the MMP9 caused the migration and invasion of A549 adenocarcinoma cells. Finally, Suzuki et al. (2012) revealed that IL-23 directly promoted the proliferation and invasiveness of colorectal carcinoma cells. In addition, the authors indicated that TGF-β production was also increased in these cells.

7.2.4 Studies Demonstrating the Antitumor Effects of IL-23

On the other hand, however, numerous findings indicate that IL-23 may exert anticancer activities as well. In 2003, Lo et al. provided the first evidence of antitumor properties of IL-23. The authors introduced an IL-23-containing vector to a murine colon adenocarcinoma cell line CT26, which showed a significant decrease in tumor growth and metastatic activity. Later, the research group headed by Shan et al. (2004, 2006) confirmed the previous findings, and observed the marked regression of tumors in nude mice transduced with the human esophageal or colon tumor cells containing the *IL-23* gene in a series of experiments. In particular, the authors demonstrated that IL-23 suppressed tumor growth, promoted the proliferation of splenocytes, prolonged the survival time of mice, enhanced

CTL activity, and number of DCs. Moreover, IL-23 was shown to upregulate the synthesis of Th1 cytokines, including TNF-α, IFN-γ, and IL-12 (Shan et al., 2006). Langowski et al. (2006) observed that the genetic deletion or antibody-mediated neutralization of IL-23 caused a significant infiltration of CTLs into the tumor, which thereby stimulated the development of the anticancer immune response. Consistent with these findings, Teng et al. (2011) discovered that mouse-neutralizing monoclonal antibodies to IL-23 suppressed the subcutaneous growth of EG7 thymoma. Similar anticancer effects of IL-23 were demonstrated by Ugai et al. (2003) in pancreatic carcinoma cells, Hu et al. (2006) in intracranial tumor-bearing mice, Wang et al. (2003) in murine colon carcinoma cells, Kaiga et al. (2007) in mice injected with fibrosarcoma cells, and Kuramoto et al. (2011) in mouse bladder carcinoma (MBT2) cells. An important investigation was conducted by Reay et al. (2009), who demonstrated that an intratumoral injection of adenovirus expressing IL-23 promoted the eradication of tumors in C57BL/6 mice inoculated with MCA205 sarcoma cells. Importantly, the authors discovered that the antitumor activities of the IL-23 were due to the activation and attraction of CD8+ T-cells, and the promotion of CD4+ T-cells. In addition, it was found that the IL-23-mediated antitumor immune response is IFN-γ-dependent, since tumor regression was not observed in IFN-γ deficient mice with established tumors (Reay et al., 2009). Interestingly, these results are consistent with the findings of Kaiga et al. (2007), who observed that IL-23 antitumor effects were absent in mice with *IFN-γ* gene knockout. In their further experiments, Reay et al. (2012) discovered an important fact that the IL-12 is required for the antitumor effects of IL-23; however, these cytokines did not show a synergistic effect in multiple tests. These findings may indicate a complex crosstalk between IL-12 and IL-23, which should be clarified in future studies.

Finally, it is necessary to mention some curious findings. Zijlmans et al. (2012) examined the expression of IL-23A and IL-23B in patients with cervical carcinoma, and showed that low expression of IL-23B is markedly associated with the worst disease-specific survival. Possibly, this correlation may be due to the fact that IL-23B is also a component of tumor-suppressive IL-12. In addition, an interesting study was performed by Jantschitsch et al. (2012), who examined the probability of developing the ultraviolet radiation-induced skin cancer in mice deficient in the *IL-23A* gene. The authors found that the loss of IL-23 promoted tumor occurrence, thereby suggesting the protective role of this cytokine in relation to skin cancer. Finally, Cocco et al. (2010a, 2012) demonstrated that IL-23 directly inhibited the proliferation of human follicular lymphoma and diffuse large B-cell lymphoma cells both in vitro and in vivo through the induction of apoptosis and inhibition of cancer cell proliferation. Moreover, the effect was more evident after simultaneous treatment with IL-23 and IL-27. It was recently suggested that procarcinogenic or anticarcinogenic activities of IL-23 are associated with the balance of STAT3 in tumor and immune cells (Engel and Neurath, 2010).

7.2.5 Inherited Variations within the *IL-12A* and *IL-12B* Genes and Cancer

Since single nucleotide polymorphisms (SNPs) of IL genes are often associated with cancer risk (Sehouli et al., 2002; Kupfer et al., 2009; Kutikhin et al., 2014; Yao et al., 2014), it is worthwhile to briefly mention about a potential role of inherited genetic variations within the *IL-12A* and *IL-12B* genes in carcinogenesis. Multiple studies have been carried out during 2004–2014 to investigate whether or not genetic polymorphisms within the *IL-12A* and *IL-12B* genes have an impact on cancer occurrence. The results from these studies are analyzed in detail in our recent article (Yuzhalin and Kutikhin, 2012); therefore, here we provide only a brief synopsis of the literature review on this issue.

The mutant C allele of the *IL-12B_* +1188A/C (rs3212227) polymorphism contributes to the development of cervical cancer, HCC, lymphoma, lung cancer, glioma, and nasopharyngeal carcinoma. However, there were no indications that this polymorphism modified lung and CRC risk in a series of experiments.

The impact of the *IL-12A_* +277G/A (rs568408) polymorphism on cancer risk could also be significant. There were several auspicious associations between rs568408 GA genotype and an elevated risk of developing cervical cancer, lung carcinoma, HCC, and gastric carcinoma. On the other hand, there were no indications regarding the impact of this SNP in the etiopathogenesis of lymphoma.

7.2.6 Summary

From the viewpoint of cancer research, IL-23 is a very "young" cytokine. The majority of studies investigating the impact of IL-23 on cancer were performed during 2011–2014, and there is already a significant amount of evidence indicating an important role of this cytokine in malignant disease. However, it should be noted that it is still unclear as to exactly which molecular mechanisms underlie procarcinogenic or anticarcinogenic effects of IL-23. We suggest that research on this issue must be carried out in the near future. In particular, interactions between IL-23 and Ki-67, as well as between IL-23 and MMPs should be clarified in further experiments. In addition, there also may be an association between IL-23 and TGF-β-driven increase in cell proliferation, according to a single report suggesting this link (Suzuki et al., 2012). No doubt, many of the mechanisms are still unknown, and therefore, in-depth investigations devoted to this problem are required.

7.3 INTERLEUKIN-27

Another member of the IL-12 family is IL-27. This cytokine is being actively studied, as it demonstrated profound anticancer activities in a series of experiments. Characterization and cloning of the IL-27 were performed in 2002 by the research group headed by Kastelein (Pflanz et al., 2002). This cytokine represents a heterodimer consisting of the exclusive p28 chain, and the IL-12p45-related Epstein–Barr virus induced 3 chain (EBI3, IL-27B), which was formerly isolated from B cells infected with the Epstein–Barr virus (Devergne et al., 1996). The receptor for IL-27 (IL-27R) comprises two different subunits, WSX-1 and gp130 (Pflanz et al., 2004), and promotes STAT-1- and STAT-3-mediated activation of the transcription factor T-bet and adhesion protein ICAM-1, thereby stimulating the synthesis of numerous proinflammatory cytokines and differentiation of Th1 cells and T regulatory (Treg) cells (Takeda et al., 2003; Trinchieri et al., 2003; Villarino et al., 2003; Hamano et al., 2003; Owaki et al., 2005; Xu et al., 2010; Shimozato et al., 2009). Simultaneously, IL-27 inhibits the differentiation of Th2 and Th17 cells, and thereby polarizes the immune response toward the Th1 pattern (Artis et al., 2004; Batten et al., 2006; Stumhofer et al., 2006; Yoshimoto et al., 2007). In addition, IL-27 plays a key role in the activation of the proliferation of naive $CD4^+$ T cells (Pflanz et al., 2002; Takeda et al., 2003; Kamiya et al., 2004; Xu et al., 2010). Multiple reports demonstrated that IL-27 upregulated the expression and release of IFN-γ, TNF-α, IL-1β, IL-10, and IL-21 and downregulated the synthesis of IL-2 and IL-17 in immune cells (Fitzgerald et al., 2007; Owaki et al., 2006; Awasthi et al., 2007; Stumhofer et al., 2007a; Villarino et al., 2006; Cao et al., 2008; Murugaiyan et al., 2009; Schneider et al., 2011; Batten et al., 2010; Liu et al., 2012). It is to be noted that several studies demonstrated that IL-27 synergizes with IL-2 and IL-12 to produce IFN-γ (Pflanz et al., 2002; Takeda et al., 2003; Kamiya et al., 2004). Importantly, IL-27 does not exert direct proinflammatory or antiinflammatory properties; instead, depending on the situation, its influence on the immune system may differ. In fact, IL-27 acts as a linker between innate and adaptive immunity, and its functioning is utterly important in various disorders, including arthritis (Adamopoulos and Pflanz, 2013), lupus erythematosus (Pan et al., 2010), autoimmune diabetes (Wang et al., 2008), atherosclerosis (Hirase et al., 2013), psoriasis (Shibata et al., 2010), and cancer. A more detailed description of the general biological effects of IL-27 is published in comprehensive review articles written by Yoshida et al. (2009) and Wojno and Hunter (2012). We now focus on the role of IL-27 in the context of cancer biology.

IL-27 demonstrated a profound anticancer response across numerous experiments. Importantly, it was found that the antitumor effects of IL-27 are due to several fundamental mechanisms. The first mechanism consists of the IL-27-mediated activation of NK cells and CTLs, which subsequently promote antitumor immune response. This mechanism was responsible for the tumor-suppressing effects of IL-27 in vitro and in vivo models of neuroblastoma (Salcedo et al., 2004), colon cancer (Hisada et al., 2004; Chiyo et al., 2004, 2005), esophageal carcinoma (Liu et al., 2008), melanoma (Oniki et al., 2006), HCC (Hu et al., 2009), and Lewis lung carcinoma (LLC) (Zhang et al., 2013). The second mechanism of IL-27-mediated anticancer response is antiangiogenic activity. Similarly to IL-12, its cousin IL-27 is able to induce the expression of antiangiogenic chemokines CXCL9 and CXCL10 (Airoldi and Ribatti, 2011). It was also observed that IL-27 downregulated the production of VEGF and a plethora of angiopoetins (Airoldi et al., 2004). Further investigations in this field showed that IL-27 suppressed the neovascularization in human B-cell malignancies (Airoldi et al., 2004), murine melanoma models (Shimizu et al., 2006), and multiple myeloma cell lines (Cocco et al., 2010b, 2011). The third mechanism consists of the direct STAT-1- and IRF1-mediated direct suppression of tumor growth by IL-27 (Yoshimoto et al., 2008). In particular, IL-27 directly inhibited proliferation in human lymphatic endothelial cells (Nielsen et al., 2013), mouse melanoma B16F10 cells (Yoshimoto et al., 2008), and multiple myeloma in vivo (Cocco et al., 2010b). Possibly, this effect may be due to the IL-27-dependent downregulation of proangiogenic cytokine IL-17 (Murugaiyan et al., 2009). Alternatively, the direct inhibition of tumors by IL-27 may be explained by the effects of Treg cells. There is a large amount of evidence that IL-27 may act as an antagonist for Tregs, which were found to be associated with numerous cancers (Wang et al., 2005; Szczepanski et al., 2009; Ersvaer et al., 2010; Shenghui et al., 2011; Polimeno et al., 2013; Wu et al., 2013). In particular, Huber et al. (2008)

reported that IL-27 suppressed the differentiation and development of Treg cells through the STAT-3 pathway. In addition, the IL-27-dependent down-regulation of IL-2 was also associated with the inhibition of Treg cells, since IL-2 is an essential factor for their differentiation (Villarino et al., 2006). Furthermore, multiple studies demonstrated that culturing naive CD4$^+$ T cells with IL-27 resulted in a reduced percentage of Treg cells (Neufert et al., 2007; Stumhofer et al., 2007b; Huber et al., 2008).

In addition, several potential mechanisms of anticancer effects of IL-27 are currently the subject of discussions. Taking into account that IL-27 is able to downregulate MMP9, as demonstrated by Airoldi et al. (2004), it could be suggested that this cytokine may be associated with decreased metastatic activity. Recently, Liu et al. (2012) inoculated mice with human pancreatic carcinoma cells transfected with human *IL-27* gene. The authors observed the upregulation of p21 and simultaneous downregulation of sur-vivin, which subsequently caused cell cycle arrest in cancer cells, thereby suggesting apoptotic activities of IL-27. Moreover, this suggestion is evi-denced by the fact that apoptotic tumor cells have been reported to secrete IL-27 in DCs (Sekar et al., 2012). Finally, it was demonstrated that IL-27 reduced lung tumorigenicity by inhibiting cyclooxygenase 2 (COX-2) and PGE$_2$ in cancer cells (Ho et al., 2009). In particular, the authors found that cancer cell migration and invasiveness were suppressed in their model. COX-2 and PGE$_2$ are closely interrelated factors, since the latter is con-verted from arachidonic acid with the assistance of the former. It is known that COX-2 and PGE$_2$ are associated with proangiogenic activity (Castelao et al., 2003; Pold et al., 2004), resistance to apoptosis (Hida et al., 2000; Castelao et al., 2003), and cancer invasiveness (Dohadwala et al., 2002; Castelao et al., 2003). Several studies reported that the elevated production of PGE$_2$ is associated with the carcinogenic activity of COX-2 (Sonoshita et al., 2001; Kawamori et al., 2003; Wang and DuBois. 2008). Moreover, high levels of COX and PGE$_2$ were found in colorectal carcinoma (Pugh and Thomas, 1994; Sano et al., 1995), childhood neuroblastoma (Rasmuson et al., 2012), pancreatic cancer (Hogendorf et al., 2012), breast carcinoma (Cordes et al., 2012), and ovarian cancer (Thill et al., 2010; Cordes et al., 2012). In addition, it was recently demonstrated that COX-2/PGE$_2$ acti-vated several factors to upregulate chemokine monokine induced by gamma interferon-7, which in turn, positively correlated with the migration and invasion of cancer cells, as well as with advanced stages of human lung can-cers (Ho et al., 2013). In addition, it is interesting to note that Treg cells are also known to express COX-2 and to produce PGE2, thereby contributing to cancer occurrence (Yuan et al., 2010); therefore, the IL-27–dependent inhibition of Treg cells may have a protective effect as well. Taking into account all the above-mentioned observations, it is clear that IL-27–mediated suppression of COX-2/PGE$_2$ may be yet another significant anticancer mechanism of this cytokine.

Despite all the advantages of IL-27, it has an important drawback nevertheless. The point is that pleiotropic activities of this cytokine have shown to cause severe immunosuppression, which significantly attenuates anticancer immunity. In particular IL-27 may inhibit the production of numerous cytokines and moreover reduce the antigen-presenting function of DCs (Young et al., 2012; Wang et al., 2007). In addition, IL-27 is known to upregulate IL-10 synthesis in Tr1 cells (Awasthi et al., 2007), and numerous reports indicated that IL-10 inhibits antitumor immune response both in vivo and in vitro. Moreover, IL-10 was shown to stimulate cancer progression (Sato et al., 2011) and assist in the escape from tumor immune surveillance (Hamidullah et al., 2012). All these indications limit the potential of IL-27 against cancer cells; therefore, further investigations are needed to learn how to use this cytokine properly.

So far, IL-27 has not been used as an immunomodulatory agent for cancer therapy. An interesting study was performed by Salcedo et al. (2009), who combined the delivery of IL-27 and IL-2 in mice bearing disseminated neuroblastoma metastasis. The authors demonstrated a significant synergistic antitumor response, thereby suggesting the usage of this combination in clinical studies. Perhaps, it would also be useful to try a IL-12/IL-27 combination as well. Currently, there are no clinical studies on IL-27, but undoubtedly, they will emerge soon, as it is clear that IL-27 is a powerful anticancer agent, which should definitely be used in the treatment of malignancies (Figure 7.2).

7.4 INTERLEUKIN-30

The discovery of the IL-30 is associated with an in–depth investigation of the p28 subunit of the IL-27. Surprisingly, it was found that this subunit is able to act as an independent cytokine, exerting both proinflammatory and anti-inflammatory properties (Pflanz et al., 2004; Stumhofer et al., 2010). To date, little is known about the regulation and biological effects of IL-30. It was recently found that the essential function of IL-30 is to block glycoprotein 130 (gp130), and thereby prevent the signaling of numerous cytokines, including IL-6, IL-11, and IL-27 (Stumhofer et al., 2010). It is known that

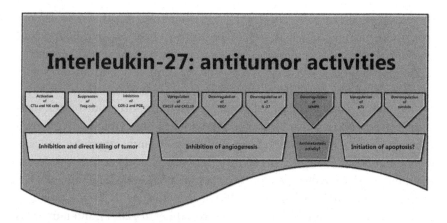

Figure 7.2 IL-27 possesses anticancer properties due to multiple mechanisms. (For color version of this figure, the reader is referred to the online version of this book.)

IFN-γ and LPS are able to induce the synthesis of IL-30 in DCs involving c-Rel, NF-κB, IRF1, IRF-3, and MyD88 (Liu et al., 2007; Molle et al., 2007). Dibra et al. (2012a) revealed that IL-30 is able to suppress liver toxicity caused by IL-12, INF-γ, and ConA. Further investigations by Dibra et al. (2012b) indicated that the simultaneous administration of anti-CD3/CD28 antibodies and CpG oligodeoxynucleotides caused the expression of IL-30 in mice splenocytes, and that MyD88 is critical in this process. IL-30 has been recently reported to inhibit biological functions of IL-27 (Shimozatio et al., 2009).

It is important to mention a recent study conducted by Di Meo et al. (2014), who examined the impact of IL-30 on prostate cancer and its effects on human prostate cancer cells. The authors found that the expression of IL-30 by prostate cancer epithelia was associated with high-grade and advanced-stage prostate cancer in a cohort of 125 patients with prostate cancer. Also, IL-30 correlated with a higher cell proliferation in either primary prostate cancer or lymph node metastasis in the same cohort of patients. In addition, IL-30 enhanced the proliferation of the hPCa human prostate cancer cell line in vitro.

Currently, multiple research groups are focused on IL-30, and hopefully, the biology of this cytokine will be illuminated in the near future.

7.5 INTERLEUKIN-35

IL-35 was initially identified by Devergne et al. in 1997. This cytokine was characterized as a heterodimeric hemopoetin that comprised IL-12 p35 chain (IL-12A) and an IL-27B (EBI3) chain. In 2007, the current nomenclature name was proposed for this cytokine. Experiments on murine models revealed that unlike other representatives of the IL-12 superfamily, which are commonly expressed on the surface of macrophages, monocytes, and DCs, IL-35 is known to be synthesized exclusively by regulatory T cells (Collison et al., 2007; Collison and Vignali, 2008). According to the results of the analysis of hematopoietic populations, several research studies speculated that IL-35 may be expressed on CD8$^+$ T cells and peripheral γδ T cells; however, the mature protein was not identified in these cells though (Devergne et al., 1997; Collison et al., 2007; Collison and Vignali, 2008). In comparison with other family representatives, the biological effects of IL-35 are different as well. In fact, IL-35 does not stimulate the differentiation Th1 or Th17 cells; instead, it inhibits the proliferation of all subsets of T cells, including Th17 cells, thereby exerting antiinflammatory properties. As written above, IL-35 is only expressed on Treg cells, which is a specific subset of CD4+ cells involved in the suppression of an immune response. Notably, Treg cells have also been found to be engaged in the regulation of an immune response to foreign antigens and in the maintenance of the natural self-tolerance (Sakaguchi, 2011). In addition, it should be noted that significantly higher percentages of Treg cells were observed in renal cell carcinoma (Polimeno et al., 2013), HCC (Wu et al., 2013), and numerous hematopoietic malignancies, including acute myeloid leukemia (Wang et al., 2005; Szczepanski et al., 2009; Ersvaer et al., 2010; Shenghui et al., 2011), chronic lymphocytic leukemia (Giannopoulos et al., 2008; D'Arena et al., 2011; Lindqvist et al., 2011; Jadidi-Niaragh et al., 2013), multiple myeloma (Beyer et al., 2006), B-cell NHL (Yang et al., 2006), and Hodgkin lymphoma (Marshall et al., 2004). In addition, it was found that a high Treg cell frequency was associated with a poor prognosis in patients with acute myeloid leukemia (Shenghui et al., 2011). However, surprisingly, the research group headed by Bardel et al. (2008) recently failed to reveal the expression patterns of IL-35 in human Treg cells, so the exact source of IL-35 is a subject of debate.

It seems that IL-35 is secreted exclusively after external stimulation, as several reports indicate that IL-35 subunit mRNAs are induced by stimulation in various human cell types. First, Li et al. (2012b) recently revealed that IL-35 is not constitutively expressed in human tissues, but it may be produced under specific stimuli. In particular, the authors demonstrated that treatment with LPS or various proinflammatory cytokines resulted in the appearance of IL-35 subunit mRNAs in human monocytes, endothelial cells, and smooth muscle cells. These findings are consistent with the results obtained by Pflanz et al. (2002), who observed IL-35 mRNA in LPS-treated human monocytes. Maaser et al. (2004) revealed that intestinal epithelial cell lines treated with TNF-α or IFN-γ had significant amounts of IL-35, and additionally, concentration of this cytokine was higher after the simultaneous administration of both TNF-α and IFN-γ. Similarly, high levels of Ebi3 and IL-12 p35 were detected by Kempe et al. (2009) in primary aortic smooth muscle cells after the simultaneous stimulation by TNF-α and IFN-γ. In addition, stimulation by IFN-γ and IL-1β induced IL-35 mRNA synthesis in immature dendritic cells and intestinal microvascular endothelial cells, respectively (van Seventer et al., 2002; Heidemann et al., 2007). Finally, Mao et al. (2013) recently found IL-35 expressed in placental trophoblasts without external stimulation.

It should be noted that the investigation of biological effects of IL-35 is associated with many difficulties. In particular, experiments on knockout mice became impossible, taking into account the fact that p35-deficient mice lack both IL-35 and IL-12, and that Ebi3-deficient mice lack both IL-35 and IL-27 (Collison and Vignali, 2008). It is clear that this circumstance caused failure to evaluate the direct impact of IL-35 on various biological processes within the body. Nevertheless, a plethora of studies were able to prove that IL-35 effectively inhibits inflammation in vivo. In particular, IL-35 markedly suppressed inflammation in the models of autoimmune diabetes (Bettini et al., 2012), colitis (Neurath, 2008; Wirtz et al., 2011), collagen-induced arthritis (Niedbala et al., 2007; Kochetkova et al., 2010), and allergic asthma (Huang et al., 2011). To date, little is known about the signaling pathways of IL-35. Li et al. (2012b) found that the promoter regions of both IL-12A and Ebi3 had binding sites for NF-κB, thereby indicating its involvement in signaling pathways of IL-35.

Several studies were performed to evaluate the role of IL-35 in cancer. An interesting investigation was conducted by Wang et al. (2013). The authors revealed that IL-35 is expressed in human cancer tissues, including melanoma, large B-cell lymphoma, and nasopharyngeal carcinoma. The authors also observed that IL-35 did not affect cancer growth and survival in vitro, but it promoted carcinogenesis in animal models. In particular, IL-35 stimulated tumor angiogenesis due to the accumulation of CD11b(+) Gr1(+) myeloid cells in a tumor microenvironment (Wang et al., 2013). In addition, anticancer immunity was inhibited by the IL-35-mediated suppression of CTL responses to tumors (Wang et al., 2013). However, in contrast to these findings, Long et al. (2013) demonstrated that the overexpression of IL-35 in human cancer cells caused cell cycle arrest at the G1 phase, thereby suppressing cell growth. Furthermore, the authors also observed that IL-35 stimulated the initiation of apoptosis due to TNF-α- and IFN-γ-mediated upregulation of Fas ligand and the simultaneous downregulation of cyclinD1, survivin, and Bcl-2. Wu et al. (2012) found that the serum levels of IL-35 were significantly increased in 55 Chinese patients with acute myeloid leukemia, and as compared to 28 subjects in complete remission or 24 healthy blood donors. Finally, Olson et al. (2012) demonstrated that IL-35 blockade inhibited human prostate tumor antigen-specific CD8+ Treg cells, thereby suggesting an impact of this cytokine on cancer progression.

Taken together, these sparse observations emphasize the importance of research devoted to IL-35 and cancer. There is still much to be done to clearly understand the impact of IL-35 on cancer development, and no doubt, further research on IL-35 and other representatives of IL-12 superfamily will shed light on how we can treat cancer and cancer biology as a whole.

REFERENCES

Abbas, A.K., Lichtman, A.H., Pillai, S., 2011. Cellular and Molecular Immunology. Elsevier, Philadelphia, PA.

Abbasi, F., Amiri, P., Sayahpour, F.A., Pirmoradi, S., Abolhalaj, M., Larijani, B., Bazzaz, J.T., Amoli, M.M., 2012. TGF-β and IL-23 gene expression in unstimulated PBMCs of patients with diabetes. Endocrine 41 (3), 430–434.

Acquaviva, J., Chen, X., Ren, R., 2008. IRF-4 functions as a tumor suppressor in early B-cell development. Blood 112 (9), 3798–3806.

Adamo, V., Franchina, T., Minciullo, P.L., Pace, E., Colonese, F., Ricciardi, G.R., Saitta, S., Ferraro, M., Spatari, G., Gangemi, S., 2011. Role of interleukin-23 circulating levels increase in resected colorectal cancer before and after chemotherapy: preliminary data and future perspectives. J. Cell. Physiol. 226 (11), 3032–3034.

Adamopoulos, I.E., Pflanz, S., 2013. The emerging role of interleukin 27 in inflammatory arthritis and bone destruction. Cytokine Growth Factor Rev. 24 (2), 115–121.

Airoldi, I., Di Carlo, E., Banelli, B., Moserle, L., Cocco, C., Pezzolo, A., Sorrentino, C., Rossi, E., Romani, M., Amadori, A., Pistoia, V., 2004. The IL-12Rbeta2 gene functions as a tumor suppressor in human B cell malignancies. J. Clin. Invest. 113 (11), 1651–1659.

Airoldi, I., Ribatti, D., 2011. Regulation of angiostatic chemokines driven by IL-12 and IL-27 in human tumors. J. Leukoc. Biol. 90 (5), 875–882.

Alatrash, G., Hutson, T.E., Molto, L., Richmond, A., Nemec, C., Mekhail, T., Elson, P., Tannenbaum, C., Olencki, T., Finke, J., Bukowski, R.M., 2004. Clinical and immunologic effects of subcutaneously administered interleukin-12 and interferon alfa-2b: Phase I trial of patients with metastatic renal cell carcinoma or malignant melanoma. J. Clin. Oncol. 22, 2891–2900.

Ansell, S.M., Witzig, T.E., Kurtin, P.J., Sloan, J.A., Jelinek, D.F., Howell, K.G., Markovic, S.N., Habermann, T.M., Klee, G.G., Atherton, P.J., Erlichman, C., 2002. Phase 1 study of interleukin-12 in combination with rituximab in patients with B-cell non-Hodgkin lymphoma. Blood 99 (1), 67–74.

Artis, D., Villarino, A., Silverman, M., He, W., Thornton, E.M., Mu, S., Summer, S., Covey, T.M., Huang, E., Yoshida, H., Koretzky, G., Goldschmidt, M., Wu, G.D., de Sauvage, F., Miller, H.R., Saris, C.J., Scott, P., Hunter, C.A., 2004. The IL-27 receptor (WSX-1) is an inhibitor of innate and adaptive elements of type 2 immunity. J. Immunol. 173 (9), 5626–5634.

Atkins, M.B., Robertson, M.J., Gordon, M., Lotze, M.T., DeCoste, M., DuBois, J.S., Ritz, J., Sandler, A.B., Edington, H.D., Garzone, P.D., Mier, J.W., Canning, C.M., Battiato, L., Tahara, H., Sherman, M.L., 1997. Phase I evaluation of intravenous recombinant human interleukin 12 in patients with advanced malignancies. Clin. Cancer Res. 3 (3), 409–417.

Awasthi, A., Carrier, Y., Peron, J.P., Bettelli, E., Kamanaka, M., Flavell, R.A., Kuchroo, V.K., Oukka, M., Weiner, H.L., 2007. A dominant function for interleukin 27 in generating interleukin 10- producing anti-inflammatory T cells. Nat. Immunol. 8 (12), 1380–1389.

Baird, A.M., Leonard, J., Naicker, K.M., Kilmartin, L., O'Byrne, K.J., Gray, S.G., 2013. IL-23 is pro-proliferative, epigenetically regulated and modulated by chemotherapy in non-small cell lung cancer. Lung Cancer 79 (1), 83–90.

Bajetta, E., Del Vecchio, M., Mortarini, R., Nadeau, R., Rakhit, A., Rimassa, L., Fowst, C., Borri, A., Anichini, A., Parmiani, G., 1998. Pilot study of subcutaneous recombinant human interleukin 12 in metastatic melanoma. Clin. Cancer. Res. 4 (1), 75–85.

Bardel, E., Larousserie, F., Charlot-Rabiega, P., Coulomb-L'Herminé, A., Devergne, O., 2008. Human CD4+ CD25+ Foxp3+ regulatory T cells do not constitutively express IL-35. J. Immunol. 181 (10), 6898–6905.

Batten, M., Li, J., Yi, S., Kljavin, N.M., Danilenko, D.M., Lucas, S., Lee, J., de Sauvage, F.J., Ghilardi, N., 2006. Interleukin 27 limits autoimmune encephalomyelitis by suppressing the development of interleukin 17-producing T cells. Nat. Immunol. 7 (9), 929–936.

Batten, M., Ramamoorthi, N., Kljavin, N.M., Ma, C.S., Cox, J.H., Dengler, H.S., Danilenko, D.M., Caplazi, P., Wong, M., Fulcher, D.A., Cook, M.C., King, C., Tangye, S.G., de Sauvage, F.J., Ghilardi, N., 2010. IL-27 supports germinal center function by enhancing IL-21 production and the function of T follicular helper cells. J. Exp. Med. 207 (13), 2895–2906.

Becskei, A., Grusby, M.J., 2007. Contribution of IL-12R mediated feedback loop to Th1 cell differentiation. FEBS Lett. 581 (27), 5199–5206.

Bettini, M., Castellaw, A.H., Lennon, G.P., Burton, A.R., Vignali, D.A., June 2012. Prevention of autoimmune diabetes by ectopic pancreatic β-cell expression of interleukin-35. Diabetes 61 (6), 1519–1526.

Beyer, M., Schultze, J.L., 2006. Regulatory T cells in cancer. Blood 108, 804–811.

Beyer, M., Kochanek, M., Giese, T., Endl, E., Weihrauch, M.R., Knolle, P.A., Classen, S., Schultze, J.L., 2006. In vivo peripheral expansion of naive CD4+CD25high FoxP3+ regulatory T cells in patients with multiple myeloma. Blood 107 (10), 3940–3949.

Boggio, K., Di Carlo, E., Rovero, S., Cavallo, F., Quaglino, E., Lollini, P.L., Nanni, P., Nicoletti, G., Wolf, S., Musiani, P., Forni, G., 2000. Ability of systemic interleukin-12 to hamper progressive stages of mammary carcinogenesis in HER2/neu transgenic mice. Cancer Res. 60 (2), 359–364.

Bouker, K.B., Skaar, T.C., Riggins, R.B., Harburger, D.S., Fernandez, D.R., Zwart, A., Wang, A., Clarke, R., 2005. Interferon regulatory factor-1 (IRF-1) exhibits tumor suppressor activities in breast cancer associated with caspase activation and induction of apoptosis. Carcinogenesis 26 (9), 1527–1535.

Bowie, M.L., Ibarra, C., Seewalt, V.L., 2008. IRF-1 promotes apoptosis in p53-damaged basal-type human mammary epithelial cells: A model for early basal-type mammary carcinogenesis. Adv. Exp. Med. Biol. 617, 367–374.

Bree, A.G., Schlerman, F.J., Kaviani, M.D., Hastings, R.C., Hitz, S.L., Goldman, S.J., 1994. Multiple effects on peripheral hematology following administration of recombinant human interleukin 12 to nonhuman primates. Biochem. Biophys. Res. Commun. 204 (3), 1150–1157.

Brunda, M.J., Luistro, L., Warrier, R.R., Wright, R.B., Hubbard, B.R., Murphy, M., Wolf, S.F., Gately, M.K., 1993. Antitumor and antimetastatic activity of interleukin 12 against murine tumors. J. Exp. Med. 178 (4), 1223–1230.

Bullwinkel, J., Baron-Lühr, B., Lüdemann, A., Wohlenberg, C., Gerdes, J., Scholzen, T., 2006. Ki-67 protein is associated with ribosomal RNA transcription in quiescent and prolif-erating cells. J. Cell. Physiol. 206 (3), 624–635.

Cao, Y., Doodes, P.D., Glant, T.T., Finnegan, A., 2008. IL-27 induces a Th1 immune response and susceptibility to experimental arthritis. J. Immunol. 180 (2), 922–930.

Castelao, J.E., Bart 3rd, R.D., DiPerna, C.A., Sievers, E.M., Bremner, R.M., 2003. Lung can-cer and cyclooxygenase-2. Ann. Thorac. Surg. 76 (4), 1327–1335.

Cavallo, F., Quaglino, E., Cifaldi, L., Di Carlo, E., Andre′, A., Bernabei, P., Musiani, P., Forni, G., Calogero, R.A., 2001. Interleukin 12-activated lymphocytes influence tumor genetic programs. Cancer Res. 61 (8), 3518–3523.

Chinnasamy, D., Yu, Z., Kerkar, S.P., Zhang, L., Morgan, R.A., Restifo, N.P., Rosenberg, S.A., March 15, 2012. Local delivery of interleukin-12 using T cells targeting VEGF receptor-2 eradicates multiple vascularized tumors in mice. Clin. Cancer Res. 18 (6), 1672–1683.

Chiyo, M., Shimozato, O., Iizasa, T., Fujisawa, T., Tagawa, M., 2004. Antitumor effects pro-duced by transduction of dendritic cells-derived heterodimeric cytokine genes in murine colon carcinoma cells. Anticancer Res. 24 (6), 3763–3767.

Chiyo, M., Shimozato, O., Yu, L., Kawamura, K., Iizasa, T., Fujisawa, T., Tagawa, M., 2005. Expression of IL-27 in murine carcinoma cells produces antitumor effects and induces protective immunity in inoculated host animals. Int. J. Cancer 115 (3), 437–442.

Cocco, C., Canale, S., Frasson, C., Di Carlo, E., Ognio, E., Ribatti, D., Prigione, I., Basso, G., Airoldi, I., 2010a. Interleukin-23 acts as antitumor agent on childhood B-acute lympho-blastic leukemia cells. Blood 116 (19), 3887–3898.

Cocco, C., Giuliani, N., Di Carlo, E., Ognio, E., Storti, P., Abeltino, M., Sorrentino, C., Ponzoni, M., Ribatti, D., Airoldi, I., 2010b. Interleukin-27 acts as multifunctional antitu-mor agent in multiple myeloma. Clin. Cancer. Res. 16 (16), 4188–4197.

Cocco, C., Morandi, F., Airoldi, I., 2011. Interleukin-27 and interleukin-23 modulate human plasma cell functions. J. Leukoc. Biol. 89 (5), 729–734.

Cocco, C., Di Carlo, E., Zupo, S., Canale, S., Zorzoli, A., Ribatti, D., Morandi, F., Ognio, E., Airoldi, I., 2012. Complementary IL-23 and IL-27 anti-tumor activities cause strong inhibition of human follicular and diffuse large B-cell lymphoma growth in vivo. Leu-kemia 26 (6), 1365–1374.

Collison, L.W., Workman, C.J., Kuo, T.T., Boyd, K., Wang, Y., Vignali, K.M., Cross, R., Sehy, D., Blumberg, R.S., Vignali, D.A., 2007. The inhibitory cytokine IL-35 contributes to regulatory T-cell function. Nature 450 (7169), 566–569.

Collison, L.W., Vignali, D.A., 2008. Interleukin-35: odd one out or part of the family? Immu-nol. Rev. 226, 248–262.

Cordes, T., Hoellen, F., Dittmer, C., Salehin, D., Kümmel, S., Friedrich, M., Köster, F., Becker, S., Diedrich, K., Thill, M., 2012. Correlation of prostaglandin metabolizing enzymes and serum PGE2 levels with vitamin D receptor and serum 25(OH)2D3 levels in breast and ovarian cancer. Anticancer Res. 32 (1), 351–357.

Croxford, A.L., Mair, F., Becher, B., 2012. IL-23: one cytokine in control of autoimmunity. Eur. J. Immunol. 42 (9), 2263–2273.

D'Arena, G., Laurenti, L., Minervini, M.M., Deaglio, S., Bonello, L., De Martino, L., De Padua, L., Savino, L., Tarnani, M., De Feo, V., Cascavilla, N., 2011. Regulatory T-cell number is increased in chronic lymphocytic leukemia patients and correlates with pro-gressive disease. Leuk. Res. 35 (3), 363–368.

Delgado, M., Ganea, D., 1999. Vasoactive intestinal peptide and pituitary adenylate cyclase-activating polypeptide inhibit interleukin-12 transcription by regulating nuclear factor kappaB and Ets activation. J. Biol. Chem. 274 (45), 31930–31940.

Daud, A.I., DeConti, R.C., Andrews, S., Urbas, P., Riker, A.I., Sondak, V.K., Munster, P.N., Sullivan, D.M., Ugen, K.E., Messina, J.L., Heller, R., 2008. Phase I trial of interleukin-12 plasmid electroporation in patients with metastatic melanoma. J. Clin. Oncol. 26 (36), 5896–5903.

Devergne, O., Hummel, M., Koeppen, H., Le Beau, M.M., Nathanson, E.C., Kieff, E., Birkenbach, M., 1996. A novel interleukin-12 p40-related protein induced by latent Epstein–Barr virus infection in B lymphocytes. J. Virol. 70 (2), 1143–1153.

Devergne, O., Birkenbach, M., Kieff, E., October 28, 1997. Epstein–Barr virus-induced gene 3 and the p35 subunit of interleukin 12 form a novel heterodimeric hematopoietin. Proc. Natl. Acad. Sci. USA 94 (22), 12041–12046.

Di Meo, S., Airoldi, I., Sorrentino, C., Zorzoli, A., Esposito, S., Di Carlo, E., 2014. Interleukin-30 expression in prostate cancer and its draining lymph nodes correlates with advanced grade and stage. Clin. Cancer. Res. 20 (3), 585–594.

Dibra, D., Cutrera, J., Xia, X., Kallakury, B., Mishra, L., Li, S., 2012a. Interleukin-30: a novel antiinflammatory cytokine candidate for prevention and treatment of inflammatory cytokine-induced liver injury. Hepatology 55 (4), 1204–1214.

Dibra, D., Cutrera, J.J., Li, S., 2012b. Coordination between TLR9 signaling in macrophages and CD3 signaling in T cells induces robust expression of IL-30. J. Immunol. 188 (8), 3709–3715.

Dohadwala, M., Batra, R.K., Luo, J., Lin, Y., Krysan, K., Pold, M., Sharma, S., Dubinett, S.M., 2002. Autocrine/paracrine prostaglandin E2 production by non-small cell lung cancer cells regulates matrix metalloproteinase-2 and CD44 in cyclooxygenase-2-dependent invasion. J. Biol. Chem. 277 (52), 50828–50833.

Engel, M.A., Neurath, M.F., 2010. Anticancer properties of the IL-12 family—focus on colorectal cancer. Curr. Med. Chem. 17 (29), 3303–3308.

Ersvaer, E., Liseth, K., Skavland, J., Gjertsen, B.T., Bruserud, Ø., 2010. Intensive chemotherapy for acute myeloid leukemia differentially affects circulating TC1, TH1, TH17 and TREG cells. BMC Immunol. 11, 38.

Fitzgerald, D.C., Zhang, G.X., El-Behi, M., Fonseca-Kelly, Z., Li, H., Yu, S., Saris, C.J., Gran, B., Ciric, B., Rostami, A., 2007. Suppression of autoimmune inflammation of the central nervous system by interleukin 10 secreted by interleukin 27-stimulated T cells. Nat. Immunol. 8 (12), 1372–1379.

Foukas, L.C., Panayotou, G., Shepherd, P.R., 2004. Direct interaction of major histocompatibility complex class II-derived peptides with class Ia phosphoinositide 3-kinase results in dose-dependent stimulatory effects. J. Biol. Chem. 279 (9), 7505–7511.

Friedmann, E., Hauben, E., Maylandt, K., Schleeger, S., Vreugde, S., Lichtenthaler, S.F., Kuhn, P.H., Stauffer, D., Rovelli, G., Martoglio, B., 2006. SPPL2a and SPPL2b promote intramembrane proteolysis of TNFalpha in activated dendritic cells to trigger IL-12 production. Nat. Cell. Biol. 8 (8), 843–848.

Gangemi, S., Minciullo, P., Adamo, B., Franchina, T., Ricciardi, G.R., Ferraro, M., Briguglio, R., Toscano, G., Saitta, S., Adamo, V., 2012. Clinical significance of circulating interleukin-23 as a prognostic factor in breast cancer patients. J. Cell. Biochem. 113 (6), 2122–2125.

Gately, M.K., Renzetti, L.M., Magram, J., Stern, A.S., Adorini, L., Gubler, U., Presky, D.H., 1998. The interleukin-12/interleukin-12-receptor system: Role in normal and pathologic immune responses. Annu. Rev. Immunol. 16, 495–521.

Gerosa, F., Baldani-Guerra, B., Lyakh, L.A., Batoni, G., Esin, S., Winkler-Pickett, R.T., Consolaro, M.R., De Marchi, M., Giachino, D., Robbiano, A., Astegiano, M., Sambataro, A., Kastelein, R.A., Carra, G., Trinchieri, G., 2008. Differential regulation of interleukin 12 and interleukin 23 production in human dendritic cells. J. Exp. Med. 205 (6), 1447–1461.

Giannopoulos, K., Schmitt, M., Kowal, M., Wlasiuk, P., Bojarska-Junak, A., Chen, J., Rolinski, J., Dmoszynska, A., 2008. Characterization of regulatory T cells in patients with B-cell chronic lymphocytic leukemia. Oncol. Rep. 20 (3), 677–682.

Goldstein, D., Laszlo, J., 1988. The role of interferon in cancer therapy: a current perspective. CA Cancer. J. Clin. 38 (5), 258–277.

Gollob, J.A., Veenstra, K.G., Parker, R.A., Mier, J.W., McDermott, D.F., Clancy, D., Tutin, L., Koon, H., Atkins, M.B., 2003. Phase I trial of concurrent twice-weekly recombinant human interleukin-12 plus low-dose IL-2 in patients with melanoma or renal cell carcinoma. J. Clin. Oncol. 21 (13), 2564–2573.

Guo, Y.Y., Wang, N.Z., Zhao, S., Hou, L.X., Xu, Y.B., Zhang, N., 2013. Increased interleukin-23 is associated with increased disease activity in patients with rheumatoid arthritis. Chin. Med. J. (Engl.) 126 (5), 850–854.

Hamano, S., Himeno, K., Miyazaki, Y., Ishii, K., Yamanaka, A., Takeda, A., Zhang, M., Hisaeda, H., Mak, T.W., Yoshimura, A., Yoshida, H., 2003. WSX-1 is required for resistance to *Trypanosoma cruzi* infection by regulation of proinflammatory cytokine production. Immunity 19 (5), 657–667.

Hamidullah, Changkija, B., Konwar, R., 2012. Role of interleukin-10 in breast cancer. Breast Cancer Res. Treat. 133 (1), 11–21.

He, S., Fei, M., Wu, Y., Zheng, D., Wan, D., Wang, L., Li, D., 2011. Distribution and clinical significance of th17 cells in the tumor microenvironment and peripheral blood of pancreatic cancer patients. Int. J. Mol. Sci. 12 (11), 7424–7437.

Hess, S.D., Egilmez, N.K., Bailey, N., Anderson, T.M., Mathiowitz, E., Bernstein, S.H., Bankert, R.B., 2003. Human CD4 T cells present within the microenvironment of human lung tumors are mobilized by the local and sustained release of IL-12 to kill tumors in situ by indirect effects of IFN-gamma. J. Immunol. 170 (1), 400–412.

Heidemann, J., Rüther, C., Kebschull, M., Domschke, W., Brüwer, M., Koch, S., Kucharzik, T., Maaser, C., 2007. Expression of IL-12-related molecules in human intestinal microvascular endothelial cells is regulated by TLR3. Am. J. Physiol. Gastrointest. Liver Physiol. 293 (6), G1315–G1324.

Heinzerling, L., Burg, G., Dummer, R., Maier, T., Oberholzer, P.A., Schultz, J., Elzaouk, L., Pavlovic, J., Moelling, K., 2005. Intratumoral injection of DNA encoding human interleukin 12 into patients with metastatic melanoma: clinical efficacy. Hum. Gene. Ther. 16 (1), 35–48.

Hida, T., Kozaki, K., Muramatsu, H., Masuda, A., Shimizu, S., Mitsudomi, T., Sugiura, T., Ogawa, M., Takahashi, T., May 2000. Cyclooxygenase-2 inhibitor induces apoptosis and enhances cytotoxicity of various anticancer agents in non-small cell lung cancer cell lines. Clin. Cancer Res. 6 (5), 2006–2011.

Hill, H.C., Conway Jr., T.F., Sabel, M.S., Jong, Y.S., Mathiowitz, E., Bankert, R.B., Egilmez, N.K., 2002. Cancer immunotherapy with interleukin 12 and granulocyte-macrophage colony-stimulating factor-encapsulated microspheres: Coinduction of innate and adaptive antitumor immunity and cure of disseminated disease. Cancer Res. 62 (24), 7254–7263.

Hirase, T., Hara, H., Miyazaki, Y., Ide, N., Nishimoto-Hazuku, A., Fujimoto, H., Saris, C.J., Yoshida, H., Node, K., August 1, 2013. Interleukin 27 inhibits atherosclerosis via immunoregulation of macrophages in mice. Am. J. Physiol. Heart Circ. Physiol. 305 (3), H420–H429.

Hisada, M., Kamiya, S., Fujita, K., Belladonna, M.L., Aoki, T., Koyanagi, Y., Mizuguchi, J., Yoshimoto, T., 2004. Potent antitumor activity of interleukin-27. Cancer Res. 64 (3), 1152–1156.

Ho, M.Y., Leu, S.J., Sun, G.H., Tao, M.H., Tang, S.J., Sun, K.H., 2009. IL-27 directly restrains lung tumorigenicity by suppressing cyclooxygenase-2-mediated activities. J. Immunol. 183 (10), 6217–6226.

Ho, M.Y., Liang, S.M., Hung, S.W., Liang, C.M., 2013. MIG-7 controls COX-2/PGE2-mediated lung cancer metastasis. Cancer Res. 73 (1), 439–449.

Hoeve, M.A., Savage, N.D., de Boer, T., Langenberg, D.M., de Waal Malefyt, R., Ottenhoff, T.H., Verreck, F.A., 2006. Divergent effects of IL-12 and IL-23 on the production of IL-17 by human T cells. Eur. J. Immunol. 36 (3), 661–670.

Hogendorf, P., Durczyński, A., Kumor, A., Strzelczyk, J., 2012. Prostaglandin E2 (PGE2) in portal blood in patients with pancreatic tumor–a single institution series. J. Invest. Surg. 25 (1), 8–13.

Hu, J., Yuan, X., Belladonna, M.L., Ong, J.M., Wachsmann-Hogiu, S., Farkas, D.L., Black, K.L., Yu, J.S., 2006. Induction of potent antitumor immunity by intratumoral injection of interleukin 23-transduced dendritic cells. Cancer Res. 66 (17), 8887–8896.

Hu, P., Hu, H.D., Chen, M., Peng, M.L., Tang, L., Tang, K.F., Matsui, M., Belladonna, M.L., Yoshimoto, T., Zhang, D.Z., Xiang, R., Ren, H., 2009. Expression of interleukins-23 and 27 leads to successful gene therapy of hepatocellular carcinoma. Mol. Immunol. 46 (8–9), 1654–1662.

Huang, C.H., Loo, E.X., Kuo, I.C., Soh, G.H., Goh, D.L., Lee, B.W., Chua, K.Y., 2011. Airway inflammation and IgE production induced by dust mite allergen-specific memory/effector Th2 cell line can be effectively attenuated by IL-35. J. Immunol. 187 (1), 462–471.

Huber, M., Steinwald, V., Guralnik, A., Brüstle, A., Kleemann, P., Rosenplänter, C., Decker, T., Lohoff, M., 2008. IL-27 inhibits the development of regulatory T cells via STAT3. Int. Immunol. 20 (2), 223–234.

Ichikawa, K., Kagamu, H., Koyama, K., Miyabayashi, T., Koshio, J., Miura, S., Watanabe, S., Yoshizawa, H., Narita, I., 2012. Epitope diversification driven by non-tumor epitope-specific Th1 and Th17 mediates potent antitumor reactivity. Vaccine 30 (43), 6190–6197.

Iida, T., Iwahashi, M., Katsuda, M., Ishida, K., Nakamori, M., Nakamura, M., Naka, T., Ojima, T., Ueda, K., Hayata, K., Nakamura, Y., Yamaue, H., 2011. Tumor-infiltrating CD4+ Th17 cells produce IL-17 in tumor microenvironment and promote tumor progression in human gastric cancer. Oncol. Rep. 25 (5), 1271–1277.

Ikeda, H., Old, L.J., Schreiber, R.D., 2002. The roles of IFN gamma in protection against tumor development and cancer immunoediting. Cytokine Growth Factor Rev. 13 (2), 95–109.

Jadidi-Niaragh, F., Ghalamfarsa, G., Yousefi, M., Tabrizi, M.H., Shokri, F., August 2013. Regulatory T cells in chronic lymphocytic leukemia: implication for immunotherapeutic interventions. Tumour Biol. 34 (4), 2031–2039.

Jahn, T., Zuther, M., Friedrichs, B., Heuser, C., Guhlke, S., Abken, H., Hombach, A.A., 2012. An IL12–IL2-antibody fusion protein targeting Hodgkin's lymphoma cells potentiates activation of NK and T cells for an anti-tumor attack. PLoS One 7 (9), e44482.

Jantschitsch, C., Weichenthal, M., Proksch, E., Schwarz, T., Schwarz, A., 2012. IL-12 and IL-23 affect photocarcinogenesis differently. J. Invest. Dermatol. 132 (5), 1479–1486.

Kaiga, T., Sato, M., Kaneda, H., Iwakura, Y., Takayama, T., Tahara, H., 2007. Systemic administration of IL-23 induces potent antitumor immunity primarily mediated through Th1-type response in association with the endogenously expressed IL-12. J. Immunol. 178 (12), 7571–7580.

Kamiya, S., Owaki, T., Morishima, N., Fukai, F., Mizuguchi, J., Yoshimoto, T., 2004. An indispensable role for STAT1 in IL-27-induced T-bet expression but not proliferation of naive CD4+ T cells. J. Immunol. 173 (6), 3871–3877.

Kanegane, C., Sgadari, C., Kanegane, H., Teruya-Feldstein, J., Yao, L., Gupta, G., Farber, J.M., Liao, F., Liu, L., Tosato, G., 1998. Contribution of the CXC chemokines IP-10 and Mig to the antitumor effects of IL-12. J. Leukoc. Biol. 64 (3), 384–392.

Kang, W.K., Park, C., Yoon, H.L., Kim, W.S., Yoon, S.S., Lee, M.H., Park, K., Kim, K., Jeong, H.S., Kim, J.A., Nam, S.J., Yang, J.H., Son, Y.I., Baek, C.H., Han, J., Ree, H.J., Lee, E.S., Kim, S.H., Kim, D.W., Ahn, Y.C., Huh, S.J., Choe, Y.H., Lee, J.H., Park, M.H., Kong, G.S., Park, E.Y., Kang, Y.K., Bang, Y.J., Paik, N.S., Lee, S.N., Kim, S.H., Kim, S., Robbins, P.D., Tahara, H., Lotze, M.T., Park, C.H., 2001. Interleukin 12 gene therapy of cancer by peritumoral injection of transduced autologous fibroblasts: outcome of a phase I study. Hum. Gene. Ther. 12 (6), 671–684.

Kawamori, T., Uchiya, N., Sugimura, T., Wakabayashi, K., 2003. Enhancement of colon carcinogenesis by prostaglandin E2 administration. Carcinogenesis 24 (5), 985–990.

Kempe, S., Heinz, P., Kokai, E., Devergne, O., Marx, N., Wirth, T., 2009. Epstein–Barr virus-induced gene-3 is expressed in human atheroma plaques. Am. J. Pathol. 175 (1), 440–447.

Kerkar, S.P., Goldszmid, R.S., Muranski, P., Chinnasamy, D., Yu, Z., Reger, R.N., Leonardi, A.J., Morgan, R.A., Wang, E., Marincola, F.M., Trinchieri, G., Rosenberg, S.A., Restifo, N.P., December 2011. IL-12 triggers a programmatic change in dysfunctional myeloid-derived cells within mouse tumors. J. Clin. Invest. 121 (12), 4746–4757.

Kerkar, S.P., Leonardi, A.J., van Panhuys, N., Zhang, L., Yu, Z., Crompton, J.G., Pan, J.H., Palmer, D.C., Morgan, R.A., Rosenberg, S.A., Restifo, N.P., July 2013. Collapse of the tumor stroma is triggered by IL-12 induction of Fas. Mol. Ther. 21 (7), 1369–1377.

Kerkar, S.P., Muranski, P., Kaiser, A., Boni, A., Sanchez-Perez, L., Yu, Z., Palmer, D.C., Reger, R.N., Borman, Z.A., Zhang, L., Morgan, R.A., Gattinoni, L., Rosenberg, S.A., Trinchieri, G., Restifo, N.P., 2010. Tumor-specific CD8+ T cells expressing interleukin12 eradicate established cancers in lymphodepleted hosts. Cancer Res. 70 (17), 6725–6734.

Kerkar, S.P., Restifo, N.P., 2012. The power and pitfalls of IL-12. Blood 119 (18), 4096–4097.

Kinnebrew, M.A., Buffie, C.G., Diehl, G.E., Zenewicz, L.A., Leiner, I., Hohl, T.M., Flavell, R.A., Littman, D.R., Pamer, E.G., 2012. Interleukin 23 production by intestinal CD103(+)CD11b(+) dendritic cells in response to bacterial flagellin enhances mucosal innate immune defense. Immunity 36 (2), 276–287.

Klinke 2nd, D.J., 2010. A multiscale systems perspective on cancer, immunotherapy, and Interleukin-12. Mol. Cancer 9, 242.

Kobayashi, M., Fitz, L., Ryan, M., Hewick, R.M., Clark, S.C., Chan, S., Loudon, R., Sherman, F., Perussia, B., Trinchieri, G., 1989. Identification and purification of natural killer cell stimulatory factor (NKSF), a cytokine with multiple biologic effects on human lymphocytes. J. Exp. Med. 170 (3), 827–845.

Kochetkova, I., Golden, S., Holderness, K., Callis, G., Pascual, D.W., 2010. IL-35 stimulation of CD39+ regulatory T cells confers protection against collagen II-induced arthritis via the production of IL-10. J. Immunol. 184 (12), 7144–7153.

Koussoulas, V., Vassiliou, S., Giamarellos-Bourboulis, E.J., Tassias, G., Kotsaki, A., Barbatzas, C., Tzivras, M., 2009. Implications for a role of interleukin-23 in the pathogenesis of chronic gastritis and of peptic ulcer disease. Clin. Exp. Immunol. 156 (1), 97–101.

Kupfer, S.S., Torres, J.B., Hooker, S., Anderson, J.R., Skol, A.D., Ellis, N.A., Kittles, R.A., 2009. Novel single nucleotide polymorphism associations with colorectal cancer on chromosome 8q24 in African and European Americans. Carcinogenesis 30 (8), 1353–1357.

Kuramoto, T., Fujii, R., Nagai, H., Belladonna, M.L., Yoshimoto, T., Kohjimoto, Y., Inagaki, T., Hara, I., 2011. IL-23 gene therapy for mouse bladder tumour cell lines. BJU Int. 108 (6), 914–921.

Kutikhin, A.G., Yuzhalin, A.E., Volkov, A.N., Zhivotovskiy, A.S., Brusina, E.B., 2014. Correlation between genetic polymorphisms within IL-1B and TLR4 genes and cancer risk in a Russian population: a case–control study. Tumour Biol. 35 (5), 4821–4830.

Kuwajima, S., Sato, T., Ishida, K., Tada, H., Tezuka, H., Ohteki, T., 2006. Interleukin 15-dependent crosstalk between conventional and plasmacytoid dendritic cells is essential for CpG-induced immune activation. Nat. Immunol. 7 (7), 740–746.

Lan, F., Zhang, L., Wu, J., Zhang, J., Zhang, S., Li, K., Qi, Y., Lin, P., 2011. IL-23/IL-23R: potential mediator of intestinal tumor progression from adenomatous polyps to colorectal carcinoma. Int. J. Colorectal Dis. 26 (12), 1511–1518.

Langowski, J.L., Zhang, X., Wu, L., Mattson, J.D., Chen, T., Smith, K., Basham, B., McClanahan, T., Kastelein, R.A., Oft, M., 2006. IL-23 promotes tumour incidence and growth. Nature 442 (7101), 461–465.

Lehtonen, A., Lund, R., Lahesmaa, R., Julkunen, I., Sareneva, T., Matikainen, S., November 7, 2003. IFN-alpha and IL-12 activate IFN regulatory factor 1 (IRF-1), IRF-4, and IRF-8 gene expression in human NK and T cells. Cytokine 24 (3), 81–90.

Lenzi, R., Rosenblum, M., Verschraegen, C., Kudelka, A.P., Kavanagh, J.J., Hicks, M.E., Lang, E.A., Nash, M.A., Levy, L.B., Garcia, M.E., Platsoucas, C.D., Abbruzzese, J.L., Freedman, R.S., 2002. Phase I study of intraperitoneal recombinant human interleukin 12 in patients with Mullerian carcinoma, gastrointestinal primary malignancies, and mesothelioma. Clin. Cancer Res. 8, 3686–3695.

Li, J., Zhang, L., Zhang, J., Wei, Y., Li, K., Huang, L., Zhang, S., Gao, B., Wang, X., Lin, P., 2013. Interleukin 23 regulates proliferation of lung cancer cells in a concentration-dependent way in association with the interleukin-23 receptor. Carcinogenesis 34 (3), 658–666.

Li, J., Lau, G., Chen, L., Yuan, Y.F., Huang, J., Luk, J.M., Xie, D., Guan, X.Y., 2012a. Interleukin 23 promotes hepatocellular carcinoma metastasis via NF-kappa B induced matrix metalloproteinase 9 expression. PLoS One 7 (9), e46264.

Li, X., Mai, J., Virtue, A., Yin, Y., Gong, R., Sha, X., Gutchigian, S., Frisch, A., Hodge, I., Jiang, X., Wang, H., Yang, X.F., 2012b. IL-35 is a novel responsive anti-inflammatory cytokine–a new system of categorizing anti-inflammatory cytokines. PLoS One 7 (3), e33628.

Liu, J., Guan, X., Ma, X., 2007. Regulation of IL-27 p28 gene expression in macrophages through MyD88- and interferon-gamma-mediated pathways. J. Exp. Med. 204 (1), 141–152.

Liu, L., Wang, S., Shan, B., Shao, L., Sato, A., Kawamura, K., Li, Q., Ma, G., Tagawa, M., 2008. IL-27-mediated activation of natural killer cells and inflammation produced antitumour effects for human oesophageal carcinoma cells. Scand. J. Immunol. 68 (1), 22–29.

Liu, L., Meng, J., Zhang, C., Duan, Y., Zhao, L., Wang, S., Shan, B., 2012. Effects on apoptosis and cell cycle arrest contribute to the antitumor responses of interleukin-27 mediated by retrovirus in human pancreatic carcinoma cells. Oncol. Rep. 27 (5), 1497–1503.

Lindqvist, C.A., Christiansson, L.H., Thörn, I., Mangsbo, S., Paul-Wetterberg, G., Sundström, C., Tötterman, T.H., Simonsson, B., Enblad, G., Frisk, P., Olsson-Strömberg, U., Loskog, A.S., 2011. Both CD4+ FoxP3+ and CD4+ FoxP3- T cells from patients with B-cell malignancy express cytolytic markers and kill autologous leukaemic B cells in vitro. Immunology 133 (3), 296–306.

Ljujic, B., Radosavljevic, G., Jovanovic, I., Pavlovic, S., Zdravkovic, N., Milovanovic, M., Acimovic, L., Knezevic, M., Bankovic, D., Zdravkovic, D., Arsenijevic, N., 2010. Elevated serum level of IL-23 correlates with expression of VEGF in human colorectal carcinoma. Arch. Med. Res. 41 (3), 182–189.

Lo, C.H., Lee, S.C., Wu, P.Y., Pan, W.Y., Su, J., Cheng, C.W., Roffler, S.R., Chiang, B.L., Lee, C.N., Wu, C.W., Tao, M.H., 2003. Antitumor and antimetastatic activity of IL-23. J. Immunol. 171 (2), 600–607.

Long, J., Zhang, X., Wen, M., Kong, Q., Lv, Z., An, Y., Wei, X.Q., 2013. IL-35 over-expression increases apoptosis sensitivity and suppresses cell growth in human cancer cells. Biochem. Biophys. Res. Commun. 430 (1), 364–369.

Lowes, M.A., Russell, C.B., Martin, D.A., Towne, J.E., Krueger, J.G., 2013. The IL-23/T17 pathogenic axis in psoriasis is amplified by keratinocyte responses. Trends Immunol. 34 (4), 174–181.

Ma, X., Trinchieri, G., 2001. Regulation of interleukin-12 production in antigen-presenting cells. Adv. Immunol. 79, 55–92.

Maaser, C., Egan, L.J., Birkenbach, M.P., Eckmann, L., Kagnoff, M.F., 2004. Expression of Epstein–Barr virus-induced gene 3 and other interleukin-12-related molecules by human intestinal epithelium. Immunology 112 (3), 437–445.

Mahvi, D.M., Henry, M.B., Albertini, M.R., Weber, S., Meredith, K., Schalch, H., Rakhmilevich, A., Hank, J., Sondel, P., 2007. Intratumoral injection of IL-12 plasmid DNA—results of a phase I/IB clinical trial. Cancer Gene Ther. 14 (8), 717–723.

Maloy, K.J., 2008. The Interleukin-23/interleukin-17 axis in intestinal inflammation. J. Intern. Med. 263 (6), 584–590.

Mao, H., Gao, W., Ma, C., Sun, J., Liu, J., Shao, Q., Song, B., Qu, X., July 2013. Human placental trophoblasts express the immunosuppressive cytokine IL-35. Hum. Immunol. 74 (7), 872–877.

Marshall, N.A., Christie, L.E., Munro, L.R., Culligan, D.J., Johnston, P.W., Barker, R.N., Vickers, M.A., 2004. Immunosuppressive regulatory T cells are abundant in the reactive lymphocytes of Hodgkin lymphoma. Blood 103 (5), 1755–1762.

Meyaard, L., Hovenkamp, E., Otto, S.A., Miedema, F., 1996. IL-12- induced IL-10 production by human T cells as a negative feedback for IL-12-induced immune responses. J. Immunol. 156, 2776–2782.

Mitsuhashi, M., Liu, J., Cao, S., Shi, X., Ma, X., 2004. Regulation of interleukin-12 gene expression and its anti-tumor activities by prostaglandin E2 derived from mammary carcinomas. J. Leukoc. Biol. 76 (2), 322–332.

Molle, C., Nguyen, M., Flamand, V., Renneson, J., Trottein, F., De Wit, D., Willems, F., Goldman, M., Goriely, S., 2007. IL-27 synthesis induced by TLR ligation critically depends on IFN regulatory factor 3. J. Immunol. 178 (12), 7607–7615.

Mortarini, R., Borri, A., Tragni, G., Bersani, I., Vegetti, C., Bajetta, E., Pilotti, S., Cerundolo, V., Anichini, A., 2000. Peripheral burst of tumor-specific cytotoxic T lymphocytes and infiltration of metastatic lesions by memory CD8.T cells in melanoma patients receiving interleukin 12. Cancer Res. 60 (13), 3559–3568.

Motzer, R.J., Rakhit, A., Thompson, J.A., Nemunaitis, J., Murphy, B.A., Ellerhorst, J., Schwartz, L.H., Berg, W.J., Bukowski, R.M., 2001. Randomized multicenter phase II trial of subcutaneous recombinant human interleukin-12 versus interferon-alpha 2a for patients with advanced renal cell carcinoma. J. Interferon. Cytokine. Res. 21 (4), 257–263.

Motzer, R.J., Bukowski, R.M., 2006. Targeted therapy for metastatic renal cell carcinoma. J. Clin. Oncol. 24 (35), 5601–5608.

Mrklić, I., Ćapkun, V., Pogorelić, Z., Tomić, S., May 2013. Prognostic value of Ki-67 proliferating index in triple negative breast carcinomas. Pathol. Res. Pract. 209 (5), 296–301.

Murphy, C.A., Langrish, C.L., Chen, Y., Blumenschein, W., McClanahan, T., Kastelein, R.A., Sedgwick, J.D., Cua, D.J., 2003. Divergent pro- and antiinflammatory roles for IL-23 and IL-12 in joint autoimmune inflammation. J. Exp. Med. 198 (12), 1951–1957.

Murugaiyan, G., Mittal, A., Lopez-Diego, R., Maier, L.M., Anderson, D.E., Weiner, H.L., 2009. IL-27 is a key regulator of IL-10 and IL-17 production by human CD4+ T cells. J. Immunol. 183 (4), 2435–2443.

Nair, R.E., Jong, Y.S., Jones, S.A., Sharma, A., Mathiowitz, E., Egilmez, N.K., 2006. IL-12. GM-CSF microsphere therapy induces eradication of advanced spontaneous tumors in HER-2/neu transgenic mice but fails to achieve long-term cure due to the inability to maintain effector T-cell activity. J. Immunother. 29 (1), 10–20.

Nakahira, M., Tomura, M., Iwasaki, M., Ahn, H.J., Bian, Y., Hamaoka, T., Ohta, T., Kurimoto, M., Fujiwara, H., 2001. An absolute requirement for STAT4 and a role for IFN-gamma as an amplifying factor in IL-12 induction of the functional IL-18 receptor complex. J. Immunol. 167 (3), 1306–1312.

Nanni, P., Nicoletti, G., De Giovanni, C., Landuzzi, L., Di Carlo, E., Cavallo, F., Pupa, S.M., Rossi, I., Colombo, M.P., Ricci, C., Astolfi, A., Musiani, P., Forni, G., Lollini, P.L., 2001. Combined allogeneic tumor cell vaccination and systemic interleukin 12 prevents mammary carcinogenesis in HER-2/neu transgenic mice. J. Exp. Med. 194, 1195–1205.

Nastala, C.L., Edington, H.D., McKinney, T.G., Tahara, H., Nalesnik, M.A., Brunda, M.J., Gately, M.K., Wolf, S.F., Schreiber, R.D., Storkus, W.J., Johns, A., 1994. Recombinant IL-12 administration induces tumor regression in association with IFN-gamma production. J. Immunol. 153 (4), 1697–1706.

Neufert, C., Becker, C., Wirtz, S., Fantini, M.C., Weigmann, B., Galle, P.R., Neurath, M.F., 2007. IL-27 controls the development of inducible regulatory T cells and Th17 cells via differential effects on STAT1. Eur. J. Immunol. 37 (7), 1809–1816.

Neurath, M.F., 2008. IL-12 family members in experimental colitis. Mucosal Immunol. 1 (Suppl. 1), S28–S30.

Niedbala, W., Wei, X.Q., Cai, B., Hueber, A.J., Leung, B.P., McInnes, I.B., Liew, F.Y., 2007. IL-35 is a novel cytokine with therapeutic effects against collagen-induced arthritis through the expansion of regulatory T cells and suppression of Th17 cells. Eur. J. Immunol. 37 (11), 3021–3029.

Nielsen, S.R., Hammer, T., Gibson, J., Pepper, M.S., Nisato, R.E., Dissing, S., Tritsaris, K., August 2013. IL-27 inhibits lymphatic endothelial cell proliferation by STAT1-regulated gene expression. Microcirculation 20 (6), 555–564.

Noguchi, Y., Jungbluth, A., Richards, E.C., Old, L.J., 1996. Effect of interleukin 12 on tumor induction by 3-methylcholanthrene. Proc. Natl. Acad. Sci. U.S.A. 93, 11798–11801.

Oppmann, B., Lesley, R., Blom, B., Timans, J.C., Xu, Y., Hunte, B., Vega, F., Yu, N., Wang, J., Singh, K., Zonin, F., Vaisberg, E., Churakova, T., Liu, M., Gorman, D., Wagner, J., Zurawski, S., Liu, Y., Abrams, J.S., Moore, K.W., Rennick, D., de Waal-Malefyt, R., Hannum, C., Bazan, J.F., Kastelein, R.A., 2000. Novel p19 protein engages IL-12p40 to form a cytokine, IL-23, with biological activities similar as well as distinct from IL-12. Immunity 13 (5), 715–725.

Olson, B.M., Jankowska-Gan, E., Becker, J.T., Vignali, D.A., Burlingham, W.J., McNeel, D.G., 2012. Human prostate tumor antigen-specific CD8+ regulatory T cells are inhibited by CTLA-4 or IL-35 blockade. J. Immunol. 189 (12), 5590–5601.

Oniki, S., Nagai, H., Horikawa, T., Furukawa, J., Belladonna, M.L., Yoshimoto, T., Hara, I., Nishigori, C., 2006. Interleukin-23 and interleukin-27 exert quite different antitumor and vaccine effects on poorly immunogenic melanoma. Cancer Res. 66 (12), 6395–6404.

Owaki, T., Asakawa, M., Morishima, N., Hata, K., Fukai, F., Matsui, M., Mizuguchi, J., Yoshimoto, T., 2005. A role for IL-27 in early regulation of Th1 differentiation. J. Immunol. 175 (4), 2191–2200.

Owaki, T., Asakawa, M., Kamiya, S., Takeda, K., Fukai, F., Mizuguchi, J., Yoshimoto, T., 2006. IL-27 suppresses CD28-mediated [correction of medicated] IL-2 production through suppressor of cytokine signaling 3. J. Immunol. 176 (5), 2773–2780.

Paladugu, M., Thakur, A., Lum, L.G., Mittal, S., Parajuli, P., 2013. Generation and immunologic functions of Th17 cells in malignant gliomas. Cancer Immunol. Immunother. 62 (1), 75–86.

Pan, H.F., Tao, J.H., Ye, D.Q., 2010. Therapeutic potential of IL-27 in systemic lupus erythematosus. Expert Opin. Ther. Targets 14 (5), 479–484.

Parihar, R., Nadella, P., Lewis, A., Jensen, R., De Hoff, C., Dierksheide, J.E., VanBuskirk, A.M., Magro, C.M., Young, D.C., Shapiro, C.L., Carson 3rd, W.E., 2004. A phase I study of interleukin 12 with trastuzumab in patients with human epidermal growth factor receptor-2-overexpressing malignancies: Analysis of sustained interferon gamma production in a subset of patients. Clin. Cancer Res. 10 (15), 5027–5037.

Pathak, S., Ma, S., Trinh, L., Eudy, J., Wagner, K.U., Joshi, S.S., Lu, R., 2011. IRF4 is a suppressor of c-Myc induced B cell leukemia. PLoS One 6 (7), e22628.

Peterson, A.C., Harlin, H., Gajewski, T.F., June 15, 2003. Immunization with Melan-A peptide-pulsed peripheral blood mononuclear cells plus recombinant human interleukin-12 induces clinical activity and T-cell responses in advanced melanoma. J Clin. Oncol. 21 (12), 2342–2348.

Pflanz, S.,Timans,J.C., Cheung,J., Rosales, R., Kanzler, H., Gilbert,J., Hibbert, L., Churakova,T., Travis, M.,Vaisberg, E., Blumenschein,W.M., Mattson,J.D.,Wagner,J.L.,To,W., Zurawski, S., McClanahan, T.K., Gorman, D.M., Bazan, J.F., de Waal Malefyt, R., Rennick, D., Kastelein, R.A., 2002. IL-27, a heterodimeric cytokine composed of EBI3 and p28 protein, induces proliferation of naive CD4(+) T cells. Immunity 16 (6), 779–790.

Pflanz, S., Hibbert, L., Mattson, J., Rosales, R., Vaisberg, E., Bazan, J.F., Phillips, J.H., McClanahan,T.K., de Waal Malefyt, R., Kastelein, R.A., 2004.WSX-1 and glycoprotein 130 constitute a signal-transducing receptor for IL-27. J. Immunol. 172 (4), 2225–2231.

Polimeno, M., Napolitano, M., Costantini, S., Portella, L., Esposito, A., Capone, F., Guerriero, E.,Trotta,A., Zanotta, S., Pucci, L., Longo, N., Perdonà, S., Pignata, S., Castello, G., Scala, S., March 15, 2013. Regulatory T cells, interleukin (IL)-6, IL-8, vascular endothelial growth factor (VEGF), CXCL10, CXCL11, epidermal growth factor (EGF) and hepatocyte growth factor (HGF) as surrogate markers of host immunity in patients with renal cell carcinoma. BJU Int. http://dx.doi.org/10.1111/bju.12068. [Epub ahead of print].

Põld, M., Zhu, L.X., Sharma, S., Burdick, M.D., Lin,Y., Lee, P.P., Põld,A., Luo,J., Krysan, K., Dohadwala, M., Mao,J.T., Batra, R.K., Strieter, R.M., Dubinett, S.M., 2004. Cyclooxygenase-2-dependent expression of angiogenic CXC chemokines ENA-78/CXC Ligand (CXCL) 5 and interleukin-8/CXCL8 in human non-small cell lung cancer. Cancer Res. 64 (5), 1853–1860.

Portielje, J.E., Kruit, W.H., Schuler, M., Beck, J., Lamers, C.H., Stoter, G., Huber, C., de Boer-Dennert, M., Rakhit,A., Bolhuis, R.L., Aulitzky,W.E., 1999. Phase I study of subcutaneously administered recombinant human interleukin 12 in patients with advanced renal cell cancer. Clin. Cancer Res. 5 (12), 3983–3989.

Pugh, S., Thomas, G.A., 1994. Patients with adenomatous polyps and carcinomas have increased colonic mucosal prostaglandin E2. Gut. 35 (5), 675–678.

Rasmuson,A., Kock,A., Fuskevåg, O.M., Kruspig, B., Simón-Santamaría,J., Gogvadze,V.,Johnsen, J.I., Kogner, P., Sveinbjörnsson, B., 2012. Autocrine prostaglandin E2 signaling promotes tumor cell survival and proliferation in childhood neuroblastoma. PLoS One 7 (1), e29331.

Reay,J., Kim, S.H., Lockhart, E., Kolls,J., Robbins, P.D., 2009.Adenoviral-mediated, intratumor gene transfer of interleukin 23 induces a therapeutic antitumor response. Cancer Gene Ther. 16 (10), 776–785.

Reay, J., Gambotto, A., Robbins, P.D., 2012. The antitumor effects of adenoviral-mediated, intratumoral delivery of interleukin 23 require endogenous IL-12. Cancer Gene Ther. 19 (2), 135–143.

Reppert, S., Boross, I., Koslowski, M.,Türeci, Ö., Koch, S., Lehr, H.A., Finotto, S., 2011. A role for T-bet-mediated tumour immune surveillance in anti-IL-17A treatment of lung cancer. Nat. Commun. 2, 600.

Rook, A.H.,Wood, G.S.,Yoo, E.K., Elenitsas, R., Kao, D.M., Sherman, M.L.,Witmer,W.K., Rockwell, K.A., Shane, R.B., Lessin, S.R.,Vonderheid, E.C., 1999. Interleukin-12 therapy of cutaneous T-cell lymphoma induces lesion regression and cytotoxic T-cell responses. Blood 94 (3), 902–908.

Sakaguchi, S., 2011. Regulatory T cells: history and perspective. Methods Mol. Biol. 707, 3–17.

Salcedo, R., Stauffer, J.K., Lincoln, E., Back,T.C., Hixon, J.A., Hahn, C., Shafer-Weaver, K., Malyguine,A., Kastelein, R.,Wigginton, J.M., 2004. IL-27 mediates complete regression of orthotopic primary and metastatic murine neuroblastoma tumors: role for CD8+ T cells. J. Immunol. 173 (12), 7170–7182.

Salcedo, R., Hixon, J.A., Stauffer, J.K., Jalah, R., Brooks,A.D., Khan,T., Dai, R.M., Scheetz, L., Lincoln, E., Back,T.C., Powell, D., Hurwitz,A.A., Sayers,T.J., Kastelein, R., Pavlakis, G.N., Felber, B.K., Trinchieri, G., Wigginton, J.M., April 1, 2009. Immunologic and therapeutic synergy of IL-27 and IL-2: enhancement of T cell sensitization, tumor-specific CTL reactivity and complete regression of disseminated neuroblastoma metastases in the liver and bone marrow. J. Immunol. 182 (7), 4328–4338.

Sarmiento, U.M., Riley, J.H., Knaack, P.A., Lipman, J.M., Becker, J.M., Gately, M.K., Chiz-zonite, R., Anderson, T.D., 1994. Biologic effects of recombinant human interleukin-12 in squirrel monkeys (*Sciureus saimiri*). Lab. Invest. 71 (6), 862–873.

Sano, H., Kawahito, Y., Wilder, R.L., Hashiramoto, A., Mukai, S., Asai, K., Kimura, S., Kato, H., Kondo, M., Hla, T., 1995. Expression of cyclooxygenase-1 and -2 in human colorectal cancer. Cancer Res. 55 (17), 3785–3789.

Sato, T., Terai, M., Tamura, Y., Alexeev, V., Mastrangelo, M.J., Selvan, S.R., 2011. Interleukin 10 in the tumor microenvironment: a target for anticancer immunotherapy. Immunol. Res. 51 (2–3), 170–182.

Sehouli, J., Mustea, A., Könsgen, D., Katsares, I., Lichtenegger, W., 2002. Polymorphism of IL-1 receptor antagonist gene: role in cancer. Anticancer Res. 22 (6A), 3421–3424.

Sekar, D., Hahn, C., Brüne, B., Roberts, E., Weigert, A., June 2012. Apoptotic tumor cells induce IL-27 release from human DCs to activate Treg cells that express CD69 and attenuate cytotoxicity. Eur. J. Immunol. 42 (6), 1585–1598.

Sgadari, C., Angiolillo, A.L., Tosato, G., 1996. Inhibition of angiogenesis by interleukin-12 is mediated by the interferon inducible protein 10. Blood 87, 3877–3882.

Shan, B., Yu, L., Shimozato, O., Li, Q., Tagawa, M., 2004. Expression of interleukin-21 and 23 in human esophageal tumors produced antitumor effects in nude mice. Anticancer Res. 24 (1), 79–82.

Shan, B.E., Hao, J.S., Li, Q.X., Tagawa, M., 2006. Antitumor activity and immune enhancement of murine interleukin-23 expressed in murine colon carcinoma cells. Cell. Mol. Immunol. 3 (1), 47–52.

Shen, C.J., Yuan, Z.H., Liu, Y.X., Hu, G.Y., 2012. Increased numbers of T helper 17 cells and the correlation with clinicopathological characteristics in multiple myeloma. J. Int. Med. Res. 40 (2), 556–564.

Shenghui, Z., Yixiang, H., Jianbo, W., Kang, Y., Laixi, B., Yan, Z., Xi, X., 2011. Elevated frequencies of CD4+CD25+CD127lo regulatory T cells is associated to poor prognosis in patients with acute myeloid leukemia. Int. J. Cancer 129 (6), 1373–1381.

Shibata, S., Tada, Y., Kanda, N., Nashiro, K., Kamata, M., Karakawa, M., Miyagaki, T., Kai, H., Saeki, H., Shirakata, Y., Watanabe, S., Tamaki, K., Sato, S., 2010. Possible roles of IL-27 in the pathogenesis of psoriasis. J. Invest. Dermatol. 130 (4), 1034–1039.

Shimizu, M., Shimamura, M., Owaki, T., Asakawa, M., Fujita, K., Kudo, M., Iwakura, Y., Takeda, Y., Luster, A.D., Mizuguchi, J., Yoshimoto, T., 2006. Antiangiogenic and antitumor activities of IL-27. J. Immunol. 176 (12), 7317–7324.

Shimozato, O., Sato, A., Kawamura, K., Chiyo, M., Ma, G., Li, Q., Tagawa, M., September 2009. The secreted form of p28 subunit of interleukin (IL)-27 inhibits biological functions of IL-27 and suppresses anti-allogeneic immune responses. Immunology 128 (Suppl. 1), e816–e825.

Schneider, R., Yaneva, T., Beauseigle, D., El-Khoury, L., Arbour, N., 2011. IL-27 increases the proliferation and effector functions of human naïve CD8+ T lymphocytes and promotes their development into Tc1 cells. Eur. J. Immunol. 41 (1), 47–59.

Sonoshita, M., Takaku, K., Sasaki, N., Sugimoto, Y., Ushikubi, F., Narumiya, S., Oshima, M., Taketo, M.M., 2001. Acceleration of intestinal polyposis through prostaglandin receptor EP2 in Apc(Delta 716) knockout mice. Nat. Med. 7 (9), 1048–1051.

Stanilov, N.S., Miteva, L.D., Dobreva, Z.G., Jovchev, J.P., Cirovski, G.M., Stanilova, S.A., 2012. Monocytes expression of IL-12 related and IL-10 genes in association with development of colorectal cancer. Mol. Biol. Rep. 39 (12), 10895–10902.

Stumhofer, J.S., Laurence, A., Wilson, E.H., Huang, E., Tato, C.M., Johnson, L.M., Villarino, A.V., Huang, Q., Yoshimura, A., Sehy, D., Saris, C.J., O'Shea, J.J., Hennighausen, L., Ernst, M., Hunter, C.A., 2006. Interleukin 27 negatively regulates the development of interleukin 17-producing T helper cells during chronic inflammation of the central nervous system. Nat. Immunol. 7 (9), 937–945.

Stumhofer, J.S., Silver, J.S., Laurence, A., Porrett, P.M., Harris, T.H., Turka, L.A., Ernst, M., Saris, C.J., O'Shea, J.J., HunteKr, C.A., 2007a. Interleukins 27 and 6 induce STAT3-mediated T cell production of interleukin 10. Nat. Immunol. 8 (12), 1363–1371.

Stumhofer, J.S., Silver, J., Hunter, C.A., 2007b. Negative regulation of Th17 responses. Semin. Immunol. 19 (6), 394–399.

Stumhofer, J.S., Tait, E.D., Quinn 3rd, W.J., Hosken, N., Spudy, B., Goenka, R., Fielding, C.A., O'Hara, A.C., Chen, Y., Jones, M.L., Saris, C.J., Rose-John, S., Cua, D.J., Jones, S.A., Elloso, M.M., Grötzinger, J., Cancro, M.P., Levin, S.D., Hunter, C.A., 2010. A role for IL-27p28 as an antagonist of gp130-mediated signaling. Nat. Immunol. 11 (12), 1119–1126.

Stritesky, G.L., Yeh, N., Kaplan, M.H., 2008. IL-23 promotes maintenance but not commitment to the Th17 lineage. J. Immunol. 181 (9), 5948–5955.

Sunderkotter, C., Steinbrink, K., Goebeler, M., Bhardwaj, R., Sorg, C., 1994. Macrophages and angiogenesis. J. Leukoc. Biol. 55 (3), 410–422.

Suzuki, H., Ogawa, H., Miura, K., Haneda, S., Watanabe, K., Ohnuma, S., Sasaki, H., Sase, T., Kimura, S., Kajiwara, T., Komura, T., Toshima, M., Matsuda, Y., Shibata, C., Sasaki, I., 2012. IL-23 directly enhances the proliferative and invasive activities of colorectal carcinoma. Oncol. Lett. 4 (2), 199–204.

Szczepanski, M.J., Szajnik, M., Czystowska, M., Mandapathil, M., Strauss, L., Welsh, A., Foon, K.A., Whiteside, T.L., Boyiadzis, M., 2009. Increased frequency and suppression by regulatory T cells in patients with acute myelogenous leukemia. Clin. Cancer Res. 15 (10), 3325–3332.

Tang, C., Iwakura, Y., 2012. IL-23 in colitis: targeting the progenitors. Immunity 37 (6), 957–959.

Takaoka, A., Hayakawa, S., Yanai, H., Stoiber, D., Negishi, H., Kikuchi, H., Sasaki, S., Imai, K., Shibue, T., Honda, K., Taniguchi, T., 2003. Integration of interferon-alpha/beta signalling to p53 responses in tumour suppression and antiviral defence. Nature 424 (6948), 516–523.

Takeda, A., Hamano, S., Yamanaka, A., Hanada, T., Ishibashi, T., Mak, T.W., Yoshimura, A., Yoshida, H., 2003. Cutting edge: role of IL-27/WSX-1 signaling for induction of T-bet through activation of STAT1 during initial Th1 commitment. J. Immunol. 170 (10), 4886–4890.

Teng, M.W., Andrews, D.M., McLaughlin, N., von Scheidt, B., Ngiow, S.F., Möller, A., Hill, G.R., Iwakura, Y., Oft, M., Smyth, M.J., 2010. IL-23 suppresses innate immune response independently of IL-17A during carcinogenesis and metastasis. Proc. Natl. Acad. Sci. USA 107 (18), 8328–8333.

Teng, M.W., von Scheidt, B., Duret, H., Towne, J.E., Smyth, M.J., March 15, 2011. Anti-IL-23 monoclonal antibody synergizes in combination with targeted therapies or IL-2 to suppress tumor growth and metastases. Cancer Res. 71 (6), 2077–2086.

Thill, M., Fischer, D., Kelling, K., Hoellen, F., Dittmer, C., Hornemann, A., Salehin, D., Diedrich, K., Friedrich, M., Becker, S., 2010. Expression of vitamin D receptor (VDR), cyclooxygenase-2 (COX-2) and 15-hydroxyprostaglandin dehydrogenase (15-PGDH) in benign and malignant ovarian tissue and 25-hydroxycholecalciferol (25(OH2)D3) and prostaglandin E2 (PGE2) serum level in ovarian cancer patients. J. Steroid Biochem. Mol. Biol. 121 (1–2), 387–390.

Trinchieri, G., Pflanz, S., Kastelein, R.A., 2003. The IL-12 family of heterodimeric cytokines: new players in the regulation of T cell responses. Immunity 19 (5), 641–644.

Ugai, S., Shimozato, O., Yu, L., Wang, Y.Q., Kawamura, K., Yamamoto, H., Yamaguchi, T., Saisho, H., Sakiyama, S., Tagawa, M., 2003. Transduction of the IL-21 and IL-23 genes in human pancreatic carcinoma cells produces natural killer cell-dependent and -independent antitumor effects. Cancer Gene Ther. 10 (10), 771–778.

van-Netten, J.P., Ashmead, B.J., Parker, R.L., Thornton, I.G., Fletcher, C., Cavers, D., Coy, P., Brigden, M.L., 1993. Macrophage-tumor cell associations: A factor in metastasis of breast cancer? J. Leukoc. Biol. 54, 360–362.

van Seventer, J.M., Nagai, T., van Seventer, G.A., 2002. Interferon-beta differentially regulates expression of the IL-12 family members p35, p40, p19 and EBI3 in activated human dendritic cells. J. Neuroimmunol. 133 (1–2), 60–71.

Villarino, A., Hibbert, L., Lieberman, L., Wilson, E., Mak, T., Yoshida, H., Kastelein, R.A., Saris, C., Hunter, C.A., 2003. The IL-27R (WSX-1) is required to suppress T cell hyperactivity during infection. Immunity 19 (5), 645–655.

Villarino, A.V., Stumhofer, J.S., Saris, C.J., Kastelein, R.A., de Sauvage, F.J., Hunter, C.A., 2006. IL-27 limits IL-2 production during Th1 differentiation. J. Immunol. 176 (1), 237–247.

Voest, E.E., Kenyon, B.M., O'Reilly, M.S., Truitt, G., D'Amato, R.J., Folkman, J., 1995. Inhibition of angiogenesis in vivo by interleukin 12. J. Natl. Cancer Inst. 87 (8), 581–586.

Volpe, E., Servant, N., Zollinger, R., Bogiatzi, S.I., Hupé, P., Barillot, E., Soumelis, V., 2008. A critical function for transforming growth factor-beta, interleukin 23 and pro-inflammatory cytokines in driving and modulating human T(H)-17 responses. Nat. Immunol. 9 (6), 650–657.

Wagner, H.J., Bollard, C.M., Vigouroux, S., Huls, M.H., Anderson, R., Prentice, H.G., Brenner, M.K., Heslop, H.E., Rooney, C.M., 2004. A strategy for treatment of Epstein–Barr virus-positive Hodgkin's disease by targeting interleukin 12 to the tumor environment using tumor antigen-specific T cells. Cancer Gene Ther. 11 (2), 81–91.

Wang, K.S., Frank, D.A., Ritz, J., 2000. Interleukin-2 enhances the response of natural killer cells to interleukin-12 through upregulation of the interleukin-12 receptor and STAT4. Blood 95 (10), 3183–3190.

Wang, Y.Q., Ugai, S., Shimozato, O., Yu, L., Kawamura, K., Yamamoto, H., Yamaguchi, T., Saisho, H., Tagawa, M., 2003. Induction of systemic immunity by expression of interleukin-23 in murine colon carcinoma cells. Int. J. Cancer 105 (6), 820–824.

Wang, X., Zheng, J., Liu, J., Yao, J., He, Y., Li, X., Yu, J., Yang, J., Liu, Z., Huang, S., 2005. Increased population of CD4(+)CD25(high), regulatory T cells with their higher apoptotic and proliferating status in peripheral blood of acute myeloid leukemia patients. Eur. J. Haematol. 75 (6), 468–476.

Wang, S., Miyazaki, Y., Shinozaki, Y., Yoshida, H., 2007. Augmentation of antigen-presenting and Th1 promoting functions of dendritic cells by WSX-1 (IL-27R) deficiency. J. Immunol. 179 (10), 6421–6428.

Wang, R., Han, G., Wang, J., Chen, G., Xu, R., Wang, L., Li, X., Shen, B., Li, Y., 2008. The pathogenic role of interleukin-27 in autoimmune diabetes. Cell. Mol. Life Sci. 65 (23), 3851–3860.

Wang, D., DuBois, R.N., 2008. Pro-inflammatory prostaglandins and progression of colorectal cancer. Cancer Lett. 267 (2), 197–203.

Wang, W.W., Wang, Z.M., Liu, Y.Y., Qin, Y.H., Shen, Q., 2010. Increased level of Th17 cells in peripheral blood correlates with the development of hepatocellular carcinoma. Zhonghua Zhong Liu Za Zhi 32 (10), 757–761.

Wang, Z., Liu, J.Q., Liu, Z., Shen, R., Zhang, G., Xu, J., Basu, S., Feng, Y., Bai, X.F., 2013. Tumor-derived IL-35 promotes tumor growth by enhancing myeloid cell accumulation and angiogenesis. J. Immunol. 190 (5), 2415–2423.

Waldner, M.J., Neurath, M.F., 2009. Gene therapy using IL 12 family members in infection, auto immunity, and cancer. Curr. Gene Ther. 9 (4), 239–247.

Watkins, S.K., Egilmez, N.K., Suttles, J., Stout, R.D., 2007. IL-12 rapidly alters the functional profile of tumor-associated and tumor infiltrating macrophages in vitro and in vivo. J. Immunol. 178 (3), 1357–1362.

Watkins, S.K., Li, B., Richardson, K.S., Head, K., Egilmez, N.K., Zeng, Q., Suttles, J., Stout, R.D., 2009. Rapid release of cytoplasmic IL-15 from tumor-associated macrophages is an initial and critical event in IL-12-initiated tumor regression. Eur. J. Immunol. 39 (8), 2126–2135.

Weiss, G.R., O'Donnell, M.A., Loughlin, K., Zonno, K., Laiberte, R.J., Sherman, M.L., 2003. Phase 1 study of the intravesical administration of recombinant human interleukin-12 in patients with recurrent superficial transitional cell carcinoma of the bladder. J. Immunother. 26, 343–348.

Wirtz, S., Billmeier, U., Mchedlidze, T., Blumberg, R.S., Neurath, M.F., 2011. Interleukin-35 mediates mucosal immune responses that protect against T-cell-dependent colitis. Gastroenterology 141 (5), 1875–1886.

Wojno, E.D., Hunter, C.A., 2012. New directions in the basic and translational biology of interleukin-27. Trends Immunol. 33 (2), 91–97.

Wu, H., Li, P., Shao, N., Ma, J., Ji, M., Sun, X., Ma, D., Ji, C., May 2012. Aberrant expression of Treg-associated cytokine IL-35 along with IL-10 and TGF-β in acute myeloid leukemia. Oncol. Lett. 3 (5), 1119–1123.

Wu, H., Chen, P., Liao, R., Li, Y.W., Yi, Y., Wang, J.X., Cai, X.Y., He, H.W., Jin, J.J., Cheng, Y.F., Fan, J., Sun, J., Qiu, S.J., September 2013. Intratumoral regulatory T cells with higher prevalence and more suppressive activity in hepatocellular carcinoma patients. J. Gastroenterol. Hepatol. 28 (9), 1555–1564.

Xia, L., Tian, D., Huang, W., Zhu, H., Wang, J., Zhang, Y., Hu, H., Nie, Y., Fan, D., Wu, K., 2012. Upregulation of IL-23 expression in patients with chronic hepatitis B is mediated by the HBx/ERK/NF-κB pathway. J. Immunol. 188 (2), 753–764.

Xin, Z., Sriram, S., 1998. Vasoactive intestinal peptide inhibits IL-12 and nitric oxide production in murine macrophages. J. Neuroimmunol. 89 (1–2), 206–212.

Xu, M., Mizoguchi, I., Morishima, N., Chiba, Y., Mizoguchi, J., Yoshimoto, T., 2010. Regulation of antitumor immune responses by the IL-12 family cytokines, IL-12, IL-23, and IL-27. Clin. Dev. Immunol. 2010.

Yao, J., Liu, L., Yang, M., 2014. Interleukin-23 receptor genetic variants contribute to susceptibility of multiple cancers. Gene 533 (1), 21–25.

Yanagida, T., Kato, T., Igarashi, O., Inoue, T., Nariuchi, H., 1994. Second signal activity of IL-12 on the proliferation and IL-2R expression of T helper cell-1 clone. J. Immunol. 152 (10), 4919–4928.

Yang, Z.Z., Novak, A.J., Stenson, M.J., Witzig, T.E., Ansell, S.M., 2006. Intratumoral CD4+CD25+ regulatory T-cell-mediated suppression of infiltrating CD4+ T cells in B-cell non-Hodgkin lymphoma. Blood 107 (9), 3639–3646.

Yoshida, H., Nakaya, M., Miyazaki, Y., 2009. Interleukin 27: a double-edged sword for offense and defense. J. Leukoc. Biol. 86 (6), 1295–1303.

Yoshimoto, T., Takeda, K., Tanaka, T., Ohkusu, K., Kashiwamura, S., Okamura, H., Akira, S., Nakanishi, K., 1998. IL-12 up-regulates IL-18 receptor expression on T cells, Th1 cells, and B cells: Synergism with IL-18 for IFN-gamma production. J. Immunol. 161 (7), 3400–3407.

Yoshimoto, T., Yoshimoto, T., Yasuda, K., Mizuguchi, J., Nakanishi, K., 2007. IL-27 suppresses Th2 cell development and Th2 cytokines production from polarized Th2 cells: a novel therapeutic way for Th2-mediated allergic inflammation. J. Immunol. 179 (7), 4415–4423.

Yoshimoto, T., Morishima, N., Mizoguchi, I., Shimizu, M., Nagai, H., Oniki, S., Oka, M., Nishigori, C., Mizoguchi, J., 2008. Antiproliferative activity of IL-27 on melanoma. J. Immunol. 180 (10), 6527–6535.

Younes, A., Pro, B., Robertson, M.J., Flinn, I.W., Romaguera, J.E., Hagemeister, F., Dang, N.H., Fiumara, P., Loyer, E.M., Cabanillas, F.F., McLaughlin, P.W., Rodriguez, M.A., Samaniego, F., 2004. Phase II clinical trial of interleukin-12 in patients with relapsed and refractory non-Hodgkin's lymphoma and Hodgkin's disease. Clin. Cancer Res. 10 (16), 5432–5438.

Young, A., Linehan, E., Hams, E., O'Hara Hall, A.C., McClurg, A., Johnston, J.A., Hunter, C.A., Fallon, P.G., Fitzgerald, D.C., 2012. Cutting edge: suppression of GM-CSF expression in murine and human T cells by IL-27. J. Immunol. 189 (5), 2079–2083.

Yuan, X.L., Chen, L., Li, M.X., Dong, P., Xue, J., Wang, J., Zhang, T.T., Wang, X.A., Zhang, F.M., Ge, H.L., Shen, L.S., Xu, D., 2010. Elevated expression of Foxp3 in tumor-infiltrating Treg cells suppresses T-cell proliferation and contributes to gastric cancer progression in a COX-2-dependent manner. Clin. Immunol. 134 (3), 277–288.

Yuzhalin, A.E., Kutikhin, A.G., 2012. Interleukin-12: clinical usage and molecular markers of cancer susceptibility. Growth Factors 30 (3), 176–191.

Zhang, L., Kerkar, S.P., Yu, Z., Zheng, Z., Yang, S., Restifo, N.P., Rosenberg, S.A., Morgan, R.A., 2011. Improving adoptive T cell therapy by targeting and controlling IL-12 expression to the tumor environment. Mol. Ther. 19 (4), 751–759.

Zhang, S., Li, J., Zhang, J., Zhang, L., Lin, P., 2012. Interleukin 23 promotes lung adenocarcinoma a549 cell migration and invasion. Zhongguo Fei Ai Za Zhi 15 (5), 253–259.

Zhang, J., Tian, H., Li, C., Cheng, L., Zhang, S., Zhang, X., Wang, R., Xu, F., Dai, L., Shi, G., Chen, X., Li, Y., Du, T., Deng, J., Liu, Y., Yang, Y., Wei, Y., Deng, H., 2013. Antitumor effects obtained by autologous Lewis lung cancer cell vaccine engineered to secrete mouse Interleukin 27 by means of cationic liposome. Mol. Immunol. 55 (3–4), 264–274.

Zijlmans, H.J., Punt, S., Fleuren, G.J., Trimbos, J.B., Kenter, G.G., Gorter, A., 2012. Role of IL-12p40 in cervical carcinoma. Br. J. Cancer 107 (12), 1956–1962.

CHAPTER 8

Interleukin-17 Superfamily and Cancer

The most exciting phrase to hear in science, the one that heralds new discoveries, is not 'Eureka!' (I found it!) but 'That's funny ...'

Isaac Asimov, American biologist (1920–1992)

8.1 INTRODUCTION

Recent discoveries in the field of immunology have brought significant modifications in the commonly accepted model of Th1/Th2 helper T cells. Not long ago, a subset of T cells that differed from both Th1 and Th2 cells has been discovered (Yao et al., 1995). During the detailed investigation, the novel subset had been demonstrated to produce a number of specific cytokines such as interleukin (IL)-21, IL-22, and IL-17, which are not normally expressed by other T cells. Since further research had revealed that IL-17 is responsible for the key features of that new T cell lineage, the whole subset of cells was termed Th17 (Yao et al., 1995). To date, the Th17 cell subset has been widely known as an essential factor linking innate and adaptive immunity. The importance of Th17 cells is definitely recognized much more today, as it has become clear that they play a vital role in activating the immune response against bacteria and fungi (Gaffen, 2009).

However, it is worth noting that strong proinflammatory effects, together with immune-mediated tissue damage, have long been established as a hallmark of Th17 cells (Steinman, 2008). Apparently due to the fact that they are crucial inflammatory mediators, Th17 cells have been found to be involved in the development of various autoimmune and inflammatory diseases such as diabetes, rheumatoid arthritis, inflammatory bowel disease, thrombocytopenia, multiple sclerosis, asthma, psoriasis, and Sjogren's syndrome (reviewed by Hemdan et al., 2010).

The problem of the role of Th17 cells in cancer biology has been much discussed in the recent literature. Nonetheless, the present understanding of this question is limited due to numerous conflicting findings and a relative lack of a consistent pattern of results (reviewed by Ji and Zhang, 2010; Hemdan et al., 2010). Most researchers now agree that there is no definitely

Interleukins in Cancer Biology
http://dx.doi.org/10.1016/B978-0-12-801121-8.00008-7

positive or negative impact of Th17 cells on malignant tumors, as numerous studies indicated not only suppressing but also supporting activities of these cells in different cancers (Greten et al., 2012). The current research in the field is focused on the clarification of subtle differences in the roles of these cells in various malignancies. Due to the fact that all the basic characteristics of Th17 cells are determined by the biological effects exerted by the IL-17 family, the majority of the contemporary studies are being concentrated on identifying the link between IL-17 and the peculiarities of the etiology and pathogenesis of Th17-modulated diseases, including cancer. Here, we give a summary of the present understanding of the place of IL-17 in tumor development.

8.2 IL-17 SUPERFAMILY IN BRIEF

8.2.1 Nomenclature and Classification

The first member of the IL-17 superfamily was discovered by Rouvier et al. (1993) and named cytotoxic T-lymphocyte antigen 8. More recently, it has been shown that there are actually six different but structurally related representatives of the one family, among which are IL-17A, IL-17B, IL-17C, IL-17D, IL-17E (also known as IL-25), and IL-17F (Gaffen, 2009). All these cytokines are homodimeric molecules composed of 155–202 amino acid residues. Most of them exhibit a significant difference in identity to one another; for instance, IL-17A shares only 17% of the amino acid residues with IL-17E but has a 50% identity to IL-17F (Iwakura et al., 2011).

All the representatives of the IL-17 superfamily exert their biological effects through corresponding receptors, namely, IL-17RA, IL-17RB, IL-17RC, IL-17RD, and IL-17RE. It is to be noted that these receptors are believed to act as either homodimers, such as IL-17RB, IL-17RC, and IL-17RD, or heterodimers, such as IL-17RA/IL-17RC, IL-17RA/IL-17RB, and IL-17RA/IL-17RE. In particular, IL-17A and IL-17F are both known to be ligands of the IL-17RA/IL-17RC heterodimer, whereas IL-17C and IL-17E bind to IL-17RA/IL-17RE and IL-17RA/IL-17RB, respectively (reviewed by Iwakura et al., 2011; Song and Qian, 2013). It is also interesting to note that all the receptors of the IL-17 superfamily possess specific conserved motifs such as an intracellular toll/interleukin-1 receptor-like domain called SEF/IL-17R (SEFIR) and an extracellular fibronectin III-like domain. It should also be noted that nowadays there is some confusion in the current nomenclature, as the functional receptor for IL-17D has not yet been identified, whereas the actual ligand for IL-17RD is still unknown (reviewed by Gaffen, 2009).

8.2.2 Cellular Sources and Targeting Cells

Different representatives of the IL-17 superfamily are to be produced by different cellular sources. As mentioned above, the vast majority of IL-17A and IL-17F are expressed by Th17 cells; however, they are also known to be produced by monocytes, γδ T cells, natural killer (NK) cells, natural killer T(NKT) cells, epithelial cells, neutrophils, B cells, and intestinal Paneth cells (Song and Quian, 2008; Takahashi et al., 2008; Li et al., 2010; Passos et al., 2010; Cua and Tato, 2010). Regarding the other members of the IL-17 family, their expression throughout the body is much more limited. While IL-17B is to be mainly produced by neurons and chondrocytes, trace concentrations of this molecule have also been found in the stomach, pancreas, small intestine, and in the spinal cord (Li et al., 2000; Moore et al., 2002). IL-17D has been found to be synthesized by $CD4^+$ T cell and B cells. In addition, low amounts of this cytokine have been detected in neurons, prostate cells, and in skeletal muscle cells (Starnes et al., 2002). IL-17E is believed to be primarily expressed by the brain, testes, prostate, and lung (Lee et al., 2001); nevertheless, it was also found in epithelial cells, dendritic cells (DCs), endothelial cells, microglial cells, macrophages, $CD4^+$ cells, $CD8^+$ T cells, mast cells, eosinophils, and in basophils (reviewed by Weaver et al., 2007; Song and Quian, 2008; Iwakura et al., 2011). Finally, IL-17C has been detected in the human spleen, thymus, testes, and prostate (reviewed by Moseley et al., 2003), and has also been shown to be synthesized by keratinocytes as well as epithelial cells of bronchi and intestines in response to various bacterial pathogens (Song and Quian, 2008; Holland et al., 2009; Song et al., 2011; Pfeifer et al., 2013).

There is a great diversity of target cells for the IL-17 family members. IL-17A and IL-17F predominantly target endothelial cells, epithelial cells, synoviocytes, muscle cells, fibroblasts, keratinocytes, T cell, B cell, and macrophages. IL-17E is known to exert its biological effects on T cells, non-B/non-T-cells, macrophages, NKT cells, epithelial cells, normal human conjunctiva cells, matrix metalloproteinase (MMP)-type 2 cells, innate type 2 helper cells, and nuocytes (reviewed by Song and Quian, 2008; Iwakura et al., 2011). Little information is available about targeting the cells of IL-17B, IL-17C, and IL-17D. Some studies showed that IL-17D may exert an inhibitory effect on myeloid progenitor cells (Starnes et al., 2002), while IL-17B and IL-17C are able to trigger the release of tumor necrosis factor

(TNF)-α and IL-1β from monocytes (Li et al., 2000). Since IL-17 members may affect numerous cells types, it is clear that the family of IL-17 receptors is expressed ubiquitously throughout the body and can be found in literally every cell type.

8.2.3 Functions

The major function of the IL-17 family is the activation of host defense against various bacteria and certain fungi. It should be pointed out that all the representatives of the family except for IL-17E have very similar biological effects. It is known that IL-17A, IL-17B, IL-17C, and IL-17D primarily act as strong proinflammatory agents, upregulating the expression of key proinflammatory cytokines, including IL-1β, IL-6, TNF-α, granulocyte colony-stimulating factor (G-CSF), and granulocyte-macrophage CSF (reviewed by Kolls and Lindén, 2004). Furthermore, they were also reported to upregulate the synthesis of a plethora of proinflammatory chemokines, such as CXCL1, CCL2, CXCL5, CXCL8, CXCL10, CCL7, CCL20, and IL-8 (Yang et al., 2008b; Chang and Dong, 2009; Reynolds et al., 2010; Xu and Cao, 2010). In addition, IL-17A and IL-17F were shown to promote neutrophil recruitment (Wu et al., 2007; Watanabe et al., 2009) and the production of certain antimicrobial peptides such as β-defensin-2, cathelicidin, S100A7, S100A8, and S100A9 (Kao et al., 2004; Liang et al., 2006). Finally, a few studies demonstrated that IL-17 may stimulate the synthesis of acute phase protein lipocalin-2 (LCN2) (Shen et al., 2005; Raffatellu et al., 2008), which was reported to play a major role in antimicrobial defense (Flo et al., 2004).

Regarding the biological effects of IL-17E, it has been found to be involved in eosinophil recruitment followed by the development of eosinophilia, altered production of antibodies, and B-lymphocyte hyperplasia (Kim et al., 2002). It was also recently reported that IL-17E can stimulate luminal Innate Immunity and enhance barrier defense mechanisms during parenteral nutrition (Heneghan et al., 2013). Additionally, IL-17E may lead to the promotion of Th2 and Th9 cell responses and suppression of Th1 and Th17 cell response development, which is critical for the proper shift of immune cell polarization during the infection (reviewed by Iwakura et al., 2011).

Remarkably, some representatives of the IL-17 family are known to have synergistic effects with other cytokines. In particular, IL-17F is able to synergize with IL-22, IL-23, or TNF-α to stimulate the production of IL-6, and IL-1β (McAllister et al., 2005; Liang et al., 2006; Cheung et al., 2008; Chang and Dong, 2009). Moreover, IL-17 has been reported to cooperate with oncostatin M, vitamin D3, B-cell-activating factor, and interferon (IFN)-γ in the activation of certain cytokines, MMPs, or antimicrobial peptides (reviewed by Onishi and Gaffen, 2010).

8.2.4 Regulation

The mechanisms of the regulation of the human form of IL-17 are diverse. Since Th17 cells are recognized as a main source of IL-17, factors that stimulate the differentiation of Th17 cells from naive T cells are generally associated with an increased production of IL-17 mRNA and protein. A series of experiments demonstrated that agents such as transforming growth factor (TGF)-β1, IL-6, IL-21, and IL-23, separately or in combination, are necessary for the differentiation of the Th17 lineage (Bettelli et al., 2006; Mangan et al., 2006; Veldhoen et al., 2006; Korn et al., 2007; Liu et al., 2007; Wei et al., 2007; Yang et al., 2008b). Therefore, these molecules may be considered as positive regulators of IL-17, acting through the STAT3 pathway and triggering transcription factors RORγT and RORα (ROR - RAR-related orphan receptor), which in turn activate the transcription of the *IL-17* gene (Ivanov et al., 2006). It was recently reported that impaired STAT3 dramatically reduced the synthesis of IL-17 (Milner et al., 2008), whereas its hyperactive form markedly enhanced the production of this cytokine in $CD4^+$ T cells (Yang et al., 2007). Among other transcription factors triggering the differentiation of Th17 cells are forkhead box P3 (Foxp3), RUNX1, and interferon regulatory factor 4 (Brüstle et al., 2007; Zhang et al., 2008b). These mediators are currently being examined for the impact on IL-17 upregulation and downregulation.

It has been recently discovered that IL-17 production may be activated by T cell receptor (TCR) (Gomez-Rodriguez et al., 2009). In particular, the authors found that TCR signaling triggers the transcription of the *IL-17A* gene through the activation of interleukin-2-inducible T-cell kinase (ITK). In turn, ITK signaling leads to the elevation of calcium ions, which eventually results in the activation of nuclear factor of activated T-cells (NFAT) and its translocation to the nucleus. Interestingly, activated NFAT binds to the IL-17A, but not to the IL-17F promoter. In addition, itk-deficient cells exhibited a significantly reduced expression of IL-17A but not IL-17F both in vivo and in vitro.

One of the most significant findings was reported by Durrant et al. (2009), who found that transcriptional factor T-bet acts as a negative regulator of IL-17A in the lung through the downstream activation of RORα4 and $RORC_2$. After that, Reppert et al. (2011) showed that T-bet inhibited IL-17A synthesis in $CD4^+$ T cells in cancer cells, thereby suppressing tumor growth in mice with lung tumors. Moreover, the authors observed that T-bet also reduced IL-17R levels in tumor-infiltrating CD4$^+$ T cells and significantly increased the proliferation of these cells as well.

Yet another pathway of IL-17 regulation involves prostaglandin E2, which has been reported to induce IL-17 production in activated T cells through the inhibition of IL-12 and IL-23 (Sheibanie et al., 2007).

8.2.5 Role in Human Disease

All the representatives of IL-17 family were found to be involved in the pathogenesis of various autoimmune diseases, suggesting a key role of these cytokines in human immunity. In short, high proinflammatory activity of IL-17 underlies its strong relationship with certain inflammatory disorders, such as rheumatoid arthritis, inflammatory bowel disease, psoriasis, autoimmune encephalomyelitis, systemic lupus erythematosus, and so forth (reviewed by Onishi and Gaffen, 2010). Furthermore, supplementary IL-17-modulated activities may have a considerable impact on a disease progression. For example, due to a marked upregulation of MMPs, IL-17 is able to cause significant damage to joints, thereby exacerbating the course of rheumatoid arthritis (Chabaud et al., 2000; Jovanovic et al., 2000, 2001; Sylvester et al., 2004; Koenders et al., 2005a, 2005b; Rifas and Arackal, 2003; Onishi and Gaffen, 2010). Further, IL-17-driven osteoclast differentiation may have an adverse effect on bones and cartilages (Moseley et al., 2003).

The overwhelming majority of the studies investigating the role of IL-17 in human disease are focused on IL-17A, IL-17F, and IL-17E. Several findings demonstrated that the abrogation of IL-17A significantly reduced antigen-induced arthritis in animal models (Bush et al., 2002; Lubberts et al., 2004). Similarly, IL-17A-deficient mice exhibited an attenuated development of experimental autoimmune encephalomyelitis and collagen-induced arthritis (Ishigame et al., 2009). In addition, for several years, great effort has been devoted to the investigation of the role of IL-17A in hepatitis (Yasumi et al., 2007). In particular, the pathological role of IL-17A was recently found in Poly I:C-induced acute hepatitis (He et al., 2013a). Furthermore, this cytokine was shown to markedly reduce liver damage through neutrophil recruitment in the experimental hepatitis model induced by *Listeria monocytogenes* (Hamada et al., 2008; Xu et al., 2010a). Finally, the hepatic or serum IL-17 concentration was associated with the severity of liver injury in animal models (Zhu et al., 2012).

There is accumulating evidence that IL-17E may have a considerable influence on the pathogenesis of certain diseases (reviewed by Reynolds et al., 2010). It was found that IL-17E therapy delayed recurrent autoimmunity and stimulated a period of remission from new-onset diabetes in the majority of treated mice (Emamaullee et al., 2009). Furthermore, several studies reported that this cytokine was suspected to exacerbate allergic rhinitis (Xu et al., 2010b) and allergic asthma (Tamachi et al., 2006; Wang et al., 2007) by provoking airway hyperresponsiveness (Ballantyne et al., 2007). On the other hand, IL-17E demonstrated protective activities in colitis (Caruso et al., 2009) and in experimental autoimmune encephalomyelitis (Kleinschek et al., 2007) by inhibiting proinflammatory cytokine production. Finally, IL-17E contributed to worm clearance in helminthic parasite infection through the activation of Th2 cytokines (Fallon et al., 2006).

There are a number of studies that link IL-17F to the development of certain diseases (reviewed by Chang and Dong, 2009). Elevated levels of IL-17F were observed in human psoriasis samples (Wilson et al., 2007) as well as in animal models of psoriasis-like skin inflammation (Ma et al., 2008). Another report showed that the combined blockade of IL-17A and IL-17F significantly attenuated the development of experimental colitis (McLean et al., 2013). Similarly, it was demonstrated that a deficiency in the *IL-17F* gene caused the inhibition of dextran sulfate sodium-induced colitis in animal models by the reduction of Th2 response (Yang et al., 2008a). Furthermore, there is some evidence to suggest a considerable role of IL-17F in chronic inflammatory and allergic lung disease (Hizawa et al., 2006).

8.3 FINDINGS DEMONSTRATING PROTUMORIGENIC ACTIVITIES OF IL-17

8.3.1 IL-17 and Tumor Growth

Tartour et al. (1999) observed a marked increase in tumor size in nude mice inoculated with two cervical cell lines transfected with a cDNA encoding the *IL-17* gene. Nevertheless, the authors failed to demonstrate the direct relationship between IL-17 and tumor proliferation in vitro. In addition, the investigators showed that IL-17 stimulated the production of IL-17 mRNA and protein in cervical cell lines. Similarly, Numasaki et al. (2005) indicated that non-small-cell cancer cell lines transfected with the *IL-17* gene grew more rapidly in comparison with controls upon transplantation in immunodeficient mice. In consistency with previous reports, Hayata et al. (2013) demonstrated that the inhibition of naturally expressed IL-17A at tumor sites prominently suppressed cancer development in mice inoculated with colon carcinoma cell line. Further, Chae et al. (2010) found that IL-17A

ablation corrected immune abnormalities and inhibited intestinal tumorigenesis in vivo. A recent study performed by Zhang et al. (2012a) showed
that IL-17RC-deficient mice developed smaller prostate tumors as compared to control IL-17RC$^{+/+}$ mice; the authors revealed that the observed
effects were due to the decreased proliferation of cancer cells. Finally, He
et al. (2010) revealed that tumor growth was substantially inhibited in IL-
17R-deficient mice with various tumors, including lymphoma, melanoma,
and prostate cancer. Further findings of He et al. (2012) demonstrated that
the blockade of IL-17 markedly reduced the progression of existing skin
tumors in animal models.

According to all the above-mentioned findings, it is clear that IL-17 is
able to promote the proliferation of cancer cells, thereby stimulating tumor
progression and development.

8.3.2 IL-17 and Angiogenesis

Early studies revealed that IL-17 may promote angiogenesis through the
upregulation of multiple growth factors, such as TGF-β, fibroblast growth
factor-β, hepatocyte growth factor, and vascular endothelial growth factor (VEGF), essential for neovascularization (Takahashi et al., 2005;
Numasaki et al., 2003, 2005; Honorati et al., 2006). Chung et al. (2013)
recently demonstrated that IL-17 largely determines the resistance to the
antitumor and antiangiogenic effects of VEGF blockade in four cancer
cell lines. Furthermore, the authors pointed out that IL-17 itself stimulated cancer progression by activating CD11b$^+$Gr1$^+$ immature myeloid
cells, which were repeatedly reported to induce tumor neovascularization
and immunosuppression (reviewed by Gabrilovich and Nagaraj, 2009;
Gabrilovich et al., 2012). Similar results were recently obtained by Wakita
et al. (2010), who showed that IL-17-deficient mice had a significantly
reduced growth of skin carcinoma in comparison with that of wild-type
animals. Moreover, the authors observed that the presence of IL-17 correlated with a marked increase in VEGF and Ang-2 transcripts in cancer
cells, thereby confirming the involvement of this cytokine in tumor
angiogenesis. Another study conducted by Nam et al. (2008) revealed that
IL-17 directly promoted the growth of cancer cells in a metastatic breast
tumor model both in vitro and in vivo. In particular, the authors found
that IL-17 exhibited a prosurvival and antiapoptotic effect on cancer cells
in a dose-dependent manner. A series of well-designed studies by Numasaki
et al. (2003, 2005) demonstrated that IL-17 dramatically stimulated tumor
neovascularization through the upregulated expression of certain

proangiogenic CXC chemokines, such as CXCL1, CXCL5, CXCL6, and CXCL8, in mice inoculated with non-small-cell lung cancer cells. A plethora of further research studies confirmed that IL-17 is able to upregulate multiple proangiogenic agents including VEGF and others (Chen et al., 2010; Gu et al., 2012; Li et al., 2012).

8.3.3 IL-17 and Metastasis

It has long been known that IL-17 has a considerable effect on the expression and release of MMPs, which in turn induce the degradation of extracellular matrix, thereby promoting cell migration and invasion followed by metastatic formation. There are a number of reports indicating a direct relationship between IL-17 and prometastatic activity in tumor models. First, He et al. (2010) clearly demonstrated that IL-17 promoted tumor growth due to the fact that myeloid-derived suppressor cells from IL-17R-deficient tumor bearing mice produced significantly lower amounts of MMP9 as compared to that produced by wild-type animals. Second, Li et al. (2011) examined the expression pattern of IL-17A in 43 clinical samples from patients with hepatocellular carcinoma. The authors found that IL-17A upregulated the expression of MMP2 and MMP9 mRNA; moreover, a significantly higher frequency of IL-17A-expressing cells was observed in metastatic tissues. According to these findings, the authors suggested that IL-17A contributed to metastasis formation through the upregulation of MMPs. Further investigation carried out by Li et al. (2012) showed that the metastasis index in IL-17-deficient mice inoculated with Lewis lung carcinoma (LLC) cells was prominently decreased as compared to that of animals with a normal expression of the *IL-17* gene. Besides, the authors indicated that IL-17 directly stimulated cell migration and invasion in three different cancer cell lines. Third, Wang et al. (2013a) indicated that the interaction between IL-17A and IL-17RA stimulated the upregulation of VEGF, MMP9, and CXCR4 in osteosarcoma tissues, and thereby markedly increased metastasis formation. Similarly, Zhang et al. (2012b) found that IL-17RC knockout profoundly decreased the expression of MMP7 in mice with prostate cancer, thus inhibiting the formation of invasive adenocarcinoma. Finally, Gu et al. (2011) recently showed that exogenous IL-17 stimulated the invasion and migration of tumor cells in two different hepatocellular carcinoma cell lines through the upregulation of IL-6, IL-8, and MMP2. All these studies clearly show that IL-17 may contribute to the formation of metastasis through the upregulation of

MMPs, which are major modulators of extracellular matrix breakdown, cell migration, invasion and ultimately, and metastatic activity.

8.3.4 IL-17 and Lipocalin

As mentioned above, several studies found that IL-17 may stimulate the synthesis of acute phase protein LCN2 (Shen et al., 2005; Raffatellu et al., 2008). In particular, IL-17 activates NF-κB and C/EBP to bind to the Lcn-2 promoter, and this results in the rapid expression of LCN2 mRNA (Shen et al., 2006). It was further found that LCN2 production is regulated synergistically by TNF-α and IL-17 at the level of its promoter (Shen et al., 2005). In addition, the suppression of NF-κB has been repeatedly shown to reduce the expression of LCN2 mRNA and protein in various cancer cell lines (Iannetti et al., 2008; Leng et al., 2009; Mahadevan et al., 2011). These observations revealed a link between IL-17 and LCN2, which is very interesting in the context of cancer biology. LCN2 was found to be markedly upregulated in solid human tumors from diverse histological origins, including in pancreatic carcinoma, brain cancer, gastric carcinoma, lung cancer, ovarian cancer, liver carcinoma, and colon cancer (reviewed by Rodvold et al., 2012). Furthermore, several findings suggested that the suppression of LCN2 abrogated cancer development and progression.

Some mechanisms have been proposed to explain a protumorigenic impact of LCN2 (reviewed by Rodvold et al., 2012). First, it is supposed that LCN2 is responsible for the stability of MMP9 through binding to this protein. Protected from proteolytic degradation, MMP9 can stimulate extracellular matrix remodeling and promote tumor cell migration (Rudd et al., 1999). Second, LNC2 has also been reported to promote cell migration in an MMP-independent manner by upregulating extracellular-signal-regulated kinase (ERK)1/ERK2 (Gwira et al., 2005). Third, LCN2 is also known to promote survival of cancer cells through the sequestration of iron, which is critical for tumor development (Richardson et al., 2009). Finally, the aberrant expression of the *LCN* gene in human cancers has been repeatedly shown to affect the response of cancer cells to hypoxia and inflammation, factors that may provoke the endoplasmic reticulum stress response (Rodvold et al., 2012).

According to the above-mentioned findings, it is feasible to continue the research on the crosstalk between IL-17 and LCN2 in order to elucidate their cumulative impact on tumorigenesis.

8.3.5 Signaling Pathways of IL-17 in Cancer

In the last 10 years, a growing interest has been devoted to the aspects of the molecular basis of the IL-17-modulated carcinogenesis. Many recent reports have shed some light on this issue; however, more studies will be needed to clarify all the peculiarities of IL–17 signaling with respect to cancer development. So far, several general mechanisms have been established.

First, Wang et al. (2009) observed that IL–17 had a considerable influence on tumor growth through the activation of STAT3 in both stromal and cancer cells in the tumor microenvironment. It was further demonstrated that IL–17-deficient mice exhibited a marked reduction in the expression of STAT3 downstream genes VEGF and MMP9, thereby suggesting a link between IL–17 and angiogenesis and metastasis. Simultaneously, Bcl-2 and Bcl-xL were upregulated in mice lacking *IL-17* gene, which may explain the antiapoptotic activities of IL–17 shown above. Further investigations by Wang et al. (2010) revealed that the loss of IL–17 leads to the inhibition of STAT3 in the tumor microenvironment, and thereby significantly decreases tumorigenesis. A link between IL–17-modulated activation of STAT3 and cancer development was also demonstrated by Wu et al. (2009), Gu et al. (2012), Li et al. (2012), Hyun et al. (2012), Huang et al. (2013), Kim et al. (2013), and Wang et al. (2013b).

Importantly, several researchers demonstrated that protumorigenic activities of IL–17 are largely due to IL-6, which is an activator of STAT3 as well (Wang et al., 2009; Gu et al., 2012; Li et al., 2012). In particular, the presence of antibodies against IL-6 abrogated IL–17-induced Stat3 activation in human cancer cells, thereby preventing tumor development (Wang et al., 2009). Another study showed that the neutralization of IL-6 significantly decreased the activity of STAT3 and the production of MMP9 induced by IL–17, and thus decreased the metastatic activity of this cytokine in adenocarcinomic human alveolar basal epithelial cells (Li et al., 2010). Gu et al. (2012) demonstrated that neutralizing monoclonal antibody against IL-6 markedly inhibited STAT3 activation and henceforth totally stopped IL–17-stimulated tumor invasion in a hepatocellular carcinoma model. Taking into account the fact that the expression of both IL-6 and STAT3 is known to be enhanced by IL–17 through a positive feedback loop (Ogura et al., 2008), the crosstalk between these cytokines seem even more complicated.

Second, there is strong evidence suggesting that IL–17 may dramatically increase the production of intracellular NO (Shalom-Barak et al., 1998). We have mentioned in previous chapters that intracellular NO has a substantial impact on cancer development progression. In short, it may lead to impaired DNA repair through the upregulation of p53, poly(adenosine diphosphate ribose) polymerase, and DNA-dependent protein kinase. Furthermore, intracellular NO is able to promote angiogenesis by upregulating VEGF (reviewed by Xu et al., 2002).

Third, it has been mentioned above that IL-17 activates NF-κB through the ERK/Jun N-terminus kinase/mitogen-activated protein kinase pathway (Shalom-Barak et al., 1998; Subramaniam et al., 1999). Recently, Huang et al. (2013) demonstrated that the IL-17-driven activation of NF-κB prevents apoptosis via the upregulation of Bcl-2, thereby enhancing tumorigenesis in the breast cancer cell line. Furthermore, the authors were able to inhibit cancer development through NF-κB blockade triggered by antibodies against IL-17.

8.4 FINDINGS DEMONSTRATING ANTICANCER ACTIVITIES OF IL-17

Paradoxically enough, despite the huge amount of research showing the direct impact of IL-17 on tumor development through several investigated mechanisms, we still cannot establish the fact that IL-17 is a solely protumorigenic cytokine. The problem is that IL-17 per se plays a great role in immunity, and is involved in dozens of immune reactions, including those associated with antitumor immune response. Due to this fact, there are a number of studies indicating clear anticancer effects of IL-17 in contrast to previous reports.

In 2001, Hirahara et al. (2001) transfected murine fibrosarcoma cells with the hIL-17 gene. The authors indicated that IL-17 exhibited a tumor-specific immune response by activating CD4$^+$ and CD8$^+$ T cells and enhancing the expression of major histocompatibility complex (MHC) class I and II antigens. It is known that an increased number of MHC molecules are associated with better processing and presenting of tumor antigens (Leone et al., 2013). Benchetrit et al. (2002) demonstrated that hematopoietic immunogenic tumors producing IL-17 exhibited a considerable reduction in tumor cell growth as compared to that exhibited by normal tumors in vivo. In addition, the researchers revealed that the observed effect was T-cell dependent. Another research conducted by Martin-Orozco et al. (2009) revealed that IL-17-deficient mice inoculated with melanoma cells had an increased number of tumor foci and larger tumors in size in comparison with that in wild-type animals. The observed results were largely due to the presence of differentiated Th17 cells, 35% of which constantly expressed IL-17. In addition, the authors found that Th17 cells enhanced the activation of DCs and tumor-specific CD8$^+$ T cells, thereby contributing to tumor suppression. Similarly, yet another evidence of IL-17-modulated activation of DCs and MHC antigens was provided by Antonysamy et al. (1999).

Kryczek et al. (2009) demonstrated that mice deficient in the *IL-17* gene had an enhanced growth of colon tumors as compared to that of wild-type animals. In addition, control mice exhibited a higher metastatic potential in comparison with that exhibited by IL-17-deficient animals. Although the authors did not indicate differences in the number of $CD4^+$ and $CD8^+$ T cells, the levels of tumor-infiltrating $IFN-\gamma^+$ T cells and $IFN-\gamma^+$ NK cells were markedly increased in control mice than in IL-17-deficient mice. Furthermore, Ngiow et al. (2010) successfully replicated these results, and showed that IL-17 had no effect on colon carcinoma tumor cells growth and metastatic potential.

Importantly, another mechanism of IL-17-mediated tumor suppression may consist of the IL-17-dependent upregulation of IL-12, which possesses strong anticancer activities (Yuzhalin and Kutikhin, 2012). It was found that the synthesis and release of IL-12 were markedly increased in human macrophages exposed to recombinant human IL-17 (Jovanovic et al., 1998).

Recent findings revealed yet another signaling pathway that seemed to be involved in cancer development. As mentioned before, Durrant et al. (2009) revealed that transcriptional factor T-bet acts as a negative regulator of IL-17A in the lung through the downstream activation of $ROR\alpha4$ and $RORC_2$. After that, Reppert et al. (2011) showed that T-bet inhibited IL-17A synthesis in $CD4^+$ T cells in cancer cells, and thereby suppressed tumor growth in mice with lung tumors. Moreover, the authors observed that T-bet also reduced IL-17R levels in tumor-infiltrating $CD4^+$ T cells and significantly increased the proliferation of these cells as well.

Recent findings of Xie et al. (2010) indicated that IL-17F had no influence on the proliferation and cell cycle of hepatocarcinoma cells in vitro. Moreover, the authors showed that IL-17F markedly inhibited vascular endothelial cell growth and downregulated the expression of IL-6, IL-8, and VEGF. Importantly, this observation is not consistent with that in previous reports. Ma et al. (2011) performed another interesting study, wherein IL-17-producing $\gamma\delta$ Th17 cells induced apoptosis in cancer cells and augmented antitumor immune response driven by cytotoxic chemotherapeutics in vivo. In addition, the inhibition of the IL-17 signaling pathway significantly reduced anticancer immunity in mice with various tumors. Finally, Hinrichs et al. (2009) showed a marked antitumor response in vivo caused by the expansion and persistence of the Th17-polarized cells. However, further analysis showed that the amount of IL-17 was diminished in these cells; thereby its role in anticancer defense seemed to be negligible.

8.5 IL-17 LEVELS IN CANCER PATIENTS

Multiple studies indicated that marked levels of IL-17 mRNA and protein were present in patients with various malignancies, including ovarian cancer (Kato et al., 2001; Rogala et al., 2012), breast cancer (Nam et al., 2008; Zhu et al., 2008; Yang et al., 2012), non-small-cell lung cancer (Liu et al., 2012; Zhang et al., 2012c; He et al., 2013b), renal cell carcinoma (Inozume et al., 2009), lung adenocarcinoma (Li et al., 2011), small-cell lung cancer (Li et al., 2012; He et al., 2013a), laryngeal squamous cell carcinoma (Meng et al., 2012a), non-small-cell lung carcinoma (Kirshberg et al., 2011), prostate cancer (Haudenschild et al., 2002), Sezary syndrome (Cirée et al., 2004), multiple myeloma (Prabhala et al., 2010; Dong et al., 2012; Lemancewicz et al., 2012; Zhang et al., 2012c), pancreatic cancer (Kuang et al., 2010; He et al., 2011), colorectal carcinoma (Le Gouvello et al., 2008; Radosavljevic et al., 2010; Cui et al., 2012), breast cancer (Lyon et al., 2008), and gastric carcinoma (Zhang et al., 2008a; Meng et al., 2012b). In addition, considerable proportions of IL-17 were observed in subjects with malignant pleural effusions (Klimatsidas et al., 2012; Xu et al., 2013) and bladder carcinoma (Doroudchi et al., 2013). On the other hand, recent findings showed that decreased amounts of IL-17 were found in patients with glioma (Hu et al., 2011), small lymphocytic lymphoma (Karmali et al., 2013), lung squamous cell carcinoma (Zhao et al., 2013), hepatocellular carcinoma (Gabitass et al., 2011; Welling et al., 2012), melanoma (Shetty et al., 2013), colorectal cancer (Wägsäter et al., 2006), esophageal cancer (Gabitass et al., 2011), Langerhans cell histiocytosis lesions (Peters et al., 2011), acute myeloid leukemia (Wróbel et al., 2003), and adenocarcinoma of the lung (Zhao et al., 2013).

There are a number of studies assessing the impact of IL-17 on cancer prognosis; nevertheless, obtained findings are somewhat inconsistent. On the one hand, it was recently revealed that an increased production of IL-17 is associated with a favorable prognosis in patients with esophageal cancer (Wang et al., 2013b) as well as with better progression-free survival in subjects with advanced epithelial ovarian cancer (Lan et al., 2013), esophageal squamous cell carcinoma (Lv et al., 2011), and glioblastoma (Cui et al., 2013). On the other hand, the presence of intratumor IL-17-expressing cells correlated with a worse prognosis in individuals with intrahepatic cholangiocarcinoma (Gu et al., 2012), hepatocellular carcinoma (Li et al., 2011), colorectal carcinoma (Liu et al., 2011), T-cell lymphoma (Krejsgaard et al., 2013), and breast cancer (Eiró et al., 2012; Chen et al., 2013). Although there was no statistically significant correlation between IL-17 levels and clinicopathological characteristics of gastric cancer (Meng et al., 2012b), some findings suggest that this cytokine may be regarded as an independent prognostic indicator for this disease (Yamada et al., 2012). Finally, Linkov et al. (2007) suggested that IL-17 may be included in the panel of tumor biomarkers for diagnosis of head and neck cancer.

8.6 INHERITED VARIATIONS WITHIN THE GENES OF IL-17 FAMILY MEMBERS AND CANCER

Multiple groups have analyzed the impact of IL-17 gene polymorphisms on the risk of various cancers (reviewed by Yuzhalin, 2011).

Shibata et al. (2010) showed that the heterozygous genotype of IL17_-197G/A polymorphism (rs2275913) correlates with a higher risk of developing gastric cancer as compared to carriers of the GG genotype (odds ratio (OR) = 1.42). Furthermore, the carriers of the AA genotype had a three times increased gastric cancer risk (OR = 3.02). This finding is consistent with the results obtained by Rafiei et al. (2013), who demonstrated that patients who were homozygous (AA) at position −197 were 2.9 times more likely to develop gastric cancer in an Iranian population. In addition, the authors found that the presence of a single A allele elevated the risk of developing gastric cancer up to 1.7-fold. Similarly, Arisawa et al. (2012) showed that the presence of the IL17_-197G/A AA genotype correlated with an increased risk for the development of both intestinal and diffuse types of gastric cancer in a Japanese population (OR = 2.38). On the contrary, Kutikhin et al. (2014) failed to establish a relationship between IL17_-197G/A polymorphism and either colorectal or gastric cancer in a Russian population.

Zhou et al. (2013) recently showed that rs2275913 and rs763780 gene polymorphisms are associated with bladder cancer in a Chinese Han population (OR = 1.37 and 1.46, respectively). In addition, the authors indicated that rs2275913 correlated with male gender, nonsmokers, and invasion of bladder cancer, whereas rs763780 correlated with the invasion of bladder cancer.

A genomewide association study was conducted by Innocenti et al. (2012), who genotyped for >550,000 gene polymorphisms to establish risk alleles for overall survival in pancreatic cancer patients treated with gemcitabine plus either bevacizumab or placebo. The authors found that the variant genotype for IL-17F_H161 (rs763780) polymorphism is associated with a worse prognosis through the suppression of antiangiogenic properties of IL-17F.

Shibata et al. (2009) did not identify any significant associations between the IL17F_+7488 A/G (rs763780) single nucleotide polymorphism (SNP) and gastric cancer risk. Nevertheless, Wu et al. (2010) found that the GA and GG genotypes of +7488 SNP correlated with an elevated gastric cancer risk as compared to the variant AA genotype (OR = 1.51 for GA and 1.61 for GG genotypes). Furthermore, the authors reported the absence of an association between the IL17_−197G/A polymorphism and gastric cancer risk (p = 0.098).

Tahara et al. (2009) reported that the IL17F_+7488T/C and IL17_−197G/A polymorphisms may be involved in CpG island hypermethylation. CpG islands are DNA regions in which a cytosine nucleotide occurs next to a guanine in the linear sequence of bases along its length. CpGs are believed to promote malignant transformation. The authors observed that CpG island hypermethylation-positive status in gastric mucosa was associated with allele variants of the *IL17* gene.

All the above-mentioned inherited variations are undoubtedly attractive for further investigations, and clarification of their role in carcinogenesis is desirable.

8.7 SUMMARY

Research devoted to IL-17 and cancer has been gaining considerable importance in recent years. Due to the great diversity of functions among IL-17 family members, it is not easy to understand their impacts on cancer cells clearly enough. Undoubtedly, this issue should be considered wider than only the role of IL-17 itself. In fact, the whole subset of IL-17-producing Th17 cells should be taken into account when investigating the role of this cytokine in tumorigenesis. In addition, IL-17 has shown multiple cooperative effects with various growth factors and with other cytokines, thereby expanding the area for further research. So far, the role of IL-17 and Th17 cells in cancer development has remained unclear, especially at the molecular level. However, the basic aspects of IL-17 immunobiology in cancer have been established and may therefore shed some light on the current state of the problem.

It appears that under different settings IL-17 may exhibit differential biological effects. On the one hand, numerous studies established proangiogenic and prometastatic activities as a hallmark of this cytokine. Specifically, these effects are due to IL-17-modulated upregulation of genes responsible for vasculogenesis (VEGF, Ang-2, CXCL1, CXCL5, CXCL6, and others), prevention of apoptosis (Bcl-2) and breakdown of extracellular matrix (MMP2, MMP7, and MMP9). On the other hand, we must bear in mind that IL-17 by itself has a great impact on the immune response of the body. Even though there are molecular mechanisms underlying protumorigenic functions, this cytokine may also stimulate lymphocytes to kill tumor cells. In particular, IL-17 is able to activate antitumor response by triggering DCs, CD4$^+$, and CD8$^+$ effector T cells, and by upregulating MHC class I and II molecules. Moreover, taking into account the fact that IL-17 has been demonstrated to stimulate tumor development by promoting angiogenesis, we must also consider that this process provides the influx of the immune cells to the site of the tumor, allowing them to invade and attack cancer cells. In spite of this functional ambiguity, however, the majority of the literature is currently demonstrating the tumor-promoting role of this cytokine, whereas only occasional reports indicate the opposite. Therefore, we may suggest that IL-17 is a rather protumorigenic cytokine than an antitumorigenic one.

Although numerous studies were performed to identify IL-17 mRNA and protein levels in cancer patients, this cytokine may not be considered as a valuable cancer biomarker so far. Even though there are multiple findings indicating high expression levels of IL-17 in some tumor types, many studies show decreased concentrations of this cytokine in other cancer types. Similarly, some researchers indicated that high serum IL-17 levels may be considered as a marker of good prognosis of patients with cancer, whereas others demonstrated the opposite. These disparities may be explained by the fact that many investigators did not specify which member of the IL-17 family was studied; therefore, the overall picture is likely to be distorted because different representatives have differential functions.

To summarize, IL-17 can either promote or suppress cancer growth and progression. No doubt, the observed inconsistency raises a number of questions for future research. More in-depth studies are necessary to shed light on understanding the impact of this cytokine on cancer biology.

REFERENCES

Antonysamy, M.A., Fanslow, W.C., Fu, F., Li, W., Qian, S., Troutt, A.B., Thomson, A.W., 1999. Evidence for a role of IL-17 in organ allograft rejection: IL-17 promotes the functional differentiation of dendritic cell progenitors. J. Immunol. 162 (1), 577–584.

Arisawa, T., Tahara, T., Shiroeda, H., Matsue, Y., Minato, T., Nomura, T., Yamada, H., Hayashi, R., Saito, T., Matsunaga, K., Fukuyama, T., Hayashi, N., Otsuka, T., Fukumura, A., Nakamura, M., Shibata, T., 2012. Genetic polymorphisms of IL17A and pri-microRNA-938, targeting IL17A 3'-UTR, influence susceptibility to gastric cancer. Hum. Immunol. 73 (7), 747–752.

Ballantyne, S.J., Barlow, J.L., Jolin, H.E., Nath, P., Williams, A.S., Chung, K.F., Sturton, G., Wong, S.H., McKenzie, A.N., 2007. Blocking IL-25 prevents airway hyperresponsiveness in allergic asthma. J. Allergy Clin. Immunol. 120 (6), 1324–1331.

Benchetrit, F., Ciree, A., Vives, V., Warnier, G., Gey, A., Sautès-Fridman, C., Fossiez, F., Haicheur, N., Fridman, W.H., Tartour, E., 2002. Interleukin-17 inhibits tumor cell growth by means of a T-cell-dependent mechanism. Blood 99 (6), 2114–2121.

Bettelli, E., Carrier, Y., Gao, W., Korn, T., Strom, T.B., Oukka, M., Weiner, H.L., Kuchroo, V.K., 2006. Reciprocal developmental pathways for the generation of pathogenic effector TH17 and regulatory T cells. Nature 441 (7090), 235–238.

Brüstle, A., Heink, S., Huber, M., Rosenplänter, C., Stadelmann, C., Yu, P., Arpaia, E., Mak, T.W., Kamradt, T., Lohoff, M., 2007. The development of inflammatory T(H)-17 cells requires interferon-regulatory factor 4. Nat. Immunol. 8 (9), 958–966.

Bush, K.A., Farmer, K.M., Walker, J.S., Kirkham, B.W., 2002. Reduction of joint inflammation and bone erosion in rat adjuvant arthritis by treatment with interleukin-17 receptor IgG1 Fc fusion protein. Arthritis Rheum. 46 (3), 802–805.

Caruso, R., Sarra, M., Stolfi, C., Rizzo, A., Fina, D., Fantini, M.C., Pallone, F., MacDonald, T.T., Monteleone, G., 2009. Interleukin-25 inhibits interleukin-12 production and Th1 cell-driven inflammation in the gut. Gastroenterology 136 (7), 2270–2279.

Chabaud, M., Garnero, P., Dayer, J.M., Guerne, P.A., Fossiez, F., Miossec, P., 2000. Contribution of interleukin 17 to synovium matrix destruction in rheumatoid arthritis. Cytokine 12, 1092–1099.

Chae, W.J., Gibson, T.F., Zelterman, D., Hao, L., Henegariu, O., Bothwell, A.L., 2010. Ablation of IL-17A abrogates progression of spontaneous intestinal tumorigenesis. Proc. Natl. Acad. Sci. USA 107 (12), 5540–5544.

Chang, S.H., Dong, C., 2009. IL-17F: regulation, signaling and function in inflammation. Cytokine 46 (1), 7–11.

Chen, W.C., Lai, Y.H., Chen, H.Y., Guo, H.R., Su, I.J., Chen, H.H., 2013. Interleukin-17-producing cell infiltration in the breast cancer tumour microenvironment is a poor prognostic factor. Histopathology 63 (2), 225–233.

Chen, X., Xie, Q., Cheng, X., Diao, X., Cheng, Y., Liu, J., Xie, W., Chen, Z., Zhu, B., 2010. Role of interleukin-17 in lymphangiogenesis in non-small-cell lung cancer: enhanced production of vascular endothelial growth factor C in non-small-cell lung carcinoma cells. Cancer Sci. 101 (11), 2384–2390.

Cheung, P.F., Wong, C.K., Lam, C.W., 2008. Molecular mechanisms of cytokine and chemokine release from eosinophils activated by IL-17A, IL-17F, and IL-23: implication for Th17 lymphocytes-mediated allergic inflammation. J. Immunol. 180, 5625–5635.

Chung, A.S.I., Wu, X., Zhuang, G., Ngu, H., Kasman, I., Zhang, J., Vernes, J.M., Jiang, Z., Meng, Y.G., Peale, F.V., Ouyang, W., Ferrara, N., September 2013. An interleukin-17-mediated paracrine network promotes tumor resistance to anti-angiogenic therapy. Nat. Med. 19 (9), 1114–1123.

Cirée, A., Michel, L., Camilleri-Bröet, S., Jean Louis, F., Oster, M., Flageul, B., Senet, P., Fossiez, F., Fridman, W.H., Bachelez, H., Tartour, E., 2004. Expression and activity of IL-17 in cutaneous T-cell lymphomas (mycosis fungoides and Sezary syndrome). Int. J. Cancer 112 (1), 113–120.

Cua, D.J., Tato, C.M., 2010. Innate IL-17-producing cells: the sentinels of the immune system. Nat. Rev. Immunol. 10 (7), 479–489.

Cui, G., Yuan, A., Goll, R., Florholmen, J., 2012. IL-17A in the tumor microenvironment of the human colorectal adenoma-carcinoma sequence. Scand. J. Gastroenterol 47 (11), 1304–1312.

Cui, X., Xu, Z., Zhao, Z., Sui, D., Ren, X., Huang, Q., Qin, J., Hao, L., Wang, Z., Shen, L., Lin, S., 2013. Analysis of CD137L and IL-17 expression in tumor tissue as prognostic indicators for glioblastoma. Int. J. Biol. Sci. 9 (2), 134–141.

Dong, S.S., Li, G.L.,Yang, J., 2012. Clinical significance of serum vascular endothelial growth factor and interleukin-17 in patients with multiple myeloma. Zhongguo Shiyan Xueyexue Zazhi 20 (2), 344–347.

Doroudchi, M., Saidi, M., Malekzadeh, M., Golmoghaddam, H., Khezri, A., Ghaderi, A., 2013. Elevated IL-17A levels in early stages of bladder cancer regardless of smoking status. Future Oncol. 9 (2), 295–304.

Durrant, D.M., Gaffen, S.L., Riesenfeld, E.P., Irvin, C.G., Metzger, D.W., 2009. Development of allergen-induced airway inflammation in the absence of T-bet regulation is dependent on IL-17. J. Immunol. 183 (8), 5293–5300.

Eiró, N., González, L., González, L.O., Fernandez-Garcia, B., Lamelas, M.L., Marín, L., González-Reyes, S., del Casar, J.M., Vizoso, F.J., 2012. Relationship between the inflammatory molecular profile of breast carcinomas and distant metastasis development. PLoS One 7 (11), e49047.

Emamaullee, J.A., Davis, J., Merani, S., Toso, C., Elliott, J.F., Thiesen, A., Shapiro, A.M., 2009. Inhibition of Th17 cells regulates autoimmune diabetes in NOD mice. Diabetes 58 (6), 1302–1311.

Fallon, P.G., Ballantyne, S.J., Mangan, N.E., Barlow, J.L., Dasvarma, A., Hewett, D.R., McIlgorm, A., Jolin, H.E., McKenzie, A.N., 2006. Identification of an interleukin (IL)-25-dependent cell population that provides IL-4, IL-5, and IL-13 at the onset of helminth expulsion. J. Exp. Med. 203 (4), 1105–1116.

Flo, T.H., Smith, K.D., Sato, S., Rodriguez, D.J., Holmes, M.A., Strong, R.K., Akira, S., Aderem, A., 2004. Lipocalin 2 mediates an innate immune response to bacterial infection by sequestrating iron. Nature 432 (7019), 917–921.

Gabitass, R.F., Annels, N.E., Stocken, D.D., Pandha, H.A., Middleton, G.W., 2011. Elevated myeloid-derived suppressor cells in pancreatic, esophageal and gastric cancer are an independent prognostic factor and are associated with significant elevation of the Th2 cytokine interleukin-13. Cancer Immunol. Immunother. 60 (10), 1419–1430.

Gabrilovich, D.I., Nagaraj, S., 2009. Myeloid-derived suppressor cells as regulators of the immune system. Nat. Rev. Immunol. 9 (3), 162–174.

Gabrilovich, D.I., Ostrand-Rosenberg, S., Bronte, V., 2012. Coordinated regulation of myeloid cells by tumours. Nat. Rev. Immunol. 12 (4), 253–268.

Gaffen, S.L., 2009. Structure and signalling in the IL-17 receptor family. Nat. Rev. Immunol. 9 (8), 556–567.

Gomez-Rodriguez, J., Sahu, N., Handon, R., Davidson, T.S., Anderson, S.M., Kirby, M.R., August, A., Schwartzberg, P.L., 2009. Differential expression of interleukin-17A and -17F is coupled to T cell receptor signaling via inducible T cell kinase. Immunity 31 (4), 587–597.

Greten, T.F., Zhao, F., Gamrekelashvili, J., Korangy, F., 2012. Human Th17 cells in patients with cancer: Friends or foe? Oncoimmunology 1 (8), 1438–1439.

Gu, F.M., Gao, Q., Shi, G.M., Zhang, X., Wang, J., Jiang, J.H., Wang, X.Y., Shi, Y.H., Ding, Z.B., Fan, J., Zhou, J., 2012. Intratumoral IL-17[+] cells and neutrophils show strong prognostic significance in intrahepatic cholangiocarcinoma. Ann. Surg. Oncol. 19 (8), 2506–2514.

Gu, F.M., Li, Q.L., Gao, Q., Jiang, J.H., Zhu, K., Huang, X.Y., Pan, J.F., Yan, J., Hu, J.H., Wang, Z., Dai, Z., Fan, J., Zhou, J., 2011. IL-17 induces AKT-dependent IL-6/JAK2/STAT3 activation and tumor progression in hepatocellular carcinoma. Mol. Cancer 10, 150.

Gwira, J.A., Wei, F., Ishibe, S., Ueland, J.M., Barasch, J., Cantley, L.G., 2005. Expression of neutrophil gelatinase-associated lipocalin regulates epithelial morphogenesis in vitro. J. Biol. Chem. 280 (9), 7875–7882.

Hamada, S., Umemura, M., Shiono, T., Tanaka, K., Yahagi, A., Begum, M.D., Oshiro, K., Okamoto, Y., Watanabe, H., Kawakami, K., Roark, C., Born, W.K., O'Brien, R., Ikuta, K., Ishikawa, H., Nakae, S., Iwakura, Y., Ohta, T., Matsuzaki, G., 2008. IL-17A produced by gammadelta T cells plays a critical role in innate immunity against listeria monocytogenes infection in the liver. J. Immunol. 181 (5), 3456–3463.

Haudenschild, D., Moseley, T., Rose, L., Reddi, A.H., 2002. Soluble and transmembrane iso-forms of novel interleukin-17 receptor-like protein by RNA splicing and expression in prostate cancer. J. Biol. Chem. 277 (6), 4309–4316.

Hayata, K., Iwahashi, M., Ojima, T., Katsuda, M., Iida, T., Nakamori, M., Ueda, K., Nakamura, M., Miyazawa, M., Tsuji, T., Yamaue, H., 2013. Inhibition of IL-17A in tumor microen-vironment augments cytotoxicity of tumor-infiltrating lymphocytes in tumor-bearing mice. PLoS One 8 (1), e53131.

He, D., Li, H., Yusuf, N., Elmets, C.A., Athar, M., Katiyar, S.K., Xu, H., 2012. IL-17 mediated inflammation promotes tumor growth and progression in the skin. PLoS. One 7 (2), e32126.

He, D., Li, H., Yusuf, N., Elmets, C.A., Li, J., Mountz, J.D., Xu, H., 2010. IL-17 promotes tumor development through the induction of tumor promoting microenvironments at tumor sites and myeloid-derived suppressor cells. J. Immunol. 184 (5), 2281–2288.

He, G., Zhang, B., Zhang, B., Qiao, L., Tian, Z., Zhai, G., Xin, X., Yang, C., Liu, P., Zhang, Y., Xu, L., 2013a. Th17 Cells and IL-17 are increased in patients with brain metastases from the primary lung cancer. Zhongguo Feiai Zazhi 16 (9), 476–481.

He, J., Lang, G., Ding, S., Li, L., 2013b. Pathological role of interleukin-17 in poly I: C-induced hepatitis. PLoS One 8 (9), e73909.

He, S., Fei, M., Wu, Y., Zheng, D., Wan, D., Wang, L., Li, D., 2011. Distribution and clinical significance of th17 cells in the tumor microenvironment and peripheral blood of pancreatic cancer patients. Int. J. Mol. Sci. 12 (11), 7424–7437.

Hemdan, N.Y., Birkenmeier, G., Wichmann, G., Abu El-Saad, A.M., Krieger, T., Conrad, K., Sack, U., 2010. Interleukin-17-producing T helper cells in autoimmunity. Autoimmun. Rev. 9 (11), 785–792.

Heneghan, A.F., Pierre, J.F., Gosain, A., Kudsk, K.A., February 19, 2013. IL-25 improves luminal innate immunity and barrier function during parenteral nutrition. Ann. Surg, 258 (6)1065–1071.

Hinrichs, C.S., Kaiser, A., Paulos, C.M., Cassard, L., Sanchez-Perez, L., Heemskerk, B., Wrzesinski, C., Borman, Z.A., Muranski, P., Restifo, N.P., 2009. Type 17 CD8+ T cells display enhanced antitumor immunity. Blood 114 (3), 596–599.

Hirahara, N., Nio, Y., Sasaki, S., Minari, Y., Takamura, M., Iguchi, C., Dong, M., Yamasawa, K., Tamura, K., 2001. Inoculation of human interleukin-17 gene-transfected Meth-A fibro-sarcoma cells induces T cell-dependent tumor-specific immunity in mice. Oncology 61 (1), 79–89.

Hizawa, N., Kawaguchi, M., Huang, S.K., Nishimura, M., 2006. Role of interleukin-17F in chronic inflammatory and allergic lung disease. Clin. Exp. Allergy 36 (9), 1109–1114.

Holland, D.B., Bojar, R.A., Farrar, M.D., Holland, K.T., 2009. Differential innate immune responses of a living skin equivalent model colonized by Staphylococcus epidermidis or Staphylococcus aureus. FEMS Microbiol. Lett. 290 (2), 149–155.

Honorati, M.C., Neri, S., Cattini, L., Facchini, A., 2006. Interleukin-17, a regulator of angio-genic factor release by synovial fibroblasts. Osteoarthritis Cartilage 14 (4), 345–352.

Hu, J., Mao, Y., Li, M., Lu, Y., 2011. The profile of Th17 subset in glioma. Int. Immunophar-macol. 11 (9), 1173–1179.

Huang, C.K., Yang, C.Y., Jeng, Y.M., Chen, C.L., Wu, H.H., Chang, Y.C., Ma, C., Kuo, W.H., Chang, K.J., Shew, J.Y., Lee, W.H., July 15, 2013. Autocrine/paracrine mechanism of interleu-kin-17B receptor promotes breast tumorigenesis through NF-κB-mediated antiapoptotic pathway. Oncogene. http://dx.doi.org/10.1038/onc.2013.268. [Epub ahead of print].

Hyun, Y.S., Han, D.S., Lee, A.R., Eun, C.S., Youn, J., Kim, H.Y., 2012. Role of IL-17A in the development of colitis-associated cancer. Carcinogenesis 33 (4), 931–936.

Iannetti, A., Pacifico, F., Acquaviva, R., Lavorgna, A., Crescenzi, E., Vascotto, C., Tell, G., Salzano, A.M., Scaloni, A., Vuttariello, E., Chiappetta, G., Formisano, S., Leonardi, A., 2008. The neutrophil gelatinase-associated lipocalin (NGAL), a NF-kappaB-regulated gene, is a sur-vival factor for thyroid neoplastic cells. Proc. Natl. Acad. Sci. U.S.A. 105 (37), 14058–14063.

Innocenti, F., Owzar, K., Cox, N.L., Evans, P., Kubo, M., Zembutsu, H., Jiang, C., Hollis, D., Mushiroda, T., Li, L., Friedman, P., Wang, L., Glubb, D., Hurwitz, H., Giacomini, K.M., McLeod, H.L., Goldberg, R.M., Schilsky, R.L., Kindler, H.L., Nakamura, Y., Ratain, M.J., 2012. A genome-wide association study of overall survival in pancreatic cancer patients treated with gemcitabine in CALGB 80303. Clin. Cancer Res. 18 (2), 577–584.

Inozume, T., Hanada, K., Wang, Q.J., Yang, J.C., 2009. IL-17 secreted by tumor reactive T cells induces IL-8 release by human renal cancer cells. J. Immunother. 32 (2), 109–117.

Ishigame, H., Kakuta, S., Nagai, T., Kadoki, M., Nambu, A., Komiyama, Y., Fujikado, N., Tanahashi, Y., Akitsu, A., Kotaki, H., Sudo, K., Nakae, S., Sasakawa, C., Iwakura, Y., 2009. Differential roles of interleukin-17A and -17F in host defense against mucoepithelial bacterial infection and allergic responses. Immunity 30 (1), 108–119.

Ivanov, I.I., McKenzie, B.S., Zhou, L., Tadokoro, C.E., Lepelley, A., Lafaille, J.J., Cua, D.J., Littman, D.R., 2006. The orphan nuclear receptor RORgammat directs the differentiation program of proinflammatory IL-17+ T helper cells. Cell 126 (6), 1121–1133.

Iwakura, Y., Ishigame, H., Saijo, S., Nakae, S., 2011. Functional specialization of interleukin-17 family members. Immunity 34 (2), 149–162.

Ji, Y., Zhang, W., 2010. Th17 cells: positive or negative role in tumor? Cancer Immunol. Immunother. 59 (7), 979–987.

Jovanovic, D.V., Di Battista, J.A., Martel-Pelletier, J., Reboul, P., He, Y., Jolicoeur, F.C., Pelletier, J.P., 2001. Modulation of TIMP-1 synthesis by antiinflammatory cytokines and prostaglandin E2 in interleukin 17 stimulated human monocytes/macrophages. J. Rheumatol. 28, 712–718.

Jovanovic, D.V., Martel-Pelletier, J., Di Battista, J.A., Mineau, F., Jolicoeur, F.C., Benderdour, M., Pelletier, J.P., 2000. Stimulation of 92-kd gelatinase (matrix metalloproteinase 9) production by interleukin-17 in human monocyte/macrophages. Arthritis Rheum. 43, 1134–1144.

Jovanovic, D.V., Di Battista, J.A., Martel-Pelletier, J., Jolicoeur, F.C., He, Y., Zhang, M., Mineau, F., Pelletier, J.P., 1998. IL-17 stimulates the production and expression of proinflammatory cytokines, IL-beta and TNF-alpha, by human macrophages. J. Immunol. 160 (7), 3513–3521.

Kao, C.Y., Chen, Y., Thai, P., Wachi, S., Huang, F., Kim, C., Harper, R.W., Wu, R., 2004. IL-17 markedly up-regulates beta-defensin-2 expression in human airway epithelium via JAK and NF-kappaB signaling pathways. J. Immunol. 173 (5), 3482–3491.

Karmali, R., Paganessi, L.A., Frank, R.R., Jagan, S., Larson, M.L., Venugopal, P., Gregory, S.A., Christopherson 2nd, K.W., 2013. Aggressive disease defined by cytogenetics is associated with cytokine dysregulation in CLL/SLL patients. J. Leukoc Biol. 93 (1), 161–170.

Kato, T., Furumoto, H., Ogura, T., Onishi, Y., Irahara, M., Yamano, S., Kamada, M., Aono, T., 2001. Expression of IL-17 mRNA in ovarian cancer. Biochem. Biophys. Res. Commun. 282 (3), 735–738.

Kim, G., Khanal, P., Lim, S.C., Yun, H.J., Ahn, S.G., Ki, S.H., Choi, H.S., 2013. Interleukin-17 induces AP-1 activity and cellular transformation via upregulation of tumor progression locus 2 activity. Carcinogenesis 34 (2), 341–350.

Kim, M.R., Manoukian, R., Yeh, R., Silbiger, S.M., Danilenko, D.M., Scully, S., Sun, J., DeRose, M.L., Stolina, M., Chang, D., Van, G.Y., Clarkin, K., Nguyen, H.Q., Yu, Y.B., Jing, S., Senaldi, G., Elliott, G., Medlock, E.S., 2002. Transgenic overexpression of human IL-17E results in eosinophilia, B-lymphocyte hyperplasia, and altered antibody production. Blood 100 (7), 2330–2340.

Kleinschek, M.A., Owyang, A.M., Joyce-Shaikh, B., Langrish, C.L., Chen, Y., Gorman, D.M., Blumenschein, W.M., McClanahan, T., Brombacher, F., Hurst, S.D., Kastelein, R.A., Cua, D.J., 2007. IL-25 regulates Th17 function in autoimmune inflammation. J. Exp. Med. 204 (1), 161–170.

Klimatsidas, M., Anastasiadis, K., Foroulis, C., Tossios, P., Bisiklis, A., Papakonstantinou, C., Rammos, K., 2012. Elevated levels of anti inflammatory IL-10 and pro inflammatory IL-17 in malignant pleural effusions. J. Cardiothorac Surg. 7, 104.

Koenders, M.I., Kolls, J.K., Oppers-Walgreen, B., van den Bersselaar, L., Joosten, L.A., Schurr, J.R., Schwarzenberger, P., van den Berg, W.B., Lubberts, E., 2005. Interleukin-17 receptor deficiency results in impaired synovial expression of interleukin-1 and matrix metalloproteinases 3, 9, and 13 and prevents cartilage destruction during chronic reactivated streptococcal cell wall-induced arthritis. Arthritis Rheum. 52, 3239–3247.

Koenders, M.I., Lubberts, E., Oppers-Walgreen, B., van den Bersselaar, L., Helsen, M.M., Di Padova, F.E., Boots, A.M., Gram, H., Joosten, L.A., van den Berg, W.B., 2005. Blocking of interleukin-17 during reactivation of experimental arthritis prevents joint inflammation and bone erosion by decreasing RANKL and interleukin-1. Am. J. Pathol. 167, 141–149.

Kolls, J.K., Lindén, A., 2004. Interleukin-17 family members and inflammation. Immunity 21 (4), 467–476.

Korn, T., Bettelli, E., Gao, W., Awasthi, A., Jäger, A., Strom, T.B., Oukka, M., Kuchroo, V.K., 2007. IL-21 initiates an alternative pathway to induce proinflammatory T(H)17 cells. Nature 448 (7152), 484–487.

Krejsgaard, T., Litvinov, I.V., Wang, Y., Xia, L., Willerslev-Olsen, A., Koralov, S.B., Kopp, K.L., Bonefeld, C.M., Wasik, M.A., Geisler, C., Woetmann, A., Zhou, Y., Sasseville, D., Odum, N., 2013. Elucidating the role of interleukin-17F in cutaneous T-cell lymphoma. Blood 122 (6), 943–950.

Kryczek, I., Wei, S., Szeliga, W., Vatan, L., Zou, W., 2009. Endogenous IL-17 contributes to reduced tumor growth and metastasis. Blood 114 (2), 357–359.

Kuang, D.M., Peng, C., Zhao, Q., Wu, Y., Chen, M.S., Zheng, L., 2010. Activated monocytes in peritumoral stroma of hepatocellular carcinoma promote expansion of memory T helper17 cells. Hepatology 51 (1), 154–164.

Kirshberg, S., Izhar, U., Amir, G., Demma, J., Vernea, F., Beider, K., Shlomai, Z., Wald, H., Zamir, G., Shapira, O.M., Peled, A., Wald, O., 2011. Involvement of CCR6/CCL20/IL-17 axis in NSCLC disease progression. PLoS One 6 (9), e24856.

Kutikhin, A.G., Yuzhalin, A.E., Volkov, A.N., Zhivotovskiy, A.S., Brusina, E.B., January 21, 2014. Correlation between genetic polymorphisms within IL-1B and TLR4 genes and cancer risk in a Russian population: a case–control study. Tumour Biol. 35 (5), 4821–4830.

Lan, C., Huang, X., Lin, S., Huang, H., Cai, Q., Lu, J., Liu, J., 2013. High density of IL-17-producing cells is associated with improved prognosis for advanced epithelial ovarian cancer. Cell Tissue Res. 352 (2), 351–359.

Le Gouvello, S., Bastuji-Garin, S., Aloulou, N., Mansour, H., Chaumette, M.T., Berrehar, F., Seikour, A., Charachon, A., Karoui, M., Leroy, K., Farcet, J.P., Sobhani, I., 2008. High prevalence of Foxp3 and IL17 in MMR-proficient colorectal carcinomas. Gut 57 (6), 772–779.

Lee, J., Ho, W.H., Maruoka, M., Corpuz, R.T., Baldwin, D.T., Foster, J.S., Goddard, A.D., Yansura, D.G., Vandlen, R.L., Wood, W.I., Gurney, A.L., 2001. IL-17E, a novel proinflammatory ligand for the IL-17 receptor homolog IL-17Rh1. J. Biol. Chem. 276 (2), 1660–1664.

Lemancewicz, D., Bolkun, L., Jablonska, E., Czeczuga-Semeniuk, E., Kostur, A., Kloczko, J., Dzieciol, J., 2012. The role of interleukin-17A and interleukin-17E in multiple myeloma patients. Med. Sci. Monit. 18 (1), BR54–59.

Leng, X., Ding, T., Lin, H., Wang, Y., Hu, L., Hu, J., Feig, B., Zhang, W., Pusztai, L., Symmans, W.F., Wu, Y., Arlinghaus, R.B., 2009. Inhibition of lipocalin 2 impairs breast tumorigenesis and metastasis. Cancer Res. 69 (22), 8579–8584.

Leone, P., Shin, E.C., Perosa, F., Vacca, A., Dammacco, F., Racanelli, V., 2013. MHC class I antigen processing and presenting machinery: organization, function, and defects in tumor cells. J. Natl. Cancer Inst. 105 (16), 1172–1187.

Li, H., Chen, J., Huang, A., Stinson, J., Heldens, S., Foster, J., Dowd, P., Gurney, A.L., Wood, W.I., 2000. Cloning and characterization of IL-17B and IL-17C, two new members of the IL-17 cytokine family. Proc. Natl. Acad. Sci. U.S.A. 97 (2), 773–778.

Li, J., Lau, G.K., Chen, L., Dong, S.S., Lan, H.Y., Huang, X.R., Li, Y., Luk, J.M., Yuan, Y.F., Guan, X.Y., 2011. Interleukin 17A promotes hepatocellular carcinoma metastasis via NF-kB induced matrix metalloproteinases 2 and 9 expression. PLoS One 6 (7), e21816.

Li, L., Huang, L., Vergis, A.L., Ye, H., Bajwa, A., Narayan, V., Strieter, R.M., Rosin, D.L., Okusa, M.D., 2010. IL-17 produced by neutrophils regulates IFN-gamma-mediated neutrophil migration in mouse kidney ischemia-reperfusion injury. J. Clin. Invest. 120 (1), 331–342.

Li, Q., Han, Y., Fei, G., Guo, Z., Ren, T., Liu, Z., 2012. IL-17 promoted metastasis of non-small-cell lung cancer cells. Immunol. Lett. 148 (2), 144–150.

Li, Y., Cao, Z.Y., Sun, B., Wang, G.Y., Fu, Z., Liu, Y.M., Kong, Q.F., Wang, J.H., Zhang, Y., Xu, X.Y., Li, H.L., 2011. Effects of IL-17A on the occurrence of lung adenocarcinoma. Cancer Biol. Ther. 12 (7), 610–616.

Liang, S.C., Tan, X.Y., Luxenberg, D.P., Karim, R., Dunussi-Joannopoulos, K., Collins, M., Fouser, L.A., 2006. Interleukin (IL)-22 and IL-17 are coexpressed by Th17 cells and cooperatively enhance expression of antimicrobial peptides. J. Exp. Med. 203 (10), 2271–2279.

Linkov, F., Lisovich, A., Yurkovetsky, Z., Marrangoni, A., Velikokhatnaya, L., Nolen, B., Winans, M., Bigbee, W., Siegfried, J., Lokshin, A., Ferris, R.L., 2007. Early detection of head and neck cancer: development of a novel screening tool using multiplexed immunobead-based biomarker profiling. Cancer Epidemiol., Biomarkers Prev. 16 (1), 102–107.

Liu, J., Duan, Y., Cheng, X., Chen, X., Xie, W., Long, H., Lin, Z., Zhu, B., 2011. IL-17 is associated with poor prognosis and promotes angiogenesis via stimulating VEGF production of cancer cells in colorectal carcinoma. Biochem. Biophys. Res. Commun. 407 (2), 348–354.

Liu, S.J., Tsai, J.P., Shen, C.R., Sher, Y.P., Hsieh, C.L., Yeh, Y.C., Chou, A.H., Chang, S.R., Hsiao, K.N., Yu, F.W., Chen, H.W., 2007. Induction of a distinct CD8 Tnc17 subset by transforming growth factor-beta and interleukin-6. J. Leukoc Biol. 82 (2), 354–360.

Lubberts, E., Koenders, M.I., Oppers-Walgreen, B., van den Bersselaar, L., Coenen-de Roo, C.J., Joosten, L.A., van den Berg, W.B., 2004. Treatment with a neutralizing anti-murine interleukin-17 antibody after the onset of collagen-induced arthritis reduces joint inflammation, cartilage destruction, and bone erosion. Arthritis Rheum. 50 (2), 650–659.

Lv, L., Pan, K., Li, X.D., She, K.L., Zhao, J.J., Wang, W., Chen, J.G., Chen, Y.B., Yun, J.P., Xia, J.C., 2011. The accumulation and prognosis value of tumor infiltrating IL-17 producing cells in esophageal squamous cell carcinoma. PLoS One 6 (3), e18219.

Lyon, D.E., McCain, N.L., Walter, J., Schubert, C., 2008. Cytokine comparisons between women with breast cancer and women with a negative breast biopsy. Nurs. Res. 57 (1), 51–58.

Ma, H.L., Liang, S., Li, J., Napierata, L., Brown, T., Benoit, S., Senices, M., Gill, D., Dunussi-Joannopoulos, K., Collins, M., Nickerson-Nutter, C., Fouser, L.A., Young, D.A., 2008. IL-22 is required for Th17 cell-mediated pathology in a mouse model of psoriasis-like skin inflammation. J. Clin. Invest. 118, 597–607.

Ma, Y., Aymeric, L., Locher, C., Mattarollo, S.R., Delahaye, N.F., Pereira, P., Boucontet, L., Apetoh, L., Ghiringhelli, F., Casares, N., Lasarte, J.J., Matsuzaki, G., Ikuta, K., Ryffel, B., Benlagha, K., Tesnière, A., Ibrahim, N., Déchanet-Merville, J., Chaput, N., Smyth, M.J., Kroemer, G., Zitvogel, L., 2011. Contribution of IL-17-producing gamma delta T cells to the efficacy of anticancer chemotherapy. J. Exp. Med. 208 (3), 491–503.

Mahadevan, N.R., Rodvold, J., Almanza, G., Pérez, A.F., Wheeler, M.C., Zanetti, M., 2011. ER stress drives lipocalin 2 upregulation in prostate cancer cells in an NF-κB-dependent manner. BMC Cancer 11, 229.

Mangan, P.R., Harrington, L.E., O'Quinn, D.B., Helms, W.S., Bullard, D.C., Elson, C.O., Hatton, R.D., Wahl, S.M., Schoeb, T.R., Weaver, C.T., 2006. Transforming growth factor-beta induces development of the T(H)17 lineage. Nature 441 (7090), 231–234.

Martin-Orozco, N., Muranski, P., Chung, Y., Yang, X.O., Yamazaki, T., Lu, S., Hwu, P., Restifo, N.P., Overwijk, W.W., Dong, C., 2009. T helper 17 cells promote cytotoxic T cell activation in tumor immunity. Immunity 31 (5), 787–798.

McAllister, F., Henry, A., Kreindler, J.L., Dubin, P.J., Ulrich, L., Steele, C., Finder, J.D., Pilewski, J.M., Carreno, B.M., Goldman, S.J., Pirhonen, J., Kolls, J.K., 2005. Role of IL-17A, IL-17F, and the IL-17 receptor in regulating growth-related oncogene-alpha and granulocyte colony-stimulating factor in bronchial epithelium: implications for airway inflammation in cystic fibrosis. J. Immunol. 175, 404–412.

McLean, L.P., Cross, R.K., Shea-Donohue, T., 2013. Combined blockade of IL-17A and IL-17F may prevent the development of experimental colitis. Immunotherapy 5 (9), 923–925.

Meng, C.D., Zhu, D.D., Jiang, X.D., Li, L., Sha, J.C., Dong, Z., Kong, H., 2012. Overexpression of interleukin-17 in tumor-associated macrophages is correlated with the differentiation and angiogenesis of laryngeal squamous cell carcinoma. Chin. Med. J. (Engl.) 125 (9), 1603–1607.

Meng, X.Y., Zhou, C.H., Ma, J., Jiang, C., Ji, P., 2012. Expression of interleukin-17 and its clinical significance in gastric cancer patients. Med. Oncol. 29 (5), 3024–3028.

Milner, J.D., Brenchley, J.M., Laurence, A., Freeman, A.F., Hill, B.J., Elias, K.M., Kanno, Y., Spalding, C., Elloumi, H.Z., Paulson, M.L., Davis, J., Hsu, A., Asher, A.I., O'Shea, J., Holland, S.M., Paul, W.E., Douek, D.C., 2008. Impaired T(H)17 cell differentiation in subjects with autosomal dominant hyper-IgE syndrome. Nature 452 (7188), 773–776.

Moore, E.E., Presnell, S., Garrigues, U., Guilbot, A., LeGuern, E., Smith, D., Yao, L., Whitmore, T.E., Gilbert, T., Palmer, T.D., Horner, P.J., Kuestner, R.E., 2002. Expression of IL-17B in neurons and evaluation of its possible role in the chromosome 5q-linked form of Charcot–Marie–Tooth disease. Neuromuscul. Disord. 12 (2), 141–150.

Moseley, T.A., Haudenschild, D.R., Rose, L., Reddi, A.H., 2003. Interleukin-17 family and IL-17 receptors. Cytokine Growth Factor Rev. 14 (2), 155–174.

Nam, J.S., Terabe, M., Kang, M.J., Chae, H., Voong, N., Yang, Y.A., Laurence, A., Michalowska, A., Mamura, M., Lonning, S., Berzofsky, J.A., Wakefield, L.M., 2008. Transforming growth factor beta subverts the immune system into directly promoting tumor growth through interleukin-17. Cancer Res. 68 (10), 3915–3923.

Ngiow, S.F., Smyth, M.J., Teng, M.W., 2010. Does IL-17 suppress tumor growth? Blood 115 (12), 2554–2557.

Numasaki, M., Fukushi, J., Ono, M., Narula, S.K., Zavodny, P.J., Kudo, T., Robbins, P.D., Tahara, H., Lotze, M.T., 2003. Interleukin-17 promotes angiogenesis and tumor growth. Blood 101 (7), 2620–2627.

Numasaki, M., Watanabe, M., Suzuki, T., Takahashi, H., Nakamura, A., McAllister, F., Hishinuma, T., Goto, J., Lotze, M.T., Kolls, J.K., Sasaki, H., 2005. IL-17 enhances the net angiogenic activity and in vivo growth of human non-small cell lung cancer in SCID mice through promoting CXCR-2-dependent angiogenesis. J. Immunol. 175 (9), 6177–6189.

Ogura, H., Murakami, M., Okuyama, Y., Tsuruoka, M., Kitabayashi, C., Kanamoto, M., Nishihara, M., Iwakura, Y., Hirano, T., 2008. Interleukin-17 promotes autoimmunity by triggering a positive-feedback loop via interleukin-6 induction. Immunity 29 (4), 628–636.

Onishi, R.M., Gaffen, S.L., 2010. Interleukin-17 and its target genes: mechanisms of interleukin-17 function in disease. Immunology 129 (3), 311–321.

Passos, S.T., Silver, J.S., O'Hara, A.C., Sehy, D., Stumhofer, J.S., Hunter, C.A., 2010. IL-6 promotes NK cell production of IL-17 during toxoplasmosis. J. Immunol. 184 (4), 1776–1783.

Peters, T.L., McClain, K.L., Allen, C.E., 2011. Neither IL-17A mRNA nor IL-17A protein are detectable in Langerhans cell histiocytosis lesions. Mol. Ther. 19 (8), 1433–1439.

Pfeifer, P., Voss, M., Wonnenberg, B., Hellberg, J., Seiler, F., Lepper, P.M., Bischoff, M., Langer, F., Schäfers, H.J., Menger, M.D., Bals, R., Beisswenger, C., 2013. IL-17C is a mediator of respiratory epithelial innate immune response. Am. J. Respir. Cell Mol. Biol. 48 (4), 415–421.

Prabhala, R.H., Pelluru, D., Fulciniti, M., Prabhala, H.K., Nanjappa, P., Song, W., Pai, C., Amin, S., Tai, Y.T., Richardson, P.G., Ghobrial, I.M., Treon, S.P., Daley, J.F., Anderson, K.C., Kutok, J.L., Munshi, N.C., 2010. Elevated IL-17 produced by TH17 cells promotes myeloma cell growth and inhibits immune function in multiple myeloma. Blood 115 (26), 5385–5392.

Radosavljevic, G., Ljujic, B., Jovanovic, I., Srzentic, Z., Pavlovic, S., Zdravkovic, N., Milovanovic, M., Bankovic, D., Knezevic, M., Acimovic, L.J., Arsenijevic, N., 2010. Interleukin-17 may be a valuable serum tumor marker in patients with colorectal carcinoma. Neoplasma 57 (2), 135–144.

Raffatellu, M., Santos, R.L., Verhoeven, D.E., George, M.D., Wilson, R.P., Winter, S.E., Godinez, I., Sankaran, S., Paixao, T.A., Gordon, M.A., Kolls, J.K., Dandekar, S., Bäumler, A.J., 2008. Simian immunodeficiency virus-induced mucosal interleukin-17 deficiency promotes Salmonella dissemination from the gut. Nat. Med. 14 (4), 421–428.

Rafiei, A., Hosseini, V., Janbabai, G., Ghorbani, A., Ajami, A., Farzmandfar, T., Azizi, M.D., Gilbreath, J.J., Merrell, D.S., 2013. Polymorphism in the interleukin-17A promoter contributes to gastric cancer. World J. Gastroenterol. 19 (34), 5693–5699.

Reppert, S., Boross, I., Koslowski, M., Türeci, Ö., Koch, S., Lehr, H.A., Finotto, S., 2011. A role for T-bet-mediated tumour immune surveillance in anti-IL-17A treatment of lung cancer. Nat. Commun. 2, 600.

Reynolds, J.M., Angkasekwinai, P., Dong, C., 2010. IL-17 family member cytokines: regulation and function in innate immunity. Cytokine Growth Factor Rev. 21 (6), 413–423.

Richardson, D.R., Kalinowski, D.S., Lau, S., Jansson, P.J., Lovejoy, D.B., 2009. Cancer cell iron metabolism and the development of potent iron chelators as anti-tumour agents. Biochim. Biophys. Acta. 1790 (7), 702–717.

Rifas, L., Arackal, S., 2003. T cells regulate the expression of matrix metalloproteinase in human osteoblasts via a dual mitogen-activated protein kinase mechanism. Arthritis Rheum. 48, 993–1001.

Rodvold, J.J., Mahadevan, N.R., Zanetti, M., 2012. Lipocalin 2 in cancer: when good immunity goes bad. Cancer Lett. 316 (2), 132–138.

Rogala, E., Nowicka, A., Bednarek, W., Barczyński, B., Wertel, I., Zakrzewski, M., Kotarski, J., 2012. Evaluation of the intracellular expression of interleukin 17 in patients with ovarian cancer. Ginekol. Pol. 83 (6), 424–428.

Rouvier, E., Luciani, M.F., Mattéi, M.G., Denizot, F., Golstein, P., 1993. CTLA-8, cloned from an activated T cell, bearing AU-rich messenger RNA instability sequences, and homologous to a herpesvirus saimiri gene. J. Immunol. 150 (12), 5445–5456.

Rudd, P.M., Mattu, T.S., Masure, S., Bratt, T., Van den Steen, P.E., Wormald, M.R., Küster, B., Harvey, D.J., Borregaard, N., Van Damme, J., Dwek, R.A., Opdenakker, G., 1999. Glycosylation of natural human neutrophil gelatinase B and neutrophil gelatinase B-associated lipocalin. Biochemistry 38 (42), 13937–13950.

Shalom-Barak, T., Quach, J., Lotz, M., 1998. Interleukin 17 induced gene expression in articular chondrocytes is associated with activation of mitogen-activated protein kinases and NF-kappaB. J. Biol. Chem. 273 (42), 27467–27473.

Sheibanie, A.F., Yen, J.H., Khayrullina, T., Emig, F., Zhang, M., Tuma, R., Ganea, D., 2007. The proinflammatory effect of prostaglandin E2 in experimental inflammatory bowel disease is mediated through the IL-23-->IL-17 axis. J. Immunol. 178 (12), 8138–8147.

Shen, F., Hu, Z., Goswami, J., Gaffen, S.L., 2006. Identification of common transcriptional regulatory elements in interleukin-17 target genes. J. Biol. Chem. 281 (34), 24138–24148.

Shen, F., Ruddy, M.J., Plamondon, P., Gaffen, S.L., 2005. Cytokines link osteoblasts and inflammation: microarray analysis of interleukin-17- and TNF-alpha-induced genes in bone cells. J. Leukoc Biol. 77 (3), 388–399.

Shetty, G., Beasley, G.M., Sparks, S., Barfield, M., Masoud, M., Mosca, P.J., Pruitt, S.K., Salama, A.K., Chan, C., Tyler, D.S., Weinhold, K.J., 2013. Plasma cytokine analysis in patients with advanced extremity melanoma undergoing isolated limb infusion. Ann. Surg. Oncol. 20 (4), 1128–1135.

Shibata, T., Tahara, T., Hirata, I., Arisawa, T., 2009. Genetic polymorphism of interleukin-17A and -17F genes in gastric carcinogenesis. Hum. Immunol. 70 (7), 547–551.

Song, X., Qian, Y., 2013. IL-17 family cytokines mediated signaling in the pathogenesis of inflammatory diseases. Cell Signal 25 (12), 2335–2347.

Song, X., Zhu, S., Shi, P., Liu, Y., Shi, Y., Levin, S.D., Qian, Y., 2011. IL-17RE is the functional receptor for IL-17C and mediates mucosal immunity to infection with intestinal pathogens. Nat. Immunol. 12 (12), 1151–1158.

Starnes, T., Broxmeyer, H.E., Robertson, M.J., Hromas, R., 2002. Cutting edge: IL-17D, a novel member of the IL-17 family, stimulates cytokine production and inhibits hemopoiesis. J. Immunol. 169 (2), 642–646.

Steinman, L., 2008. A rush to judgment on Th17. J. Exp. Med. 205 (7), 1517–1522.

Subramaniam, S.V., Cooper, R.S., Adunyah, S.E., 1999. Evidence for the involvement of JAK/STAT pathway in the signaling mechanism of interleukin-17. Biochem. Biophys. Res. Commun. 262 (1), 14–19.

Sylvester, J., Liacini, A., Li, W.Q., Zafarullah, M., 2004. Interleukin-17 signal transduction pathways implicated in inducing matrix metalloproteinase-3, -13 and aggrecanase-1 genes in articular chondrocytes. Cell Signal 16, 469–476.

Tahara, T., Shibata, T., Nakamura, M., Yamashita, H., Yoshioka, D., Okubo, M., Yonemura, J., Maeda, Y., Maruyama, N., Kamano, T., Kamiya, Y., Fujita, H., Nakagawa, Y., Nagasaka, M., Iwata, M., Hirata, I., Arisawa, T., 2009. Effect of polymorphisms of IL-17A, -17F and MIF genes on CpG island hyper-methylation (CIHM) in the human gastric mucosa. Int. J. Mol. Med. 24 (4), 563–569.

Takahashi, H., Numasaki, M., Lotze, M.T., Sasaki, H., 2005. Interleukin-17 enhances bFGF-, HGF- and VEGF-induced growth of vascular endothelial cells. Immunol. Lett. 98 (2), 189–193.

Takahashi, N., Vanlaere, I., de Rycke, R., Cauwels, A., Joosten, L.A., Lubberts, E., van den Berg, W.B., Libert, C., 2008. IL-17 produced by Paneth cells drives TNF-induced shock. J. Exp. Med. 205 (8), 1755–1761.

Tamachi, T., Maezawa, Y., Ikeda, K., Kagami, S., Hatano, M., Seto, Y., Suto, A., Suzuki, K., Watanabe, N., Saito, Y., Tokuhisa, T., Iwamoto, I., Nakajima, H., 2006. IL-25 enhances allergic airway inflammation by amplifying a TH2 cell-dependent pathway in mice. J. Allergy Clin. Immunol. 118 (3), 606–614.

Tartour, E., Fossiez, F., Joyeux, I., Galinha, A., Gey, A., Claret, E., Sastre-Garau, X., Couturier, J., Mosseri, V., Vives, V., Banchereau, J., Fridman, W.H., Wijdenes, J., Lebecque, S., Sautès-Fridman, C., 1999. Interleukin 17, a T-cell-derived cytokine, promotes tumorigenicity of human cervical tumors in nude mice. Cancer Res. 59 (15), 3698–3704.

Veldhoen, M., Hocking, R.J., Atkins, C.J., Locksley, R.M., Stockinger, B., 2006. TGFb in the context of an inflammatory cytokine milieu supports de novo differentiation of IL-17-producing T cells. Immunity 24, 179–189.

Wägsäter, D., Löfgren, S., Hugander, A., Dimberg, J., 2006. Expression of interleukin-17 in human colorectal cancer. Anticancer Res. 26 (6B), 4213–4216.

Wakita, D., Sumida, K., Iwakura,Y., Nishikawa, H., Ohkuri,T., Chamoto, K., Kitamura, H., Nishimura, T., 2010. Tumor-infiltrating IL-17-producing gammadelta T cells support the progression of tumor by promoting angiogenesis. Eur. J. Immunol. 40 (7), 1927–1937.

Wang, B., Li, L., Liao,Y., Li, J.,Yu, X., Zhang,Y., Xu, J., Rao, H., Chen, S., Zhang, L., Zheng, L., 2013b. Mast cells expressing interleukin 17 in the muscularis propria predict a favorable prognosis in esophageal squamous cell carcinoma. Cancer Immunol. Immunother. 62 (10), 1575–1585.

Wang, L.,Yi,T., Kortylewski, M., Pardoll, D.M., Zeng, D.,Yu, H., 2009. IL-17 can promote tumor growth through an IL-6-Stat3 signaling pathway. J. Exp. Med. 206 (7), 1457–1464.

Wang, L.,Yi,T., Zhang,W., Pardoll, D.M.,Yu, H., 2010. IL-17 enhances tumor development in carcinogen-induced skin cancer. Cancer Res. 70 (24), 10112–10120.

Wang, M.,Wang, L., Ren,T., Xu, L.,Wen, Z., 2013a. IL-17A/IL-17RA interaction promoted metastasis of osteosarcoma cells. Cancer Biol.Ther. 14 (2), 155–163.

Wang, Y.H., Angkasekwinai, P., Lu, N., Voo, K.S., Arima, K., Hanabuchi, S., Hippe, A., Corrigan, C.J., Dong, C., Homey, B.,Yao, Z.,Ying, S., Huston, D.P., Liu,Y.J., 2007. IL-25 augments type 2 immune responses by enhancing the expansion and functions ofTSLP-DC-activated Th2 memory cells. J. Exp. Med. 204 (8), 1837–1847.

Watanabe, H., Kawaguchi, M., Fujishima, S., Ogura, M., Matsukura, S.,Takeuchi, H., Ohba, M., Sueki, H., Kokubu, F., Hizawa, N., Adachi, M., Huang, S.K., Iijima, M., 2009. Functional characterization of IL-17F as a selective neutrophil attractant in psoriasis. J. Invest. Dermatol. 129 (3), 650–656.

Weaver, C.T., Hatton, R.D., Mangan, P.R., Harrington, L.E., 2007. IL-17 family cytokines and the expanding diversity of effector T cell lineages. Annu. Rev. Immunol. 25, 821–852.

Wei, L., Laurence, A., Elias, K.M., O'Shea, J.J., 2007. IL-21 is produced by Th17 cells and drives IL-17 production in a STAT3-dependent manner. J. Biol. Chem. 282 (48), 34605–34610.

Welling,T.H., Fu, S.,Wan, S., Zou,W., Marrero, J.A., 2012. Elevated serum IL-8 is associated with the presence of hepatocellular carcinoma and independently predicts survival. Cancer Invest. 30 (10), 689–697.

Wilson, N.J., Boniface, K., Chan, J.R., McKenzie, B.S., Blumenschein,W.M., Mattson, J.D., Basham, B., Smith, K., Chen, T., Morel, F., Lecron, J.C., Kastelein, R.A., Cua, D.J., McClanahan,T.K., Bowman, E.P., de Waal Malefyt, R., 2007. Development, cytokine profile and function of human interleukin 17-producing helper T cells. Nat. Immunol. 8, 950–957.

Wróbel,T., Mazur, G., Jazwiec, B., Kuliczkowski, K., 2003. Interleukin-17 in acute myeloid leukemia. J. Cell Mol. Med. 7 (4), 472–474.

Wu, Q., Martin, R.J., Rino, J.G., Breed, R.,Torres, R.M., Chu, H.W., 2007. IL-23-dependent IL-17 production is essential in neutrophil recruitment and activity in mouse lung defense against respiratory Mycoplasma pneumoniae infection. Microbes Infect. 9 (1), 78–86.

Wu, S., Rhee, K.J., Albesiano, E., Rabizadeh, S.,Wu, X.,Yen, H.R., Huso, D.L., Brancati, F.L., Wick, E., McAllister, F., Housseau, F., Pardoll, D.M., Sears, C.L., 2009. A human colonic commensal promotes colon tumorigenesis via activation of T helper type 17 T cell responses. Nat. Med. 15 (9), 1016–1022.

Wu, X., Zeng, Z., Chen, B.,Yu, J., Xue, L., Hao,Y., Chen, M., Sung, J.J., Hu, P., 2010. Association between polymorphisms in interleukin-17A and interleukin-17F genes and risks of gastric cancer. Int. J. Cancer 127 (1), 86–92.

Xie,Y., Sheng,W., Xiang, J.,Ye, Z.,Yang, J., 2010. Interleukin-17F suppresses hepatocarcinoma cell growth via inhibition of tumor angiogenesis. Cancer Invest. 28 (6), 598–607.

Xu, C.H., Zhan, P.,Yu, L.K., Zhang, X.W., September 26, 2013. Diagnostic value of pleural interleukin 17 and carcinoembryonic antigen in lung cancer patients with malignant pleural effusions. Tumour Biol. 35 (2), 1599–1603.

Xu, S., Han,Y., Xu, X., Bao,Y., Zhang, M., Cao, X., 2010a. IL-17A-producing gammadeltaT cells promote CTL responses against Listeria monocytogenes infection by enhancing dendritic cell cross-presentation. J. Immunol. 185 (10), 5879–5887.

Xu, G., Zhang, L.,Wang, D.Y., Xu, R., Liu, Z., Han, D.M.,Wang, X.D., Zuo, K.J., Li, H.B., 2010b. Opposing roles of IL-17A and IL-25 in the regulation of TSLP production in human nasal epithelial cells. Allergy 65 (5), 581–589.

Xu, W., Liu, L.Z., Loizidou, M., Ahmed, M., Charles, I.G., 2002. The role of nitric oxide in cancer. Cell Res. 12 (5–6), 311–320.

Yamada, Y., Saito, H., Ikeguchi, M., 2012. Prevalence and clinical relevance of Th17 cells in patients with gastric cancer. J. Surg. Res. 178 (2), 685–691.

Yang, L., Qi,Y., Hu, J., Tang, L., Zhao, S., Shan, B., 2012. Expression of Th17 cells in breast cancer tissue and its association with clinical parameters. Cell Biochem. Biophys. 62 (1), 153–159.

Yang, X.O., Chang, S.H., Park, H., Nurieva, R., Shah, B., Acero, L.,Wang,Y.H., Schluns, K.S., Broaddus, R.R., Zhu, Z., Dong, C., 2008. Regulation of inflammatory responses by IL-17F. J. Exp. Med. 205 (5), 1063–1075.

Yang, X.O., Nurieva, R., Martinez, G.J., Kang, H.S., Chung,Y., Pappu, B.P., Shah, B., Chang, S.H., Schluns, K.S.,Watowich, S.S., Feng, X.H., Jetten, A.M., Dong, C., 2008. Molecular antagonism and plasticity of regulatory and inflammatory T cell programs. Immunity 29 (1), 44–56.

Yang, X.O., Panopoulos, A.D., Nurieva, R., Chang, S.H.,Wang, D.,Watowich, S.S., Dong, C., 2007. STAT3 regulates cytokine-mediated generation of inflammatory helper T cells. J. Biol. Chem. 282 (13), 9358–9363.

Yao, Z., Painter, S.L., Fanslow, W.C., Ulrich, D., Macduff, B.M., Spriggs, M.K., Armitage, R.J., 1995. Human IL-17: a novel cytokine derived from T cells. J. Immunol. 155 (12), 5483–5486.

Yasumi,Y., Takikawa,Y., Endo, R., Suzuki, K., 2007. Interleukin-17 as a new marker of severity of acute hepatic injury. Hepatol. Res. 37 (4), 248–254.

Yuzhalin, A., 2011. The role of interleukin DNA polymorphisms in gastric cancer. Hum. Immunol. 72 (11), 1128–1136.

Yuzhalin, A.E., Kutikhin, A.G., 2012. Interleukin-12: clinical usage and molecular markers of cancer susceptibility. Growth Factors 30 (3), 176–191.

Zhang, B., Rong, G.,Wei, H., Zhang, M., Bi, J., Ma, L., Xue, X.,Wei, G., Liu, X., Fang, G., 2008. The prevalence of Th17 cells in patients with gastric cancer. Biochem. Biophys. Res. Commun. 374 (3), 533–537.

Zhang, F., Meng, G., Strober, W., 2008. Interactions among the transcription factors Runx1, RORgammat and Foxp3 regulate the differentiation of interleukin 17-producing T cells. Nat. Immunol. 9 (11), 1297–1306.

Zhang, Q., Liu, S., Ge, D., Zhang, Q., Xue,Y., Xiong, Z., Abdel-Mageed, A.B., Myers, L., Hill, S.M., Rowan, B.G., Sartor, O., Melamed, J., Chen, Z., You, Z., 2012a. Interleukin-17 promotes formation and growth of prostate adenocarcinoma in mouse models. Cancer Res. 72 (10), 2589–2599.

Zhang, X.L., Zhang, W.H., Fan, X.H.,Wei, F., Zhang, M., 2012b. Serum level of IL-17 in patients with multiple myeloma and its clinical significance. Zhongguo Shiyan Xueyexue Zazhi 20 (4), 930–932.

Zhang, G.Q., Han, F., Fang, X.Z., Ma, X.M., 2012c. Expression of CD4(+) and IL-17, Foxp3 in non-small cell lung cancer and their correlation with microvessel density. Zhonghua Zhongliu Zazhi 34 (8), 596–599.

Zhao, L.,Yang, J.,Wang, H.P., Liu, R.Y., 2013. Imbalance in the Th17/Treg and cytokine environment in peripheral blood of patients with adenocarcinoma and squamous cell carcinoma. Med. Oncol. 30 (1), 461.

Zhou, B., Zhang, P., Wang, Y., Shi, S., Zhang, K., Liao, H., Zhang, L., 2013. Interleukin-17 gene polymorphisms are associated with bladder cancer in a Chinese Han population. Mol. Carcinog. 52 (11), 871–878.

Zhu, L., Chen, T., Lu, Y., Wu, D., Luo, X., Ning, Q., 2012. Contribution of IL-17 to mouse hepatitis virus strain 3-induced acute liver failure. J. Huazhong Univ. Sci. Technol., Med. Sci. 32 (4), 552–556.

Zhu, X., Mulcahy, L.A., Mohammed, R.A., Lee, A.H., Franks, H.A., Kilpatrick, L., Yilmazer, A., Paish, E.C., Ellis, I.O., Patel, P.M., Jackson, A.M., 2008. IL-17 expression by breast-cancer-associated macrophages: IL-17 promotes invasiveness of breast cancer cell lines. Breast Cancer Res. 10 (6), R95.

CHAPTER 9

The Rest of Interleukins

The further one goes, the less one knows.

Laozi, Chinese Philosopher (6th century BC)

9.1 INTERLEUKIN-8 AND CANCER

9.1.1 Interleukin-8 Biology in Brief

Interleukin (IL)-8, also known as CXCL8, is a CXC-type chemokine originally identified as a leukocyte chemoattractant (Matsushima et al., 1992; Rollins, 2009). IL-8 is secreted by a wide range of cell types, including leukocytes, fibroblasts, endothelial cells and malignant cancer cells (Rollins, 2009). The IL-8 gene encodes a precursor protein of 99 amino acids, which, upon processing, yields active proteins of either 77 amino acids in nonimmune cells or 72 amino acids in monocytes and macrophages (Strieter et al., 1989; Brat et al., 2005). IL-8 mediates its effects via binding to two heterotrimeric G protein-coupled receptors, CXCR1 and CXCR2 (Brat et al., 2005). Following ligand-induced activation, CXCR1/2 becomes phosphorylated, desensitized, and internalized (Waugh and Wilson, 2008). A number of signaling pathways may be activated downstream of CXCR1/2, including mitogen-activated protein kinase (MAPK), Phosphoinositide 3-kinase (PI3K), protein kinase C (PKC), focal adhesion kinase (FAK), and Src. IL-8 signaling activates a wide range of transcription factors such as nuclear factor kappa B (NFκB), activator protein-1 (AP-1), hypoxia inducible factor 1 (HIF-1), and signal transducer and activator of transcription 3 (STAT3), and androgen receptor (Waugh and Wilson, 2008). IL-8 signaling is normally under strict regulation, with minimal IL-8 and CXCR1/2 expression in normal tissue (Hoffmann et al., 2002), and it may be enhanced by inflammatory signals, reactive oxygen species, death receptors, and steroid hormones (Shi et al., 2001; Hoffmann et al., 2002; Imamura et al., 2004; Waugh and Wilson, 2008). It may also be induced as a result of numerous environmental stresses within the tumor microenvironment including hypoxia, acidosis, hyperglycemia, cytotoxic chemotherapies, and radiation (Shi et al., 2001). In addition, tumor cells harboring oncogenic mutations or mutations within tumor suppressor genes may cause increased IL-8 or

CXCR1/2 expression (Sparmann and Bar-Sagi, 2004). The regulation of IL-8 expression mainly occurs at the transcriptional level; nevertheless, post-transcriptional regulation may also take place through the stabilization of mRNA transcripts, with steady-state mRNA levels being proportional to IL-8 secretion (Shi et al., 2001; Hoffmann et al., 2002). Translational regula-tion of IL-8 is also possible (Siddiqui et al., 1999; Yu et al., 2003). IL-8 binds with high specificity to CXCR1 (Holmes et al., 1991) and with less speci-ficity to CXCR2 (Brat et al., 2005) expressed on stromal, endothelial, and tumor cells. Considering the fact that CXCR1 and CXCR2 receptors are expressed on cancer cells, endothelial cells, monocytes, basophils, T-lympho-cytes neutrophils, and tumor-associated macrophages, it can be suggested that the synthesis and secretion of IL-8 from tumor cells affect the tumor microenvironment (Brat et al., 2005). The two receptors share a 78% homol-ogy (Murphy, 1994). However, differences in their N-terminal domains result in different binding specificities (Murphy, 1994; Hu et al., 2013).

Various signaling pathways may induce IL-8 expression in cancers (Lin et al., 2004). For instance, the RAS–RAF signaling pathway activates the NF-κB transcription factor, which, in turn, results in the production of numerous cytokines such as IL-8 (Mantovani et al., 2006). Moreover, there is persistent NF-κB activation in malignancies promoting growth, angio-genesis, and metastasis, which are associated with chronic inflammation (Terzic et al., 2010; Greten et al., 2004). In addition to NF-κB, AP-1 also controls the expression of IL-8 (Karin et al., 2002), and epidermal growth factor receptor (EGFR) may regulate IL-8 production or expression as well (Zhang et al., 2012). Once the expression of IL-8 has been induced, it acti-vates NF-κB and launches the inflammatory cycle (Pikarsky et al., 2004). The transcription of IL-8 requires NF-κB that works along with AP-1 and elements of nuclear factor induced by IL-6 (Brat et al., 2005; Wang et al., 2012). The interaction between IL-8 and EGFR promotes cell proliferation via transactivation of the receptor by the activation of a disintegrin and matrix metalloproteinases (MMPs) (Joh et al., 2005). IL-8 may induce EGFR phosphorylation and the processing of EGFR ligands, which may further bind and stimulate EGFR in paracrine and autocrine manners to induce cell proliferation (Joh et al., 2005).

9.1.2 IL-8 and Vital Processes Underlying Cancer

Research on the role of IL-8 in cancer has been hampered by the lack of a homologous gene in the mouse, the common animal model for human cancer studies, and by the functional overlap between various chemokines

(Ren et al., 2003). Therefore, our knowledge about the IL-8 gene and its regulation has been obtained mostly from investigations on cultured or isolated cells (Ren et al., 2003). The impact of IL-8 on tumor development and progression has been well documented in a wide range of cancer cells (Singh et al., 2006; Araki et al., 2007; Yao et al., 2007; Merritt et al., 2008; Singh et al., 2009). Clinical data on IL-8 efficacy are based on the association between high serum levels and poor cancer prognosis (Ueda et al., 1994; Yuan et al., 2005). IL-8 seems to be a promising prognostic and predictive cancer biomarker. It is known that IL-8 levels are elevated in cancer-associated nonvascular extracellular fluids, such as pleural effusion, ascites, cyst fluid, cerebrospinal fluid, urine, saliva, interstitial fluid, and cervicovaginal secretions (Kotyza, 2012). Higher IL-8 levels are typically found in high-grade peritumoral fluids rather than low-grade tumors and benign conditions (Kotyza, 2012). It has been originally identified as a chemoattractant for neutrophils that release angiogenic growth factors, thereby promoting angiogenesis. According to the recent data, IL-8 increases the proliferation, survival, and migration of endothelial cells; facilitates survival, epithelial–mesenchymal transition (EMT), and further migration of cancer cells; and activates immune response at the tumor site (Vandercappellen et al., 2008). Moreover, in response to stress, stromal cells also produce IL-8, which affects the invasiveness and/or metastatic potential of cancer cells (Inoue et al., 2000; Mukaida, 2003). In recent years, it was also demonstrated that a link exists between IL-8, tumor EMT, and tumor stemness (Palena et al., 2012). Certain studies identified IL-8 as an essential factor for the induction and maintenance of the mesenchymal and stem-like phenotype of aggressive, metastatic carcinoma cells (Palena et al., 2012). IL-8 released by tumor cells undergoing EMT is able to maintain the mesenchymal, invasive phenotype of tumor cells that have undergone EMT via an autocrine loop (Palena et al., 2012). Moreover, it exerts a paracrine effect on adjacent epithelial tumor cells to induce EMT, enhance angiogenesis, and attract immune cells to the site of the tumor, and thus creates an inflammatory environment, and promotes metastasis (Palena et al., 2012). Depletion of IL-8 reduces the stemness and tumorigenicity of colon cancer cells (Hwang et al., 2011). Endothelial cells are able to proliferate and migrate in response to IL-8 signaling, leading to neovascularization (Li et al., 2003). The increased secretion of IL-8 by tumor cells undergoing EMT can also lead to enhanced recruitment of neutrophils, which may exert protumorigenic and prometastatic functions (Waugh and Wilson, 2008). Tumor progression can be assisted by tumor-associated neutrophils via the secretion of MMPs, which are able to remodel the extracellular matrix (ECM) and favor tumor migration (Gregory and Houghton, 2011). Tumor stroma, consisting of fibroblasts, endothelial cells, and immune cells, can also secrete IL-8 in response to various stress factors. IL-8 released by the stroma can directly influence tumor cell proliferation (Schadendorf et al., 1993), migration, invasion, and EMT (De Larco et al., 2001; Bates et al., 2004; Fernando et al., 2011), and can also help tumor cells to avoid stress-induced apoptosis (Maxwell et al., 2007). IL-8 contributes to the production and secretion of MMP-2 and MMP-9 (Li et al., 2005; Coppe et al., 2008), modifying invasiveness and/or ECM remodeling in normal physiological conditions and in cancer progression. In human colon cancer cell lines, the constitutive expression of IL-8 has shown to determine the metastatic potential and overall postoperative survival (Li et al., 2001). Highly metastatic melanoma cells express higher levels of IL-8 mRNA than do low metastatic cells, and this increased mRNA expression directly correlates with IL-8 protein secretion (Singh et al., 1994). Undifferentiated highly metastatic cell lines produce much more IL-8 than do their differentiated lower metastatic counterparts (De Larco et al., 2003). In addition, the stable and selective overexpression of IL-8 is associated with a drug-resistant phenotype (Duan et al., 1999). On the contrary, depleting intracellular IL-8 in androgen-independent prostate cancer has increased the cytotoxic activity of multiple chemotherapeutic drugs (Singh and Lokeshwar, 2009). Since tumor cells are usually surrounded by fibroblasts, dendritic cells, tumor-associated macrophages, and other cells of lymphoid origin, IL-8 produced by tumor cells could act on one or more of these cells, and produce other cytokines, growth factors, and/or MMPs. Neutrophil chemotaxis and activation are the major physiological roles of IL-8 (Zeilhofer and Schorr, 2000). It has been demonstrated that the inhibition of neutrophil recruitment to the tumor site via IL-8 or CXCR1/2 inhibition can reduce tumor growth in vivo (Farooq et al., 2009; Tazzyman et al., 2011; Jamieson et al., 2012).

9.1.3 IL-8 Expression and Cancer

Previous studies have revealed that highly metastatic solid tumors such as prostate, breast, melanoma, and ovarian cancer constitutively express IL-8 (Xu and Filder, 2000; Xie, 2001; Huang et al., 2002). In IL-8 transgenic mice, the high expression of IL-8 has promoted colon cancer development, confirming a significant role of IL-8 in gastrointestinal tumorigenesis (Asfaha et al., 2013). In cancer models of the liver, pancreas, colorectum, and melanoma, IL-8 functions as an autocrine growth factor (Schadendorf et al.,

1993; Miyamoto et al., 1998; Brew et al., 2000; Zhu et al., 2004; Li et al., 2005a; Li et al., 2005b). An increased expression of IL-8 and its receptors has been detected in many types of cancer including prostate (Murphy et al., 2005), colorectal (Li et al., 2001), and non-small-cell lung cancer (Yuan et al., 2000). IL-8 signaling has also been shown to promote migration and invasion in melanoma (Wang et al., 1990), colon (Wilson et al., 1999), and gastric cancer (Kuai et al., 2012). Many types of human carcinomas, including breast, colon, cervical, gastric, lung, and ovarian cancers, among others, express high levels of IL-8 relative to normal tissues (Waugh and Wilson, 2008). In addition, multiple clinical studies on melanoma, as well as on breast, ovarian, prostate, and colon cancer, have shown a direct correlation between serum IL-8 levels and disease progression (Xie, 2001). It has also been shown that the level of IL-8 and polymorphisms within the gene encoding IL-8 may be considered as predictive and prognostic biomarkers for vascular endothelial growth factor (VEGF)-targeted therapy in renal cell carcinoma (Funakoshi et al., 2013). IL-8 is upregulated in breast cancer compared with normal breast tissue and a high IL-8 level correlates with poor prognosis (Benoy et al., 2004; Singh et al., 2013). An elevated serum IL-8 level is associated with the worse outcomes, a higher tumor load, the presence of liver or lymph node involvement, and with an early metastatic spread (Benoy et al., 2004). Moreover, IL-8 may promote breast cancer progression by regulating breast cancer stem cells activity; increasing cell invasion, angiogenesis, and metastasis; and it is particularly upregulated in HER2-positive cancers (Singh et al., 2013; Chin and Wang, 2014). IL-8 was found to be highly overexpressed in ER$^-$ breast cancers; however, it is able to elevate the invasiveness and metastatic potential of both ER$^-$ and ER$^+$ breast cancer cells (Todorovic-Rakovic et al., 2013). Serum IL-8 levels have been associated with prostate cancer stage, with the greatest levels detected in patients with metastatic prostate cancer (Veltri et al., 1999). Schauer et al. have detected that reactive stroma initiates at focal sites of benign prostatic hyperplasia that overexpress IL-8 and have increased deposition of tenascin-C (Schauer et al., 2008). These findings have been confirmed using different in vivo rodent models, which have shown that upregulated IL-8 expression in prostate epithelial cells induced a tenascin-C positive reactive stroma with markers almost identical to those observed in prostate cancer (Schauer et al., 2009; Schauer et al., 2011). In addition, it has been suggested that IL-8 is involved in neoplastic activities of salivary glands and the oral cavity, and salivary IL-8 may be used as a biomarker for the early detection of head and neck squamous cell carcinomas (Schapher et al., 2011; Lee et al., 2011).

Furthermore, IL-8 may promote the development of lung, endometrial, and pancreatic cancer as well (Zhang et al., 2012; Ewington et al., 2012; Chen et al., 2012; Li et al., 2012). Measurement of urinary IL-8 seems to be a promising marker for assessing therapeutic response in bladder cancer (Mertens et al., 2013). Based on current urine-based assays, IL-8 has been identified as a prominent urinary biomarker for the detection of bladder cancer (Urquidi et al., 2012). A significant association of high IL-8 expression level in gastric mucosa with a risk of developing gastric cancer has been reported (Yamada et al., 2013), and it has been hypothesized that the IL-8 serum level may be a marker of gastric cancer (Macri et al., 2006). Furthermore, the elevated expression of IL-8 mRNA in tissue extracts from gastric cancer patients has been correlated with a poor prognosis of the disease (Lee et al., 2004). It has been reported that IL-8 overexpression increases the vascularity of human gastric malignancies and that IL-8-transfected cells have produced rapidly growing, highly vascular neoplasms while control cells have not (Lee et al., 2004). In contrast, the inhibition of IL-8 decreases angiogenesis in gastric cancer (Kitadai et al., 1998). IL-8 has also been linked with cell adhesion and migration in gastric cancer (Kitadai et al., 1998). These processes are mediated via NF-κB and Akt signals, and a number of adhesion molecules are involved, including intercellular adhesion molecule-1, vascular cell adhesion molecule-1, and CD44 (Kuai et al., 2012).

9.1.4 Inherited Variations Within the IL-8 Gene and Cancer

It has been observed that *IL-8* gene polymorphisms are associated with the risk of developing gastric cancer (reviewed by Yuzhalin, 2011). A common single nucleotide polymorphism at −251 bp (251-bp upstream of the IL-8 transcription start site) has been associated with elevated plasma levels of IL-8 (Hull et al., 2000) and with IL-8 promoter activities (Lee et al., 2005; Ohyauchi et al., 2005). It has been supposed that *IL-8-251 A/T* genotype may correlate with an increased risk of developing breast and prostate cancer (McCarron et al., 2002; Snoussi et al., 2006) and with a risk of tumor recurrence (Gordon et al., 2006). One research group (Taguchi et al., 2005) has found the association of the *IL-8-251 A/T* genotype with a higher expression of IL-8 protein, severe neutrophil infiltration, and increased risk of atrophic gastritis and gastric cancer. *IL-8-251* A/T and *IL-8-251* A/A genotypes may correlate with enhanced MMP-9 and angiopoietin-1 production in gastric malignant tumors of *Helicobacter pylori*-infected Koreans (Song et al., 2010). Another group (Felipe et al., 2012) has revealed that patients with the *IL-8-251* A/T genotype have an increased risk of developing gastric cancer in a Brazilian population. However, the association of IL-8 polymorphisms and gastric cancer is controversial, and a *meta*-analysis of epidemiological studies has revealed an overall lack of association between IL-8-251 gene polymorphisms and risk of developing gastric cancer (Liu et al., 2010). Surprisingly, another *meta*-analysis has found the AA genotype to be associated with the overall risk of developing gastric cancer, particularly in Asian populations and with the intestinal-type gastric cancer (Xue et al., 2012). The results of another *meta*-analysis demonstrated that the carriage of the −251A allele correlates with a 12–21% increased risk of developing cancer in total, particularly of breast cancer, gastric cancer, and nasopharyngeal cancer (Wang et al., 2012). However, the authors found that −251A allele carriers may have reduced risk of prostate cancer (Wang et al., 2012). Interestingly, African and Asian populations, but not the European population, were at a higher risk of developing cancer, which may suggest significant differences in the distribution of risk allele across various ethnicities (Wang et al., 2012).

According to the above-mentioned findings, the exact impact of inherited variations within the IL-8 gene on gastric cancer remains obscured due to inconsistent data. Nonetheless, it is clear that the −251 gene polymorphism plays a pivotal role in gastric cancer development and requires follow-up investigation. In addition, certain functional polymorphisms within the IL-8 gene, such as IL-8_+396T/G (rs2227307) and IL-8_+781C/T (rs2227306), have not been investigated at all. Undoubtedly, these potential molecular biomarkers should be included in further case–control studies.

9.1.5 IL-8 Inhibitors: A New Way to Treat Cancer?

Multiple inhibitors of IL-8 expression regulating the IL-8 downstream signals are known. For instance, polyphenols derived from natural products that include resveratrol, apigenin, and anthocyanins inhibit IL-8 (Manna et al., 2000; Goswami and Das, 2009; Speciale et al., 2010; Wang and Huang, 2013). Since resveratrol inhibits NF-κB (Manna et al., 2000), its suppressive effect on IL-8 secretion may be closely associated with its NF-κB inhibitory activity; however, it may also be due to the modulation of regulatory enzymes such as MAPK (Goswami and Das, 2009). Apigenin, one of the most common flavonoids, increases IκBα expression, and thus inhibits NF-κB activation and decreases IL-8 expression (Wang and Huang, 2013). Cyanidin-3-glucoside, which is abundant in anthocyanins, inactivates NF-κB by inhibiting the phosphorylation of IκB (Speciale et al., 2010). Rebamipide (2-(4-chlorobenzoylamino)-3-(2(1H) quinolinon-4-yl) propionic acid; OPC-12,759), a mucosal-protective antiulcer agent, may inhibit IL-8 in gastric cancer by the regulation of phospholipase D expression (Kang et al., 2013). Moreover, rebamipide inhibits the growth of gastric cancer cells (Tarnawski et al., 2005). Gefitinib (Iressa™, ZD1839), an orally active, quinazoline-derived agent, inhibits EGFR-tyrosine kinase, epidermal growth factor (EGF) signals, and IL-8 production in gastric cancer cells (Ciardiello et al., 2001; Hirata et al., 2002; Kishida et al., 2005). Conjugated linoleic acids produced by *Lactobacillus acidophilus* also reduce the activation of NF-κB and IL-8 expression in *H. pylori*-infected gastric epithelial cells (Hwang et al., 2012). Inhibition of IL-8 with small interfering RNA has lowered the adhesion, migration, and invasion potential in cancer cells (Kitadai et al., 1998). IL-8 small interfering RNA (IL-8siRNA) has been validated to suppress the IL-8 expression in colon cancer cells (Ning et al., 2011). In mouse models of ovarian cancer, liposomes containing IL-8 siRNA decreased tumor weight compared with empty control liposomes (Merritt et al., 2008). Anti-IL-8-monoclonal antibody has successfully reduced tumor growth, angiogenesis, and metastasis of human melanoma in vivo (Zigler et al., 2008) and inhibits tumor growth in orthotopic bladder cancer xenografts via the downregulation of matrix metalloproteases and NF-kB (Mian et al., 2003). Several microRNAs (miR), which are central regulators of various vital processes, have been found to regulate *IL-8* gene expression (Li et al., 2012). Recently, a research group has detected that miR-146a decreases the expression of IL-8 via lowered NF-κB activity, which reduces the metastatic potential of cancer cells (Bhaumik et al., 2008). In addition, it has been observed that miR-146a may negatively affect the release of IL-1β-induced IL-8 (Perry et al., 2009). The overexpression of miR-155, which plays a significant role in the immune response, has also reduced the *H. pylori*-induced IL-8 expression (Tang et al., 2010; Lee et al., 2013). MyD88 protein has been proposed for IL-8 regulation among a number of targets of miR-155, and it has been suggested that miR-155 may downregulate MyD88 through the inhibition of translation (Janssens and Beyaert, 2002). Toll-like receptors activate MyD88 leading to the nuclear translocation of NF-κB, and thus transcriptionally regulate IL-8 (Chen et al., 2007). Finally, small molecule inhibitors targeting IL-8 receptors (CXCR1 and CXCR2) have been synthesized to suppress prostate and colon cancer (Liu et al., 2012; Ning et al., 2012). Inhibition of these receptors decreases cell migration and invasion, while increasing apoptosis in cancer cells (Singh et al., 2010). Another research group (Liu et al., 2012) has developed a derivative of the human cytokine IL-8, G31P, with a high affinity for human CXCR1 and CXCR2. G31P treatment has significantly reduced prostate cancer cell viability, adhesion, and migration capacity (Liu et al., 2012). Moreover, G31P has inhibited tumor tissue vascularization, which has been associated with the decreased expression of VEGF and NF-κB in orthotopic xenograft tissues (Liu et al., 2012). Another small molecule inhibitor targeting CXCR2 is SCH-527123 (Ning et al., 2012). This drug is able to suppress CXCR2-mediated signal transduction via decreased phosphorylation of the NF-κB, MAPK, and Akt pathways in colon cancer cells (Ning et al., 2012). The antitumor activity of SCH-527123 is performed via the inhibition of cancer cell growth, motility, and angiogenesis (Ning et al., 2012). In addition, targeting IL-8 or CXCR2 may also increase chemosensitivity to chemotherapeutics since it has also been shown that IL-8/CXCR2 signaling promotes resistance to chemotherapeutics such as oxaliplatin through NF-κB activity (Wilson et al., 2008). In various human malignancies, high levels of IL-8 in serum or at local sites are associated with aggressive disease and poor initial response to drugs including oxaliplatin, 5-fluorouracil, paclitaxel, and camptothecin (Bellocq et al., 1998; Kuniyasu et al., 2000; Haraguchi et al., 2002; McCarron et al., 2002; Rial et al., 2009; Kantola et al., 2012). In contrast, paclitaxel, camptothecin, and erlotinib elevate IL-8 transcription and secretion in cancer cells (Collins et al., 2000; Wilson et al., 2012; Gales et al., 2013).

9.2 IL-14 AND CANCER

IL-14 is a cytokine that has been originally cloned from a Burkitt lymphoma cell line (Ambrus and Fauci, 1985). Before DNA cloning, IL-14 was designated as a high molecular weight B cell growth factor (Leca et al., 2008). Purified IL-14 has been demonstrated to enhance B cell proliferation and expand a subpopulation of memory B cells (Ambrus et al., 1990; Ambrus et al., 1993). More recently, the role of IL-14 in antibody formation has been investigated in a transgenic mouse model wherein IL-14 was predominantly expressed in the B cell compartment (Shen et al., 2006). Furthermore, IL-14 transgenic mice have demonstrated an increased number of B1, B2, and germinal center B cells and enhanced antibody responses to T-dependent and T-independent antigens (Shen et al., 2006). IL-14 has two biological isoforms, namely, IL-14α and IL-14β (Peng et al., 2009).

There is a significant lack of articles devoted to the role of IL-14 in cancer. In 1995, a research group (Ford et al., 1995) observed that IL-14 mRNA was constitutively expressed in the freshly isolated lymphoma cells that also expressed the receptor for IL-14 (IL14R). In this study, cell lines developed from these patients produced IL-14 in vitro and antisense oligos to IL-14 blocked their growth in vitro (Ford et al., 1995). The authors concluded that the autocrine or paracrine production of IL-14 may play a significant role in the progression of aggressive B cell non-Hodgkin lymphoma (Ford et al., 1995). In 2006, the same research group showed that 95% of IL-14α-transgenic mice developed CD5+ B cell lymphomas, consistent with the lymphomas observed in elderly patients with Sjögren's syndrome and systemic lupus erythematosus (Shen et al., 2006; Ford et al., 2007).

The role of IL-14 in human cancer remains obscured, although existing data indicate that there is every reason to believe that this cytokine may be involved in tumor development and progression. Further in-depth studies are required to shed light on the impact of IL-14 on cancer.

9.3 IL-16 AND CANCER

Since its identification in 1982 by Center and Cruikshank, IL-16 has been characterized as a regulator of a number of cellular processes including cell recruitment and activation (Center and Cruikshank, 1982; Cruikshank and Center, 1982). IL-16 is generated as a precursor molecule that is cleaved following cell activation into a promolecule and mature, secreted, component (Richmond et al., 2014). In lymphocytes, pro-IL-16, the N-terminal domain of the precursor molecule, acts as a transcriptional repressor with regulatory effects on cell cycle progression, while mature IL-16, the C-terminal domain, is secreted from the cell as a ligand for CD4 with chemoattractant, growth factor, and differentiation factor capabilities on a variety of hematopoietic cell types involved in an inflammatory response (Richmond et al., 2014). It is well established that the primary receptor for IL-16 is CD4, which is expressed on many hematopoietic and neuronal cells (Cruikshank et al., 1987; Center et al., 1996). However, another research group has shown that CD9 is also able to transmit IL-16-induced migratory and differentiation signaling in mast cells (Qi et al., 2006).

According to the recent study conducted by Yellapa et al. (2013), IL-16-expressing cells were observed more frequently in patients with ovarian cancer as compared to that in patients with benign ovarian tumors and in healthy control subjects. Moreover, the concentration of serum IL-16 was significantly higher in ovarian cancer patients in comparison to that in those with benign ovarian tumors and healthy controls (Yellapa et al., 2013). Furthermore, an increase in tissue expression and serum levels of IL-16 in ovarian cancer patients positively correlated with the degree of tumor vasculature, suggesting the involvement of this cytokine in angiogenesis (Yellapa et al., 2013). In addition, the authors found that serum levels of IL-16 rose significantly even before ovarian tumors become detectable in animal models (Yellapa et al., 2012; Yellapa et al., 2013).

Atanackovic et al. (2012) indicated that IL-16 is markedly overexpressed in the bone marrow of myeloma patients as compared to that in healthy blood donors. Moreover, the authors demonstrated that myeloma cell lines and primary tumor cells from myeloma patients constitutively expressed IL-16 and its receptors CD4 and/or CD9 and spontaneously secreted soluble IL-16 (Atanackovic et al., 2012). Silencing of IL-16 has decreased the proliferative activity of myeloma cells by about 80% compared with untreated cells, and a monoclonal antibody blocking IL-16 or its receptors had a comparably strong growth-inhibiting effect on the tumor cells (Atanackovic et al., 2012). Similarly, IL-16 has been reported to be overexpressed in primary effusion lymphoma cells line BCBL-1 (Arguello et al., 2006).

Comperat et al. (2010) examined whether or not the tissue expression of IL-16 is a valuable prognostic factor of survival in 304 patients with prostate cancer. The authors found that IL-16 expression in prostate cancer tissue has been significantly associated with tumor aggressiveness and biochemical relapse of the disease. More importantly, the expression of IL-16 correlated with high Gleason score and was established as an independent factor for survival in prostate cancer patients (Comperat et al., 2010).

Gao et al. (2009a) found that IL-16 serum levels have been significantly elevated in 376 patients with colorectal carcinoma or in 220 subjects with gastric cancer, in comparison with that in 480 age- and sex-matched healthy controls.

Nakajima et al. (2009) demonstrated that IL-16 administration has increased the expression of murine double minute 2 (MDM2) protein and cell proliferation in *H. pylori*-coincubated human gastric carcinoma cell line AGS. It is to be noted that MDM2 overexpression was observed in various cancers, and it is also known to bind tumor suppressor protein p53 (Iwakuma and Lozano, 2003). Based on these findings, the authors proposed that IL-16 may be considered as a risk factor of *H. pylori*-induced gastric cancer (Nakajima et al., 2009).

Liebrich et al. (2007) examined the presence of IL-16-expressing macrophages and microglial cells in 50 primary brain tumor specimens, consisting of three protoplasmatic astrocytomas, 21 fibrillary astrocytomas, seven anaplastic astrocytomas, and 19 glioblastoma multiforme. The authors observed a marked increase in parenchymal IL-16-positive cells in grade II astrocytomas, with a further increase on transition from grade II to III astrocytomas. Interestingly, there were no IL-16-positive cells in the brains of four normal rat control brains.

Finally, IL-16 protein has been repeatedly associated with an increased stage of multiple myeloma and other malignant tumors, correlating with poor survival (Kovacs, 2001; Alexandrakis et al., 2004). However, in the study conducted by Kovasc (2001), IL-16 levels were overexpressed together with IL-12, which is known to be an antitumor cytokine (Yuzhalin and Kutikhin, 2012); therefore, the exact role of IL-16 has not been fully explained in this study.

There is evidence suggesting the involvement of inherited variations within the IL-16 gene in cancer risk. In particular, it was recently reported that rs4778889 CC and rs11556218 GG genotypes are associated with an increased risk of developing noncardia gastric cancer in a Chinese population (Zhang and Wang, 2013). On the contrary, previous results obtained from Zhu et al. (2010) and Azimzadeh et al. (2011) indicated that the CC genotype of the rs4778889 polymorphism correlated with a decreased colorectal cancer risk and renal cancer risk, respectively.

In addition, a series of studies performed by Azimzadeh et al. (2011, 2012) revealed an association between the CC genotype and C allele of the rs1131445 polymorphism and TG genotype of the rs11556218 polymorphism and colorectal cancer risk in an Iranian population.

Moreover, rs7175701 and rs11556218 polymorphisms have been shown to be markedly associated with prostate cancer risk (Batai et al., 2012). The TG and GG genotypes and G allele of the rs11556218 polymorphism as well as TT genotype of the rs4072111 polymorphism have been associated with a significantly increased risk of developing hepatitis B virus-related hepatocellular carcinoma (HCC) (Li et al., 2011). A number of studies (Gao et al., 2009a,b; Qin et al., 2013) have identified the TG genotype and G allele of the rs11556218 polymorphism as a risk factor for developing nasopharyngeal carcinoma, colorectal cancer, and gastric cancer. In addition, the G allele of the rs11556218 polymorphism has been associated with increased serum IL-16 levels in nasopharyngeal carcinoma patients (Qin et al., 2013).

However, in the recent meta-analysis of seven eligible studies pooling 1678 cases and 1937 controls, the rs11556218 T/G polymorphism of the IL-16 gene was markedly associated with an elevated cancer risk in Asian populations, while rs4778889 and rs4072111 polymorphisms showed no association with cancer risk (Zhao et al., 2013).

In conclusion, serum and tumor tissue IL-16 levels along with certain polymorphisms within the *IL-16* gene may be considered as a promising predictive and diagnostic biomarker of many malignant tumors.

9.4 IL-32 AND CANCER

The first report on the molecule has been published by a research group (Dahl et al., 1992) that has identified a protein that was highly expressed in activated T- and NK-cells, and therefore, it was called NK4. Nonetheless, at that time and for the next 13 years, the biological function of NK4 was not known. In 2005, the NK4 gene was found as one of the most upregulated genes (Kim et al., 2005). Researchers (Kim et al., 2005) have detected that the recombinant form of the NK4 protein may induce several proinflammatory cytokines, and therefore NK4 has been renamed to IL-32. However, the structure of IL-32 has not matched the sequence homology observed in most of the known cytokines (Kim et al., 2005). IL-32 mRNA has been predominantly found in immune tissues and cells, and also in nonimmune cells such as in epithelial cells (Kim et al., 2005). IL-32 occurs in four major splice variant isoforms of the mRNA, namely, IL-32α, IL-32β, IL-32γ, and IL-32δ (Kim et al., 2005); nevertheless, IL-32β seems to be most abundant (Goda et al., 2006). Overexpression of endogenous IL-32γ has caused cell death, which, however, has not occurred with the IL-32α isoform (Heinhuis et al., 2012a). The differences among IL-32 isoforms have been described in several reports (Choi et al., 2009; Heinhuis et al., 2011, 2012b). The level of IL-32 can be altered in monocytes, macrophages, or endothelial cells both on mRNA and protein levels by exposure to a various stimuli such as lipopolysaccharide (LPS), muramyl dipeptide, double-stranded RNA (poly I:C), and several cytokines such as tumor necrosis factor-alpha (TNF-α) and interferon-gamma (Netea et al., 2005; Hasegawa et al., 2011; Schenk et al., 2012).

A recent investigation performed by Nold-Petry et al. (2014) revealed that IL-32 may possess angiogenic properties. The authors showed that small interfering RNA-mediated silencing of IL-32 negated the 58% proliferation of epithelial cells that occurred within 24h in scrambled-transfected controls. Further investigation of molecular mechanisms demonstrated that proangiogenic effects of IL-32 that are VEGF independent are due to integrin αVβ3.

The level of IL-32 expression has been positively associated with tumor size, number of lymph node metastases, and tumor stage (Park et al., 2013). Breast cancer-derived MDA-MB-231 cells exogenously expressing IL-32 have been characterized by a higher migration and invasion capacity associated with an increased expression of the EMT markers vimentin and Slug, and also VEGF (Park et al., 2013). In addition, the IL-32 may also play a role in the migration and invasion of breast cancer cells under the conditions of normoxia and hypoxia (Park et al., 2013).

However, certain groups implicate IL-32 as an antitumor agent. Yun et al. (2013) demonstrated that IL-32 inhibits tumor growth through the increase in the number of cytotoxic lymphocytes. Also, the authors found that the antitumor activities of this cytokine were due to the inactivation of NF-κB and STAT3 pathways through changing of cytokine levels in tumor tissues. Similarly, Kang et al. (2012) found that IL-32α was overexpressed in the tissue and serum of patients with hepatocellular carcinoma as compared to that in the normal serum from healthy controls. Furthermore, the authors demonstrated that the suppression of IL-32α in hepatocellular carcinoma decreased the expression of phospho-p38 MAPK, NF-κB, and antiapoptotic protein Bcl-2 and induced the expression of proapoptotic proteins as well as p53 and p53 upregulated modulator of apoptosis (PUMA) resulting in the inhibition of cell growth and induction of intrinsic apoptosis.

According to the recent study conducted by Plantinga et al. (2013), IL-32 was overexpressed in thyroid tumor tissue samples from 139 patients with epithelial cell-derived thyroid carcinoma. Furthermore, the authors found that carriers of an IL-32 genetic variant associated with an increased IL-32γ gene expression and a higher production of proinflammatory cytokines had a higher risk of developing thyroid cancer. In addition, Plantinga et al. indicated a twofold increase in IL-32γ mRNA and protein levels after stimulation with LPS. It is interesting, however, that LPS administration did not alter the expression of IL-32β.

Ishigami et al. (2013) established IL-32 as an independent prognostic marker for gastric carcinoma. In their study, the authors examined a cohort of 182 gastric cancer patients who received curative gastrectomy. It was found that IL-32-positive gastric cancer patients had a higher tumor depth and a higher number of lymph node metastases. In addition, lymphatic invasion and venous invasion in the IL-32-positive group were more severe as compared to that in the IL-32-negative group.

The overexpression of IL-32 mRNA has also been detected in malignant esophageal tissue, and the plasma level of IL-32 has been elevated in 65 patients with esophageal cancer (Yousif et al., 2013). In addition, the IL-32 expression in gastric cancer tissues has been significantly higher than in *H. pylori*-uninfected gastric mucosa (Seo et al., 2008; Sakitani et al., 2012).

IL-32 also plays an important role in regulating the stem cell-like properties that promote tumorigenesis of colorectal cancer stem cells (Chang et al., 2011). It has been found that IL-32 mRNA levels in primary adherent cells from patients with myelodysplastic syndromes may be 14-fold to 17-fold higher than in controls (Marcondes et al., 2008; Marcondes et al., 2009). Furthermore, IL-32 expression has been strongly upregulated in most lung adenocarcinomas, large-cell carcinomas, and small-cell lung cancers (Sorrentino et al., 2009). Overexpression of IL-32 in lung adenocarcinoma has significantly correlated with the clinical staging and metastasis (Zeng et al., 2014). Moreover, IL-32-facilitated cell migration and invasion in vitro have been mediated through the transactivation of the nuclear transcription factor (NF)-κB signaling pathway and the subsequent upregulation of MMP-2 and MMP-9 expression (Zeng et al., 2014). Expression levels of IL-32 by both tumor-infiltrating lymphocytes and tumor cells have correlated with a high intratumoral microvessel density and poor clinical outcome (Sorrentino et al., 2009). IL-32 has been weakly expressed by pancreatic duct cells, but a strong expression of IL-32 has been demonstrated in the pancreatic cancer cell lines (Nishida et al., 2009). Then, another research group has identified a positive association of IL-32 levels with human breast cancer and glioblastoma multiforme (Kobayashi and Lin, 2009).

Finally, IL-32 overexpression has been associated with high recurrence rates and low survival rates in patients with clear cell renal cell carcinoma and head and neck squamous cell carcinoma (Lee et al., 2012; Guenin et al., 2013). However, other researchers have found that IL-32γ may potentiate TNF-α-induced cell growth inhibition through the activation of p38 MAPK pathways (Park et al., 2012), and it has been observed that IL-32γ may inhibit cancer cell growth through the inactivation of NF-κB and STAT3 signals (Oh et al., 2011). To conclude, it can be suggested that serum and tumor tissue IL-32 levels can soon become promising diagnostic and prognostic biomarkers of cancer.

9.5 IL-34 AND CANCER

IL-34 has been recently discovered as the second ligand for colony-stimulating factor-1 receptor (CSF-1R) (Lin et al., 2008; Nakamichi et al., 2013). Although it lacks appreciable similarity with any other proteins,

IL-34 strongly binds to CSF-1R and promotes the differentiation, proliferation, and survival of monocytes, macrophages, and osteoclasts (Lin et al., 2008; Wei et al., 2010; Chen et al., 2011). Recently, two investigations described immunological phenotypes of IL-34-deficient mice (Greter et al., 2012; Wang et al., 2012). IL-34 is expressed in neurons and keratinocytes and a deficiency of IL-34 declines the populations of Langerhans cells and microglia, whereas monocytes, macrophages, and dendritic cells are largely unaffected by IL-34 deficiency (Greter et al., 2012; Wang et al., 2012). IL-34 does not control the recruitment of blood monocytic cells and their differentiation into Langerhans cells in inflammation but is crucial for their maintenance in situ (Greter et al., 2012; Wang et al., 2012). In addition, IL-34 contributes to the maintenance of microglia in specific areas of the adult brain (Greter et al., 2012; Wang et al., 2012) such as cortex, olfactory nucleus, and hippocampus. However, the role of IL-34 in cancer remains obscure.

9.6 SUMMARY

To conclude this section, it could be said that IL-8 is one of the most significant regulators of cancer development. First, it has been repeatedly associated with the proliferation, survival, and migration of endothelial cells. Second, IL-8 was found to facilitate the survival, EMT and further migration of cancer cells. Third, multiple tumors, including breast, liver, pancreatic, gastric, colon, cervical, prostate, lung, and ovarian, were shown to overexpress IL-8 as compared to normal tissues. Finally, the use of IL-8 inhibitors is potentially a new way to treat cancer, and the investigation of this issue is being continued.

Serum and tumor tissue IL-16 and IL-32 levels along with certain polymorphisms within the IL-16 gene may be considered as promising predictive and diagnostic biomarkers of many malignant tumors. Regarding the impact of IL-14 and IL-34 on human cancer, a lack of studies does not enable us to draw any conclusions. Further in-depth studies are needed to evaluate the role of these agents in tumor biology.

REFERENCES

Alexandrakis, M.G., Passam, F.H., Kyriakou, D.S., Christophoridou, A.V., Perisinakis, K., Hatzivasili, A., Foudoulakis, A., Castanas, E., 2004. Serum level of interleukin-16 in multiple myeloma patients and its relationship to disease activity. Am. J. Hematol. 75 (2), 101–106.

Ambrus Jr., J.L., Chesky, L., Stephany, D., McFarland, P., Mostowski, H., Fauci, A.S., 1990. Functional studies examining the subpopulation of human B lymphocytes responding to high molecular weight B cell growth factor. J. Immunol. 145 (12), 3949–3955.

Ambrus Jr., J.L., Fauci, A.S., 1985. Human B lymphoma cell line producing B cell growth factor. J. Clin. Invest. 75 (2), 732–739.

Ambrus Jr., J.L., Pippin, J., Joseph, A., Xu, C., Blumenthal, D., Tamayo, A., Claypool, K., McCourt, D., Srikiatchatochorn, A., Ford, R.J., 1993. Identification of a cDNA for a human high-molecular-weight B-cell growth factor. Proc. Natl. Acad. Sci. U.S.A. 90 (13), 6330–6334.

Araki, S., Omori, Y., Lyn, D., Singh, R.K., Meinbach, D.M., Sandman, Y., Lokeshwar, V.B., Lokeshwar, B.L., 2007. Interleukin-8 is a molecular determinant of androgen independence and progression in prostate cancer. Cancer Res. 67 (14), 6854–6862.

Arguello, M., Paz, S., Hernandez, E., Corriveau-Bourque, C., Fawaz, L.M., Hiscott, J., Lin, R., 2006. Leukotriene A4 hydrolase expression in PEL cells is regulated at the transcriptional level and leads to increased leukotriene B4 production. J. Immunol. 176 (11), 7051–7061.

Asfaha, S., Dubeykovskiy, A.N., Tomita, H., Yang, X., Stokes, S., Shibata, W., Friedman, R.A., Ariyama, H., Dubeykovskaya, Z.A., Muthupalani, S., Ericksen, R., Frucht, H., Fox JG, Wang, T.C., 2013. Mice that express human interleukin-8 have increased mobilization of immature myeloid cells, which exacerbates inflammation and accelerates colon carcinogenesis. Gastroenterology 144 (1), 155–166.

Atanackovic, D., Hildebrandt, Y., Templin, J., Cao, Y., Keller, C., Panse, J., Meyer, S., Reinhard, H., Bartels, K., Lajmi, N., Sezer, O., Zander, A.R., Marx, A.H., Uhlig, R., Zustin, J., Bokemeyer, C., Kröger, N., 2012. Role of interleukin 16 in multiple myeloma. J. Natl. Cancer Inst. 104 (13), 1005–1020.

Azimzadeh, P., Romani, S., Mohebbi, S.R., Kazemian, S., Vahedi, M., Almasi, S., Fatemi, S.R., Zali, M.R., 2011. Interleukin-16 (IL-16) gene polymorphisms in Iranian patients with colorectal cancer. J. Gastrointestin. Liver Dis. 20 (4), 371–376.

Azimzadeh, P., Romani, S., Mohebbi, S.R., Mahmoudi, T., Vahedi, M., Fatemi, S.R., Zali, N., Zali, M.R., 2012. Association of polymorphisms in microRNA-binding sites and colorectal cancer in an Iranian population. Cancer Genet. 205 (10), 501–507.

Batai, K., Shah, E., Murphy, A.B., Newsome, J., Ruden, M., Ahaghotu, C., Kittles, R.A., 2012. Fine-mapping of IL16 gene and prostate cancer risk in African Americans. Cancer Epidemiol. Biomarkers Prev. 21 (11), 2059–2068.

Bates, R.C., DeLeo 3rd, M.J., Mercurio, A.M., 2004. The epithelial–mesenchymal transition of colon carcinoma involves expression of IL-8 and CXCR-1-mediated chemotaxis. Exp. Cell. Res. 299 (2), 315–324.

Bellocq, A., Antoine, M., Flahault, A., Philippe, C., Crestani, B., Bernaudin, J.F., Mayaud, C., Milleron, B., Baud, L., Cadranel, J., 1998. Neutrophil alveolitis in bronchioloalveolar carcinoma: induction by tumor-derived interleukin-8 and relation to clinical outcome. Am. J. Pathol. 152 (1), 83–92.

Benoy, I.H., Salgado, R., Van Dam, P., Geboers, K., Van Marck, E., Scharpé, S., Vermeulen, P.B., Dirix, L.Y., 2004. Increased serum interleukin-8 in patients with early and metastatic breast cancer correlates with early dissemination and survival. Clin. Cancer Res. 10 (21), 7157–7162.

Bhaumik, D., Scott, G.K., Schokrpur, S., Patil, C.K., Campisi, J., Benz, C.C., 2008. Expression of microRNA-146 suppresses NF-kappaB activity with reduction of metastatic potential in breast cancer cells. Oncogene 27 (42), 5643–5647.

Brat, D.J., Bellail, A.C., van Meir, E.G., 2005. The role of interleukin-8 and its receptors in gliomagenesis and tumoral angiogenesis. Neuro-Oncol. 7 (2), 122–133.

Brew, R., Erikson, J.S., West, D.C., Kinsella, A.R., Slavin, J., Christmas, S.E., 2000. Interleukin-8 as an autocrine growth factor for human colon carcinoma cells in vitro. Cytokine 12 (1), 78–85.

Center, D.M., Cruikshank, W., 1982. Modulation of lymphocyte migration by human lymphokines. I. Identification and characterization of chemoattractant activity for lymphocytes from mitogen-stimulated mononuclear cells. J. Immunol. 128 (6), 2563–2568.

Center, D.M., Kornfeld, H., Cruikshank, W.W., 1996. Interleukin 16 and its function as a CD4 ligand. Immunol. Today 17 (10), 476–481.

Chang, C.J., Chien, Y., Lu, K.H., Chang, S.C., Chou, Y.C., Huang, C.S., Chang, C.H., Chen, K.H., Chang, Y.L., Tseng, L.M., Song, W.S., Wang, J.J., Lin, J.K., Huang, P.I., Lan, Y.T., 2011. Oct4-related cytokine effects regulate tumorigenic properties of colorectal cancer cells. Biochem. Biophys. Res. Commun. 415 (2), 245–251.

Chen, X.M., Splinter, P.L., O'Hara, S.P., LaRusso, N.F., 2007. A cellular micro-RNA, let-7i, regulates Toll-like receptor 4 expression and contributes to cholangiocyte immune responses against *Cryptosporidium parvum* infection. J. Biol. Chem. 282 (39), 28929–28938.

Chen, Y., Shi, M., Yu, G.Z., Qin, X.R., Jin, G., Chen, P., Zhu, M.H., 2012. Interleukin-8, a promising predictor for prognosis of pancreatic cancer. World J. Gastroenterol. 18 (10), 1123–1129.

Chen, Z., Buki, K., Vääräniemi, J., Gu, G., Väänänen, H.K., 2011. The critical role of IL-34 in osteoclastogenesis. PLoS One 6 (4), e18689.

Chin, A.R., Wang, S.E., 2014. Cytokines driving breast cancer stemness. Mol. Cell. Endocrinol. 382 (1), 598–602.

Choi, J.D., Bae, S.Y., Hong, J.W., Azam, T., Dinarello, C.A., Her, E., Choi, W.S., Kim, B.K., Lee, C.K., Yoon, D.Y., Kim, S.J., Kim, S.H., 2009. Identification of the most active interleukin-32 isoform. Immunology 126 (4), 535–542.

Ciardiello, F., Caputo, R., Bianco, R., Damiano, V., Fontanini, G., Cuccato, S., De Placido, S., Bianco, A.R., Tortora, G., 2001. Inhibition of growth factor production and angiogenesis in human cancer cells by ZD1839 (Iressa), a selective epidermal growth factor receptor tyrosine kinase inhibitor. Clin. Cancer Res. 7 (5), 1459–1465.

Collins, T.S., Lee, L.-F., Ting, J.P.-Y., 2000. Paclitaxel up-regulates interleukin-8 synthesis in human lung carcinoma through an NF-κB- and AP-1-dependent mechanism. Cancer Immunol. Immunother. 49 (2), 78–84.

Compérat, E., Roupret, M., Drouin, S.J., Camparo, P., Bitker, M.O., Houlgatte, A., Cancel-Tassin, G., Cussenot, O., 2010. Tissue expression of IL16 in prostate cancer and its association with recurrence after radical prostatectomy. Prostate 70 (15), 1622–1627.

Coppé, J.P., Patil, C.K., Rodier, F., Sun, Y., Muñoz, D.P., Goldstein, J., Nelson, P.S., Desprez, P.Y., Campisi, J., 2008. Senescence-associated secretory phenotypes reveal cell-nonautonomous functions of oncogenic RAS and the p53 tumor suppressor. PLoS Biol. 6(12, article e301).

Cruikshank, W., Center, D.M., 1982. Modulation of lymphocyte migration by human lymphokines. II. Purification of a lymphotactic factor (LCF). J. Immunol. 128 (6), 2569–2574.

Cruikshank, W.W., Berman, J.S., Theodore, A.C., Bernardo, J., Center, D.M., 1987. Lymphokine activation of T4+ T lymphocytes and monocytes. J. Immunol. 138 (11), 3817–3823.

Dahl, C.A., Schall, R.P., He, H.L., Cairns, J.S., 1992. Identification of a novel gene expressed in activated natural killer cells and T cells. J. Immunol. 148 (2), 597–603.

De Larco, J.E., Wuertz, B.R., Rosner, K.A., Erickson, S.A., Gamache, D.E., Manivel, J.C., Furcht, L.T., 2001. A potential role for interleukin-8 in the metastatic phenotype of breast carcinoma cells. Am. J. Pathol. 158 (2), 639–646.

De Larco, J.E., Wuertz, B.R., Yee, D., Rickert, B.L., Furcht, L.T., 2003. Atypical methylation of the interleukin-8 gene correlates strongly with the metastatic potential of breast carcinoma cells. Proc. Natl. Acad. Sci. U.S.A. 100 (24), 13988–13993.

Duan, Z., Feller, A.J., Penson, R.T., Chabner, B.A., Seiden, M.V., 1999. Discovery of differentially expressed genes associated with paclitaxel resistance using cDNA array technology: analysis of interleukin (IL) 6, IL-8, and monocyte chemotactic protein 1 in the paclitaxel-resistant phenotype. Clin. Cancer Res. 5 (11), 3445–3453.

Ewington, L., Taylor, A., Sriraksa, R., Horimoto, Y., Lam, E.W., El-Bahrawy, M.A., 2012. The expression of interleukin-8 and interleukin-8 receptors in endometrial carcinoma. Cytokine 59 (2), 417–422.

Farooq, S.M., Stillie, R., Svensson, M., Svanborg, C., Strieter, R.M., Stadnyk, A.W., 2009. Therapeutic effect of blocking CXCR2 on neutrophil recruitment and dextran sodium sulfate-induced colitis. J. Pharmacol. Exp. Ther. 329 (1), 123–129.

Felipe, A.V., Silva, T.D., Pimenta, C.A., Kassab, P., Forones, N.M., 2012. Interleukin-8 gene polymorphism and susceptibility to gastric cancer in a Brazilian population. Biol. Res. 45 (4), 369–374.

Fernando, R.I., Castillo, M.D., Litzinger, M., Hamilton, D.H., Palena, C., 2011. IL-8 signaling plays a critical role in the epithelial–mesenchymal transition of human carcinoma cells. Cancer Res. 71 (15), 5296–5306.

Ford, R., Tamayo, A., Martin, B., Niu, K., Claypool, K., Cabanillas, F., Ambrus Jr., J., 1995. Identification of B-cell growth factors (interleukin-14; high molecular weight-B-cell growth factors) in effusion fluids from patients with aggressive B-cell lymphomas. Blood 86 (1), 283–293.

Ford, R.J., Shen, L., Lin-Lee, Y.C., Pham, L.V., Multani, A., Zhou, H.J., Tamayo, A.T., Zhang, C., Hawthorn, L., Cowell, J.K., Ambrus Jr., J.L., 2007. Development of a murine model for blastoid variant mantle-cell lymphoma. Blood 109 (11), 4899–4906.

Funakoshi, T., Lee, C.H., Hsieh, J.J., December 4, 2013. A systematic review of predictive and prognostic biomarkers for VEGF-targeted therapy in renal cell carcinoma. Cancer Treat. Rev. http://dx.doi.org/10.1016/j.ctrv.2013.11.008. pii: S0305-7372(13)00261-2, (Epub ahead of print).

Gales, D., Clark, C., Manne, U., Samuel, T., 2013. The chemokine CXCL8 in carcinogenesis and drug response. ISRN Oncol. 2013, 859154.

Gao, L.B., Liang, W.B., Xue, H., Rao, L., Pan, X.M., Lv, M.L., Bai, P., Fang, W.L., Liu, J., Liao, M., Zhang, L., 2009a. Genetic polymorphism of interleukin-16 and risk of nasopharyngeal carcinoma. Clin. Chim. Acta 409 (1–2), 132–135.

Gao, L.B., Rao, L., Wang, Y.Y., Liang, W.B., Li, C., Xue, H., Zhou, B., Sun, H., Li, Y., Lv, M.L., Du, X.J., Zhang, L., 2009b. The association of interleukin-16 polymorphisms with IL-16 serum levels and risk of colorectal and gastric cancer. Carcinogenesis 30 (2), 295–299.

Goda, C., Kanaji, T., Kanaji, S., Tanaka, G., Arima, K., Ohno, S., Izuhara, K., 2006. Involvement of IL-32 in activation-induced cell death in T cells. Int. Immunol. 18 (2), 233–240.

Gordon, M.A., Gil, J., Lu, B., Zhang, W., Yang, D., Yun, J., Schneider, S., Groshen, S., Iqbal, S., Press, O.A., Rhodes, K., Lenz, H.J., 2006. Genomic profiling associated with recurrence in patients with rectal cancer treated with chemoradiation. Pharmacogenomics 7 (1), 67–88.

Goswami, S.K., Das, D.K., 2009. Resveratrol and chemoprevention. Cancer Lett. 284 (1), 1–6.

Gregory, A.D., Houghton, A.M., 2011. Tumor-associated neutrophils: new targets for cancer therapy. Cancer Res. 71 (7), 2411–2416.

Greten, F.R., Eckmann, L., Greten, T.F., Park, J.M., Li, Z.W., Egan, L.J., Kagnoff, M.F., Karin, M., 2004. IKKβ links inflammation and tumorigenesis in a mouse model of colitis-associated cancer. Cell. 118 (3), 285–296.

Greter, M., Lelios, I., Pelczar, P., Hoeffel, G., Price, J., Leboeuf, M., Kündig, T.M., Frei, K., Ginhoux, F., Merad, M., Becher, B., 2012. Stroma-derived interleukin-34 controls the development and maintenance of Langerhans cells and the maintenance of microglia. Immunity 37 (6), 1050–1060.

Guenin, S., Mouallif, M., Hubert, P., Jacobs, N., Krusy, N., Duray, A., Ennaji, M.M., Saussez, S., Delvenne, P., January 28, 2013. Interleukin-32 expression is associated with a poorer prognosis in head and neck squamous cell carcinoma. Mol. Carcinog., (Epub ahead of print).

Haraguchi, M., Komuta, K., Akashi, A., Matsuzaki, S., Furui, J., Kanematsu, T., 2002. Elevated IL-8 levels in the drainage vein of resectable Dukes' C colorectal cancer indicate high risk for developing hepatic metastasis. Oncol. Rep. 9 (1), 159–165.

Hasegawa, H., Thomas, H.J., Schooley, K., Born, T.L., 2011. Native IL-32 is released from intestinal epithelial cells via a non-classical secretory pathway as a membrane-associated protein. Cytokine 53 (1), 74–83.

Heinhuis, B., Koenders, M.I., van de Loo, F.A., Netea, M.G., van den Berg, W.B., Joosten, L.A., 2011. Inflammation-dependent secretion and splicing of IL-32{gamma} in rheumatoid arthritis. Proc. Natl. Acad. Sci. U.S.A. 108 (12), 4962–4967.

Heinhuis, B., Koenders, M.I., van den Berg, W.B., Netea, M.G., Dinarello, C.A., Joosten, L.A., 2012a. Interleukin 32 (IL-32) contains a typical α-helix bundle structure that resembles focal adhesion targeting region official adhesion kinase-1. J. Biol. Chem. 287 (8), 5733–5743.

Heinhuis, B., Netea, M.G., van den Berg, W.B., Dinarello, C.A., Joosten, L.A., 2012b. Interleukin-32: a predominantly intracellular proinflammatory mediator that controls cell activation and cell death. Cytokine 60 (2), 321–327.

Hirata, A., Ogawa, S., Kometani, T., Kuwano, T., Naito, S., Kuwano, M., Ono, M., 2002. ZD1839 (Iressa) induces antiangiogenic effects through inhibition of epidermal growth factor receptor tyrosine kinase. Cancer Res. 62 (9), 2554–2560.

Hoffmann, E., Dittrich-Breiholz, O., Holtmann, H., Kracht, M., 2002. Multiple control of interleukin-8 gene expression. J. Leukocyte Biol. 72 (5), 847–855.

Holmes, W.E., Lee, J., Kuang, W.J., Rice, G.C., Wood, W.I., 1991. Structure and functional expression of a human interleukin-8 receptor. Science 253 (5025), 1278–1280.

Hu, W., Wang, J., Luo, G., Luo, B., Wu, C., Wang, W., Xiao, Y., Li, J., 2013. Proteomics-based analysis of differentially expressed proteins in the CXCR1-knockdown gastric carcinoma MKN45 cell line and its parental cell. Acta Biochim. Biophys. Sin. (Shanghai) 45 (10), 857–866.

Huang, S., Mills, L., Mian, B., Tellez, C., McCarty, M., Yang, X.D., Gudas, J.M., Bar-Eli, M., 2002. Fully humanized neutralizing antibodies to interleukin-8 (ABX-IL8) inhibit angiogenesis, tumor growth, and metastasis of human melanoma. Am. J. Pathol. 161 (1), 125–134.

Hull, J., Thomson, A., Kwiatkowski, D., 2000. Association of respiratory syncytial virus bronchiolitis with the interleukin 8 gene region in UK families. Thorax 55 (12), 1023–1027.

Hwang, S.W., Kim, N., Kim, J.M., Huh, C.S., Ahn, Y.T., Park, S.H., Shin, C.M., Park, J.H., Lee, M.K., Nam, R.H., Lee, H.S., Kim, J.S., Jung, H.C., Song, I.S., 2012. Probiotic suppression of the H. pylori-induced responses by conjugated linoleic acids in a gastric epithelial cell line. Prostaglandins Leukot. Essent. Fatty Acids 86 (6), 225–231.

Hwang, W.L., Yang, M.H., Tsai, M.L., Lan, H.Y., Su, S.H., Chang, S.C., Teng, H.W., Yang, S.H., Lan, Y.T., Chiou, S.H., Wang, H.W., 2011. SNAIL regulates interleukin-8 expression, stem cell-like activity, and tumorigenicity of human colorectal carcinoma cells. Gastroenterology 141 (1), 279–291. 291.e1–5.

Imamura, R., Konaka, K., Matsumoto, N., Hasegawa, M., Fukui, M., Mukaida, N., Kinoshita, T., Suda, T., 2004. Fas ligand induces cell-autonomous NF-kappaB activation and interleukin-8 production by a mechanism distinct from that of tumor necrosis factor-alpha. J. Biol. Chem. 279 (45), 46415–46423.

Inoue, K., Slaton, J.W., Eve, B.Y., Kim, S.J., Perrotte, P., Balbay, M.D., Yano, S., Bar-Eli, M., Radinsky, R., Pettaway, C.A., Dinney, C.P., 2000. Interleukin 8 expression regulates tumorigenicity and metastases in androgen-independent prostate cancer. Clin. Cancer Res. 6 (5), 2104–2119.

Ishigami, S., Arigami, T., Uchikado, Y., Setoyama, T., Kita, Y., Sasaki, K., Okumura, H., Kurahara, H., Kijima, Y., Harada, A., Ueno, S., Natsugoe, S., 2013. IL-32 expression is an independent prognostic marker for gastric cancer. Med. Oncol. 30 (2), 472.

Iwakuma, T., Lozano, G., 2003. MDM2, an introduction. Mol. Cancer Res. 1 (14), 993–1000.

Jamieson,T., Clarke, M., Steele, C.W., Samuel, M.S., Neumann, J., Jung, A., Huels, D., Olson, M.F., Das, S., Nibbs, R.J.B., Sansom, O.J., 2012. Inhibition of CXCR2 profoundly suppresses inflammation-driven and spontaneous tumorigenesis. J. Clin. Invest. 122 (9), 3127–3144.

Janssens, S., Beyaert, R., 2002. A universal role for MyD88 in TLR/IL-1R-mediated signaling. Trends. Biochem. Sci. 27 (9), 474–482.

Joh, T., Kataoka, H., Tanida, S., Watanabe, K., Ohshima, T., Sasaki, M., Nakao, H., Ohhara, H., Higashiyama, S., Itoh, M., 2005. *Helicobacter pylori*-stimulated interleukin-8 (IL-8) promotes cell proliferation through transactivation of epidermal growth factor receptor (EGFR) by disintegrin and metalloproteinase (ADAM) activation. Dig. Dis. Sci. 50 (11), 2081–2089.

Kang, D.W., Hwang, W.C., Park, M.H., Ko, G.H., Ha, W.S., Kim, K.S., Lee, Y.C., Choi, K.Y., Min, D.S., 2013. Rebamipide abolishes *Helicobacter pylori* CagA-induced phospholipase D1 expression via inhibition of NFκB and suppresses invasion of gastric cancer cells. Oncogene 32 (30), 3531–3542.

Kang, Y.H., Park, M.Y., Yoon, D.Y., Han, S.R., Lee, C.I., Ji, N.Y., Myung, P.K., Lee, H.G., Kim, J.W., Yeom, Y.I., Jang, Y.J., Ahn, D.K., Kim, J.W., Song, E.Y., 2012. Dysregulation of overexpressed IL-32α in hepatocellular carcinoma suppresses cell growth and induces apoptosis through inactivation of NF-κB and Bcl-2. Cancer Lett. 318 (2), 226–233.

Kantola, T., Klintrup, K., Väyrynen, J.P., Vornanen, J., Bloigu, R., Karhu, T., Herzig, K.H., Näpänkangas, J., Mäkelä, J., Karttunen, T.J., Tuomisto, A., Mäkinen, M.J., 2012. Stage-dependent alterations of the serum cytokine pattern in colorectal carcinoma. Br. J. Cancer 107 (10), 1729–1736.

Karin, M., Cao, Y., Greten, F.R., Li, Z.W., 2002. NF-kappaB in cancer: from innocent bystander to major culprit. Nat. Rev. Cancer 2 (4), 301–310.

Kim, S.H., Han, S.Y., Azam, T., Yoon, D.Y., Dinarello, C.A., 2005. Interleukin-32: a cytokine and inducer of TNFalpha. Immunity 22 (1), 131–142.

Kishida, O., Miyazaki, Y., Murayama, Y., Ogasa, M., Miyazaki, T., Yamamoto, T., Watabe, K., Tsutsui, S., Kiyohara, T., Shimomura, I., Shinomura, Y., 2005. Gefitinib (Iressa, ZD1839) inhibits SN38-triggered EGF signals and IL-8 production in gastric cancer cells. Cancer Chemother. Pharmacol. 55 (6), 584–594.

Kitadai, Y., Haruma, K., Sumii, K., Yamamoto, S., Ue, T., Yokozaki, H., Yasui, W., Ohmoto, Y., Kajiyama, G., Fidler, I.J., Tahara, E., 1998. Expression of interleukin-8 correlates with vascularity in human gastric carcinomas. Am. J. Pathol. 152 (1), 93–100.

Kobayashi, H., Lin, P.C., 2009. Molecular characterization of IL-32 in human endothelial cells. Cytokine 46 (3), 351–358.

Kotyza, J., 2012. Interleukin-8 (CXCL8) in tumor associated non-vascular extracellular fluids: its diagnostic and prognostic values. A review. Int. J. Biol. Markers 27 (3), 169–178.

Kovacs, E., 2001. The serum levels of IL-12 and IL-16 in cancer patients. Relation to the tumour stage and previous therapy. Biomed. Pharmacother. 55 (2), 111–116.

Kuai, W.-X., Wang, Q., Yang, X.-Z., Zhao, Y., Yu, R., Tang, X.-J., 2012. Interleukin-8 associates with adhesion, migration, invasion and chemosensitivity of human gastric cancer cells. World J. Gastroenterol. 18 (9), 979–985.

Kuniyasu, H., Yasui, W., Shinohara, H., Yano, S., Ellis, L.M., Wilson, M.R., Bucana, C.D., Rikita, T., Tahara, E., Fidler, I.J., 2000. Induction of angiogenesis by hyperplastic colonic mucosa adjacent to colon cancer. Am. J. Pathol. 157 (5), 1523–1535.

Leca, N., Laftavi, M., Shen, L., Matteson, K., Ambrus Jr., J., Pankewycz, O., 2008. Regulation of human interleukin 14 transcription in vitro and in vivo after renal transplantation. Transplantation 86 (2), 336–341.

Lee, H.J., Liang, Z.L., Huang, S.M., Lim, J.S., Yoon, D.Y., Lee, H.J., Kim, J.M., 2012. Overexpression of IL-32 is a novel prognostic factor in patients with localized clear cell renal cell carcinoma. Oncol. Lett. 3 (2), 490–496.

Lee, K.D., Lee, H.S., Jeon, C.H., 2011. Body fluid biomarkers for early detection of head and neck squamous cell carcinomas. Anticancer Res. 31 (4), 1161–1167.

Lee, K.E., Khoi, P.N., Xia, Y., Park, J.S., Joo, Y.E., Kim, K.K., Choi, S.Y., Jung, Y.D., 2013. *Helicobacter pylori* and interleukin-8 in gastric cancer. World J. Gastroenterol. 19 (45), 8192–8202.

Lee, K.H., Bae, S.H., Lee, J.L., Hyun, M.S., Kim, S.H., Song, S.K., Kim, H.S., 2004. Relationship between urokinase-type plasminogen receptor, interleukin-8 gene expression and clinicopathological features in gastric cancer. Oncology 66 (3), 210–217.

Lee, W.P., Tai, D.I., Lan, K.H., Li, A.F., Hsu, H.C., Lin, E.J., Lin, Y.P., Sheu, M.L., Li, C.P., Chang, F.Y., Chao, Y., Yen, S.H., Lee, S.D., 2005. The -251T allele of the interleukin-8 promoter is associated with increased risk of gastric carcinoma featuring diffuse-type histopathology in Chinese population. Clin. Cancer Res. 11 (18), 6431–6441.

Li, A., Dubey, S., Varney, M.L., Dave, B.J., Singh, R.K., 2003. IL-8 directly enhanced endothelial cell survival, proliferation, and matrix metalloproteinases production and regulated angiogenesis. J. Immunol. 170 (6), 3369–3376.

Li, A., Varney, M.L., Singh, R.K., 2005. Constitutive expression of growth regulated oncogene (gro) in human colon carcinoma cells with different metastatic potential and its role in regulating their metastatic phenotype. Clin. Exp. Metastasis. 21 (7), 571–579.

Li, A., Varney, M.L., Singh, R.K., 2001. Expression of interleukin 8 and its receptors in human colon carcinoma cells with different metastatic potentials expression of interleukin 8 and its receptors in human colon carcinoma cells with different metastatic potentials 1. Clin. Cancer Res. 7 (10), 3298–3304.

Li, A., Varney, M.L., Valasek, J., Godfrey, M., Dave, B.J., Singh, R.K., 2005. Autocrine role of interleukin-8 in induction of endothelial cell proliferation, survival, migration and MMP-2 production and angiogenesis. Angiogenesis 8 (1), 63–71.

Li, N., Xu, X., Xiao, B., Zhu, E.D., Li, B.S., Liu, Z., Tang, B., Zou, Q.M., Liang, H.P., Mao, X.H., 2012. *H. pylori* related proinflammatory cytokines contribute to the induction of miR-146a in human gastric epithelial cells. Mol. Biol. Rep. 39 (4), 4655–4661.

Li, S., Deng, Y., Chen, Z.P., Huang, S., Liao, X.C., Lin, L.W., Li, H., Peng, T., Qin, X., Zhao, J.M., 2011. Genetic polymorphism of interleukin-16 influences susceptibility to HBV-related hepatocellular carcinoma in a Chinese population. Infect. Genet. Evol. 11 (8), 2083–2088.

Li, X.J., Peng, L.X., Shao, J.Y., Lu, W.H., Zhang, J.X., Chen, S., Chen, Z.Y., Xiang, Y.Q., Bao, Y.N., Zheng, F.J., Zeng, M.S., Kang, T.B., Zeng, Y.X., Teh, B.T., Qian, C.N., 2012. As an independent unfavorable prognostic factor, IL-8 promotes metastasis of nasopharyngeal carcinoma through induction of epithelial–mesenchymal transition and activation of AKT signaling. Carcinogenesis 33 (7), 1302–1309.

Liebrich, M., Guo, L.H., Schluesener, H.J., Schwab, J.M., Dietz, K., Will, B.E., Meyermann, R., 2007. Expression of interleukin-16 by tumor-associated macrophages/activated microglia in high-grade astrocytic brain tumors. Arch. Immunol. Ther. Exp. (Warsz) 55 (1), 41–47.

Lin, H., Lee, E., Hestir, K., Leo, C., Huang, M., Bosch, E., Halenbeck, R., Wu, G., Zhou, A., Behrens, D., Hollenbaugh, D., Linnemann, T., Qin, M., Wong, J., Chu, K., Doberstein, S.K., Williams, L.T., 2008. Discovery of a cytokine and its receptor by functional screening of the extracellular proteome. Science 320 (5877), 807–811.

Lin, Y., Huang, R., Chen, L., Li, S., Shi, Q., Jordan, C., Huang, R.P., 2004. Identification of interleukin-8 as estrogen receptor-regulated factor involved in breast cancer invasion and angiogenesis by protein arrays. Int. J. Cancer 109 (4), 507–515.

Liu, L., Zhuang, W., Wang, C., Chen, Z., Wu, X.T., Zhou, Y., 2010. Interleukin-8 -251 A/T gene polymorphism and gastric cancer susceptibility: a meta-analysis of epidemiological studies. Cytokine 50 (3), 328–334.

Liu, X., Peng, J., Sun, W., Yang, S., Deng, G., Li, F., Cheng, J.W., Gordon, J.R., 2012. G31P, an antagonist against CXC chemokine receptors 1 and 2, inhibits growth of human prostate cancer cells in nude mice. Tohoku J. Exp. Med. 228 (2), 147–156.

Macrì, A., Versaci, A., Loddo, S., Scuderi, G., Travagliante, M., Trimarchi, G., Teti, D., Famulari, C., 2006. Serum levels of interleukin 1beta, interleukin 8 and tumour necrosis factor alpha as markers of gastric cancer. Biomarkers 11 (2), 184–193.

Manna, S.K., Mukhopadhyay, A., Aggarwal, B.B., 2000. Resveratrol suppresses TNF-induced activation of nuclear transcription factors NF-kappa B, activator protein-1, and apoptosis: potential role of reactive oxygen intermediates and lipid peroxidation. J. Immunol. 164 (12), 6509–6519.

Mantovani, A., Bonecchi, R., Locati, M., 2006. Tuning inflammation and immunity by chemokine sequestration: decoys and more. Nat. Rev. 6 (12), 907–918.

Marcondes, A.M., Mhyre, A.J., Stirewalt, D.L., Kim, S.H., Dinarello, C.A., Deeg, H.J., 2008. Dysregulation of IL-32 in myelodysplastic syndrome and chronic myelomonocytic leukemia modulates apoptosis and impairs NK function. Proc. Natl. Acad. Sci. U.S.A. 105 (8), 2865–2870.

Marcondes, A.M., Ramakrishnan, A., Deeg, H.J., 2009. Myeloid malignancies and the marrow microenvironment: some recent studies in patients with MDS. Curr. Cancer Ther. Rev. 5 (4), 310–314.

Matsushima, K., Baldwin, E.T., Mukaida, N., 1992. Interleukin-8 and MCAF: novel leukocyte recruitment and activating cytokines. Chem. Immunol. 51, 236–265.

Maxwell, P.J., Gallagher, R., Seaton, A., Wilson, C., Scullin, P., Pettigrew, J., Stratford, I.J., Williams, K.J., Johnston, P.G., Waugh, D.J., 2007. HIF-1 and NF-kappaB-mediated upregulation of CXCR1 and CXCR2 expression promotes cell survival in hypoxic prostate cancer cells. Oncogene 26 (52), 7333–7345.

McCarron, S.L., Edwards, S., Evans, P.R., Gibbs, R., Dearnaley, D.P., Dowe, A., Southgate, C., Easton, D.F., Eeles, R.A., Howell, W.M., 2002. Influence of cytokine gene polymorphisms on the development of prostate cancer. Cancer Res. 62 (12), 3369–3372.

Merritt, W.M., Lin, Y.G., Spannuth, W.A., Fletcher, M.S., Kamat, A.A., Han, L.Y., Landen, C.N., Jennings, N., De Geest, K., Langley, R.R., Villares, G., Sanguino, A., Lutgendorf, S.K., Lopez-Berestein, G., Bar-Eli, M.M., Sood, A.K., 2008. Effect of interleukin-8 gene silencing with liposome-encapsulated small interfering RNA on ovarian cancer cell growth. J. Natl. Cancer Inst. 100 (5), 359–372.

Mertens, L.S., Neuzillet, Y., Horenblas, S., van Rhijn, B.W., 2013. Biomarkers for assessing therapeutic response in bladder cancer. Arch. Esp. Urol. 66 (5), 495–504.

Mian, B.M., Dinney, C.P., Bermejo, C.E., Sweeney, P., Tellez, C., Yang, X.D., Gudas, J.M., McConkey, D.J., Bar-Eli, M., 2003. Fully human anti-interleukin 8 antibody inhibits tumor growth in orthotopic bladder cancer xenografts via down-regulation of matrix metalloproteases and nuclear factor-kappaB. Clin. Cancer Res. 9 (8), 3167–3175.

Miyamoto, M., Shimizu, Y., Okada, K., Kashii, Y., Higuchi, K., Watanabe, A., 1998. Effect of interleukin-8 on production of tumor-associated substances and autocrine growth of human liver and pancreatic cancer cells. Cancer Immunol. Immunother. 47 (1), 47–57.

Mukaida, N., 2003. Pathophysiological roles of interleukin-8/CXCL8 in pulmonary diseases. Am. J. Physiol. Lung Cell. Mol. Physiol. 284 (4), L566–L577.

Murphy, C., McGurk, M., Pettigrew, J., Santinelli, A., Mazzucchelli, R., Johnston, P.G., Montironi, R., Waugh, D.J.J., 2005. Nonapical and cytoplasmic expression of interleukin-8, CXCR1, and CXCR2 correlates with cell proliferation and microvessel density in prostate cancer. Clin. Cancer Res. 11 (11), 4117–4127.

Murphy, P.M., 1994. The molecular biology of leukocyte chemoattractant receptors. Annu. Rev. Immunol. 12, 593–633.

Nakajima, N., Ito, Y., Yokoyama, K., Uno, A., Kinukawa, N., Nemoto, N., Moriyama, M., 2009. The expression of murine double minute 2 (MDM2) on *Helicobacter pylori*-infected intestinal metaplasia and gastric cancer. J. Clin. Biochem. Nutr. 44 (2), 196–202.

Nakamichi, Y., Udagawa, N., Takahashi, N., 2013. IL-34 and CSF-1: similarities and differences. J. Bone Miner. Metab. 31 (5), 486–495.

Netea, M.G., Azam, T., Ferwerda, G., Girardin, S.E., Walsh, M., Park, J.S., Abraham, E., Kim, J.M., Yoon, D.Y., Dinarello, C.A., Kim, S.H., 2005. IL-32 synergizes with nucleotide oligomerization domain (NOD) 1 and NOD2 ligands for IL-1beta and IL-6 production through a caspase 1-dependent mechanism. Proc. Natl. Acad. Sci. U.S.A. 102 (45), 16309–16314.

Ning, Y., Labonte, M.J., Zhang, W., Bohanes, P.O., Gerger, A., Yang, D., Benhaim, L., Paez, D., Rosenberg, D.O., Nagulapalli Venkata, K.C., Louie, S.G., Petasis, N.A., Ladner, R.D., Lenz, H.J., 2012. The CXCR2 antagonist, SCH-527123, shows antitumor activity and sensitizes cells to oxaliplatin in preclinical colon cancer models. Mol. Cancer Ther. 11 (6), 1353–1364.

Ning, Y., Manegold, P.C., Hong, Y.K., Zhang, W., Pohl, A., Lurje, G., Winder, T., Yang, D., LaBonte, M.J., Wilson, P.M., Ladner, R.D., Lenz, H.J., 2011. Interleukin-8 is associated with proliferation, migration, angiogenesis and chemosensitivity in vitro and in vivo in colon cancer cell line models. Int. J. Cancer 128 (9), 2038–2049.

Nishida, A., Andoh, A., Inatomi, O., Fujiyama, Y., 2009. Interleukin-32 expression in the pancreas. J. Biol. Chem. 284 (26), 17868–17876.

Nold-Petry, C.A., Rudloff, I., Baumer, Y., Ruvo, M., Marasco, D., Botti, P., Farkas, L., Cho, S.X., Zepp, J.A., Azam, T., Dinkel, H., Palmer, B.E., Boisvert, W.A., Cool, C.D., Taraseviciene-Stewart, L., Heinhuis, B., Joosten, L.A., Dinarello, C.A., Voelkel, N.F., Nold, M.F., 2014. IL-32 promotes angiogenesis. J. Immunol. 192 (2), 589–602.

Oh, J.H., Cho, M.C., Kim, J.H., Lee, S.Y., Kim, H.J., Park, E.S., Ban, J.O., Kang, J.W., Lee, D.H., Shim, J.H., Han, S.B., Moon, D.C., Park, Y.H., Yu, D.Y., Kim, J.M., Kim, S.H., Yoon, D.Y., Hong, J.T., 2011. IL-32γ inhibits cancer cell growth through inactivation of NF-κB and STAT3 signals. Oncogene 30 (30), 3345–3359.

Ohyauchi, M., Imatani, A., Yonechi, M., Asano, N., Miura, A., Iijima, K., Koike, T., Sekine, H., Ohara, S., Shimosegawa, T., 2005. The polymorphism interleukin 8 -251 A/T influences the susceptibility of Helicobacter pylori related gastric diseases in the Japanese population. Gut 54 (3), 330–335.

Palena, C., Hamilton, D.H., Fernando, R.I., 2012. Influence of IL-8 on the epithelial–mesenchymal transition and the tumor microenvironment. Future Oncol. 8 (6), 713–722.

Park, E.S., Yoo, J.M., Yoo, H.S., Yoon, D.Y., Yun, Y.P., Hong, J., December 19, 2012. IL-32γ enhances TNF-α-induced cell death in colon cancer. Mol. Carcinog. (Epub ahead of print).

Park, J.S., Choi, S.Y., Lee, J.H., Lee, M., Nam, E.S., Jeong, A.L., Lee, S., Han, S., Lee, M.S., Lim, J.S., Yoon do, Y., Kwon, Y., Yang, Y., 2013. Interleukin-32β stimulates migration of MDA-MB-231 and MCF-7cells via the VEGF-STAT3 signaling pathway. Cell Oncol. (Dordr) 36 (6), 493–503.

Peng, X., Zhou, C., Wei, D., Luo, Z., Zhang, C., 2009. Characteristics of a novel monoclonal antibody against interleukin-14alpha. Hybridoma (Larchmt) 28 (4), 235–239.

Perry, M.M., Williams, A.E., Tsitsiou, E., Larner-Svensson, H.M., Lindsay, M.A., 2009. Divergent intracellular pathways regulate interleukin-1beta-induced miR-146a and miR-146b expression and chemokine release in human alveolar epithelial cells. FEBS Lett. 583 (20), 3349–3355.

Pikarsky, E., Porat, R.M., Stein, I., Abramovitch, R., Amit, S., Kasem, S., Gutkovich-Pyest, E., Urieli-Shoval, S., Galun, E., Ben-Neriah, Y., 2004. NF-kappaB functions as a tumour promoter in inflammation-associated cancer. Nature 431 (7007), 461–466.

Plantinga, T.S., Costantini, I., Heinhuis, B., Huijbers, A., Semango, G., Kusters, B., Netea, M.G., Hermus, A.R., Smit, J.W., Dinarello, C.A., Joosten, L.A., Netea-Maier, R.T., 2013. A promoter polymorphism in human interleukin-32 modulates its expression and influences the risk and the outcome of epithelial cell-derived thyroid carcinoma. Carcinogenesis 34 (7), 1529–1535.

Qi, J.C., Wang, J., Mandadi, S., Tanaka, K., Roufogalis, B.D., Madigan, M.C., Lai, K., Yan, F., Chong, B.H., Stevens, R.L., Krilis, S.A., 2006. Human and mouse mast cells use the tetraspanin CD9 as an alternate interleukin-16 receptor. Blood 107 (1), 135–142.

Qin, X., Peng, Q., Lao, X., Chen, Z., Lu,Y., Lao, X., Mo, C., Sui, J.,Wu, J., Zhai, L.,Yang, S., Li, S., Zhao, J., March, 2013.The association of interleukin-16 gene polymorphisms with IL-16 serum levels and risk of nasopharyngeal carcinoma in a Chinese population. Tumour Biol. 35(3), 1917–1924.

Ren,Y., Poon, R.T., Tsui, H.T., Chen, W.H., Li, Z., Lau, C.,Yu, W.C., Fan, S.T., 2003. Interleukin-8 serum levels in patients with hepatocellular carcinoma: correlations with clinicopathological features and prognosis. Clin. Cancer Res. 9 (16 Pt 1), 5996–6001.

Rial, N.S., Lazennec, G., Prasad, A.R., Krouse, R.S., Lance, P., Gerner, E.W., 2009. Regulation of deoxycholate induction of CXCL8 by the adenomatous polyposis coli gene in colorectal cancer. Int. J. Cancer 124 (10), 2270–2280.

Richmond, J.,Tuzova, M., Cruikshank,W., Center, D., 2014. Regulation of cellular processes by interleukin-16 in homeostasis and cancer. J. Cell. Physiol. 229 (2), 139–147.

Rollins, B.J., 2009. Where the confusion began: cloning the first chemokine receptors. J. Immunol. 183 (5), 2893–2894.

Sakitani, K., Hirata,Y., Hayakawa,Y., Serizawa, T., Nakata, W.,Takahashi, R., Kinoshita, H., Sakamoto, K., Nakagawa, H.,Akanuma, M.,Yoshida, H., Maeda, S., Koike, K., 2012. Role of interleukin-32 in Helicobacter pylori-induced gastric inflammation. Infect. Immun. 80 (11), 3795–3803.

Schadendorf, D., Moller, A., Algermissen, B., Worm, M., Sticherling, M., Czarnetzki, B.M., 1993. IL-8 produced by human malignant melanoma cells in vitro is an essential autocrine growth factor. J. Immunol. 151 (5), 2667–2675.

Schapher, M., Wendler, O., Gröschl, M., 2011. Salivary cytokines in cell proliferation and cancer. Clin. Chim. Acta 412 (19–20), 1740–1748.

Schauer, I.G., Ressler, S.J., Rowley, D.R., 2009. Keratinocyte-derived chemokine induces prostate epithelial hyperplasia and reactive stroma in a novel transgenic mouse model. Prostate 69 (4), 373–384.

Schauer, I.G., Ressler, S.J.,Tuxhorn, J.A., Dang,T.D., Rowley, D.R., 2008. Elevated epithelial expression of interleukin-8 correlates with myofibroblast reactive stroma in benign prostatic hyperplasia. Urology 72 (1), 205–213.

Schauer, I.G., Rowley, D.R., 2011.The functional role of reactive stroma in benign prostatic hyperplasia. Differentiation 82 (4–5), 200–210.

Schenk, M., Krutzik, S.R., Sieling, P.A., Lee, D.J.,Teles, R.M., Ochoa, M.T., Komisopoulou, E., Sarno, E.N., Rea,T.H., Graeber,T.G., Kim, S., Cheng, G.,Modlin, R.L., 2012. NOD2 triggers an interleukin-32-dependent human dendritic cell program in leprosy. Nat. Med. 18 (4), 555–563.

Seo, E.H., Kang, J., Kim, K.H., Cho, M.C., Lee, S., Kim, H.J., Kim, J.H., Kim, E.J., Park, D.K., Kim, S.H., Choi,Y.K., Kim, J.M., Hong, J.T.,Yoon, D.Y., 2008. Detection of expressed IL-32 in human stomach cancer using ELISA and immunostaining. J. Microbiol. Biotechnol. 18 (9), 1606–1612.

Shen, L., Zhang, C.,Wang,T., Brooks, S., Ford, R.J., Lin-Lee,Y.C., Kasianowicz, A., Kumar, V., Martin, L., Liang, P., Cowell, J.,Ambrus Jr., J.L., 2006. Development of autoimmunity in IL-14alpha-transgenic mice. J. Immunol. 177 (8), 5676–5686.

Shi, Q., Xiong, Q., Le, X., Xie, K., 2001. Regulation of interleukin-8 expression by tumor-associated stress factors. J. Interf. Cytok. Res. 21 (8), 553–566.

Siddiqui, R.A., Akard, L.P., Garcia, J.G., Cui,Y., English, D., 1999. Chemotactic migration triggers IL-8 generation in neutrophilic leukocytes. J. Immunol. 162 (2), 1077–1083.

Singh, B., Berry, J.A.,Vincent, L.E., Lucci,A., 2006. Involvement of IL-8 in COX-2-mediated bone metastases from breast cancer. J. Surg. Res. 134 (1), 44–51.

Singh, J.K., Simões, B.M., Howell, S.J., Farnie, G., Clarke, R.B., 2013. Recent advances reveal IL-8 signaling as a potential key to targeting breast cancer stem cells. Breast Cancer Res. 15 (4), 210.

Singh, R.K., Gutman, M., Radinsky, R., Bucana, C.D., Fidler, I.J., 1994. Expression of interleukin 8 correlates with the metastatic potential of human melanoma cells in nude mice.
Cancer Res. 54 (12), 3242–3247.

Singh, R.K., Lokeshwar, B.L., 2009. Depletion of intrinsic expression of Interleukin-8 in
prostate cancer cells causes cell cycle arrest, spontaneous apoptosis and increases the
efficacy of chemotherapeutic drugs. Mol. Cancer 8, 57.

Singh, S., Sadanandam, A., Varney, M.L., Nannuru, K.C., Singh, R.K., 2010. Small interfering
RNA-mediated CXCR1 or CXCR2 knock-down inhibits melanoma tumor growth
and invasion. Int. J. Cancer 126 (2), 328–336.

Singh, S., Varney, M., Singh, R.K., 2009. Host CXCR2-dependent regulation of melanoma
growth, angiogenesis, and experimental lung metastasis. Cancer Res. 69 (2), 411–415.

Snoussi, K., Mahfoudh, W., Bouaouina, N., Ahmed, S.B., Helal, A.N., Chouchane, L., 2006.
Genetic variation in IL-8 associated with increased risk and poor prognosis of breast
carcinoma. Hum. Immunol. 67 (1–2), 13–21.

Song, J.H., Kim, S.G., Jung, S.A., Lee, M.K., Jung, H.C., Song, I.S., 2010. The interleukin-8-251
AA genotype is associated with angiogenesis in gastric carcinogenesis in *Helicobacter
pylori*-infected Koreans. Cytokine 51 (2), 158–165.

Sorrentino, C., Di Carlo, E., 2009. Expression of IL-32 in human lung cancer is related to
the histotype and metastatic phenotype. Am. J. Respir. Crit. Care Med. 180 (8),
769–779.

Sparmann, A., Bar-Sagi, D., 2004. Ras-induced interleukin-8 expression plays a critical role
in tumor growth and angiogenesis. Cancer Cell. 6 (5), 447–458.

Speciale, A., Canali, R., Chirafisi, J., Saija, A., Virgili, F., Cimino, F., 2010. Cyanidin-3-O-
glucoside protection against TNF-α-induced endothelial dysfunction: involvement of
nuclear factor-κB signaling. J. Agric. Food Chem. 58 (22), 12048–12054.

Strieter, R.M., Kunkel, S.L., Showell, H.J., Remick, D.G., Phan, S.H., Ward, P.A., Marks,
R.M., 1989. Endothelial cell gene expression of a neutrophil chemotactic factor by
TNF-α, LPS, and IL-1β. Science 243 (4897), 1467–1469.

Taguchi, A., Ohmiya, N., Shirai, K., Mabuchi, N., Itoh, A., Hirooka, Y., Niwa, Y., Goto, H.,
2005. Interleukin-8 promoter polymorphism increases the risk of atrophic gastritis
and gastric cancer in Japan. Cancer Epidemiol. Biomarkers Prev. 14 (11 Pt 1),
2487–2493.

Tang, B., Xiao, B., Liu, Z., Li, N., Zhu, E.D., Li, B.S., Xie, Q.H., Zhuang, Y., Zou, Q.M.,
Mao, X.H., 2010. Identification of MyD88 as a novel target of miR-155, involved in
negative regulation of *Helicobacter pylori*-induced inflammation. FEBS Lett. 584 (8),
1481–1486.

Tarnawski, A., Pai, R., Chiou, S.K., Chai, J., Chu, E.C., 2005. Rebamipide inhibits gastric
cancer growth by targeting survivin and Aurora-B. Biochem. Biophys. Res. Commun.
334 (1), 207–212.

Tazzyman, S., Barry, S.T., Ashton, S., Wood, P., Blakey, D., Lewis, C.E., Murdoch, C., 2011. Inhibition of neutrophil infiltration into A549 lung tumors *in vitro* and *in vivo* using a CXCR2-
specific antagonist is associated with reduced tumor growth. Int. J. Cancer 129 (4), 847–858.

Terzić, J., Grivennikov, S., Karin, E., Karin, M., 2010. Inflammation and colon cancer. Gastroenterology 138 (6), 2101. e5–2114.e5.

Todorović-Raković, N., Milovanović, J., 2013. Interleukin-8 in breast cancer progression. J.
Interferon. Cytokine Res. 33 (10), 563–570.

Ueda, T., Shimada, E., Urakawa, T., 1994. Serum levels of cytokines in patients with colorectal cancer: possible involvement of interleukin-6 and interleukin-8 in hematogenous
metastasis. J. Gastroenterol. 29 (4), 423–429.

Urquidi, V., Chang, M., Dai, Y., Kim, J., Wolfson, E.D., Goodison, S., Rosser, C.J., 2012. IL-8
as a urinary biomarker for the detection of bladder cancer. BMC Urol. 12, 12.

Vandercappellen, J., van Damme, J., Struyf, S., 2008. The role of CXC chemokines and their
receptors in cancer. Cancer Lett. 267 (2), 226–244.

Veltri, R.W., Miller, M.C., Zhao, G., Ng, A., Marley, G.M., Wright Jr., G.L., Vessella, R.L., Ralph, D., 1999. Interleukin-8 serum levels in patients with benign prostatic hyperplasia and prostate cancer. Urology 53 (1), 139–147.

Wang, J.M., Taraboletti, G., Matsushima, K., van Damme, J., Mantovani, A., 1990. Induction of haptotactic migration of melanoma cells by neutrophil activating protein/ interleukin-8. Biochem. Biophys. Res. Commun. 169 (1), 165–170.

Wang, N., Zhou, R., Wang, C., Guo, X., Chen, Z., Yang, S., Li, Y., 2012. -251 T/A polymorphism of the interleukin-8 gene and cancer risk: a HuGE review and meta-analysis based on 42 case-control studies. Mol. Biol. Rep. 39 (3), 2831–2841.

Wang, Q., Huber, N., Noel, G., Haar, L., Shan, Y., Pritts, T.A., Ogle, C.K., 2012. NF-κβ inhibition is ineffective in blocking cytokine-induced IL-8 production but P38 and STAT1 inhibitors are effective. Inflamm. Res. 61 (9), 977–985.

Wang, Y., Szretter, K.J., Vermi, W., Gilfillan, S., Rossini, C., Cella, M., Barrow, A.D., Diamond, M.S., Colonna, M., 2012. IL-34 is a tissue-restricted ligand of CSF1R required for the development of Langerhans cells and microglia. Nat. Immunol. 13 (8), 753–760.

Wang, Y.C., Huang, K.M., 2013. In vitro anti-inflammatory effect of apigenin in the *Helicobacter pylori*-infected gastric adenocarcinoma cells. Food Chem. Toxicol. 53, 376–383.

Waugh, D.J.J., Wilson, C., 2008. The interleukin-8 pathway in cancer. Clin. Cancer Res. 14, 6735–6741.

Wei, S., Nandi, S., Chitu, V., Yeung, Y.G., Yu, W., Huang, M., Williams, L.T., Lin, H., Stanley, E.R., 2010. Functional overlap but differential expression of CSF-1 and IL-34 in their CSF-1 receptor-mediated regulation of myeloid cells. J. Leukoc. Biol. 88 (3), 495–505.

Wilson, A.J., Byron, K., Gibson, P.R., 1999. Interleukin-8 stimulates the migration of human colonic epithelial cells *in vitro*. Clin. Sci. (London) 97 (3), 385–390.

Wilson, C., Maxwell, P.J., Longley, D.B., Wilson, R.H., Johnston, P.G., Waugh, D.J.J., 2012. Constitutive and treatment-induced CXCL8-signalling selectively modulates the efficacy of anti-metabolite therapeutics in metastatic prostate cancer. PLoS One 7 (5), e36545.

Wilson, C., Wilson, T., Johnston, P.G., Longley, D.B., Waugh, D.J., 2008. Interleukin-8 signaling attenuates TRAIL- and chemotherapy-induced apoptosis through transcriptional regulation of c-FLIP in prostate cancer cells. Mol. Cancer Ther. 7 (9), 2649–2661.

Xie, K., 2001. Interleukin-8 and human cancer biology. Cytokine Growth Factor Rev. 12 (4), 375–391.

Xu, L., Fidler, I.J., 2000. Interleukin 8: an autocrine growth factor for human ovarian cancer. Oncol. Res. 12 (2), 97–106.

Xue, H., Liu, J., Lin, B., Wang, Z., Sun, J., Huang, G., 2012. A meta-analysis of interleukin-8 -251 promoter polymorphism associated with gastric cancer risk. PLoS One 7 (1), e28083.

Yamada, S., Kato, S., Matsuhisa, T., Makonkawkeyoon, L., Yoshida, M., Chakrabandhu, T., Lertprasertsuk, N., Suttharat, P., Chakrabandhu, B., Nishiumi, S., Chongraksut, W., Azuma, T., 2013. Predominant mucosal IL-8 mRNA expression in non-cagA Thais is risk for gastric cancer. World J. Gastroenterol. 19 (19), 2941–2949.

Yao, C., Lin, Y., Chua, M.S., Ye, C.S., Bi, J., Li, W., Zhu, Y.F., Wang, S.M., 2007. Interleukin-8 modulates growth and invasiveness of estrogen receptor-negative breast cancer cells. Int. J. Cancer 121 (9), 1949–1957.

Yellapa, A., Bahr, J.M., Bitterman, P., Abramowicz, J.S., Edassery, S.L., Penumatsa, K., Basu, S., Rotmensch, J., Barua, A., 2012. Association of interleukin 16 with the development of ovarian tumor and tumor-associated neoangiogenesis in laying hen model of spontaneous ovarian cancer. Int. J. Gynecol. Cancer 22 (2), 199–207.

Yellapa, A., Bitterman, P., Sharma, S., Guirguis, A.S., Bahr, J.M., Basu, S., Abramowicz, J.S., Barua, A., March, 2013. Interleukin 16 (IL-16) expression changes in association with ovarian malignant transformation. Am. J. Obstet. Gynecol. 210 (3), 272. e1-10.

Yousif, N.G., Al-Amran, F.G., Hadi, N., Lee, J., Adrienne, J., 2013. Expression of IL-32 modulates NF-κB and p38 MAP kinase pathways in human esophageal cancer. Cytokine 61 (1), 223–227.

Yu, Y., Zeng, H., Lyons, S., Carlson, A., Merlin, D., Neish, A.S., Gewirtz, A.T., 2003. TLR5-mediated activation of p38 MAPK regulates epithelial IL-8 expression via posttranscriptional mechanism. Am. J. Physiol. Gastr. L. 285 (2), G282–G290.

Yuan, A., Chen, J.J., Yao, P.L., Yang, P.C., 2005. The role of interleukin-8 in cancer cells and microenvironment interaction. Front Biosci. 10, 853–865.

Yuan, A., Yang, P.C., Yu, C.J., Chen, W.J., Lin, F.Y., Kuo, S.H., Luh, K.T., 2000. Interleukin-8 messenger ribonucleic acid expression correlates with tumor progression, tumor angiogenesis, patient survival, and timing of relapse in non-small-cell lung cancer. Am. J. Res. Crit. Care 162 (5), 1957–1963.

Yun, H.M., Oh, J.H., Shim, J.H., Ban, J.O., Park, K.R., Kim, J.H., Lee, D.H., Kang, J.W., Park, Y.H., Yu, D., Kim, Y., Han, S.B., Yoon, D.Y., Hong, J.T., 2013. Antitumor activity of IL-32β through the activation of lymphocytes, and the inactivation of NF-κB and STAT3 signals. Cell Death Dis. 4, e640.

Yuzhalin, A., 2011. The role of interleukin DNA polymorphisms in gastric cancer. Hum. Immunol. 72 (11), 1128–1136.

Yuzhalin, A.E., Kutikhin, A.G., 2012. Interleukin-12: clinical usage and molecular markers of cancer susceptibility. Growth Factors 30 (3), 176–191.

Zeilhofer, H.U., Schorr, W., 2000. Role of interleukin-8 in neutrophil signaling. Curr. Opin. Hematol. 7 (3), 178–182.

Zeng, Q., Li, S., Zhou, Y., Ou, W., Cai, X., Zhang, L., Huang, W., Huang, L., Wang, Q., 2014. Interleukin-32 contributes to invasion and metastasis of primary lung adenocarcinoma via NF-kappaB induced matrix metalloproteinases 2 and 9 expression. Cytokine 65 (1), 24–32.

Zhang, T., Wang, H., 2013. Variants of interleukin-16 associated with gastric cancer risk. Asian Pac. J. Cancer Prev. 14 (9), 5269–5273.

Zhang, Y., Wang, L., Zhang, M., Jin, M., Bai, C., Wang, X., 2012. Potential mechanism of interleukin-8 production from lung cancer cells: an involvement of EGF-EGFR-PI3K-Akt-Erk pathway. J. Cell. Physiol. 227 (1), 35–43.

Zhao, Y., Tao, L., Wang, B., Nie, P., Tang, Y., Zhu, M., March, 2013. Interleukin-16 Gene Polymorphisms rs4778889, rs4072111, rs11556218, and Cancer Risk in Asian Populations: A Meta-Analysis. Genet. Test. Mol. Biomarkers 18 (3), 174–182.

Zhu, J., Qin, C., Yan, F., Wang, M., Ding, Q., Zhang, Z., Yin, C., 2010. IL-16 polymorphism and risk of renal cell carcinoma: association in a Chinese population. Int. J. Urol. 17 (8), 700–707.

Zhu, Y.M., Webster, S.J., Flower, D., Woll, P.J., 2004. Interleukin-8/CXCL8 is a growth factor for human lung cancer cells. Br. J. Cancer 91 (11), 1970–1976.

Zigler, M., Villares, G.J., Lev, D.C., Melnikova, V.O., Bar-Eli, M., 2008. Tumor immunotherapy in melanoma: strategies for overcoming mechanisms of resistance and escape. Am. J. Clin. Dermatol. 9 (5), 307–311.

CHAPTER 10

Concluding Remarks

Cancer is a dreadful disease and it kills millions of individuals throughout the world a year (Jemal et al., 2011; Siegel et al., 2012). The incidence rate in countries with economies in transition and developing countries is especially high due to very limited medical infrastructure as well as a lack of screening, early diagnosis, and advanced treatment options (El-Basmy et al., 2012; Kutikhin et al., 2012; Zhivotovskiy et al., 2012; Perez-Santos and Anaya-Ruiz, 2013; Moore, 2013; Pandey and Chandravati, 2013).

The main objective of this book is to illuminate the state of the art in the field of interleukins (ILs) and tumor biology. This monograph addresses a number of issues. First, we intended to overview all known ILs, and characterize them and describe their role in biological processes within the body. Undoubtedly, many researchers would agree that it is not convenient to seek out information about a particular molecule among hundreds of published scientific articles. Second, the central question to be examined in this monograph was to summarize, review, and discuss the impact of all known ILs on cancer. In the last 15 years, a growing interest has been devoted to this broad topic. The search query for the combination of words "interleukin" and "cancer" in the PubMed database has >47,000 available results. Such an abundance of information can be confusing, so we have tried to present as briefly and as clearly as possible all available up-to-date information on this issue to outline the state of the art in the field. Finally, our goal was to create in the mind of the reader an understanding of ILs as a single harmoniously functioning machine that maintains the viability of the entire immune system. Cancer is an extremely complicated multistep process; nevertheless, the anticancer immune response coordinated by ILs and other cytokines is effective in many cases.

More than 38 ILs have been identified to date; however, only a few of them can be considered exclusively as anticancer agents. Among these are IL-1 receptor (IL-1R), IL-2, IL-12, and IL-27. IL-1R antagonist constrains the destructive influence of IL-1β on the body through three main mechanisms: (1) blockade of IL-1 signaling, (2) inhibition of metastasis formation due to the reduction of adherence between tumor and endothelial cells, and (3) suppression of angiogenesis in tumors. In the future, it is very likely that great efforts will be focused on the study of the clinical use of IL-1Ra for

Interleukins in Cancer Biology
http://dx.doi.org/10.1016/B978-0-12-801121-8.00010-5

IL-1β blockade (Dinarello, 2010). IL-2 possesses profound antitumor activities and has been extensively used as an anticancer drug for the treatment of kidney cancers and of some other malignancies (Antony and Dudek, 2010). Additionally, this cytokine is being administered for the treatment of systemic autoimmune diseases, chronic viral infections, and as adjuvants for vaccines. We suggest that further studies on IL-2 should examine the clinical effectiveness of this cytokine in combination with other promising anticancer ILs. Despite the fact that IL-12 has shown profound anticancer properties, such as upregulation of interferon-γ, inhibition of angiogenesis and various immunostimulatory effects, IL-12-based immunotherapy failed to demonstrate significant improvements in the course of disease in patients with different cancers. Nevertheless, this cytokine showed promising results during gene therapy (Yuzhalin and Kutikhin, 2012). IL-27 demonstrated a profound anticancer response across multiple studies; however, this cytokine may cause severe immunosuppression that can contribute to cancer development (Murugaiyan and Saha, 2013). Thus, further research should be performed to compensate the side effects caused by this cytokine. Possibly, the combination of IL-27 with other cytokines could help in achieving this goal.

One the other hand, some of the ILs, such as IL-1β, IL-3, IL-6, IL-8, IL-17, and IL-19 are obviously procarcinogenic. IL-1β contributes to the development and progression of malignant tumors through enhanced angiogenesis, increased proinflammatory and pyrogenic activity, and inducible nitric oxide synthase (iNOS)-dependent stimulation of NO generation. Further research devoted to this cytokine should definitely be associated with IL-1Ra, which deactivates IL-1β, and thereby neutralizes its tumorigenic properties (Dinarello, 2010). IL-3 is a crucial factor that controls the regulation of proliferation, apoptosis inhibition, and survival of hematopoietic cells (Broughton et al., 2012). Numerous studies demonstrated that this cytokine exacerbated hematopoetic cancers; therefore, further research should be focused specifically on this cancer type. It is of interest that the IL-3 receptor is currently being tested as an aim for targeted therapy, and some promising results have been obtained so far (Frankel et al., 2008). Multiple investigations showed that IL-6 plays a great role in the development and progression and malignant tumors through the promotion of tumor proliferation, angiogenesis, proapoptotic, and prometastatic activities. Furthermore, numerous studies identified IL-6 as a marker of poor prognosis in patients with various cancers. In addition, IL-6 modulates the resistance to different chemotherapy drugs. Inhibitors of IL-6 signaling pathway have long been examined in patients with malignant tumors (reviewed by Ataie-Kachoie et al., 2013).

IL-8 has a considerable influence on tumorigenesis through the promotion of survival, epithelial–mesenchymal transition, and migration of cancer cells. It is suggested that the use of IL-8 inhibitors is potentially a new way to treat cancer and that the investigation of this problem is being continued (reviewed by Waugh and Wilson, 2008). Despite the fact that IL-17 is considered to have both protumorigenic and antitumorigenic properties, the majority of published reports reveal the tumor-promoting impacts of this cytokine, whereas only occasional studies argue the opposite (Chang and Dong, 2011). In particular IL-17 was found to upregulate genes responsible for angiogenesis, such as vascular endothelial growth factor (VEGF), angiopoietin-2, CXCL1, CXCL5, and CXCL6. In addition, this cytokine plays a role in the prevention of apoptosis and breakdown of extracellular matrix, which can promote uncontrollable cell division and metastasis formation, respectively. The only study devoted to IL-19 found that this cytokine promotes cancer development and progression through matrix metalloproteinase (MMP)- and fibronectin-modulated formation of metastasis, transforming growth factor beta (TGF)-β-driven increase in cell proliferation, and CXCR 4-dependent activation of angiogenesis (Hsing et al., 2008). However, these findings are still to be replicated in the future.

Interestingly, some ILs, such as IL-5, IL-10, IL-18, IL-23, and IL-33 have demonstrated both procarcinogenic and anticarcinogenic activities, and therefore, their impact on cancer is ambiguous. Of these "double-edged sword" cytokines, IL-10 is one of the most attractive candidates for cancer therapy. This cytokine is able to provide an efficient anticancer immune response through the suppression of cyclooxygenase-2/prostaglandin E2 and activation of NK cells. On the other hand, however, IL-10-mediated immunosuppression may significantly weaken the immunity, which may lead to the development of tumors (Sato et al., 2011). More interestingly, the crosstalk between IL-10 and certain modulators such as programed cell death ligands, TGF-β, VEGF, iNOS, and E-selectin seem to have a decisive role in what type of activity, protumorigenic or antitumorigenic, the cytokine will ultimately exert. Thus, the question of interactions between IL-10 and these molecules should be addressed to further studies.

It is also necessary to mention that many ILs are still poorly investigated in the context of cancer research. Among these cytokines are IL-25, IL-26, IL-28A, IL-28B, IL-29, IL-30, IL-31, IL-35, IL-36, IL-37, and IL-38. Some of them, such as IL-30 and IL-31, have been shown to elicit a considerable effect on tumor biology in a few studies; therefore, more in-depth investigations are required in order to identify whether or not they are involved in tumorigenesis.

It is clear that ILs can either contribute to tumor development and exacerbate the disease, or activate the immune response properly, so that cancer cells are attacked and eliminated by leukocytes. Based on the analysis of studies described in the book, several common ways of IL-mediated tumor development can be pointed out in brief.

One of the most obvious mechanisms of IL-driven carcinogenesis includes a chronic inflammation and a proinflammatory response. The link between proinflammatory environment and elevated cancer risk has long been known. Originally intended to eliminate pathogenic microorganisms within the body, inflammation heavily damages normal cells, thereby increasing the risk of getting mutations associated with cancer. Proinflammatory ILs such as IL-1α, IL-6, IL-8, IL-18, and IL-20 possesses strong pyrogenic activities, which enables them to promote systemic inflammation and subsequently leads to cancer occurrence.

Certain ILs are major regulators of cell cycle control, which enables them to directly induce the proliferation of target cells. In turn, increased proliferation can serve as a stimulating factor to malignant transformation of cells. Furthermore, these ILs can also promote cancer progression by elevating the rate of proliferation in existing tumors. For example, recent investigations suggest that IL-16 plays a crucial role in the regulation of lymphocytic cancer cell proliferation (reviewed by Richmond et al., 2014). Another case in point is IL-3, which was repeatedly shown to stimulate the proliferation of various normal and cell lineages through the activation of mitogenic signals, involving Raf, MEK1, extracellular-signal-regulated kinase 1 (ERK1), and ERK2. IL-modulated cancer cell proliferation is usually associated with the activation of cyclins D1 and B, c-Myc, c-Jun, c-Foc, p21, and cdc2.

In addition to the stimulation of cell proliferation, ILs often promote the survival of cancer cells, mostly due to the activation of several antiapoptotic proteins, including Bcl family members (Bcl-xL, Bcl-2, and Mcl-1) and survivin. In particular, cancer cell survival is known to be stimulated by IL-3 (Blalock et al., 1999), IL-4 (Vella et al., 2004), IL-6 (Neiva et al., 2014), IL-8 (Maxwell et al., 2007), IL-17 (Numasaki et al., 2003, 2005), IL-21 (Ménoret et al., 2008), IL-26 (You et al., 2013), IL-29 (Maher et al., 2008), and IL-32 (Kang et al., 2012).

Yet another mechanism of the IL-mediated promotion of malignant growth includes the stimulation of tumor neovascularization. Formation of new vessels is critical for cancer development, as growing tumors require more and more oxygen supply. In addition, angiogenesis is essentially required for the formation of metastasis, which underlies the link between certain ILs and cancer progression. It is known that various ILs upregulate the expression of fibroblast growth factor (FGF), VERF, and certain angiopoetins, which are major regulators of angiogenic activity. In particular, the activation of signal transducer and activator of transcription 3, one of the most common triggers of angiogenesis in cancer cells, is under the control of IL-5, IL-6, IL-9, IL-10, IL-11, IL-12, IL-21, IL-22, and IL-27 (reviewed by Siveen et al., 2014).

Finally, various ILs are known to be involved in cell motility and invasiveness, thereby having a considerable effect on metastatic formation. It is known that ILs are able to modulate the remodeling of basement membranes and extracellular matrix through the upregulation of the expression of certain proteolytic enzymes, such as MMPs. The major examples of this are IL-1β, IL-6, IL-8, IL-17, IL-18, IL-19, IL-23, and IL-32. Although IL-13Rα2, IL-20, and IL-30 have demonstrated clear prometastatic activities in a few studies, it is not clear whether or not they act through the MMP pathway or some alternative mechanism.

Throughout the chapters, it is clearly seen that the findings obtained from multiple in vivo and in vitro studies are not always consistent. Furthermore, sometimes, the results are completely opposite, which confuse research workers and disable them to draw any conclusions. The possible reasons for these disparities may be due to errors in study design. The most common mistakes include an inadequate sample size, inappropriate choice of species and their strains, failure to minimize variation within the sample, maintain the purity of experiment, incorrect statistical analysis, or misinterpretation of statistical results. Among these, the inability to minimize variation is one of the most crucial factors. Speaking in general terms, all the variables may be divided into two groups: fixed effects and random effects. The conceptual distinction between them is that the former are more likely to be controlled by the research worker, whereas the latter are beyond the control of the investigator. In animal experiments, fixed effects that may affect the outcome of an experiment may include physical characteristics of an animal house (i.e., temperature, light, noise, availability, and type of bedding or nesting cover, cage design, and size), quality of husbandry (i.e., type of diet, quality of food, and water, number of animals in cage), competence of staff (quality of surgery and other procedures, route of injections, etc.), and characteristics of animals themselves (strain, sex, etc.). Considering random effects, we should take into account factors such as differences in body weight; presence of the infectious agents; variation of the genotype within the outbred stock; and contamination of food, water, blood, or other samples. To minimize the random effects, it is more feasible to prefer isogenic strains to outbred stocks. The latter are phenotypically more diverse due to the fact that they are genetically heterogeneous; therefore, these animals are not likely to exhibit a low level of variability during the study. With regards to clinical studies, the sources of variation may include differences in age, sex, ethnic, racial, and clinicopathological characteristics. Additionally, the prevalence of the pathogen burden (such as *Helicobacter pylori*) relevant to the disease under investigation in the case and control groups may also distort the results. Of course, the major role belongs to factors such as any differences in statistical analysis, stratification, methods of diagnostics of cancer or chronic inflammatory conditions, and methods used in the particular study, as well as chance. Importantly, stratification of the study population by chronic inflammation status as well as infectious agent status must be conducted in further investigations to distinguish the impact of chronic inflammatory conditions from the contribution of other mechanisms to the association between cause (abundance of certain cytokine in cell culture/animal/patient) and effect (features of tumor development, clinical outcome, cancer risk, prognosis, etc.).

It is certainly true that our present understanding of tumor biology is far from complete, as multiple molecular pathways and etiologic factors of this disease remain poorly investigated. A wide variety of cancer types partially explains the fact that the behavior of malignant neoplasms is incredibly complex and unpredictable. At early stages, cancer develops without apparent signs or symptoms, which makes this disease particularly dangerous. However, the study of ILs shows us that proper governance of the capabilities of the human body can lead to effective cancer management.

Undoubtedly, the cutting edge of biomedical research focused on ILs will soon lead us to breakthroughs for therapeutic interventions in the field of cancer and autoimmune diseases. Further research on ILs will provide new and robust data for the understanding of their impact on carcinogenesis and lead to major breakthroughs in cancer treatment.

REFERENCES

Antony, G.K., Dudek, A.Z., 2010. Interleukin 2 in cancer therapy. Curr. Med. Chem. 17 (29), 3297–3302.
Ataie-Kachoie, P., Pourgholami, M.H., Morris, D.L., 2013. Inhibition of the IL-6 signaling pathway: a strategy to combat chronic inflammatory diseases and cancer. Cytokine Growth Factor Rev. 24 (2), 163–173.

Blalock, W.L., Weinstein-Oppenheimer, C., Chang, F., Hoyle, P.E., Wang, X.Y., Algate, P.A., Franklin, R.A., Oberhaus, S.M., Steelman, L.S., McCubrey, J.A., 1999. Signal transduction, cell cycle regulatory, and anti-apoptotic pathways regulated by IL-3 in hematopoietic cells: possible sites for intervention with anti-neoplastic drugs. Leukemia 13 (8), 1109–1166.

Broughton, S.E., Dhagat, U., Hercus, T.R., Nero, T.L., Grimbaldeston, M.A., Bonder, C.S., Lopez, A.F., Parker, M.W., 2012. The GM-CSF/IL-3/IL-5 cytokine receptor family: from ligand recognition to initiation of signaling. Immunol. Rev. 250 (1), 277–302.

Chang, S.H., Dong, C., 2011. Signaling of interleukin-17 family cytokines in immunity and inflammation. Cell. Signalling 23 (7), 1069–1075.

Dinarello, C.A., 2010. Why not treat human cancer with interleukin-1 blockade? Cancer Metastasis Rev. 29 (2), 317–329.

El-Basmy, A., Al-Mohannadi, S., Al-Awadi, A., 2012. Some epidemiological measures of cancer in Kuwait: national cancer registry data from 2000–2009. Asian Pac. J. Cancer Prev. 13 (7), 3113–3118.

Frankel, A., Liu, J.S., Rizzieri, D., Hogge, D., 2008. Phase I clinical study of diphtheria toxin–interleukin 3 fusion protein in patients with acute myeloid leukemia and myelodysplasia. Leuk. Lymphoma 49 (3), 543–553.

Hsing, C.H., Chiu, C.J., Chang, L.Y., Hsu, C.C., Chang, M.S., 2008. IL-19 is involved in the pathogenesis of endotoxic shock. Shock 29 (1), 7–15.

Jemal, A., Bray, F., Center, M.M., Ferlay, J., Ward, E., Forman, D., 2011. Global cancer statistics. Ca–Cancer J. Clin. 61 (2), 69–90.

Kang, Y.H., Park, M.Y., Yoon, D.Y., Han, S.R., Lee, C.I., Ji, N.Y., Myung, P.K., Lee, H.G., Kim, J.W., Yeom, Y.I., Jang, Y.J., Ahn, D.K., Kim, J.W., Song, E.Y., 2012. Dysregulation of overexpressed IL-32α in hepatocellular carcinoma suppresses cell growth and induces apoptosis through inactivation of NF-κB and Bcl-2. Cancer Lett. 318 (2), 226–233.

Kutikhin, A.G., Yuzhalin, A.E., Brailovskiy, V.V., Zhivotovskiy, A.S., Magarill, Y.A., Brusina, E.B., 2012. Analysis of cancer incidence and mortality in the industrial region of South-East Siberia from 1991 through 2010. Asian Pac. J. Cancer Prev. 13 (10), 5189–5193.

Maher, S.G., Sheikh, F., Scarzello, A.J., Romero-Weaver, A.L., Baker, D.P., Donnelly, R.P., Gamero, A.M., 2008. IFNalpha and IFNlambda differ in their antiproliferative effects and duration of JAK/STAT signaling activity. Cancer Biol. Ther. 7 (7), 1109–1115.

Maxwell, P.J., Gallagher, R., Seaton, A., Wilson, C., Scullin, P., Pettigrew, J., Stratford, I.J., Williams, K.J., Johnston, P.G., Waugh, D.J., 2007. HIF-1 and NF-kappaB-mediated upregulation of CXCR1 and CXCR2 expression promotes cell survival in hypoxic prostate cancer cells. Oncogene 26 (52), 7333–7345.

Ménoret, E., Maïga, S., Descamps, G., Pellat-Deceunynck, C., Fraslon, C., Cappellano, M., Moreau, P., Bataille, R., Amiot, M., 2008. IL-21 stimulates human myeloma cell growth through an autocrine IGF-1 loop. J. Immunol. 181 (10), 6837–6842.

Moore, M.A., 2013. Overview of cancer registration research in the Asian Pacific from 2008–2013. Asian Pac. J. Cancer Prev. 14 (8), 4461–4484.

Murugaiyan, G., Saha, B., 2013. IL-27 in tumor immunity and immunotherapy. Trends Mol. Med. 19 (2), 108–116.

Neiva, K.G., Warner, K.A., Campos, M.S., Zhang, Z., Moren, J., Danciu, T.E., Nör, J.E., February 17, 2014. Endothelial cell-derived interleukin-6 regulates tumor growth. BMC Cancer 14 (1), 99. [Epub ahead of print].

Numasaki, M., Fukushi, J., Ono, M., Narula, S.K., Zavodny, P.J., Kudo, T., Robbins, P.D., Tahara, H., Lotze, M.T., 2003. Interleukin-17 promotes angiogenesis and tumor growth. Blood 101 (7), 2620–2627.

Numasaki, M., Watanabe, M., Suzuki, T., Takahashi, H., Nakamura, A., McAllister, F., Hishinuma, T., Goto, J., Lotze, M.T., Kolls, J.K., Sasaki, H., 2005. IL-17 enhances the net angiogenic activity and in vivo growth of human non-small cell lung cancer in SCID mice through promoting CXCR-2-dependent angiogenesis. J. Immunol. 175 (9), 6177–6189.

Pandey, S., Chandravati, 2013. Breast screening in North India: a cost-effective cancer prevention strategy. Asian Pac. J. Cancer Prev. 14 (2), 853–857.

Perez-Santos, J.L., Anaya-Ruiz, M., 2013. Mexican breast cancer research output, 2003–2012. Asian Pac. J. Cancer Prev. 14 (10), 5921–5923.

Richmond, J., Tuzova, M., Cruikshank, W., Center, D., 2014. Regulation of cellular processes by interleukin-16 in homeostasis and cancer. J. Cell. Physiol. 229 (2), 139–147.

Sato, T., Terai, M., Tamura, Y., Alexeev, V., Mastrangelo, M.J., Selvan, S.R., 2011. Interleukin 10 in the tumor microenvironment: a target for anticancer immunotherapy. Immunol. Res. 51 (2–3), 170–182.

Siegel, R., Naishadham, D., Jemal, A., 2012. Cancer statistics, 2012. Ca–Cancer J. Clin. 62 (1), 10–29.

Siveen, K.S., Sikka, S., Surana, R., Dai, X., Zhang, J., Kumar, A.P., Tan, B.K., Sethi, G., Bishayee, A., 2014. Targeting the STAT3 signaling pathway in cancer: role of synthetic and natural inhibitors. Biochim. Biophys. Acta 1845 (2), 136–154.

Vella, V., Mineo, R., Frasca, F., Mazzon, E., Pandini, G., Vigneri, R., Belfiore, A., 2004. Interleukin-4 stimulates papillary thyroid cancer cell survival: implications in patients with thyroid cancer and concomitant Graves' disease. J. Clin. Endocrinol. Metab. 89 (6), 2880–2889.

Waugh, D.J., Wilson, C., 2008. The interleukin-8 pathway in cancer. Clin. Cancer Res. 14 (21), 6735–6741.

You, W., Tang, Q., Zhang, C., Wu, J., Gu, C., Wu, Z., Li, X., 2013. IL-26 promotes the proliferation and survival of human gastric cancer cells by regulating the balance of STAT1 and STAT3 activation. PLoS One 8 (5), e63588.

Yuzhalin, A.E., Kutikhin, A.G., 2012. Interleukin-12: clinical usage and molecular markers of cancer susceptibility. Growth Factors 30 (3), 176–191.

Zhivotovskiy, A.S., Kutikhin, A.G., Azanov, A.Z., Yuzhalin, A.E., Magarill, Y.A., Brusina, E.B., 2012. Colorectal cancer risk factors among the population of South-East Siberia: a case–control study. Asian Pac. J. Cancer Prev. 13 (10), 5183–5188.

Further Reading

Books

Balkwill, F.R., 2000. The Cytokine Network. Oxford UP, Oxford. Print.

Bock, G., Marsh, J., 1987. Tumour Necrosis Factor and Related Cytotoxins. Wiley, Chichester. Print.

Caligiuri, M.A., Lotze, M.T., 2007. Cytokines in the Genesis and Treatment of Cancer. Humana, Totowa, NJ. Print.

Chadwick, D., Goode, J., 2004. Cancer and Inflammation. John Wiley & Sons, Hoboken, NJ. Print.

Festing, M.F., 2011. The Design of Animal Experiments: Reducing the Use of Animals in Research through Better Experimental Design. Royal Soc. of Medicine, London. Print.

Fitzgerald, K.A., 2001. The Cytokine Factsbook. Academic, San Diego. Print.

Forni, G., 1994. Cytokine-induced Tumor Immunogenicity: From Exogenous Molecules to Gene Therapy. Academic, London. Print.

Heppner, G.H., Edward Bittar, E., 1996. Advances in Oncobiology. Jai, Greenwich, CT. Print.

Kutikhin, A.G., Yuzhalin, A.E., Brusina, E.B., 2013. Infectious Agents and Cancer. Springer, Dordrecht. Print.

Litwack, G., 2006. Interleukins. Elsevier/Academic, Amsterdam. Print.

Löwy, I., 1996. Between Bench and Bedside: Science, Healing, and Interleukin-2 in a Cancer Ward. Harvard UP, Cambridge, MA. Print.

O'Neill, L.A.J., Bowie, A., 2001. Interleukin Protocols. Humana, Totowa, NJ. Print.

Oppenheim, J.J., Feldmann, M., Durum, S.K., 2001. Cytokine Reference: A Compendium of Cytokines and Other Mediators of Host Defense. Academic, San Diego. Print.

Parham, P., Janeway, C., 2009. The Immune System. Garland Science, London. Print.

Robins, R.A., Robert, C.R., 2001. Cancer Immunology. Kluwer Academic, Dordrecht. Print.

Thomson, A.W., Lotze, M.T., 2003. The Cytokine Handbook: Vol-1. Academic, London. Print.

Wagstaff, J., 1993. The Role of Interleukin-2 in the Treatment of Cancer Patients. Kluwer Academic, Dordrecht. Print.

Weinberg, R.A., 2014. The Biology of Cancer. Garland Science, Taylor & Francis Group, New York. Print.

General Review Articles

Baeriswyl, V., Christofori, G., 2009. The angiogenic switch in carcinogenesis. Semin. Cancer Biol. 19 (5), 329–337.

Dunn, G.P., Koebel, C.M., Schreiber, R.D., 2006. Interferon's, immunity and cancer immunoediting. Nat. Rev. Immunol. 6 (11), 836–848.

Hanahan, D., Weinberg, R.A., 2011. Hallmarks of cancer: the next generation. Cell 144 (5), 646–674.

Kutikhin, A.G., Yuzhalin, A.E., 2012. C-type lectin receptors and RIG-I-like receptors: new points on the oncogenomics map. Cancer Manage. Res. 4, 39–53.

Kutikhin, A.G., Yuzhalin, A.E., 2012. Inherited variation in pattern recognition receptors and cancer: dangerous liaisons? Cancer Manage. Res. 4, 31–38.

Lauta, V.M., 2003. A review of the cytokine network in multiple myeloma: diagnostic, prognostic, and therapeutic implications. Cancer 97 (10), 440–452.

Lippitz, B.E., 2013. Cytokine patterns in patients with cancer: a systematic review. Lancet Oncol. 14 (6), e218–e228.

Newton, K., Dixit, V.M., 2012. Signaling in innate immunity and inflammation. Cold Spring Harbor Perspect. Biol. 4 (3). pii: a006049.

Nicolini, A., Carpi, A., Rossi, G., 2006. Cytokines in breast cancer. Cytokine Growth Factor Rev. 17 (5), 325–337.

Yoshimoto, T., Morishima, N., Okumura, M., Chiba, Y., Xu, M., Mizuguchi, J., 2009. Interleukins and cancer immunotherapy. Immunotherapy 1 (5), 825–844.

Yuzhalin, A., 2011. The role of interleukin DNA polymorphisms in gastric cancer. Hum. Immunol. 72 (11), 1128–1136.

Yuzhalin, A.E., Kutikhin, A.G., 2012. Integrative systems of genomic risk markers for cancer and other diseases: future of predictive medicine. Cancer Manage. Res. 4, 131–135.

Interleukin-specific Articles

Andorsky, D.J., Timmerman, J.M., 2008. Interleukin-21: biology and application to cancer therapy. Expert Opin. Biol. Ther 8 (9), 1295–1307.

Antony, G.K., Dudek, A.Z., 2010. Interleukin 2 in cancer therapy. Curr. Med. Chem. 17 (29), 3297–3302.

Ara, T., Declerck, Y.A., 2010. Interleukin-6 in bone metastasis and cancer progression. Eur. J. Cancer 46 (7), 1223–1231.

Atanackovic, D., Hildebrandt, Y., Templin, J., Cao, Y., Keller, C., Panse, J., Meyer, S., Reinhard, H., Bartels, K., Lajmi, N., Sezer, O., Zander, A.R., Marx, A.H., Uhlig, R., Zustin, J., Bokemeyer, C., Kröger, N. 2012. Role of interleukin 16 in multiple myeloma. J. Natl. Cancer Inst. 104 (13), 1005–1020.

Bhatia, M., Davenport, V., Cairo, M.S., 2007. The role of interleukin-11 to prevent chemotherapy-induced thrombocytopenia in patients with solid tumors, lymphoma, acute myeloid leukemia and bone marrow failure syndromes. Leuk. Lymphoma 48 (1), 9–15.

Chen, Y.Y., Li, C.F., Yeh, C.H., Chang, M.S., Hsing, C.H., 2013. Interleukin-19 in breast cancer. Clin. Dev. Immunol. 2013, 294–320.

Croxford, A.L., Mair, F., Becher, B., 2012. IL-23: one cytokine in control of autoimmunity. Eur. J. Immunol. 42 (9), 2263–2273.

Dinarello, C.A., 2010. Why not treat human cancer with interleukin-1 blockade? Cancer Metastasis Rev. 29 (2), 317–329.

Grosfeld, J.L., Du, X., Williams, D.A., 1999. Interleukin-11: its biology and prospects for clinical use. JPEN J. Parenter. Enteral Nutr. 23 (5 Suppl.), S67–S69.

Harrison, C., 2013. Cancer: IL-22: linking inflammation and cancer. Nat. Rev. Drug Discovery 12 (7), 504.

Hunter, C.A., Kastelein, R., 2012. Interleukin-27: balancing protective and pathological immunity. Immunity 37 (6), 960–969.

Joshi, B.H., Hogaboam, C., Dover, P., Husain, S.R., Puri, R.K., 2006. Role of interleukin-13 in cancer, pulmonary fibrosis, and other T(H)2-type diseases. Vitam. Horm. 74, 479–504.

Kioi, M., Husain, S.R., Croteau, D., Kunwar, S., Puri, R.K., 2006. Convection-enhanced delivery of interleukin-13 receptor-directed cytotoxin for malignant glioma therapy. Technol. Cancer Res. Treat. 5 (3), 239–250.

Klinke 2nd, D.J., 2010. A multiscale systems perspective on cancer, immunotherapy, and interleukin-12. Mol. Cancer 9, 242.

Knoops, L., Renauld, J.C., 2004. IL-9 and its receptor: from signal transduction to tumorigenesis. Growth Factors 22 (4), 207–215.

Kotyza, J., 2012. Interleukin-8 (CXCL8) in tumor associated non-vascular extracellular fluids: its diagnostic and prognostic values. A review. Int. J. Biol. Markers 27 (3), 169–178.

Kreis, S., Philippidou, D., Margue, C., Behrmann, I., 2008. IL-24: a classic cytokine and/or a potential cure for cancer? J. Cell. Mol. Med. 12 (6A), 2505–2510.

Kutikhin, A.G., Yuzhalin, A.E., Volkov, A.N., Zhivotovskiy, A.S., Brusina, E.B., January 21, 2014. Correlation between genetic polymorphisms within IL-1B and TLR4 genes and cancer risk in a Russian population: a case-control study. Tumour Biol. [Epub ahead of print].

Lee, S.J., Cho, S.C., Lee, E.J., Kim, S., Lee, S.B., Lim, J.H., Choi, Y.H., Kim, W.J., Moon, S.K. 2013. Interleukin-20 promotes migration of bladder cancer cells through extracellular signal-regulated kinase (ERK)-mediated MMP-9 protein expression leading to nuclear factor (NF-κB) activation by inducing the up-regulation of p21(WAF1) protein expression. J. Biol. Chem. 288 (8), 5539–5552.

Lundström, W., Fewkes, N.M., Mackall, C.L., 2012. IL-7 in human health and disease. Semin. Immunol. 24 (3), 218–224.

Mosser, D.M., Zhang, X., 2008. Interleukin-10: new perspectives on an old cytokine. Immunol. Rev. 226, 205–218.

Murugaiyan, G., Saha, B., 2009. Protumor vs antitumor functions of IL-17. J. Immunol. 183 (7), 4169–4175.

Nakashima, H., Husain, S.R., Puri, R.K., 2012. IL-13 receptor-directed cancer vaccines and immunotherapy. Immunotherapy 4 (4), 443–451.

Nowak, E.C., Noelle, R.J., 2010. Interleukin-9 as a T helper type 17 cytokine. Immunology 131 (2), 169–173.

Ochoa, M.C., Mazzolini, G., Hervas-Stubbs, S., de Sanmamed, M.F., Berraondo, P., Melero, I., 2013. Interleukin-15 in gene therapy of cancer. Curr. Gene Ther. 13 (1), 15–30.

Renauld, J.C., Kermouni, A., Vink, A., Louahed, J., Van Snick, J., 1995. Interleukin-9 and its receptor: involvement in mast cell differentiation and T cell oncogenesis. J. Leukocyte Biol. 57 (3), 353–360.

Richmond, J., Tuzova, M., Cruikshank, W., Center, D., Feb, 2013. Regulation of cellular processes by interleukin-16 in homeostasis and cancer. J. Cell. Physiol. 229 (2), 139–147. http://dx.doi.org/10.1002/jcp.24441.

Sato, T., Terai, M., Tamura, Y., Alexeev, V., Mastrangelo, M.J., Selvan, S.R., 2011. Interleukin 10 in the tumor microenvironment: a target for anticancer immunotherapy. Immunol. Res. 51 (2–3), 170–182.

Srivastava, S., Salim, N., Robertson, M.J., 2010. Interleukin-18: biology and role in the immunotherapy of cancer. Curr. Med. Chem. 17 (29), 3353–3357.

Trinchieri, G., 2003. Interleukin-12 and the regulation of innate resistance and adaptive immunity. Nat. Rev. Immunol. 3 (2), 133–146.

Yuzhalin, A.E., Kutikhin, A.G., 2012. Interleukin-12: clinical usage and molecular markers of cancer susceptibility. Growth Factors 30 (3), 176–191.

List of Human Interleukins

Interleukin (IL)	Other/Previous Names	Structure	Molecular Weight (kDa)	Cellular Sources	Receptor	Protein Length (Mature Form)	Main Function
IL-1α	LAF, IL1, IL-1A; IL1F1, IL1-Alpha	Monomer	15	Fibroblasts, monocytes, neutrophils, macrophages, epithelial, dendritic, endothelial cells, NK cells, B cells	IL-1RI, IL-1RII	115	Profound proinflammatory and pyrogenic activities. May also have metabolic and hematopoietic activities
IL-1β	IL1B, IL1-Beta; IL1F2	29	15	Th-2 cells	IL-2RA, IL-2RB, IL-2RG	267	Pro-inflammatory activities. Promotes cell proliferation, differentiation, and apoptosis
IL-2	T cell growth factor (TCGF), IL2	Monomer	15	CD4+ T cells, naive CD8+ T cells, dendritic cells	IL-2R	133	A growth factor for antigen-stimulated T cells and is one of key molecules performing T-cell clonal expansion after antigen recognition A growth factor for cytotoxic T cells at late stages of the immune reaction

IL-3	Multipotential colony-stimulating factor (MCSF), hematopoietic growth factor, P-cell-stimulating factor, mast-cell growth factor (MCGF), IL3	Monomer	32	Activated T cells, mast cells, basophils, eosinophils	IL-3R	152	Generation and maintenance of multipotent hematopoietic stem cells and their differentiation to myeloid progenitor cells
IL-4	B cell growth factor 1 (BCGF-1), BCGF1, B cell stimulatory factor 1 (BSF-1), BSF1, IL4	Monomer	16	Macrophages, dendritic cells, mast cells, NK cells, NKT cells, basophils, eosinophils, T lymphocytes	Type I and type II IL-4R	137	Stimulation of activated B-cell and T-cell proliferation and differentiation
IL-5	T cell-replacing factor (TRF), eosinophil differentiation factor (EDF), IL5	Dimer	15	Eosinophils, basophils, CD4+ Th2 lymphocytes, CD34+ progenitor cells, mast cells, invariant natural killer T cells, Reed Sternberg cells	IL-5R	134	Has a profound impact on differentiation, activation, survival, and proliferation of eosinophils, T cells and B cells

Continued

—Cont'd

Interleukin (IL)	Other/Previous Names	Structure	Molecular Weight (kDa)	Cellular Sources	Receptor	Protein Length (Mature Form)	Main Function
IL-6	B-cell differentiation factor (BCDF), B-cell stimulatory factor 2 (BSF2), hepatocyte growth factor (HGF), HSF, IFNB2, IL6	Monomer	28	T cells, B cells, macrophages, neutrophils, monocytes, keratinocytes, fibroblasts, endothelial cells, epithelial cells, osteoblasts, chondrocytes, adipocytes, and mesangial cells	IL-6R/gp130	184	Pro-inflammatory activities. Involved in the development of chronic inflammation, antigen-specific immune responses, regulation of host defense mechanisms, hematopoiesis, osteoclastogenesis, and skeletal muscle growth
IL-7	IL7	Monomer	25	Stromal cells, keratinocytes, dendritic cells, hepatocytes, neurons, epithelial cells	IL-7R	153	Hematopoietic growth factor, essential for T cell production, maturation and expansion
IL-8	CXCL8, neutrophil chemotactic factor, GCP-1, GCP1, LECT, LUCT, LYNAP, MDNCF, MONAP, NAF, NAP-1, NAP1	Monomer or dimer	8	Leukocytes, fibroblasts, endothelial cells, malignant cancer cells	CXCR1, CXCR2	77 in non-immune cells; 72 in monocytes and macrophages	Leukocyte chemoattractant, increases the proliferation, survival and migration of endothelial cells, and activates immune response at the tumor site

IL-9	p40, mast cell growth-enhancing activity	Monomer	32–39	T lymphocytes, mast cells	IL-9R	127	Promotes T cell growth and Th17 development, affects B cell development and functioning, enhances growth and functioning of mast cells, enhances hematopoiesis, potentiates allergic inflammation in the airway epithelial cells, induce airway mucus production
IL-10	Cytokine synthesis inhibitory factor (CSIF), IL10	Homodimer	20	Monocytes, macrophages, T regulatory cells, Th1 cells, Th2 cells, B cells, DCs, mast cells, eosinophils, and keratinocytes	IL-10R1/IL-10R2	178	Downregulation of all major pro-inflammatory cytokines, such as IL-1, IL-2, IL-6, IL-8, IL-12, IFN-γ and TNF-α in NK cells and macrophages, up regulation of anti-inflammatory cytokines, including IL-1RA and soluble TNF-α receptor, suppression of proliferation and function of T cells and differentiation and activity of DCs, downregulation of MHC class I in DCs and B cells, stimulation of proliferation and cytotoxicity of NK cells

Continued

—Cont'd

Interleukin (IL)	Other/Previous Names	Structure	Molecular Weight (kDa)	Cellular Sources	Receptor	Protein Length (Mature Form)	Main Function
IL–11	Adipogenesis inhibitory factor (AGIF), oprelvekin, IL11	Monomer	23	Lymphocytes, B-cells, macrophages, endothelial cells, hematopoietic cells, chondrocytes, osteoclasts, synoviocytes, trophoblasts and fibroblasts	IL–11R/ gp130	178	Anti-inflammatory and immunomodulatory effects, plays role in bone cell proliferation and differentiation
IL–12	Cytotoxic lymphocyte maturation factor 1 (CLMF1), natural killer cell stimulatory factor 1 (NKSF1), p35, IL12	Heterodimer	35/40	T cells, macrophages, human B-lymphoblastoid and dendritic cells	IL–12R–b1/ IL–12R–b2	219/364	Plays role in differentiation of naive T cells into Th1 cells, anti-angiogenic and pro-apoptotic activity
IL–13	ALRH, BHR1, P600, IL13	Monomer	12.5	Macrophages, dendritic cells, mast cells, NKT, NK cells, basophils, eosinophils, and T lymphocytes	IL–13R	114	Similar to IL–4, mediator of allergic inflammation

IL-14	High molecular weight B cell growth factor, alpha-taxilin (TXLN), IL14	Monomer	53	Follicular dendritic cells, germinal T-cells	IL-14R	468	Enhances B cell proliferation and expands a subpopulation of memory B cells
IL-15	IL15	Monomer	14–15	Monocytes/macrophages and dendritic cells	IL-15R	21; 48	Stimulation of T cell proliferation, the generation of cytotoxic T lymphocytes, stimulation of immunoglobulin production by B cells and the generation and persistence of NK cells
IL-16	Lymphocyte chemoattractant factor, neuronal interleukin 16 (NIL16), PRIL16, IL16	Homo-tetramer	56	CD8+ T lymphocytes	CD4, CD9	520	Chemoattractant, growth factor, and other activities on lymphocytes, monocytes, and eosinophils
IL-17A IL-17B IL-17C IL-17D IL-17F	IL17A IL17B IL17C IL17D IL17F		35 41 40 52 44	Th17 cells, CD8 T cells, B cells, NK cells, γδ T cells, Neutrophils, epithelial cells, NKT cell, LTi-like cells, Paneth cells Chondrocytes and neuron	IL-17RA, IL-17RB, IL-17RC, IL-17RD and IL-17RE	155 180 197 202 153	Activation of host defense against various bacteria and certain fungi. Activation of proliferation of naive CD4+ T cells. Promote neutrophil recruitment, and production of certain antimicrobial peptides

Continued

—Cont'd

Interleukin (IL)	Other/Previous Names	Structure	Molecular Weight (kDa)	Cellular Sources	Receptor	Protein Length (Mature Form)	Main Function
IL–18	Interferon-gamma-inducing factor (IGIF), IL–1g, IL1F4, IL18	Monomer	18	Th1 cells, NK cells, macrophages, dendritic cells, astrocytes, microglial cells	IL–18Rα, IL–18β	163	Proinflammatory activities. Modulation of Th1 differentiation, suppression of osteoclast proliferation, stimulation of NK-mediated cytotoxicity. Upregulation of IFN-γ, TNF-α, IL–1β, IL–8
IL–19	Melanoma differentiation association like protein, MDA1, NG.1, ZMDA1, IL–10C, IL19	Monomer	21	B cells, monocytes, macrophages, epithelial cells, endothelial cells, keratinocytes, smooth muscle cells, fetal membranes, synovial tissue	IL–20R1/IL–20R2	177	Both pro- and anti-inflammatory activities. Upregulation of IL–6 and TNF-α. Proapoptotic activities
IL–20	Zcyto10, IL–10D, IL20	Monomer	18	Epithelial and endothelial cells, activated keratinocytes and monocytes	IL–22R1/IL–20R2	176	Regulates proliferation and differentiation of keratinocytes during inflammation. Pro-inflammatory activity in mesangial cells, keratinocytes, endothelial cells, synovial fibroblasts, and renal epithelial cells

IL-21	Zα-11, IL21	?	16	CD4+ T cells, Th17 cells, natural killer T (NKT) cells	IL-21R	131	Regulates activity and proliferation of NK and cytotoxic T cells
IL-22	IL-10-related T-cell-derived inducible factor, Zcyto18, TIFIL-23, IL18	Monomer	20	Th1 cells, Th17 cells, Th22 cells, Tc17 cells, Tc22 cells, cd T cells, NKT cells, lymphoid tissue inducer (LTi) cells, certain NK cell subsets, mast cells, splenocytes	IL-22R	179	Upregulation of IL-6, G-CSF, and TNF, maintains tissue homeostasis, supports tissue repair and wound healing. Plays role in anti-microbial defense of the body. Has been implicated in the development of inflammatory disease
IL-23	IL23P19; P19; SGRF, IL23	Monomer	20	Various immune cells	IL-23R	189	Plays a role in inflammatory response against infection. Promotes synthesis of MMP9, IL-1, IL-6, IL-17, and TNF-α
IL-24	IL24, IL-4-induced secreted protein, C49A, FISP; IL10B, melanocyte-associated MDA7, MOB5, ST16	Monomer	23	Activated monocytes, macrophages, T helper 2 (Th2) cells, keratinocytes	IL-20R1/IL-20R2 and IL-22R1/IL-20R2	206	Inhibition of tumor growth due to anti-angiogenic, pro-apoptotic activities. Promotion of senescence and autophagy

Continued

—Cont'd

Interleukin (IL)	Other/Previous Names	Structure	Molecular Weight (kDa)	Cellular Sources	Receptor	Protein Length (Mature Form)	Main Function
IL-25	IL-17E, IL25	Monomer	34	Type 2 helper T cells, mast cells		161	Upregulation of IL-4, IL-5, IL-13. Stimulation of eosinophils. Proinflammatory activities favoring Th2-type immune response
IL-26	AK155, IL26	Can act as monomer and dimer	20	NK cells, activated T cells, macrophage-like synoviocytes from rheumatoid arthritis joints, peripheral mononuclear blood cells	IL-20R1/ IL-10R2	171	Pro-inflammatory, pro-survival and antiproliferative activities
IL-27	p28, IL27	Heterodimer	27	Activated monocytes, DCs, macrophages, endothelial cells	IL27RA/ gp130	243	Modulation of the activity of B and T cells

IL-28A	IFN-γ1, IL28A, ZCYTO20	Monomer	22	Immune cells, including Th1, NK, and NKT-cell subsets	IL-28RA/IL-10R2	200	Promotion of promote Th1 immune skewing, antimicrobial and anti-viral functions, suppression of Th2 and Th17 responses, upregulation of MHC I, MIG/CXCL9, IP-10/CXCL10, TAC/CXCL11, TLR3, downregulation of IL-4, IL-5, IL-6, IL-10, IL-13
IL-28B	IFN-γ2, IL28B, ZCYTO22	Monomer	22	Immune cells, including Th1, NK, and NKT-cell subsets	IL-28RA/IL-10R2	196	Antimicrobial and anti-viral functions, suppression of Th2 and Th17 responses, upregulation of MHC I, downregulation of IL-4, IL-5, IL-6, IL-10, IL-13
IL-29	IFN-γ3, IL29	Monomer	22	Immune cells, including Th1, NK, and NKT-cell subsets	IL-28RA/IL-10R2	200	Antimicrobial and anti-viral functions, suppression of Th2 and Th17 responses, upregulation of MHC I, TNF, IL-12p40, down-regulation of IL-4, IL-5, IL-6, IL-10, IL-13

Continued

—Cont'd

Interleukin (IL)	Other/Previous Names	Structure	Molecular Weight (kDa)	Cellular Sources	Receptor	Protein Length (Mature Form)	Main Function
IL–30	IL27p28, p28, IL30	Monomer	28				Blockade of gp130, thereby preventing signaling of numerous cytokines, including IL–6, IL–11, and IL–27
IL–31	IL31	Monomer	18	Skin-homing activated CD4+ T cells and activated CD8+ T cells but neither in resting nor in activated NK cells, monocytes and B cells. Normally expressed in skin. Small amounts of IL–31 mRNA were identified in testis, skeletal muscle, bone marrow, colon, small intestine, kidney, thymus, and trachea	IL–31RA/ OSMR	164	Play a role in pathogenesis of various autoimmune diseases
IL–32	NK4, IL32	Monomer	19	Found not only in immune tissues and cells, but also in epithelial cells	IL–32R	171	Pro-inflammatory cytokine that can induce cells of the immune system to secrete inflammatory cytokines

IL-33	C9orf26, DVS27, IL1F11, NF-HEV, NFEHEV, IL33	Monomer	30	Has been found expressed in almost all tissues and organs, especially in endothelial and epithelial cells	IL-1RL1	270	Triggers anti-inflammatory Th1-polarized immune response by expressing IL-4, IL-5, IL-6, IL-13 in immune cells and increasing production of immunoglobulins
IL-34	C16orf77, IL34	Homodimer	39	Neurons and keratinocytes. Small amounts of IL-34 were found in thymus, liver, small intestine, colon, prostate gland, lung, heart, brain, kidney, testes, and ovary	CSF-1R	241	Maintains populations of Langerhans cells and microglia, enhances growth and survival of immune cells
IL-35	IL35	Heterodimer	18	Treg cells			Anti-inflammatory properties, inhibits the proliferation of all subsets of T cells, including Th17 cells
IL-36	Fil1e, Il1e, Il1f6, Il1h1, IL36				IL-36R	160	Pro-inflammatory activities. Acts synergically with IL-12 to promote polarization of Th1

Continued

—Cont'd

Interleukin (IL)	Other/Previous Names	Structure	Molecular Weight (kDa)	Cellular Sources	Receptor	Protein Length (Mature Form)	Main Function
IL-37	FIL1Z, IL1F7, IL1H4, IL1RP1, IL37	Monomer	24	Expressed in lung, heart, brain, stomach, spleen, prostate, pancreas, liver, and kidney	SIGIRR, IL-18Rα	218	Anti-inflammatory activities. Natural suppressor of innate inflammatory and immune responses. Downregulates TNF α, IL-1α, IL-6, MIP-2, and IL-10
IL-38	FIL1T, IL1HY2, IL38	Monomer	17	Expressed in skin and in proliferating B-cells of the tonsil	IL-36R	152	Anti-inflammatory activities. Inhibits the synthesis of IL-8, IL-17A, and IL-22

INDEX

Note: Page numbers followed by 'f' indicate figures; 't', tables.

Printed in the United States
By Bookmasters